ALLE ZEIT WACH 1842

Helmut Thomä Horst Kächele

# Psychoanalytic Practice

## 1 Principles

With the Collaboration of
Andreas Bilger Manfred Cierpka Hans-Joachim Grünzig
Roderich Hohage Lisbeth Klöß Julian Christopher Kübler
Lisbeth Neudert Rainer Schors Hartmut Schrenk
Brigitte Thomä

Translated by M. Wilson and D. Roseveare
Foreword by R. S. Wallerstein

Springer-Verlag
Berlin Heidelberg New York Paris London Tokyo

Professor Dr. Helmut Thomä
Professor Dr. Horst Kächele
Abteilung Psychotherapie der Universität
Am Hochsträss 8, D-7900 Ulm
Federal Republic of Germany

*Translators:*
Dr. Michael Wilson
Max-Wolf-Straße 16, D-6900 Heidelberg
David Roseveare
Eselsgrundweg 6, D-6900 Heidelberg

Title of the original German edition:
Lehrbuch der psychoanalytischen Therapie, Band 1 Grundlagen
© Springer-Verlag Berlin Heidelberg 1985
ISBN-13:978-3-642-71432-0 / 0-387-15386-1

ISBN-13:978-3-642-71432-0 e-ISBN-13:978-3-642-71430-6
DOI: 10.1007/978-3-642-71430-6

Library of Congress Cataloging-in-Publication Data. Thomä, Helmut. Psychoanalytic practice. Translation of: Lehrbuch der psychoanalytischen Therapie. Bibliography: p. Includes indexes. Contents: 1. Principles. 1. Psychoanalysis. I. Kächele, Horst, 1944- II. Title. [DNLM: 1. Psychoanalytic Therapy. WM 460.6 T452L]
RC504.T4613 1986 616.89'17 86-28042
ISBN-13:978-3-642-71432-0 (U.S.: v. 1)



2119/3140-543210

# Foreword

A basic issue for all those essaying to write comprehensive texts on the nature of psychoanalysis, whether oriented primarily to the exposition of the theory or of the technique of psychoanalysis, — within the American literature the books by Brenner and by Greenson come to mind as exemplars of the two categories — is that of the relationship of the theory to the technique and the practice. This issue is however not always brought into explicit focus in this literature and thereby its problematic nature as a fundamental and not yet satisfactorily resolved dilemma of our discipline is often glossed over, or even bypassed completely, as if we could comfortably assume that Freud had, uniquely in the world's intellectual history, fully succeeded in creating a science and a discipline in which the theory (the understanding) and the therapy (i. e., the cure) were inherently together and truly the same, but two sides of the same coin.

It is the achievement of Helmut Thomä and Horst Kächele, the authors of this book presenting within two volumes — this first one on theory and a second imminent companion volume on clinical interaction and application — an overall statement on what psychoanalysis is (or should be) all about, that they have more than others kept this central problematic of the relationship of theory to practice in the center of the reader's conceptual field and have organized their presentation of the phenomena of our field, of its concepts and its data, accordingly. The heart of the problematic to which I am referring is caught in one short paragraph in Chap. 7: "As for psychoanalysis, one can see that while the theories are predominantly concerned with the determinants of *genesis*, the rules of technique are oriented toward achieving the necessary and sufficient conditions for *change*: psychoanalytic technique is not *simply* application of theory" (p. 218, emphasis added). From this distinction and inevitable tension, all else follows — though it is of course also an oversimplification and something of an injustice for me to focus the overall thrust of this so very comprehensive book in *just* this way, or to imply that the whole range of conceptual problems of our field is caught up in the effort at the delineation of the interplay — and the dialectic — between theoretical and clinical therapeutic development.

Nonetheless, it is an important perspective and one that I feel *is* central to the authors' thinking; and for my part I would indicate two (to me) necessary consequences of this conceptual disjunction of theory from technique with the problem that then emerges of the conditions and the parameters of their relatedness — as against the conventional psychoanalytic assumption of the conceptual unity of theory and technique which conceals and papers over these very questions at the heart of our discipline, how a theory of how the mind functions can relate to a technique to alter that functioning in desired directions. The first consequence to which I would draw attention runs like a quiet but insistent leitmotif throughout the book, the call at many points for empirical research into the psychoanalytic process and its outcomes that is designed to elucidate the conditions and the parameters of the relationship of theory to technique, research with which the authors have themselves long been identified, and of which they are actually the leading continental European representatives alongside a small band of fellow investigators in the United States and in Great Britain. In this they join forces solidly with the pragmatic and empirical tradition in the Anglo-Saxon (scientific) intellectual world.

A second consequence of this conceptual disjunction emerges even more softly but still unmistakably in the book, the inevitable consideration of the relationship of psychoanalysis qua therapy to the whole range of psychoanalytic psychotherapies, varyingly expressive and supportive, which represent applications of the same psychoanalytic theoretical understanding of the organization and functioning of the mind to the varieties of psychopathological formations presented in our consulting rooms via an array of differentiated expressive and supportive technical interventions, i.e., one theory, but various techniques conceptualized within it. This message emerges most explicitly, as one would expect, in Chap. 6 on the initial interview(s) with all its focus on the problem of diagnosis and of case formulation and the shift expressed there from the concept of "analyzability" to the preferred concept of "treatability," ending in "a *diagnostic phase of therapy,* which is not a trial analysis in the conventional sense followed by the decision regarding suitability, but rather has the purpose of finding out what changes can be achieved under what therapeutic conditions. The wide scope of the current forms of psychoanalytic therapy allows room for many ideas, which do not even have to be restricted to the field of psychoanalysis in the stricter sense" (p. 188).

With this statement, the authors align themselves with a tradition very familiar in the American psychoanalytic world, a tradition articulated in the various American panel discussions of the early 1950s around the similarities and differences between psychoanalysis proper and the array of psychoanalytic or psychodynamic or psychoanalytically oriented psychotherapies — varyingly expressive and supportive — that were brought into focus in the important contributions to these issues of E. Bibring and Stone and Gill and Rangell along with the more discrepant voices of Alexander and Fromm-Reichmann. This concern with the broadened scope of psychoanalytically informed psychotherapies tailored specifically to the internal psychological requirements of the patients and the sociopolitical exigencies of the external surround also makes more understandable the authors' willing placement and portrayal of *psychoanalytic therapy* within the constraints of the West German insurance reimbursement system, which limits the therapy to 240 or at most 300 hours for all but the small minority who go on past that point on their private resources.

And for the American English-speaking audience this book carries an additional, perhaps not explicitly intended, message. For a long time the American psychoanalytic world lived within the comfortable feeling that the metapsychological ego psychology paradigm brought to its fruition in the work of Hartmann, Kris, Loewenstein, Rapaport, Jacobson, Waelder, Fenichel and a host of others represented *the* main stream of psychoanalytic development from Freud through Anna Freud and into the psychoanalytic transplantation from Vienna to America (of course also to Great Britain) with the accession of Hitler to power. It has only been within recent years that American psychoanalysis has become more fully appreciative of the true diversity of theoretical perspectives within psychoanalysis, not only the Kleinian which had long been looked at as a unique theoretical aberration existing within the psychoanalytic corpus, but also the Bionian, the Lacanian, the English object relational, and now from within the American scene itself, the rise of Kohutian self psychology to shake what had once been the monolithic hegemony in America of the so-called "classical" ego psychological metapsychology paradigm. In this pluralistic and therefore relativistic psychoanalytical world in which we now all live, this book by Thomä and Kächele is nonetheless a reaffirmation of the still established place of ego psychology as an encompassing psychological world view, delineated here not from a parochially American and English language literature standpoint but drawing more broadly upon similar developments and thinking deeply within the German language orbit and to a lesser degree within other language literatures as well. Much as there are today all the diverse overall theoretical perspectives within organized psychoanalysis that have been indicated, they have also each broken loose from their origins and confines within a particular geographic and language setting and are thus more widely counterposed against each other within each regional and national center of psychoanalytic activity worldwide. (For within the same German psychoanalytic and intellectual world in which Thomä and Kächele present a natural science and an empirical research-linked ego psychological paradigm there also exists at the same time a vigorous psychoanalytic (and philosophical) hermeneutic perspective identified with such names as Habermas and Lorenzer.) It is, of course, ultimately all to the good of psychoanalysis both as science and discipline that each of its perspectives in theory and in practice should flourish in confrontation with and in side-by-side interaction with each of the others within each cultural and linguistic tradition.

All of this amounts to more than enough reason to happily introduce this book, which has already been published so successfully in the German-speaking psychoanalytic world, to its natural audience in the English-speaking psychoanalytic world. For it is indeed far more than a carrying of coals to Newcastle. A last note on a tour de force that pervades the book: The reference to the salient related literature is so very fresh and recent and so comprehensive in its coverage — at least for the English and German languages — in *each* chapter that it seems as if each of them was the very last one completed and barely so just as the book was going to press. Every reader knows that this is not always so.

October 1986 Robert S. Wallerstein, M.D.

# Preface

This is the first of a two-volume study of psychoanalytic therapy which is being presented in both English and German. Volume 1 covers the principles of the psychoanalytic method, while Volume 2, which will follow within a year, deals with the psychoanalytic dialogue. The two volumes, although forming a coherent whole, are organized separately, and each contains its own list of references and index.

Although psychoanalysis has grown to be far more than only a method of treatment, "it has not abandoned its *home-ground* and it is still linked to its contact with *patients* for increasing its depth and for its further development." These words of Freud's (1933 a, p. 151, emphasis added) provide the point of departure for our introduction to the principles of the psychoanalytic method.

Psychoanalysis has spread more and more in recent decades, and since the 1950s numerous psychodynamic offshoots have branched off the mainstream. The problem which Freud (1933 a, p. 152) touched on with the metaphor of the dilution of psychoanalysis has reached almost incomprehensible dimensions. In this situation, giving this English edition a title which is simply a translation of the German — Textbook of Psychoanalytic Therapy — might be misleading, as it might make the reader think of diluted forms of the psychoanalytic method. To avoid misunderstandings, the English edition of Volume 1 has thus been entitled *Psychoanalytic Practice: Principles.* We understand "psychoanalytic therapy" as referring to the classical application of the *psychoanalytic method* to patients as defined by Freud (1905 a, 1923 a, 1927 a).

The origin and development of this book are very closely linked to the department of psychotherapy at the University of Ulm, which was established in 1967 and formed the basis of the Ulm psychoanalytic institute. The senior author, as head of the department, was able to draw on the experience of a long professional career, which had its beginnings in Stuttgart. The years at the Psychosomatic Hospital of the University of Heidelberg provided the clinical foundation for psychoanalytic thought; this institution, directed by A. Mitscherlich, was an intellectual home which exerted a constant attraction, always inviting me to return from abroad. A year on a Fulbright scholarship at the

Yale Psychiatric Institute in 1955-1956 pointed the way, and another year of research and further training, this time in London in 1962 with the support of the American Foundations' Fund for Research in Psychiatry, proved decisive.

This text is rooted in research on the psychoanalytic process and its results. We are grateful to the German Research Foundation for its continuous support since 1970, which made it possible for the junior author to combine clinical training and research in Ulm from the outset. The direct and indirect influence of professional criticism, from within and without, on our clinical thinking and activity should not be underestimated. This book would not exist in its present form if research had not opened our eyes to many problems.

The network of contacts out of which this book has developed is so extensive that we cannot possibly acknowledge all those who have over the years provided us with emotional and intellectual support. We want to express our gratitude to everyone who has made a direct contribution, and would like to emphasize especially that the book would not have attained its present form if our colleagues in Ulm had not given us frequent guidance, contributed to drafts of some sections, and suggested amendments.

Our special thanks go to fellow psychoanalysts and to colleagues from other fields who have read individual sections or chapters at some stage. Their constructive comments have given us great encouragement in preparing particular passages. The exchange of ideas has also often forced us to formulate our own positions more precisely or to make revisions. Yet, of course, we alone bear responsibility for the final text. We would like to thank the following people for their critical comments on drafts of various sections: Hermann Beland, Christopher T. Bever, Claus Bischoff, Werner Bohleber, Clemens de Boor, Johannes Cremerius, Sibylle Drews, Erhard Effer, Ulrich Ehebald, Wolfram Ehlers, Martha Eicke-Spengler, Friedrich Wilhelm Eickhoff, Franz Rudolf Faber, Klaus Grawe, Johannes Grunert, Ursula Grunert, Rudolf Haarstrick, John S. Kafka, Reimer Karstens, Otto F. Kernberg, Gisela Klann-Delius, Martha Koukkou-Lehmann, Rainer Krause, Martin Löw-Beer, Ulrike May, Adolf Ernst Meyer, Emma Moersch, Friedrich Nienhaus, Peter Novak, Michael Rotmann, Almuth Sellschopp, Ernst Konrad Specht, Ernst Ticho, Gertrud Ticho, Margret Toennesmann, Ingeborg Zimmermann.

We were supported far more than we could reasonably have demanded, through highs and lows, by Rosemarie Berti, Ingrid Freischlad, Doris Gaissmaier, Annemarie Silberberger, and Brigitte Gebhardt. While the possibilities offered today by word processing make it easier to produce numerous modified and improved drafts, this technology places increased demands on the intelligence and organization of a busy secretariat. That the inevitable friction nevertheless always resulted in excellent and increasingly effective cooperation is due to the commitment of our assistants. Hartmut Schrenk coordinated the work within our department and between the staff of Springer-Verlag and the authors. We are also grateful to him and Claudia Simons for their painstaking preparation of the references. The author and subject index was prepared by Michael Hölzer.

From the very beginning there was a conducive and collegial atmosphere between the authors and Toni Graf-Baumann, the editor responsible for psychoanalysis at Springer-Verlag.

We would also like to express our gratitude to our translators, Michael Wilson and David Roseveare. Their task was formidable and they have mastered it well. Our discussions with the translators exposed a number of ambiguities and obscurities in the original German version. We believe that most of them have been resolved in the English edition. The help of our friend Neil Cheshire of Bangor University, North Wales, in the process of clarification is much appreciated.

This translation has been generously supported by a grant from the Breuninger Foundation, Stuttgart. We wish to express our special thanks to Dr. Helga Breuninger for her continuous interest in our work and her dedicated support of psychoanalytic research.

We now hand over this text on psychoanalytic practice to the reader, in the fervent hope that it will be of benefit to those for whom it has ultimately been written: the patients.

Ulm, September 1986

Helmut Thomä
Horst Kächele

# Contents

# Introduction

## Historical Backround

As German authors of a textbook on psychoanalysis, we believe that some comments on the dissolution of psychoanalysis in our country during the 1930s and its new beginning are appropriate.

Both as a method of treatment and as theory, psychoanalysis thrives off the fact that it directs the cognitive processes at the rediscovery of an object which assumes a new form the instant it is rediscovered, i.e., the instant it reaches consciousness through interpretive illumination. In personal life history and in the therapeutic process, as well as in the psychosocial sciences in general, Heraclitus' dictum that you cannot step twice into the same river is of great significance: Object-finding is not only a *re*discovery, but also a *new* discovery. The reader familiar with Freud's works will not miss the allusion to Freud's formulation that "the finding of an object is in fact a refinding of it" (1905d, p. 222). Psychoanalysis has become part of our intellectual history and can thus be rediscovered, even though historical circumstances can lead, and in Germany did lead, to an interruption of this tradition. During the Third Reich, the works of Freud were inaccessible to most Germans, and the science he had founded was outlawed. Jewish psychoanalysts shared the fate of all Jews in Nazi Germany and the occupied territories of Europe. Freud, at his advanced age, was able to save himself and his immediate family by going into exile in England. His sisters, who could not accompany him, died in a concentration camp. All generations of German psychoanalysts bear the burden of history in a way which goes beyond the general consequences of the holocaust as expressed by the President of the Federal Republic of Germany, R. von Weizsäcker (1985), in his speech marking the 40th anniversary of the end of World War II. Although modern psychoanalysis is, of course, independent today of its founder, and as a science stands apart from any religious creed (not to speak of racist weltanschauungen), nevertheless an analyst is necessarily born into a Jewish genealogy and acquires his professional identity through identification with Freud's work. This situation produces numerous difficulties, reaching deep into the unconscious, which German psychoanalysts have attempted to resolve in one way or another since 1945.

These problems become more comprehensible if we consider the ideas which Klauber presented in 1976 at a symposium on the identity of the psychoanalyst called by the Executive Council of the International Psychoanalytical Association (Joseph and Widlöcher 1983). Klauber (1981) convincingly demonstrated the lasting consequences which the identification with the intellectual father of psychoanalysis has had on his students and thus on the history of psychoanalysis. Freud himself described the consequences of identificatory acceptance in *Mourning and Melancholia* (1917e) and in *Transience* (1916a). Klauber believes that psychoanalysts have not been able fully to accept Freud's death. The unconscious processes associated with this lead on the one hand to a restriction of our own thinking, and on the other hand to the inability to perceive how transient all scientific, philosophical, and religious ideas are, Freud's theories among them. Klauber's interpretation provides an explanation for the fact that rigidity and revolt run parallel in the history of psychoanalysis, and also that the question of the psychoanalyst's identity has been the focus of interest for quite some time. The fact that the identity of the psychoanalyst was chosen as the theme for the IPA symposium itself shows that analysts feel they can no longer rely on their identification with Freud. Not the least of the reasons why psychoanalysis undergoes changes is that original contributions by psychoanalysts themselves have demonstrated the transient nature of some of Freud's ideas. Klauber's fundamental reflections, which we have summarized here, make it clear why the psychoanalytic profession, more than any other, is concerned with its identity (Cooper 1984a; Thomä 1983c).

The concept of identity introduced by Erikson (1959), with its social psychological implications, sheds light on the insecurity of German psychoanalysts from 1933 to the present. Their dilemma, when thought through to its conclusion at the level of the unconscious, amounts to the fact that they seek to identify with the ideas of a man whose fellow Jews were murdered by Germans. We shall return to the question of formulating some aspects of this conflict in specifically Eriksonian terms, but first, in order to be able to grasp other, comparatively superficial aspects of the problems German analysts experience with identification, it is necessary to take a short look at the dismantling of psychoanalytic institutions in Germany in the 1930s.

After the closure of the distinguished Berlin Psychoanalytic Institute and of the German Psychoanalytic Society, along with its study groups in the southwest, in Leipzig, and in Hamburg, the few remaining, non-Jewish psychoanalysts sought ways to maintain their professional existence. On the one hand, they turned to private practice; on the other, they retained a measure of independence within the German Institute for Psychological Research and Psychotherapy (Deutsches Institut für psychologische Forschung und Psychotherapie), founded in 1936, which was led by M.H. Göring (a cousin of Hermann Göring) and called, for short, the Göring Institute. The training of young psychoanalysts continued there, although the Institute's goals exerted considerable pressure on them. The aim of bringing all schools of depth psychology (Freudians, Adlerians, Jungians) under one roof, namely an institute located in Berlin with branches in other cities (e.g., Munich, Stuttgart and, later, Vienna) was to promote Aryan psychotherapy (*deutsche Seelenheilkunde*; Göring 1934) and create a standard psychotherapy. The testimony of Dräger (1971), Baumeyer (1971), Kemper (1973), Riemann (1973), Bräutigam (1984), and Scheunert (1985) as well as the study by Lockot (1985) illuminate various aspects of the influence of the historical circumstances on the working conditions at the Institute.

Cocks (1983, 1984), in his historical studies, reaches the conclusion that the gathering of the different schools at one institute had long-term consequences and side effects which, in his estimation, are on the whole positive. Yet it cannot be pointed out too strongly that these completely unintended effects can in principle be judged as positive only if they are absolutely independent of the *ideologically* determined psychotherapy which was the official aim. Even though evil may be the father of good, doubts remain about the offspring; we may think, in the words of the prophets Jeremiah (31, 29) and Ezekiel (18, 2),[1] "The fathers have eaten sour grapes, and the children's teeth are set on edge." A psychoanalytic point of view, indeed, would suggest precisely that ideologies become intimately connected with unconscious processes, and in this way survive and even take on new substance. Lifton (1985) has correctly pointed out that Cocks paid too little attention to this question; and it is to the credit of Dahmer (1983) and others that this problem has recently been brought into the open.

The incorporation of all psychotherapists employing depth psychology into one institute led to the development of communities of interests, and to a consensus on various issues between advocates of different approaches. The pressures of the time strengthened the bonds between them. The idea of a synopsis — a synoptic psychotherapy, an amalgamation of the important aspects from all the schools — survived even longer. The foundation, in 1949, of the German Society for Psychotherapy and Depth Psychology (Deutsche Gesellschaft für

---

[1] It is important to say a word about the context of this quotation. The prophets refer to the new covenant between the Lord and the houses of Israel and Judah, to the effect that "ye shall not have occasion any more to use this proverb in Israel" (Ezekiel 18, 3). The new covenant makes everybody responsible for his own sins only: "But every one shall die for his own iniquity: every man that eateth the sour grape, his teeth shall be set on edge" (Jeremiah 31, 30). Thus the Mosaic law as stated in Exodus (20, 5) is dissolved: "For I the Lord thy God am a jealous God, visiting the iniquity of the fathers upon the children unto the third and fourth generations of them that hate me." (See Lamentations 5, 7: "Our fathers have sinned, and are not; and we have borne their iniquities.")

Psychotherapie und Tiefenpsychologie, later renamed to include psychosomatics) has had considerable positive consequences right up to the present day. For instance, professional interests are pursued jointly. The annual congresses provide a forum for analytically oriented psychotherapists. It is one thing, however, to follow common interests based on agreements regarding general principles in depth psychology; it is quite another to apply a method of investigation and treatment consistently and to develop, test, and retest a theory.

The idea of synopsis springs from a yearning for unity which takes on numerous forms. Viewed scientifically, the efforts to achieve a synoptic psychotherapy and an amalgamation of schools were naive, and involved the underestimation of group-dynamic processes (Grunert 1984). Current research into general and specific factors in psychotherapy is helping to identify both the common features and the differences of the various approaches. Of course, it is necessary to define the methods used and the basic theories; and an eclectic approach to practice therefore places the highest demands on professional knowledge and ability. Moreover, the disparate elements not only have to be compatible, they also have to be capable of integration, above all by the patient.

The numerous consequences of the long years of isolation became apparent after the war. Groups formed around H. Schultz-Hencke and C. Müller-Braunschweig. Schultz-Hencke, who had gone his own way even before 1933, believed he had developed psychoanalysis further during the years of isolation. As Thomä (1963, 1969, 1986) has shown, the restricted understanding of transference in this neopsychoanalytic approach had lasting effects just at the time when extension of the theory and practice of transference was beginning in the international scientific community. On the other hand, Schultz-Hencke's criticism of libido theory and metapsychology at the first postwar congress of the International Psychoanalytical Association, held in Zurich, would today cause no sensation, and would actually be shared by many analysts. At that time, however, concepts and theories were even stronger markers of one's psychoanalytic identity than today.

The emigrant Jewish psychoanalysts and the members of the International Psychoanalytical Association placed their confidence in Müller-Braunschweig, who had remained faithful to Freud's teachings and who did not claim to have developed them further during the years of isolation or to have given them a new language. Substantive, personal, and group-dynamic differences led to a polarization, and Schultz-Hencke was the prime candidate for the role of scapegoat. In 1950 Müller-Braunschweig founded the German Psychoanalytic Association (Deutsche Psychoanalytische Vereinigung, DPV) with nine original members, all in Berlin, while the majority of the nearly 30 psychoanalysts in Germany after the war remained in the existing German Psychoanalytic Society (Deutsche Psychoanalytische Gesellschaft, DPG). This split proved to be a fateful turning point: only the new German Psychoanalytic Association was recognized as an affiliate of the International Psychoanalytical Association. The traditional German Psychoanalytic Society, originally founded in 1910, is no longer a component society of the International Psychoanalytical Association, but instead is affiliated with the American Academy of Psychoanalysis.

Berlin not only provided the setting for the division into two professional groups; the demolished city was also the center of the *reconstruction* of psychoanalysis after 1945. A decisive factor in the recognition of the German Psychoanalytic Association by the International Psychoanalytical Association was that the Berlin Psychoanalytic Institute, whose membership was identical to that of the German Psychoanalytic Association, commenced the training of analysts. German psychoanalysts of the first postwar generation could gain membership in the International Psychoanalytical Association only through this Institute. At first there was only one West German member of the International Psychoanalytical Association outside Berlin, F. Schottlaender in Stuttgart.

The later official recognition of psychoanalysis by the public health insurance organizations also began in Berlin. The Institute for Psychogenic Illnesses (Institut für psychogene Erkrankungen) was founded in Berlin in 1946 under the direction of W. Kemper and H. Schultz-Hencke. It was the first psychotherapeutic outpatient clinic to be financially sponsored by a semistate organization, the later General Communal Health Insurance (Allgemeine Ortskrankenkasse) of Berlin. This was a foundation stone for the acceptance of psychoanalytic therapy by all public health insurance organizations. Nonmedical psychoanalysts were always active at this clinic, and were able later, after the introduction of a professional standard for practicing psychologists at the German Institute for Psychological Research and Psychotherapy (Deutsches Institut für psychologische Forschung und Psychotherapie), to participate without any major obstacles in the treatment of patients. Psychoanalysts without medical qualifications have had the right to treat patients within the framework of the public health insurance system since 1967.

In West Germany the Psychosomatic Hospital of the University of Heidelberg was founded in 1950 on the initiative of V. von Weizsäcker and with the support of the Rockefeller Foundation. Under the direction of A. Mitscherlich, it grew into an institution in which psychoanalytic training, treatment, and research were united under one roof. Thus for the first time in the history of German universities, psychoanalysis was able to establish itself in the way Freud (1919j) had envisaged in a paper which was originally published only in Hungarian and has remained relatively unknown (Thomä 1983b). The subsequent founding of the Sigmund Freud Institute in Frankfurt, a public institution, was due to the efforts of Mitscherlich, supported by T.W. Adorno and M. Horkheimer.

Many of the first generation of psychoanalysts in Germany after the war began as self-taught practitioners. Their training analyses were relatively short. They shared intellectual curiosity and an enthusiasm (even love) for Freud's works, whose recognition they fought for zealously. This kind of access to psychoanalysis is characteristic of productive pioneering times (A. Freud 1983). Something that made a profound impression on the postwar generation was the fact that German-speaking psychoanalysts living abroad put aside personal feelings and offered their assistance, despite having been forced to flee from oppression in Nazi Germany, and even despite the murder of members of their families.

One significant event symbolizes this help from abroad and at home: a series of lectures on "Freud in the Present" (Adorno and Dirks 1957). These lectures were organized to commemorate the hundredth anniversary of Freud's birth. E.H. Erikson presented the first lecture on May 6, 1956, in the presence of the then President of the Federal Republic of Germany, Theodor Heuss. Eleven American, English, and Swiss psychoanalysts held the series of lectures at the Universities of Frankfurt and Heidelberg during the summer term of 1956. These lectures resulted from initiatives by Adorno, Horkheimer, and Mitscherlich, and received substantial support from the government of the state of Hesse.

The further development of psychoanalysis in West Germany was influenced very positively by the fact that full-time training was made possible at several locations, as A. Freud (1971) demanded for up-to-date psychoanalytic training. The German Research Foundation (Deutsche Forschungsgemeinschaft) began to support the new generation of analysts by providing financial support for training and supervisory analyses as a result of a report it had commissioned, entitled *Denkschrift zur Lage der ärztlichen Psychotherapie und psychosomatischen Medizin* (Görres et al. 1964). Intensive supervision, case discussions with numerous European and American psychoanalysts representing nearly all schools of psychoanalysis, and periods spent working abroad made it possible for German psychoanalysts of the postwar generation to overcome the deficit in knowledge created during the Nazi period and attain an international standard of work by the mid-1960s (Thomä 1964). Making numerous identifications during the transfer of knowledge appears to have deleterious consequences only if the identifications remain unrelated to each other and are not integrated with Freud's work in a scientific manner by means of critical discussion.

The rapid growth of psychoanalysis in West Germany can be seen in the fact that the two psychoanalytic organizations, the German Psychoanalytic Association (DPV) and the German Psychoanalytic Society (DPG), currently have a total of about 650 members. Considerable interest in psychoanalysis is also shown by those in neighboring disciplines, although genuine interdisciplinary cooperation is limited to a few locations. The number of doctors and psychologists seeking psychoanalytic training is very large in comparison to other countries. Psychoanalysts head departments of psychotherapy and psychosomatics at many German universities; if Freud's paradigm can be permanently established and extended at the universities, there is a good chance that the urgently necessary intensification of psychoanalytic research will take place. The significance of the medical application of psychoanalysis goes far beyond its specific technique of treatment, and Balint's ideas on this topic have been accepted more widely by physicians in Germany than anywhere else. There are more Balint groups in Germany than in other countries; participants examine their therapeutic activity from interactional points of view in order to achieve a type of doctor-patient relationship which has a favorable influence on the course of the illness.

Despite the internationally recognized reestablishment of psychoanalysis in Germany since 1945, many more German analysts have problems with their professional identity than do their colleagues in other countries. Most of them are insecure and show an orthodox and submissive attitude toward representatives of the International Psychoanalytical Association regardless of the latters' personal feelings (whether positive or negative) about the standards of German psychoanalytic training (Richter 1985; Rosenkötter 1983). Viewed against the background of historical events, however, it is hardly surprising that German psychoanalysts are unusually vulnerable to the unconscious processes interpreted by Klauber. Many cannot do enough to idealize the work of Freud, others strive to affirm their own identity, while others again make a point of questioning it (prophylactically, no doubt, since they fear being criticized for arrogant independence). All this is symptomatic of that form of ontogenetic identity crisis which Erikson has characterized as "autonomy *versus* shame and doubt" (Erikson 1959). They cannot comfortably mark off their own professional identities in the usual way through theoretical criticism of Freud (the founding father), because this feels like a symbolic identification with those who rejected him politically and racially and persecuted him and his people; hence the ambivalence between subservient orthodoxy and a "neurotic" reaction formation against it. Again, even though there may be legitimate scientific reasons for seeking an agreed "synoptic" theory of depth psychology (which could be corroborated by different schools of practice and would avoid ill-founded idiosyncrasies), German analysts cannot sympathize with this project without feeling that they are selling out to the Nazis' malevolently motivated "Aryan psychotherapy."

But such preoccupations serve to chain creative and critical potential to the past and to make the solution of current problems in psychoanalysis more difficult. Doubt, however, as an impetus for change and progress, must not be restricted to the past and to historical questions regarding which components of Freud's teachings were sacrificed here or there in the course of accommodating to political circumstances or for other unscientific reasons. The incrimination of real and intellectual parents and grandparents, and the demonstration of their personal and political lapses, can also be employed outside psychoanalytic therapy as a form of resistance to the mastering of current tasks. A promising basis for a fruitful new beginning appears most likely to emerge from a comparison between past and present problems. Freud reaches an encouraging conclusion in his reflections on the *transience* of beauty, art, and intellectual achievement. He states that mourning is at some point exhausted and the loss is accepted, and that young people then "replace the lost objects by fresh ones equally or still more precious" (Freud 1916a, p. 307).

**Signpost**

After a survey in Chap. 1 of the problems currently facing psychoanalysis, the remaining chapters of this volume are organized into three sections. The first of these, comprising Chaps. 2-5, covers the fundamental concepts and theories of the psychoanalytic technique of treatment, such as transference and the analytic relationship, countertransference, resistance, and dream interpretation. We begin by paying special attention to transference, the hub of psychoanalytic therapy. The analyst's contribution to all manifestations of transference depends not only on his countertransference, but also on his theory of the origin of neuroses and psychosomatic illnesses.

In the second section (Chaps. 6-8), we describe and critically discuss the necessary steps in the initiation and the conducting of psychoanalytic treatment. Chapter 6 deals with the initial interview and the influence of third parties on the psychoanalytic process, and Chap. 7 covers the rules which analysts employ and follow. Chapter 8 is particularly extensive, since the means, ways, and goals to which this chapter is devoted are great in number. Means, ways, and goals are interrelated in the psychoanalytic process, and we do not agree that interpretation is the only means, or that the way is the goal. We also do not wish to commit ourselves to a specific, limited goal.

The third section begins with Chap. 9, in which we discuss the usefulness of models of the psychoanalytic process in the classification of the clinical descriptions which we have presented in the discussion of means, ways, and goals. The relationship between theory and practice forms the silent background to the whole book, and is the focus of attention in Chap. 10. This issue constitutes one of the greatest and most significant problems in both the theory and the practice of psychoanalysis.

The foundations of psychoanalytic technique have traditionally been sought in the general and specific theory of neurosis. In light of the divergence resulting from pluralism and of the increase in knowledge on the autonomy of treatment problems, however, we are not able to derive psychoanalytic practice from a generally accepted theory of the origin and course of psychic illnesses. Such ideal assumptions have always been illusory in view of the complex relationship between theory and practice.

The goal of our discussion of the theory of therapy and its most important concepts is to safeguard the application of the psychoanalytic technique to a broad spectrum of psychic and psychosomatic illnesses. In preparing the manuscript, our exposition of the central concepts eventually reached such proportions that no room was left for detailed presentation of actual cases within the confines of a single volume. Not being ones to do half a job, we will be introducing various types of psychoanalytic dialogues in a second companion volume, where they will be discussed thoroughly with reference to the points of view presented in this first volume. We believe that dividing *principles* and *practice* into two volumes does better justice to each than squeezing them both into one book, where lack of space would prevent us from developing our themes sufficiently to show that the principles and the practice legitimate each other. For the moment the theoretical arguments will have to speak for themselves.

At this juncture we would like to devote a few words to Chap. 1, where we introduce the problems facing psychoanalysis. After consideration of the *current state of psychoanalysis* and examination of our own practice, we have arrived at a *position* which now determines our views on problems of theory and practice. Our leitmotif, the *analyst's contribution* to the psychoanalytic process, pervades the whole book. The remarks on our position, our choice of leitmotif, and our assessment of the state of psychoanalysis supplement each other.

In the section on the *crisis of theory* we review the consequences of the controversy over whether psychoanalysis is to be comprehended as an *explanatory* or an *understanding* science. We show that the criticism of metapsychology has a much greater relevance to practice than is generally thought. There are numerous indications that Freud's paradigm will emerge renewed from the crisis. In order to demonstrate these tendencies clearly, we discuss the current state of psychoanalysis from several points of view. The last section of the first chapter deals with *convergences*. We discern within psychoanalysis many attempts at integration, or at least serious scientific endeavors to resolve differences of opinion more clearly than before. We hope that the argumentative style of this book will contribute to integration. Finally, we cannot fail to observe the convergence of psychoanalysis and neighboring disciplines, which might eventually lead to the establishment of a greater degree of unity than could be expected based on the numerous divergences evident in the current situation. As an example of the stimulus provided by interdisciplinary cooperation, we discuss the significance of some aspects of neonatological research for psychoanalytic practice.

In calling these remarks "Signpost," we are alluding to the passage from Wittgenstein which we quote in Sect. 7.1. In this passage, Wittgenstein refers to the numerous functions that a signpost may have, depending on the position and the goals of the traveller. Like a signpost, our remarks here cannot indicate everything the traveller will find when he arrives at his destination, or how it will compare with the expectations he has formed over a long period of time. We must ask indulgence for our decision to restrict ourselves to only a few definite recommendations and instead to urge critical contemplation of means, ways, and goals. This approach represents an alliance of our personal style with the conviction that it is more favorable, in the long term, to examine the function of rules from the very outset, rather than to let them dictate the way we should go.

One recommendation we would make to the less experienced traveller is to begin with the chapters which we consider less difficult. It is probably a good idea to start by reading about our general position and the leitmotif of the book, the analyst's contribution to the psychoanalytic process (Sects. 1.1, 1.2). The chapter on rules (Chap. 7) is particularly important for the psychoanalytic method, although the rules only come to life when considered in the context of transference, countertransference, and resistance in the analytic situation. It might also seem natural to start with the initial interview and the role of third parties (Chap. 6). So we could go on, but we do not wish this signpost to deter the reader from going his own way. One last word: our use of the generic masculine in the text was dictated by convenience — we find it clumsy always to say "he/she" or "(s)he" and so on.

# 1 Psychoanalysis: The Current State

## 1.1 Our Position

In the course of this book we will refer to Freud's writings frequently and at length. We would therefore like to begin by outlining our understanding of his work and our general position within psychoanalysis. Extensive quotation from Freud serves several purposes. The most important is that, despite some outstanding efforts at systematization, it remains true today that "the best way of understanding psycho-analysis is still by tracing its origin and development" (Freud 1923a, p. 235). The assimilation of the classic texts is the prerequisite for understanding the present problems in psychoanalysis and finding modern solutions.

Our aim with this volume is to create a *historically oriented systematic description of psychoanalysis.* We seek the springs which have fed the psychoanalytic stream, employing quotations to demonstrate lines of development which have led to current views. The passages we cite therefore serve as a means to an end: we ground and defend our opinions in a process of discursive interaction with Freud's positions. The contradictions which appear in Freud's work and have been repeated in various forms over the decades bear witness to the openness of psychoanalysis: "it ... gropes its way forward by the help of experience, is always incomplete and always ready to correct or modify its theories" (Freud 1923a, p. 253). Its firm foundation is laid in the following three passages:

In psychoanalysis there has existed from the very first an *inseparable bond between cure and research.* Knowledge brought therapeutic success. It was impossible to treat a patient without learning something new; it was impossible to gain fresh insight without perceiving its beneficent results. Our analytic procedure is the only one in which this precious conjunction is assured. It is only by carrying on our analytic *pastoral work* that we can deepen our dawning *comprehension* of the human mind. This prospect of scientific gain has been the proudest and happiest feature of analytic work. (1927a, p. 256, emphasis added)

Analyses which lead to a favourable conclusion in a short time are of value in ministering to the therapeutist's self-esteem and substantiate the *medical importance* of psycho-analysis; but they remain for the most part insignificant as regards the *advancement of scientific knowledge.* Nothing new is learnt from them. In fact they only succeed so quickly because everything that was necessary for their accomplishment was already known. Something new can only be gained from analyses that present special difficulties, and to the overcoming of these a great deal of time has to be devoted. Only in such cases do we succeed in descending into the deepest and most primitive strata of mental development and in gaining from there solutions for the problems of the later formations. And we feel afterwards that, strictly speaking, *only an analysis which has penetrated so far deserves the name.* (1918b, p. 10, emphasis added)

I have told you that psycho-analysis began as a method of treatment; but I did not want to commend it to your interest as a method of treatment but on account of the the *truths it contains,* on account of the information it gives us about what concerns human beings most of all — their own nature — and on account of the connections it discloses between the most different of their activities. As a method of treatment it is one among many, though, to be sure, *primus inter pares.* If it was without therapeutic value it would not have been discovered, as it was, in connection with sick people and would not have gone on developing for more than thirty years. (1933a, pp. 156-157, emphasis added)

As these passages show, Freud drew up the blueprint for a classical building, which will, however, never reach completion — and not merely because every analyst finds building material in each analysis, even if it has been used before, but as a matter of principle.

The three fundamental theses expressed in these passages contain the essential components of a causal understanding of therapy. Freud countenances no loosening of the inseparable bond. The analyst cannot be satisfied with therapeutic success alone. He wants to elucidate the genesis of psychic disorders and, above all, find out how they change in the course of therapy — or why they do not. The failures always represent the biggest challenges. The assertion that there is an inseparable bond between cure and research requires that both the determinants of genesis and change and those of failure in therapy be made the object of scientific investigation. Psychoanalysis has advanced beyond symptom-oriented suggestion therapy. Making no attempt at explanation and no effort to draw general conclusions from the specific material gained would be equivalent to a relapse into mere pragmatism or "a boundless course of experimentation" (Freud 1933a, p. 153). Freud expressed the concern that "the therapy will...destroy the science" (1927a, p.254). He believed that his strict (impartial) rules of investigation and treatment produced the best scientific conditions for the reconstruction of the patient's earliest memories, and that uncovering the amnesia created the optimal conditions for therapy (1919e, p. 183). We know today that realization of the inseparable bond demands more than the abandonment of crude suggestion and adherence to standardized rules of treatment. Even Freud insisted on the creation of the most favorable circumstances for change in each individual analytic situation, i.e., he recognized the need for patient-oriented flexibility (1910d, p. 145).

The creation of a therapeutic situation is a prerequisite for gaining insight into unconscious psychic connections. Freud underestimated the scientific value of demonstrating therapeutic change and clarifying the curative factors. At one point he wrote: "a psycho-analysis is not an impartial scientific investigation, but a therapeutic measure. Its essence is not to prove anything, but merely to alter something" (1909b, p. 104). The validity of opposing these two items is questionable. The main concern of modern research into therapy is to show that changes occur in the course of psychoanalytic treatment and to clarify the relationship between these changes and the theories adhered to by the analyst. Many problems have to be solved if this is to be achieved. For Freud the establishment of *causal* connections had priority; this is the principle on which classical psychoanalysis was founded and which distinguished it from suggestion therapy. Freud discussed this principle in his commentary on the expert opinion prepared by the Innsbruck Faculty of Medicine in the Halsmann case (1931 d). Philipp Halsmann was charged with the murder of his father, and the defense pleaded that he was not responsible, referring to the Oedipus complex as a mitigating factor. The issue to be clarified was thus the causal relationship between the Oedipus complex and the alleged patricide. Freud stated that "it is a far cry from [the Oedipus complex] to the causation of such a deed. Precisely because it is *always present*, the Oedipus complex is not suited to provide a decision on the question of guilt" (1931 d, p. 252, emphasis added). The place of patricide in this example could be taken by another action or a symptom. Moreover, there is only a minimal increase in the discriminatory (specific) power of explanation if the system of pathology based on such a unitary perspective is replaced by a two-class system (oedipal vs preoedipal). Freud illustrates his point with the following anecdote:

> There was a burglary. A man who had a jemmy in his possession was found guilty of the crime. After the verdict had been given and he had been asked if he had anything to say, he begged to be sentenced for adultery at the same time — since he was carrying the tool for that on him as well. (1931 d, p. 252)

Global pseudoexplanations say no more than does the myth of man's fall from grace in theology. Just as with all claims that the world's ills can be cured by making changes in one or two areas, a strong fascination is exerted by the idea that psychic disturbances have a standard oedipal or preoedipal etiology and that there is a corresponding two-class therapy with a polarization between relationship and interpretation (Cremerius 1979). This idea equates the deepest strata with the earliest and most powerful pathogenic factors, which appear to explain everything. Various schools violate the central idea of the classical approach, in the name of their respective standardizations, when they fail to produce or even to attempt to produce the necessary evidence, or alternatively regard it as already provided. Psychoanalysis is constantly under construction if the attempt is made to translate the principles contained in the three passages we cite above into practice. Previously gained knowledge must continually be tested. The descent to the deepest, pathogenic strata must be justified by the solution of those present problems which in turn depend on deep-rooted pathogenic factors.

It can be inferred from Freud's theses that analyses which remain on familiar territory proceed more rapidly than those which break new ground. The analyst's mastery of his craft — the meaningful communication of his knowledge, ability, and experience — must even lead to an acceleration of therapy. The self-esteem of both analyst and patient grows when success is forecast and achieved. Indeed, many short therapies — whether in terms of duration or number of sessions — achieve lasting change, and thus cannot be dismissed as mere cures of symptoms or of transference. Analyses which lead to a favorable conclusion in a short time do not, however, count for much today, and are hardly calculated to raise the analyst's professional prestige. The tendency is rather to relate the quality of an analysis to its duration, although it is quite another matter whether the knowledge gained fulfills therapeutic and theoretical criteria.

Freud's work can be cited in support of different approaches. It cannot be overlooked that Freud was led, in his therapeutic and scientific thinking, by the idea of one day being able to eliminate all other influences and arrive at pure interpretation. The utopian vision of pure interpretation pleaded for by Eissler (1958), in his dispute with Loewenstein (1958), would solve enormous practical and theoretical problems, and it is hard to resist its fascination. We would also gladly go along with it, if experience had not taught us better. In this context, Freud (1919a, p. 162) asked whether it suffices to make the repressed material conscious and to uncover the resistances: "Are we to leave it to the patient to deal alone with the resistances we have pointed out to him? Can we give him no other help in this besides the stimulus he gets from the transference?" We could easily add to these questions but we feel that the need to do so is eliminated by Freud's own next question: "Does it not seem natural that we should help him in another way as well, by putting him into the mental situation most favourable to the solution of the conflict which is our aim?" According to the point of view of the standard technique, further consideration of the structuring of the analytic situation is unnecessary. It is claimed that following the rules which have been laid down creates the optimal conditions for the recognition of unconscius components of conflicts. In this case, with patients who are suitable for analysis in the first place, additional assistance by means of flexible structuring of the analytic situation would be superfluous, as the external framework — frequency of sessions, use of the couch, etc. — has already proved its worth so convincingly that critical reconsideration is superfluous. In fact, however, the art of psychoanalytic interpretation, the core of the technique, is dependent on many factors, the neglect of which would limit both the theoretical power and the therapeutic efficacy of the psychoanalytic method.

The variations of the psychoanalytic method which Freud recommended must be the goal everywhere the effort is made to adapt the method to the circumstances of individual patients or typical patient groups. Whereas the indications for the standard technique became increasingly narrow, and patients were sought who were suitable for the method, a flexible application of the method led to modifications permitting widespread use of psychoanalytic therapy. The standard technique necessitates a *selective* approach to indications — the patient has to adjust himself to the method. The modified techniques permit an *adaptive* setting of indications (Baumann 1981) — the treatment is altered to suit the patient. This reestablishes a comprehensive understanding of therapy and should benefit patients of all ages and social backgrounds with a broad spectrum of psychic and psychosomatic illness. The increase in life expectancy has also led to a relaxation of the restriction of the indication for psychoanalysis to patients not above middle age; this restriction was recommended by Freud, but questioned as early as 1920 by Abraham. The application of an adaptive indication for the psychoanalytic method in older people went hand in hand with an extension of the psychoanalytic theory: The typical crises and conflicts of each phase of life — adolescence, adulthood, middle age, old age — are accorded their due importance, alongside early childhood, in the understanding of the pathogenesis of psychic and psychosomatic illnesses (Erikson 1959; Greenspan and Pollock 1980a, b, 1981; Lidz 1968). Especially in geriatric patients, the adaptive indication involves modification of the psychoanalytic technique (Steury and Blank 1981; Radebold 1982). As we describe in more detail in Sect. 6.6, in some countries Freud's expectation has been fulfilled, and patients from all strata of society enjoy the benefits of psychoanalytic treatment (Strotzka 1969a, b, 1980).

Classical scientific theories are not ancient monuments and should not be given the protection accorded monuments. Valenstein (1979) was unable to find a convincing definition of "classical" psychoanalysis, and demonstrated, with the aid of the meanings given for "classical" in *Webster's Dictionary*, why this is the case. According to one *Webster's* definition, a self-contained and recognized theory, method, or body of ideas can generally be described as "classical" when new developments or a fundamental change in viewpoint has narrowed its area of validity. A second definition is also instructive. In retrospect, every form or system is termed "classical" which, in comparison with subsequent modifications or more radical derivations, remains credible and valid over a period of time. This definition is interesting in light of the fact that Freud himself spoke of the *classical* method only in the context of dream interpretation — in retrospect and in fairly incidental fashion — and also mentioned modifications. Besides the classical method of having the dreamer give associations to the separate portions of the dream, various other possibilities are open (1933a, p. 11). We can, for instance, "direct the dreamer to begin by looking out for the 'day's residues' in the dream; ... if we follow these constructions, we often arrive with one blow at the transition from the apparently far remote dream-world to the real life of the patient." Moreover, the term "classical treatment technique" did not originate with Freud, but was first used when modifications were introduced. Ferenczi was instrumental in giving the classical technique its name. Disturbed by the reaction of renowned analysts, including Freud, to his innovations, which for therapeutic purposes ranked experiencing higher than remembering, he wrote in a letter that he was returning repentantly to "our classical technique" (Thomä 1983a). Thus was born a term which in the early 1920s was used to refer to the therapeutically unsatisfactory preference for remembering and intellectual reconstruction (Ferenczi and Rank 1924). Whatever forms the classical technique may have assumed in the ensuing decades, it has stayed true to its origins: it thrives off the confrontation with deviations which is not supported by empirical investigations of different procedures using well-defined criteria. The admiration generally accorded to anything termed "classical" is an obstacle to investigation of the roles that classical and new elements of style have played in the continuous development of treatment technique. The *neoclassical* style is characterized not by innovations, but rather by particularly orthodox adherence to externally defined rules (Stone 1981a).

There is considerable tension between Freud's classical work and any application. This tension is characterized by problems in the relationship between theory and practice, which we discuss in Chap. 10. The danger that practical applications of the technique will fail to express Freud's central ideas, or even run counter to their development, is especially great if rules are followed for their own sake and if their function is not continually tested. For these reasons we distinguish between the terms "classical," "neoclassical," "orthodox," etc. Since Freud found no justification for labeling one course of action the classical method of dream interpretation, we will forgo speaking of the classical technique and content ourselves with concentrating on standards in the application of rules.

Although Freud's classical work is always represented in some form in every analyst's ideas, it cannot be translated into therapy in a way that would justify speaking of *the* classical technique. It is absolutely necessary, however, to follow and to standardize rules. The rules of treatment go back to Freud's recommendations and advice concerning technique, and are integrated in the *standard technique.* Therapeutic and theoretical considerations necessarily lead to *variations* and *modifications* of the system of rules, be it in the interest of patients with particular conditions (hysteria, phobia, compulsive neurosis, certain psychosomatic conditions, etc.) or of an individual analysand. In the *orthodox* technique, on the other hand, the expediency of these rules is not questioned, and patients are selected as suitable for analysis on the basis of their ability to follow the rules strictly. At the other end of the spectrum is *wild* psychoanalysis, which begins with insufficiently grounded deviations from moderately reliable standards and ends with the wildest aberrations and confusions (Freud 1910k). Yet despite its antitherapeutic offshoots, "wild" analysis is now worthy of differentiated consideration (Schafer 1985).

The growing number of publications dealing with Freud's practice (Beigler 1975; Cremerius 1981b; Kanzer and Glenn 1980) facilitate the critical reappraisal of the history of the psychoanalytic treatment technique. The solutions to modern problems cannot, however, be found in naive identification with the natural and humane behavior of Freud, who when necessary provided patients with meals or loaned or gave them money. The extension of the theory of transference has led analysts to pay particular attention to the various aspects of the analytic relationship and its interpretation. In our view, today more than ever before we are duty bound to comply with the demand which Freud raised in the afterword to *The Question of Lay Analysis* (1927a, p. 257), where he stressed that all practical applications should avail themselves of psychological concepts and be oriented on scientific psychoanalysis. That appropriate consideration should be given to the findings of research in the same area, but using other methods, is self-evident. Especially in its nontherapeutic applications, scientific psychoanalysis is dependent on interdisciplinary cooperation (see Wehler 1971, 1972).

Similarly, the treating analyst cannot ignore the modern methods of research on the process and outcome of psychotherapy. The crucial question is what distinguishes and characterizes *scientific* psychoanalysis. As authors of a book on psychoanalytic therapy, we can leave it to scholars in the respective fields to decide which of the practical applications of the psychoanalytic method to religious and cultural history, mythology, and literature satisfy the criteria of scientific psychoanalysis and of the respective discipline. In the therapeutic application of the psychoanalytic method, the question of what constitutes scientific psychoanalysis can be answered by referring to Freud's three fundamental theses contained in the passages quoted at the beginning of this chapter. The more strictly rules are laid down and the less their impact on therapy is investigated scientifically, the greater the danger of creating orthodoxy. It is obvious that orthodoxy cannot be reconciled with a scientific approach. For these reasons, we speak simply of the "psychoanalytic technique," or "analytic technique" for short. However, we never forget the rules which have been standardized over the years. Pragmatic and scientific action is rule-directed. Since rules lay down "how something is produced" (Habermas 1981, vol. 2 p. 31), their influence on psychoanalytic phenomena and their occurrence in the psychoanalytic process must constantly be borne in mind. If there were no danger of the classical psychoanalytic method becoming equated with a few external rules, we would not be so hesitant to use the term "classical technique," for in our ears too "classical" sounds better than "standard." It should be clear enough from our somewhat labored comments that it is no easy matter to preserve the intellectual tradition in treatment technique and to continue it in self-critical fashion. Considering therapeutic action from the point of view of how something is produced, the responsibility lies with the person who applies rules in one way or another. Freud expressed recommendations and gave advice.

## 1.2 The Psychoanalyst's Contribution

Our leitmotif is the conviction that the *analyst's contribution to the therapeutic process* should be made the focus of attention. We examine everything systematically from this point of view — acting out, regression, transference, resistance. The analyst influences every phenomenon felt or observed in the analytic situation.

The course of therapy depends on the influence exerted by the analyst. Naturally there are other factors as well, such as those determining the course and indeed the type of disease, the circumstances which led to its genesis, and the events in the here-and-now which constantly precipitate and reinforce it. Illnesses which are psychic in origin deteriorate under such conditions, and it is precisely here that the analyst has the opportunity to exert therapeutic influence, in the sense of new experience effecting change. An analyst is both affected personally and involved professionally in the dyadic process, and it thus seems natural to speak of therapeutically effective interaction. An interactional model conceived on the basis of *three-person psychology* is needed in order to depict the therapeutic process comprehensively (Rickman 1957; Balint 1968).

Viewing oedipal conflicts on the basis of a general psychological theory of human relationships, the third party is always present, even if not physically. This latent presence of the third party distinguishes the analytic situation from all other two-person relationships. The consequences that the bracketing out of the third party has on the theory and practice of psychoanalysis have never been given anything approximating adequate consideration. The unaccustomed deprivation in the analytic situation may not only encourage fantasies, but also greatly affect their content; for this reason, the comparison of psychoanalytic theories must always take the respective treatment techniques into consideration. How the third party (father, mother, or partner) appears in the dyad, which can be more accurately called a "triad minus one," and how the dyad reorganizes itself as a triad (or not) depends essentially on the analyst. In addition to the inevitable partnership conflicts in the course of treatment, some conflicts are determined by the problems specific to the triad minus one (Chap. 6).

In order to arrive at a genuine understanding of what happens in the therapeutic process, we must examine the analyst's behavior and *his contribution to the creation and maintenance* of the therapeutic situation. This programmatic demand, made by Balint in 1950, has not yet been satisfied, and according to Modell (1984a) has been forgotten. In most case reports, at least, the analyst's part — what he thought and did, what lay behind his choice of interpretations — is not described adequately. It is therefore not a sign of exaggerated therapeutic ambition on our part when, in agreement with Freud, we affirm that the analyst's task is to structure the therapeutic situation in such a way that the patient has the best possible conditions for solving his conflicts, recognizing their unconscious roots, and thus ridding himself of his symptoms. We thus acknowledge that the analyst must exercise a profound influence. The patient's freedom is not restricted, but rather enlarged, in that he is encouraged to take part in critical discussion.

Every rule must be considered from the point of view of whether it assists or hinders self-knowledge and *problem solving*, and the analyst should not be reluctant to make modifications accordingly. It thus becomes clear that we do not regard the theory and rules of psychoanalytic technique as holy writ. On the contrary, the impact of the rules on the therapy must be grounded in *every case*. We prefer a problem-oriented approach which is far removed from the prescriptive "cookbook" style. For example, the analyst can no longer prescribe the fundamental rule in the belief that *free associations* will then simply begin, uninfluenced by other factors. All efforts at standardization may have, in addition to the desired effects, unforeseen side effects of a positive or a negative nature which may assist or hinder the therapeutic process.

In his diagnostic and therapeutic activity, the analyst orients himself on psychoanalytic theory as a *systematized psycho(patho)logy of conflict*. Kris (1975 [1947], p. 6) characterized psychoanalysis as the study of "human behavior viewed as conflict." Binswanger (1955 [1920]) had already viewed this as the psychoanalytic paradigm in the history of science which is embodied in Freud's deceptively simple words: "We seek not merely to describe and to classify phenomena, but to understand them as signs of an interplay of forces in the mind" (1916/17, p. 67). The comprehensive significance of psychoanalytic theory lies in the fact that it views human life from its first day onward under the aspect of the impact of conflict on the subject's personal well-being and interaction with others. If, however, conflicts and their role in the origin of psychic or psychosomatic illnesses are defined as wholly *intrapsychic* — and not also interpersonal — the scope of the theory and the associated treatment technique is restricted.

Despite Hartmann's (1950) warning against reductionist theories, the history of the psychoanalytic technique is characterized by one-sidedness, and the different schools of psychoanalysis themselves are clear evidence of this. Hartmann speaks of a "genetic fallacy" if "the actual function is equated with its history, or rather reduced to its genetic precursors, as if genetic continuity were inconsistent with change of function" (1955, p. 221). However, adherents of reductionist theories are not only "very fond of selecting one portion of the truth [and] putting it in the place of the whole," but also tend to see the whole truth in this portion and dispute the rest, "which is no less true" (Freud 1916/17, p. 346). In this passage Freud is discussing the causation of neuroses, and arrives at the hypothesis of "complemental series," with the psychic conflict at their core. Reductionist theories must be criticized not only on grounds of their incompleteness and one-sidedness, but also, and above all, because they pass off provisional hypotheses as already proven. The same criticism must be directed at the claim that the psychoanalytic theory represents the whole truth and has to be protected against one-sidedness. Freud's thesis of the inseparable bond makes it necessary to apply scientific criteria to the complexity which necessarily relativize the claim to truth and make one proposition more likely to be accurate than another, or even refute one of them altogether. The fact that the whole is more than the sum of its parts is also true of complemental series. They confront the student directly with the complexity of the genesis of conflicts. To name two examples, Balint criticized the one-sided intrapsychic model of conflict and the claim that interpretation is the only instrument of therapy, and Kohut's self psychology originated in his dissatisfaction with the neoclassical technique and its theoretical basis, the intrapsychic oedipal conflicts.

The formation of schools within psychoanalysis is always a result of numerous dissatisfactions and other factors, and new schools have great hopes reposed in them — until they rigidify into new one-sidedness. Our emphasis on the decisive importance of the analyst's contribution to the therapeutic process is intended to help eliminate the development of schools by encouraging a critical approach to theory and practice. Our starting point is Freud's comprehensive theory of conflict, not the components of *intrapsychic* conflicts in a particular group of patients, as described for example by Brenner (1979b). Such restrictions have led to countermovements, the most recent example being Kohut's self psychology. The curtailment of the comprehensive model of conflict in psychoanalytic theory corresponded to neglect of the two-person relationship in practice. If the comprehensive psychoanalytic theory of conflict is reestablished in its full scope, it can incorporate descriptions of ego defects or self defects without difficulty, as shown by Wallerstein (1983), Modell (1984), and Treurniet (1983). Naturally we cannot stop at this general statement; if we were to do so, Goldberg's assertion that "if everything is conflict, conflict is nothing" (1981, p. 632) would apply. However, the psychoanalytic theory of conflict has never stopped at commonplaces, regardless of its scope with respect to pathogenesis.

The structural theory of psychoanalysis highlighted oedipal conflicts and their role in the genesis of neuroses. This theory by no means leads inevitably to attention being restricted to intra- or interpsychic conflicts within and between superego, ego ideal, ego, and id. As we will show in more detail in the discussion of the relationship of various forms of resistance to defense mechanisms (Chap. 4), the formation of structure is embedded in object relationships. In his writings on structural theory and ego psychology, Freud described the consequences of the internalization of object relationships, i.e., the processes of identification with both parents during the oedipal phase, as a model for other identifications — both in the preoedipal phase and in adolescence. One need only think of Freud's fundamental statement that identification represents the earliest form of emotional bond (1921c, p. 107).

In recent decades particularly clear descriptions of these identifications during ego and self development have been given within the framework of structural theory by Jacobson (1964) for the preoedipal phase and by Erikson (1959) for adolescence. The adherents of the ego psychology school of psychoanalysis described identifications in the framework of oedipal and preoedipal object relationships; these descriptions, however, did not lead to the extension of psychoanalysis implicit in structural theory. On the contrary, the psychoanalytic technique became rather restricted by the intrapsychic conflict model and the one-person psychology of the standard technique. The reason is that both object relationships and the resulting identifications are, like all of structural theory, founded on the basis of the economic principle of instinct discharge. This "principle of constancy," which Freud adopted from Fechner, is the basis of psychoanalytic theory and influences everything else: "The nervous system is an apparatus which has the function of getting rid of the stimuli which reach it, or of reducing them to the lowest possible level; or which, if it were feasible, would maintain itself in an altogether unstimulated condition" (Freud 1915c, p. 120). In our opinion, however, Modell was accurate in making the following statement in the prefatory note to his essay "The Ego and the Id: Fifty Years Later":

> Object relations are not discharge phenomena. Freud's concept of instinct as something arising from within the interior of the organism does not apply to the observation that the formation of object relations is a process of caring encompassing two people (a process that does not include climaxes or peaks of discharge). Further, the concept of instinct itself has not received its necessary backing from contemporary biology .... I believe, as does Bowlby, that object relations have their analog in the attachment behaviors of other species. (Modell 1984, pp. 199-200)

A comprehensive psychoanalytic psychopathology of conflict can nowadays proceed on the assumption that there are no disturbances of object relationships independent of disturbances in self-feeling.

It is advisable to supplement explanatory psychoanalytic theory, by means of which the psychopathology of conflict has been systematized, with a *systematic approach to problem solving*, i.e., a theory of therapy. The object of therapy is to master conflicts, under conditions more favorable than those which acted as midwife at the birth of the conflicts concerned. (We choose this metaphor in order to highlight the interpersonal nature of the determinants of pathogenesis.) It is thus astonishing that the development of a systematic approach to problem solving, to which the analyst makes a considerable contribution on the basis of his "change knowledge" (Kaminski 1970), limped behind the explanatory theory of psychoanalysis. A plausible model of therapy, such as that of Sampson and Weiss (1983), which places emphasis on the here-and-now mastering of old traumas that have retained their psychodynamic effectiveness, was a long time coming. This was the case although Waelder had already created conditions favorable for such a model in his article on the principle of multiple function (1936), where he raised problem solving to the status of a comprehensive ego function: "The ego always faces problems and seeks to find their solution" (p. 46). Accordingly, the processes in the ego can be designated as the attempted solution of problems; the ego of an individual is characterized by a number of specific methods of solution (pp. 46-47). At the same time, Waelder drew attention to the problems associated with the art of psychoanalytic interpretation, and was perhaps the very first to speak of *psychoanalytic hermeneutics.*

On the basis of what we have said so far, our understanding of therapy can be delineated as follows: The unfolding and structuring of transference are promoted by interpretations and take place within the special therapeutic *relationship* (working alliance). The patient has an increased degree of sensitivity as a result of earlier experience, and, on the basis of his unconscious expectations, initially takes particular note of everything that serves to foster repetition and create a *perceptual identity* (Freud 1900a). The new experiences the patient has in the analytic situation enable him to achieve solutions to previously insoluble problems. The analyst assists the patient in gaining self-knowledge and overcoming unconscious resistance by providing interpretations; in the process the patient may spontaneously achieve surprising insights. Since psychoanalytic interpretations are ideas which originate in the analyst, they can also be described as ways of seeing things, as opinions. As insights, they may have a lasting therapeutic effect if they stand up to the patient's critical examination or correspond at all to his "expectations," to his inner reality. These insights then intervene in experiencing and change it in the course of the working through, which continues in the patient's daily life. The patient perceives the changes subjectively, but they can also be demonstrated by alterations in his behavior and by the disappearance of his symptoms.

This conception of therapy implies that the value of the psychoanalytic method should be judged by the changes resulting from therapy. Yet although structural change may be the goal, it may be thwarted by unfavorable conditions of one kind or another. Under no circumstances can the psychoanalyst evade answering the following questions:

1. How does the analyst view the connection between the assumed structure (as a theoretical proposition) and the patient's symptoms?
2. Which internal changes (experienced by the patient) and which external changes indicate which structural changes?
3. In light of the answers to both of these questions, can the selected mode of therapy be justified?

We agree with Brenner (1976, p. 58) that "symptomatic improvement is a necessary criterion, though not in itself a sufficient one, for validation of a line of interpretation and the conjecture(s) on which it is based."

Interpretation, the characteristic feature of the psychoanalytic technique, is part of a complex network of relationships. It has no value on its own, and neither do rules of treatment; the analyst's psychic reality, his countertransference, and his theory become part of the analytic situation. The ability to go from general knowledge to the individual case, and vice versa, is a feature of psychoanalysis as well as of other practical disciplines.

The need to cater properly for the uniqueness of every patient makes the practical application of psychoanalysis a skill, a *techne*, a craft which one must learn in order to be able to practice according to the rules, which, however, can serve only as general recommendations. Despite the modern connotations of the word "technology," we are not afraid to use the term "psychoanalytic technology," as employed by the psychoanalytically trained philosopher Wisdom (1956). Soulless technique and alienation are one thing; psychoanalytic skill is located on quite another level of *techne*. Psychoanalysts are neither "psychotechnicians" nor "analysts" in the sense that they take the psyche apart and leave the synthesis (healing) to take care of itself. We are not deterred by misunderstandings of our attitude to therapy which may be occasioned by our use of the word "technology," for analysts follow technological principles in making their interpretations – in their skillful searching, in their heuristics, and so on, right up to the patient's "aha" experience. As a *hermeneutic technology*, the psychoanalytic method has a complicated relationship to theory (see Chap. 10).

Particularly relevant for the art of psychoanalytic interpretation is knowledge of teleological and dramaturgic actions:

> *Teleological actions* can be judged under the aspect of effectiveness. The rules of action embody technically and strategically useful knowledge, which can be criticized in reference to truth claims and can be improved through a feedback relation with the growth of empirical-theoretical knowledge. This knowledge is stored in the form of technologies and strategies. (Habermas 1985, vol. 1, p. 333)

In adapting these ideas into a form useful for the psychoanalytic technique, it must obviously be borne in mind that goal-oriented actions, a consideration in philosophical theories of action since the time of Aristotle (Bubner 1976), are not to be restricted to purposive rationality as conceived by Max Weber. It would be a fundamental misunderstanding of our position to think that our emphasis on change as the aim of therapy implies fixed goals. True, communication in psychoanalytic interpretation cannot be aimless, but the goals are not fixed, and are shaped by the patient's spontaneity, by his free associations, and by his critical examination of the analyst's ideas and of their overt or latent goals. In this process new ways and goals emerge as if of themselves, but are actually determined by the conditions which bring about various forms of the psychoanalytic process.

## 1.3 Crisis of Theory

For quite some time, psychoanalysis has been in a phase of "revolution and almost anarchy" (A. Freud 1972a, p. 152). Almost all of the concepts governing theory and technique are under attack from some direction. A. Freud refers in particular to the criticism of free association, of interpretation of dreams (which has had to cede its leading role to interpretation of transference), and of transference, which is no longer understood as a phenomenon arising spontaneously in the patient's behavior and thinking, but as one induced by the analyst's interpretations (1972a, p. 152). Meanwhile the controversies within psychoanalysis have become even more intense. Not even the cornerstones of psychoanalytic practice — transference and resistance — occupy their old positions. With regard to these essential components of psychoanalysis, Freud wrote:

> It may thus be said that the theory of psycho-analysis is an attempt to account for two striking and unexpected facts of observation which emerge whenever an attempt is made to trace the symptoms of a neurotic back to their sources in his past life: the facts of transference and of resistance. Any line of investigation which recognizes these two facts and takes them as the starting-point of its work has a right to call itself psycho-analysis, even though it arrives at results other than my own. (1914d, p. 16)

Obviously there are significant repercussions on theory and technique if one of these cornerstones is shifted, or if the psychoanalytic method has to rest on many different cornerstones in order to meet the demands imposed by practical experience.

If the signs of far-reaching change are looked at from the viewpoint of the history of science set out by Kuhn (1962), good reasons can be given for the fact that psychoanalysis was late in entering its phase of normal science, and good arguments to support the view that a process of evolution is taking place or that a change of paradigm is imminent (Spruiell 1983; Rothstein 1983; Ferguson 1981; Thomä 1983c). Widely diverging views are held together by their common connection to Freud's work. Yet it is clear that analysts can acknowledge the facts of transference and resistance and also accept other basic assumptions of psychoanalysis, such as unconscious mental processes and the evaluation of sexuality and of the Oedipus complex (Freud 1923a, p. 247), and nevertheless achieve varying results with the psychoanalytic method of investigation and treatment. This demonstrates once more the great complexity of the relationship between psychoanalytic technique and psychoanalytic theory. The innovative ferment which made its mark in the idea of "crisis of identity" (Gitelson 1964; Joseph and Wildlöcher 1983) has its counterpart in psychoanalytic orthodoxy. As a reaction to the sweeping criticism from within and without, and as an expression of concern for the essentials of psychoanalysis such orthodoxy is understandable, but for resolving conflicts it is no more suitable than some neurotic reaction would be. In fact, rigidity and anarchy determine and reinforce each other, which is why A. Freud (1972a) mentioned them both in the same breath.

The practice of psychoanalysis is not the only sphere characterized by change and innovation. The "speculative superstructure," as Freud (1925d, p. 32) termed its metapsychology, has also become shaky in recent decades. Many writers view the abandonment of this superstructure, which Freud erected in the attempt to define psychoanalysis as a science, as heralding a new era. Some believe that psychoanalytic interpretation could in this way be freed from Freud's alleged "scientistic self-misunderstanding" (Habermas 1971) and return to its home among the hermeneutic disciplines. Others are of the opinion that the abandonment of metapsychology could at last lead to full recognition of the role of the clinical theory of psychoanalysis, which is less inferential and thus better suited to serve as a guide to practice that can be empirically tested. However, the various stories forming the building of psychoanalytic theory cannot be cleanly separated. The girders supporting metapsychology also run through the lower floors, some more visible in the walls than others. Metapsychological assumptions are also contained in the less inferential clinical theory, and influence the analyst even when he believes that he is listening without a trace of prejudice, i.e., that he has given himself over to his evenly suspended attention. "Even at the stage of description it is not possible to avoid applying certain abstract ideas to the material in hand, ideas derived from somewhere or other but certainly not from the new observations alone" (Freud 1915c, p. 117).

In the secondary working through of the material he has gained in a single session or during the course of a therapy, the analyst will also concern himself with the relationship of his ideas to psychoanalytic theory. Freud believed that this task was not satisfactorily accomplished until a psychic process had been described dynamically, topographically, and economically:

> We see how we have gradually been led into adopting a third point of view in our account of psychical phenomena. Besides the dynamic and the topographical points of view, we have adopted the *economic* one. This endeavours to follow out the vicissitudes of amounts of excitation and to arrive at least at some *relative* estimate of their magnitude.
>
> It will not be unreasonable to give a special name to this whole way of regarding our subject-matter, for it is the consummation of psycho-analytic research. I propose that when we have succeeded in describing a psychical process in its dynamic, topographical and economic aspects, we should speak of it as a *metapsychological* presentation. We must say at once that in the present state of our knowledge there are only a few points at which we shall succeed in this. (Freud 1915e, p. 181)

In order to show the clinical significance of this approach, Freud gave a description of "the process of repression in the three transference neuroses which are familiar to us." Since repression is "the corner-stone on which the whole structure of psycho-analysis rests" (1914d, p. 16), it becomes clear that for Freud the metapsychological explanations were of fundamental importance. His aim in preparing a metapsychology was "to clarify and carry deeper the theoretical assumptions on which a psycho-analytic system could be founded" (Freud 1917d, p. 222). According to Laplanche and Pontalis:

> Rather than treating as metapsychological works all the theoretical studies involving concepts and hypotheses intrinsic to these three points of view, it might be preferable to reserve this

description for texts which are more basic in that they develop or expound the hypotheses which underpin psycho-analytic psychology ... (1973, p. 250)

These authors regarded the following as "the *strictly* metapsychological texts" in Freud's work: "Project for a Scientific Psychology" (1950 a; written in 1895), Chap. 7 of *The Interpretation of Dreams* (1900 a), "Formulations on the Two Principles of Mental Functioning" (1911 b), *Beyond the Pleasure Principle* (1920 g), *The Ego and the Id* (1923 b), and *An Outline of Psycho-Analysis* (1940 a). Thus, right up to his last period, Freud sought the foundations of psychoanalytic theory in the metapsychological points of view, in the "dynamic, topographical, and economic aspects" (1915 e, p. 181). On the other hand, the psychoanalytic method remained in the realm of depth psychology. Through systematic use of the new method, Freud made discoveries which made it possible to investigate the influence of unconscious psychic processes on an individual's fate and on pathogenesis.

The analytic method and the language of theory are on different levels. Freud still sought to explain the psychic apparatus in terms of drive economy in the posthumously published *An Outline of Psycho-Analysis*, although at the same time he stressed that what lies between "the two terminal points of our knowledge" – between the processes in the brain and nervous system and our acts of consciousness – is unknown to us. An increase in the knowledge on this relationship "would at the most afford an exact localization of the processes of consciousness and would give us *no help towards understanding them*" (1940 a, p. 144, emphasis added). Freud had various ideas about psychic connections. In seeking physical, biological, cerebral, and neurophysiological explanations for human behavior in the concept of instinct and in instinct theory, he stayed faithful to his first love (Sulloway 1979); the explanatory model of depth psychology, however, is oriented on the context of meaning, the investigation of which leads to motivation analysis, which in turn leads to unconscious causes and reasons. If these causes and reasons are included, the understanding of the context of meaning is extended to such a degree that meaningful explanations can be given for phenomena which previously appeared senseless, even for delusional experiencing and action. Jaspers (1963) used the term "as-if understanding" to describe this hybrid of explanation and understanding which also characterizes the everyday use of these words. This as-if understanding was introduced (as higher level clinical hypotheses) into the debate on theory in the U.S. by Rubinstein (1967). Thus, in the psychoanalytic method the doubly rooted explanation is linked in complex fashion with understanding. We regard the "as-if" as a mark of distinction.

Freud's various ideas on psychic connections are the source of the contradictions and the powerful tensions which pervade his work and give rise to the current crisis of theory. With the assistance of the psychoanalytic method he arrived at theoretical conceptions which he attempted to describe in metapsychological terms and ultimately trace back to biological processes, while simultaneously developing a theory of depth psychology that remained immanent to the method, i.e., rested on the experience gathered in the analytic situation and did not borrow its ideas from turn-of-the-century biology and physics. During the same period in which he gave a metapsychological explanation for repression with reference to energy cathexis, Freud wrote, in *The Unconscious*:

It is clear in any case that this question — whether the latent states of mental life, whose existence is undeniable, are to be conceived of as conscious mental states or as physical ones — threatens to resolve itself into a verbal dispute. We shall therefore be better advised to focus our attention on what we know with certainty of the nature of these debatable states. As far as their physical characteristics are concerned, they are totally inaccessible to us: no physiological concept or chemical process can give us any notion of their nature. On the other hand, we know for certain that they have abundant points of contact with conscious mental processes; with the help of a certain amount of work they can be transformed into, or replaced by, conscious mental processes, and all the categories which we employ to describe conscious mental acts, such as ideas, purposes, resolutions and so on, can be applied to them. Indeed, we are obliged to say of some of these latent states that the only respect in which they differ from conscious ones is precisely in the absence of consciousness. Thus we shall not hesitate to treat them as objects of psychological research, and to deal with them in the most intimate connection with conscious mental acts.

The stubborn denial of a psychical character to latent mental acts is accounted for by the circumstance that most of the phenomena concerned have not been the subject of study outside psycho-analysis. Anyone who is ignorant of pathological facts, who regards the parapraxes of normal people as accidental, and who is content with the old saw that dreams are froth (*Träume sind Schäume*) has only to ignore a few more problems of the psychology of consciousness in order to spare himself any need to assume an unconscious mental activity. Incidentally, even before the time of psycho-analysis, hypnotic experiments, and especially post-hypnotic suggestion, had tangibly demonstrated the existence and mode of operation of the mental unconscious. (1915e, pp. 168-169)

According to Freud's *Introductory Lectures* (1916/17, p. 21), "psycho-analysis must keep itself free from any hypothesis that is alien to it, whether of an anatomical, chemical or physiological kind, and must operate entirely with purely psychological auxiliary ideas." It is in the context of this famous statement that Freud wrote that psychoanalysis "tries to give psychiatry its missing psychological foundation" and "hopes to discover the common ground on the basis of which the convergence of physical and mental disorder will become intelligible." Yet the actually dominant but hidden idea, important as early as in Freud's "Project for a Scientific Psychology" (1950a) from the year 1895, was Freud's intention to develop a scientific psychology, i.e., to describe psychic processes as quantitatively determined states of material components. It remained Freud's hope that the metapsychological structure of psychoanalysis, i.e., its superstructure, could one day "be set upon its organic foundation" (1916/17, p. 389).

Depth psychological auxiliary concepts concern especially unconscious psychic processes. Together with the psychology and psychopathology of conflict that Freud founded, they form the basis on which the coincidence of somatic and psychic disturbances can be understood. In recent decades psychoanalysis has adopted other auxiliary ideas from developmental and cognitive psychology. Furthermore, one consequence of the discussion of theories of science has been that the psychoanalytic method and the detectable psychic phenomena associated with it have moved to the center of interest and become a focus for the testing of theory. These developments have led to a fundamental crisis of the entire theoretical structure of psychoanalysis. The task of our time is to renew the theory of psychoanalysis, which has previously taken the form of metapsychology and has thus been based on a weak grounding which is substantively and methodologically alien to it.

It is no accident that the crisis of metapsychology, pervading all of clinical theory, became manifest during the systematic preparation of research to test hypotheses. In the clinical or experimental testing of theories one cannot start from metapsychological speculations which consist of a jumble of ideological postulates derived from natural philosophy, profound metaphorical statements about mankind, and brilliant observations and theories on the origin of mental illness. One of the major contributors to the process of clarification was Rapaport (1967), who systematized psychoanalytic theory and sought to establish a scientific foundation for its translation into practice. His encyclopedic knowledge is reflected in *The Structure of Psychoanalytic Theory* (1960), where he elaborated the existing system of metapsychological assumptions in such a way that its weaknesses became visible. He himself mentioned this almost in passing while discussing the (in his opinion low) chances for survival of some of the system's central concepts (1960, p. 124). Rapaport and Gill (1959) expanded metapsychology to include the genetic and adaptive points of view that were implied in Freud's writings and that had already been elaborated by Hartmann et al. (1949) and Erikson (1959). It is clear that genetic (developmental) approaches, as well as adaptation, contain psychosocial elements which are far removed from the biological assumptions of the economic principle.

When, after Rapaport's death, his colleagues and students looked back in retrospect and then continued with their original scientific work, it became obvious that far-reaching changes are necessary in order to transform metapsychological concepts into theories which can be tested. Thus Holt (1967 a), editor of the volume in honor of Rapaport, proposed abandoning concepts of energy, such as cathexis and libido, and also the explanatory terms ego, superego, and id (Gill and Klein 1964). A number of Rapaport's colleagues, e.g., Gill, G. Klein, Schafer, and Spence, are among the most vociferous critics of metapsychology. It would be foolish to interpret their deviations from Rapaport psychoanalytically, as some of their critics have. Such ad hominem arguments hinder further clarification of the actual reasons why Rapaport's extensive work introduced a new epoch. The fruit of his attempt at systemization can be seen in the fact that clinical research has been encouraged, very largely due to the efforts of renowned analysts from his school. The metapsychological explanations were, as is now clear, beyond the range of the psychoanalytic method. The accuracy of metapsychology cannot be demonstrated with the help of this method, as the economic principle relates to processes in the central nervous system that are only accessible to physiological investigation. The strength of the influence which metapsychological considerations have nonetheless exerted on therapeutic action over a period of decades is connected with the fact that many concepts are used metaphorically throughout the clinical theory of psychoanalysis. Attempts were then made to differentiate various levels of theory formation with regard to their clinical and experimental testability.

In response to criticism from philosophers, Waelder outlined various levels of the psychoanalytic theory, and the concepts associated with them, in his essay "Psychoanalysis, Scientific Method and Philosophy" (1962):

1. *Individual clinical interpretation* (individual "historical" interpretation, Freud 1916/17, p.270). This is the level of observation, i.e., of the material which the analyst gathers from his patient and which is usually not accessible to others. The analyst then seeks to interpret the individual data with respect to their interconnections and their relationship to other behavior patterns or to conscious and unconscious contents.
2. *Clinical generalization* (Freud's typical symptoms). On the basis of the individual data and the interpretations of them, the analyst makes generalizations which lead to specific statements relating to patient groups, symptom development, and age groups.
3. *Clinical theory.* The clinical interpretations and the generalizations permit the formulation of theoretical concepts which may already be contained in or may result from the interpretations, e.g., repression, defense, recurrence of repressed material, and regression.
4. Beyond the clinical theory of psychoanalysis, yet not clearly separated from it, lie abstract concepts such as cathexis, psychic energy, Eros, and Thanatos: psychoanalytic metapsychology. Freud's personal philosophy can be seen especially in metapsychology and in the ideas behind it (see Wisdom 1970).

This scheme demonstrates a hierarchy of psychoanalytic theories, varying in empirical content, which have to be taken into account in any scientific assessment.

Waelder believes that the higher the level of abstraction, the lower the relevance for psychoanalytic practice. If this were true, and if clinical theory could be separated from metapsychological assumptions and viewed as an independent system, the crisis of theory could be clearly defined. In reality it is not easy to discern which ideas belong to the speculative superstructure and which are indispensable in order to put observations into context, whether in the sense of understanding or of explanation. The psychoanalytic method is directed particularly toward the recognition of unconscious psychic processes. Observation of how unconscious and preconscious wishes and intentions are expressed in parapraxes and symptoms — the return of the repressed — belongs both to the lowest level of the building and to a higher one. The analyst, however, does not look down from the higher story but rather takes one of the metapsychological points of view which Waelder located there and also uses it on the ground floor. The topographical and structural points of view, i.e., the division of the psychic apparatus into unconscious, preconscious, and conscious or id, ego, and superego, illustrates the existence of stairs connecting the floors which can be used in both directions.

Waelder's description has been revised, in our opinion rightly, by Farrell (1981), who characterizes the relationship between the low and the high levels of theory by saying that psychoanalytic concepts are "Janus-faced in their functioning." He describes the necessarily twofold function of concepts on all stories as follows: In his daily work, the analyst does not use the concepts to spell out the details of the psychic apparatus, but rather to order the material produced by his patients. Here the concepts function on the lower level. But when he concerns himself with theory, he uses concepts such as regression and repression to clarify how a patient's psychic apparatus works. Farrell writes that simple statements about connections belong to the lower level: for example, saying that a person who suffers a frustration tends to regress to an earlier stage of development. As an example of repression, Farrell mentions the regular observation of a connection between the sexual anxieties of adult patients, their forgotten (repressed) experiences in childhood, and the revival of these experiences in therapy. The analyst uses such generalizations to help bring order into the patient's communication (material). The patterned ordering explains the material in the "weak sense":

> But, if an analyst is concerned to explain why and how this sort of material is produced at all, then he will use regression and repression to help him to specify and describe the states of affairs in the system that these concepts are referring to. They then function in the High Level theory. (Farrell 1981, p.38)

Thus the concepts are already Janus-faced on the lower level and refer to the theory of the unconscious. However, when making descriptive statements on the *observable sequence* of events, the analyst can neglect the *idea of a connection* if he is concerned purely with registering data. Thus, although association studies are guided by the idea that there are connections between the different elements, in the collection of data it is initially important only to register the complete sequence of individual associations. Thus, observations in the psychoanalytic situation must first be registered descriptively.

Since for many analysts metapsychology is connected both with the scientific status of psychoanalysis as an explanatory theory and with the claim that therapy has a causal approach, the crisis affects the analyst both as a scientist and as a therapist. One way for him to escape this dilemma is to forgo explanatory theories entirely and content himself with psychoanalytic interpretation, which plays the leading role in practice. In the German-speaking countries the contrasting of the "understanding" (*verstehende*) humanities and social sciences with the explanatory sciences dates back to Dilthey and Rickert, and Hartmann (1927) believed he had clearly shown psychoanalysis to be a science. Later, however, the debate was rekindled in the English-speaking world. Klauber (1968) referred to the English historian Collingwood (1946) as one of the first proponents of the understanding approach. Home (1966) and Rycroft (1966) argued along the same line. North American analysts were quick to adopt the ideas of the French philosopher Ricoeur, who described Freud as a hermeneuticist. The term "scientistic self-misunderstanding," coined by Habermas (1971) to describe a fallacy to which Freud had fallen victim, became a catchphrase. Habermas was referring to metapsychological explanations, although without contesting that psychoanalysts need an explanatory theory as well as generalizations in order to be able to treat patients in depth, i.e., to proffer interpretations.

At this juncture, we would like to reiterate some remarks on hermeneutics from one of our previous publications (Thomä and Kächele 1975, pp.51-52).

The term is derived from the Greek word *hermeneuo* (I explain my thoughts in words, expound, interpret, translate). It is often falsely assumed that there is an etymological link between hermeneutics and Hermes, the messenger (and thus interpreter) of the gods. However, the similarity between the words is coincidental; *hermeneuo* goes back to a root with the approximate meaning "speak." The term "hermeneutics" was coined in the early seventeenth century to describe the procedure of interpreting texts. The development of hermeneutics was strongly influenced by the exegesis of the Bible. The dispute between theologians and advocates of hermeneutics is shown, for example, in Schleiermacher's principle (1959 [1819], pp. 86-87) that misunderstanding generally precedes understanding. Understanding thus turns out to be an epistemological problem: we have to know a little about an item, i.e., have a preunderstanding, before we can study it.

The hermeneutic approach was expressed most clearly in the humanities and in the branches of philology concerned with the interpretation of texts, where the fundamental question is that of the sense, i.e., the meaning, of the text concerned. There is a direct line from philological, theological, and historical hermeneutics to the understanding form of psychology. The demand that one feel and think oneself into the text, or into the situation of the other, links the understanding form of psychology to the humanities. The ability to reconstruct the experiences of the other is one of the preconditions which must be fulfilled if psychoanalytic treatment is to take its course. Introspection and empathy are essential features of the complementary technical rules of free association and evenly suspended attention. The sentence "Every understanding is already an identification of the self and the object, a reconciliation of those separated outside this understanding; that which I do not understand remains foreign and different to me" could have been written by a psychoanalyst interested in empathy (e.g., Greenson 1960; Kohut 1959), but in fact comes from Hegel (Apel 1955, p. 170). Kohut (1959, p. 464) stresses that Freud harnessed introspection and empathy as scientific instruments for systematic observation and exploration. Gadamer writes that interpretation begins

> where the meaning of a text cannot be immediately understood. One must interpret in all cases where one does not trust the immediate manifestation of a phenomenon. Thus the psychologist does not accept a patient's statements about his life at face value, but inquires as to what is going on in the patient's unconscious. In the same way, the historian interprets the recorded facts in order to discover the true meaning which they express but also conceal. (1965, p. 319)

Gadamer seems to have in mind a psychologist practicing psychoanalysis; his description characterizes the psychodynamic approach. It is precisely the incomprehensible, the apparently senseless element of psychopathological phenomena which the psychoanalytic method traces back to its origins and renders comprehensible. It is more than an incidental problem of detail that, according to Gadamer, distorted or cryptic texts create one of the most difficult hermeneutic problems. Philological hermeneutics probably encounters a barrier here similar to the one that cannot be crossed by a purely understanding form of psychology, i.e., one which lacks an explanatory theory.

Returning to our main line of argument, one's assessment of the crisis of theory and its spread through the various floors of psychoanalysis depends quite crucially on the role one attributes to metapsychology. Provocative article titles convey the impression of an explosive discussion. "Metapsychology Is Not Psychology" argues Gill (1976). "Two Theories or One?" asks Klein (1970), criticizing libido theory. "Metapsychology — Who Needs It?" asks Meissner (1981). Frank (1979) discusses the books by Klein (1976), Gill and Holzman (1976), and Schafer (1976), and seems from his title to come close to resignation: "Two Theories or One? Or None?" Modell (1981) answers the question "Does Metapsychology Still Exist?" with "yes and no": the characteristic metapsychological points of view are misleading and should thus be abandoned. All that Modell leaves of traditional metapsychology is the hollow idea. Finally, Brenner (1980) believes that the aberrations and confusions of his colleagues are clarified by his exegesis of Freud's relevant texts. He states that metapsychology is to be equated with Freud's theory of unconscious processes and with the whole of depth psychology (p. 196).

Freud's metapsychological texts can be interpreted in various ways, and these different readings lie at the root of the current controversies. Every serious psychoanalytic discussion still begins with the exegesis of Freud's work, but matters cannot rest there. It should have become clear by this point that the reason why the crisis of theory affects the psychoanalytic method is that it influences what ideas the analyst brings to the material and how far they assist understanding, and possibly even explanation. In the context of discovery, the ideas Freud had formed on the basis of the observation of fits of hysteria and other psychopathological syndromes enabled him to arrive at unexpected, unique explanations of unconscious processes. He then developed a method in order to be able to test his ideas against further observation. No one can act without a theory. In an important paper, Wisdom (1956, p. 13) writes, "Hence, when confronted with a problem, a theory must come first." In the same passage, Wisdom makes it clear that the various techniques of psychoanalysis are attempts to solve practical and theoretical problems.

How analysts answer the explosive questions which have been raised obviously depends on what they understand by metapsychology and how they interpret Freud's writings on the topic. Our own studies have convinced us that Rapaport and Gill's (1959) interpretation of metapsychology and its position in Freud's work is even-handed, giving equal weight to the various metapsychological points of view. Later, however, Gill (1976) in particular ascribed the central position to Freud's economic (biological) approach to explanation. There are various reasons for the differences in opinion on this point. For one thing the relevant passages can be interpreted in different ways; for another, in their application by analysts, all metapsychological points of view naturally also have some relationship to the patient's experiencing. In this respect metapsychology is also psychology. Finally, the dynamic and the topographical points of view seem closer to experiencing and to human conflicts than do the economic ideas about quantitative processes which the individual is not aware of. In our opinion, however, this description of metapsychology disguises the fact that Freud not only stayed true to the economic point of view, but also tried to base the theory on man's instinctual nature and on biology, and also expected that quantitative factors would later provide solutions to problems which were not yet resolved. This is the manner in which "the fallacious use of quantitative concepts in dynamic psychology" (Kubie 1947) came about.

No change is necessary, of course, if metapsychology is emptied of its specific contents, as proposed by Meissner (1981). He distances himself from metapsychology, seeing it as nothing more than a guiding idea, something that every scientist needs in addition to his method — an incontestable banality. Modell (1981) also strips metapsychology of its physicalistic features, seeing Freud's "Witch Metapsychology" as a symbol for fruitful speculation and fantasying. Like Mephisto in Goethe's *Faust* (Part I, Witches' Kitchen) one has to ask, "Is this the way to deal with witches?" In what context did Freud seek assistance in the "witch's primer"? In *Analysis Terminable and Interminable* (1937c), he was trying to get closer to answering the question of whether it is possible "by means of analytic therapy to dispose of a conflict between an instinct and the ego, or of a pathogenic instinctual demand upon the ego, permanently and definitively" (p.224). He sought help from the witch: "We can only say: *'So muss denn doch die Hexe dran!'* — the Witch Metapsychology. Without metapsychological speculation and theorizing — I had almost said 'phantasying' — we shall not get another step forward" (1937c, p.225). After consulting the witch, Freud believed he had found the answer in quantitative elements of the strength of the instinct, or in the "relation between the strength of the instinct and the strength of the ego" (1937c, pp.225-226). Freud explained the experiencing of pleasure and unpleasure by means of the economic principle. He assumed that the psychic and somatic experiences of pleasure and unpleasure originate in the cathexis of affective ideas by psychic energy: pleasure consists in the discharge of this energy. Cathexis and discharge are the regulatory mechanisms whose existence Freud assumed. The Witch Metapsychology thus leads us not into the realm of imagination but to real quantities, albeit ones that Freud localized where the psychoanalytic method can never reach: in the biological substrate, in cerebral neurophysiological processes — in short, in the body.

Brenner (1980) claims to have attained true exegesis, as a result of which metapsychology is equated with the psychology of the unconscious and with the whole of psychoanalytic psychology. It is undisputed that Freud stressed the quantitative, economic factors throughout his work, not just in his late texts. This emphasis is attributed to the influence of Brücke and thus of the Helmholtz school — as if identifying the origin of the economic principle would do anything to change the fact that the decisive factors in psychoanalytic theory, and thus obviously also in the theory of the unconscious, are discharge and cathexis, i.e., the economic or energetic point of view. Even Brenner has to concede that Freud's claim was to explain psychic phenomena dynamically, topographically, and economically. Rapaport and Gill (1959, p.153) described these assumptions as the foundation of psychoanalytic theory. This refers, in Freud's words, to "the dynamic relations between the agencies of the mental apparatus which have been recognized — or (if that is preferred) inferred or conjectured — by us" (1937c, p.226). If we add the genetic and adaptive points of view, the five metapsychological points of view together cover the entire spectrum of psychoanalytic theory.

The problem is now not how many hypotheses are formulated, and on what level of abstraction, but which theoretical assumptions are capable of being tested by means of the psychoanalytic method or psychological experiments. In his discussion of the relationship between theory and method, Brenner fails to consider one important problem: the elements which Freud borrowed from biology restricted the understanding of depth psychology and of psychoanalytic explanations, or even deformed these explanations, as shown by Modell (1981). This problem has led to the criticism of the economic point of view of metapsychology and thus of all the theoretical assumptions which are in any way connected with it. The information gathered by means of the psychoanalytic method is influenced to a high degree by the ideas which the analyst conveys. Therefore, it is not a matter of indifference what we call the forces which are ascribed a role in psychic dynamics (Rosenblatt and Thickstun 1977). By contrast, Brenner (1980, p.211) believes it makes no difference whether one speaks of psychic energy or motivational impulse, or uses instead a symbol such as *abc.* However, since the unconscious is accessible to the psychoanalytic method only to the degree to which instinct is represented in the psyche, it is of crucial importance whether we use anonymous symbols or speak in terms of significant, purposive motives.

Modell (1981, p.392) stresses that clinical theory is not explained by metapsychology, but rather derived from it. To support his argument he cites the example of A. Freud's book *The Ego and the Mechanisms of Defence* (1937), which could not have been written if Freud had not revised metapsychology and provided a new model in which unconscious forces are regarded as part of the ego. Despite all the modifications he made, Freud adhered to the idea of *materialistic* monism; at the same time, in his exploration of human psychic life he was very conscious of the role played by method. In other words, he had a dualistic approach to the *psychological* exploration of unconscious processes and to the origin and consequences of repression. His genius overcame metapsychological pseudoexplanations and paved the way for the great discoveries he described in the 1920s in *The Ego and the Id* (1923 b) and *Group Psychology and the Analysis of the Ego* (1921 c).

At the same time, his attempt to provide a metapsychological foundation for psychic life culminated in *Beyond the Pleasure Principle* (1920 g). His pseudoscientific (metapsychological) explanations retained a high degree of prestige, despite his declaration that the scientific form of psychoanalysis is that which rests on ideas borrowed from psychology (1927 a, p.257), and his demand (expressed in a letter to V. von Weizsäcker in 1932) that analysts learn "to restrict themselves to psychological modes of thinking" (von Weizsäcker 1977 [1954], p.125). This is the reason why Gill's title "Metapsychology Is Not Psychology" sent out such shock waves.

The current crisis arises from the criticism expressed by psychoanalysts who have not allowed themselves to take the easy way out. One of these is Gill. After his extension of metapsychology together with Rapaport (Rapaport and Gill 1959), his reassessment with Pribram (Pribram and Gill 1976) of Freud's

*Project for a Scientific Psychology* (1950a) marked a turning point in his thought. As can be seen from Weiner's (1979) review of Pribram and Gill's article and Holt's (1984) essay in honor of Gill's life and work, abandonment of the idea that the economic point of view is a fundamental principle of metapsychology became inescapable. The method of depth *psychology* is not capable of making statements on neuro*physiological* or other biological processes. Freud nevertheless repeatedly returned to the economic point of view and to speculative assumptions about the distribution of energy in the organism, for reasons which we will now describe.

The psychoanalyst is continually dealing with processes which relate to a person's bodily experiencing. The patient's subjective theories on his physical condition are anthropomorphic, i.e., they reflect infantile conceptions about the body. Not only does the language of metapsychology preserve obsolete biological ideas, its metaphors raise patient's fantasies about their bodies, i.e., about their conscious and unconscious images of themselves, to an abstract level. Gill (1977) pointed out that metapsychology is full of images which betray their origin in infantile notions concerning sexuality. By means of the metapsychological system, Freud wanted to *explain projections* that previously had led to the development of metaphysical ideas.

When we realize that infantile notions and obsolete biological beliefs are woven into the fabric of metapsychological metaphors, it becomes easier to understand why these concepts have retained such vitality even though they have become untenable as components of a scientific theory. If, like Gill, one adheres to Freud's definitions and their specific contents, metapsychology can no longer be accepted as a scientific theory. If, however, the definition is left to the individual analyst, each one can begin anew but still leave everything as it was. In this way, Modell (1981) includes all universal psychological phenomena — e.g., repetition, identification and internalization, origin and development of the Oedipus complex, development of superego and ego-ideal — in metapsychology. He believes that processes which are common to all people, i.e., allow the highest degree of generalization, are by definition biological.

We believe it is inappropriate to define universal phenomena, such as identifications, ego conflicts, incest wishes, and the incest taboo, as biological simply because they occur in all cultures, albeit with contents which vary widely from one culture to the next. These *psychosocial processes* presuppose a capacity for symbolization, which is normally by no means ascribed to biology. However the incest taboo in the oedipal triangle may have come into being, we prefer the psychosocial and sociocultural approach employed by Parsons (1964, pp. 57ff.) to biological hypotheses which suggest that the early *Homo sapiens* had some kind of notion of the genetic advantages of exogamy and avoidance of incest.

It must be stressed that psychosocial and sociocultural phenomena have a measure of autonomy; neither their origin nor their modification can be reduced to biological processes. In this context, and in contrast to Rubinstein (1980), we regard Popper and Eccles' (1977) admittedly speculative argumentation in favor of an interactionist view of the body-soul problem as extraordinarily fruitful for psychoanalysis. Popper and Eccles ascribe powerful evolutionary influence to psychic processes when they assume that man, after learning to speak and developing an interest in language, set off down the path leading to development of his brain and his intellect.

We are interested here not in the effect of man's psychic inner life on his evolution, or in Popper and Eccles' speculations thereon, but in another implication of philosophical interactionism: the liberation of psychoanalysis, as a psychosocial science, from the restrictions imposed by materialistic monism in its role as the fundamental principle of metapsychology. The philosophical and neurophysiological arguments which Popper and Eccles use are heuristically productive, and also much less speculative than Rubinstein (1980) assumes. Kandel's (1979, 1983) neurophysiological—better, psychoneurophysiological—experiments on a species of snail imply an interactionism, and thus provide substantiation for the view that the psyche has an independent role of its own. Systematic sensory stimulation of the organs of touch in these snails leads to structural changes in brain cells in the corresponding cerebral region. In short, these pioneering experiments can be interpreted as showing that cognitive (psychic) processes bring about structural (cellular) alterations (see Reiser 1985).

We may summarize by saying that the criticism of metapsychology, as expressed by Gill, Holt, G. Klein, and Schafer, is convincing. Modell believes the problem can be defused simply by criticizing Freud's obsolete biological principles of explanation. He cites the example of the concretization of the concept of energy, saying that it led to an incorrect theory of the discharge of affects. We are of the opinion that the root of the crisis lies in the confusion of biology and psychology, arising from Freud's materialistic monism, which ultimately amounts to an isomorphism of the psychic and the somatic. We thus argue for a theory of psychoanalysis based primarily on ideas borrowed from psychology and psychodynamics. There are methodological reasons for this approach, as it is the only one which provides a foundation for the performance of studies on psychophysiological correlations. It must be said, however, that such investigations are often inspired by the utopian notion of being able to use neurophysiological experiments to test psychological theories. The fact is overlooked that the neurophysiological methods and the psychological theories refer to completely different objects. It is thus meaningless to ask whether psychological and neurophysiological theories are compatible or incompatible.

It has been clear for some time that psychoanalysis will emerge transformed from the crisis of theory, above all because analysts will no longer have to trouble themselves with pseudoscientific metapsychological explanations of energy transformations, etc. Increasingly, the analytic situation, which is the basis of the knowledge, practical scope, and empirical significance of the psychoanalytic method, is being subjected to scientific study (Hermann 1963).

This research has great practical relevance, because it relates to the most important area of application of the method—to therapy. It has only recently begun to become clear that the crisis has taken this turn. Initially, it appeared that abandoning metapsychology would necessarily involve giving up any claim to an explanatory theory. Many analysts equated causal explanations with science, and saw such explanations in psychoanalysis as being rooted in metapsychology, which, however, lacks all the characteristics of a verifiable scientific theory. Habermas' (1971) criticism of Freud's "scientistic self-misunderstanding," referring to the latter's metapsychological pseudoexplanations, has become a catchword and has led many to overlook the fact that Habermas attaches great importance both to interpretation and to the explanatory theory of unconscious processes. We have discussed these problems in detail in a previous publication on the methodological difficulties of clinical psychoanalytic research (Thomä and Kächele 1975), where we attempted to forge a link between the prominent role of interpretation in therapeutic work, which shows the psychoanalytic method to be a special form of hermeneutics, and Freud's claim to have systematized explanations of human experiencing, action, and behavior in psychoanalytic theory. However, since the explanatory theory of psychoanalysis had been equated with metapsychology, and Rapaport's broadly based attempt at systematization had led to the realization that these ideas cannot be verified scientifically either in the analytic situation or in experiments, the turn to hermeneutics by analysts both inside and outside Rapaport's circle seemed to offer a way out.

We will now elucidate this turn to hermeneutics with reference to the work of G. Klein, the researcher who linked hermeneutics to clinical theory. In contrast to Waelder's (1962) multistory building, Klein distinguishes two theory systems which differ in regard to the kind of questions they raise. He at first elaborated this distinction in relation to sexuality (1969), and then generalized it (1970, 1973). Klein separates clinical theory and metapsychology, and differentiates them, with reference to the break in Freud's dream interpretation, by means of the why-and-how question. Clinical theory is centered on the question of meaning, purpose, and intent. Because the idea of the scientific foundation of psychoanalysis has become associated with metapsychological pseudoexplanations, Klein seems to have arrived at a dichotomy in which understanding is assigned to analytic practice, and the problem of explanation is avoided or bypassed. The issue here is whether motivational explanations have an epistemological status which differs in principle from that of causal explanations.

The philosophical arguments as to whether cause and reason are categorically different, and whether causal explanations differ from justifications of human thought and actions, are balanced. The logic of psychoanalytic explanations, and their position between description, motivational context, and functional context constitute a problem in itself and cannot be dealt with here (Rubinstein 1967; Sherwood 1969; Eagle 1973; Moore 1980). The discussion about reason and cause has not reached a conclusion (Beckerman 1977; Wollheim and Hopkins 1982; Grünbaum 1984). With regard to therapeutic practice, there is reference to both motivational explanations and contexts of meaning. We would like to illustrate this point with an excerpt from our earlier publication:

> With regard to symptoms, constructions take the form of explanatory hypotheses .... they thus become theoretical statements from which singular prognoses can be derived. Generally speaking, these prognoses identify the conditions causally responsible for the neurotic state

and claim that the therapeutic process must dissolve these conditions in order to induce change. (Thomä and Kächele 1975, p. 86)

This thesis contains nothing other than Freud's theory of repression, which Habermas also accepts. In contrast to Habermas and (even more strongly) Lorenzer (1974), however, we adhere to the idea that the verification of change can and must go beyond subjective intuition. If this were not so, hermeneutic understanding would remain exposed to the risk of *folie à deux*. Like Freud, we assume the existence of a causal connection between a particular determinant — the repression of an instinctual impulse — and the consequences — the return of the repressed material in the form of a symptom. Freud framed this thesis in metapsychological terms:

But we have arrived at the term or concept of the unconscious along another path, by considering certain experiences in which mental *dynamics* play a part. We have found — that is, we have been obliged to assume — that very powerful mental processes or ideas exist (and here a quantitative or *economic* factor comes into question for the first time) which can produce all the effects in mental life that ordinary ideas do (including effects that can in their turn become conscious as ideas), though they themselves do not become conscious. It is unnecessary to repeat in detail here what has been explained so often before. It is enough to say that at this point psycho-analytic theory steps in and asserts that the reason why such ideas cannot become conscious is that a certain force opposes them, that otherwise they could become conscious, and that it would then be apparent how little they differ from other elements which are admittedly physical. The fact that in the technique of psycho-analysis a means has been found by which the opposing force can be removed and the ideas in question made conscious renders this theory irrefutable. The state in which the ideas existed before being made conscious is called by us *repression*, and we assert that the force which instituted the repression and maintains it is perceived as *resistance* during the work of analysis. (1923 b, p. 14)

The force of resistance described here in metapsychological terms can, we believe, be substantiated psychodynamically and investigated analytically without reference to the "economic factor." In the wake of the resolution resulting from the interpretative work, the conditions maintaining the repression (and thus the symptoms) are changed. Eventually, the specific unconscious causes of the repression may become ineffective. This change may resolve the processes determined by the causal nexus, but not the nexus itself; as emphasized by Grünbaum (1984), the resolution actually confirms the suspected role of the nexus. We will not, at this juncture, go into the question of empirical proof and the problem of checking hypotheses in the analytic situation (see Chap. 10). This explanatory scheme is insufficient to answer the question of why the unconscious conditions express themselves in the form of symptoms. The energetic model, which has provided a pseudoexplanation, should be replaced by a more appropriate model.

Our concern here is to demonstrate that the *explanatory theory* of psychoanalysis refers to unconscious psychic processes which become accessible to *interpretation*. Any systematic research into the psychoanalytic situation must therefore embrace understanding as well as explanation. Particularly important is the determination of what ideas the analyst has in mind when he makes empathic interpretations. In our opinion, special attention must be paid to how the analyst's preliminary theoretical concept influences his actions. It is particularly unfortunate, in this context, that the economic principle of metapsychology continues to survive in depth hermeneutics — in the work of Habermas (1971), Ricoeur (1969), and especially Lorenzer (1974) — as our current state of knowledge clearly shows it to be inappropriate, and thus unsuitable as a framework for interpretations (see Thomä et al. 1976).

Many analysts nonetheless find it very difficult to give up metapsychology. Over the years, the metaphors of metapsychology have taken on *psychodynamic* meanings far removed from the original physical meanings. For example, Fechner's principle of constancy, which is contained in the economic point of view, turned into the Nirvana principle. Even the profound human truth expressed in Nietzsche's (1973 [1893]) verse "All pleasure seeks eternity....wants deep, deep eternity" can be understood as an anthropomorphic expression of the constancy principle and discharge theory.

Precisely these experiences, which G. Klein called "vital pleasures," are those which have a physical foundation like no other experiences. Hunger and sexuality have a quality which for good reason is termed "instinct" and is differentiated as a phenomenon from other experiences. The sexual climax is an exquisite bodily experience, and at the same time one is beside oneself with joy. The ecstasy seems to touch eternity and to lose it again at the peak, only to seek it anew and find it again in longing. At the same time prosaic processes of positive and negative feedback (i.e., motivational processes at conscious and unconscious levels) take place that are not contained in Freud's instinct theory, which he constructed on the model of the reflex arc. Thus Holt (1976), after a detailed positive appraisal of the clinical data provided by the libido theory, i.e., by human psychosexual development, comes to the conclusion that instinct is dead as a *metapsychological* concept and must be replaced by *wish*. His careful study presents convincing clinical and experimental findings in support of his position. We cannot go into detail here, but we would like to point out that Holt's use of Freud's wish theory adequately covers all elements of *psychosexuality*. The psychoanalytic theory of motivation and meaning that is currently being constructed can be regarded as a positive development with respect to the crisis of theory only if it is capable of linking observed and known phenomena to unconscious processes more convincingly, in terms of both understanding and explanation, than the previous and current theoretical hotchpotch.

And indeed, in philosophical and psychoanalytic studies with such provocative titles as "What Is Left of Psychoanalytic Theory?" (Wisdom 1984) and "The Death and Transfiguration of Metapsychology" (Holt 1981), some psychodynamic principles concerning the significance of the dynamic unconscious are stressed more clearly than in the opaque hotchpotch of metapsychology. Finally one returns — transformed — to Freud's earliest findings about man's unconscious psychic life: In the beginning was the wish. Instinctual wishes are the motive forces in our lives. The search for pleasure and the avoidance of unpleasure are the most powerful motives of human action, especially if these principles are equipped with extensive contents of pleasurable and unpleasurable experience. The pleasure-unpleasure principle is a regulatory schema of the first order. Psychoanalysis would thus lose its depth if its motivation theory did not start with the dynamic unconscious. Here, however, we come up against a major difficulty of method, as pointed out by Wisdom:

> For the unconscious [i.e., the dynamic unconscious which cannot be made conscious even by means of interpretations] is more like a root of a tree, and however much you develop the root into actual shoots, it can never be identified with the sum of the shoots that break through the soil. The unconscious always has more potential and is more than its manifestations. Its scientific status is like those high-level concepts in physics which are *never* open to checking by direct observation. (1984, p.315)

As early as *The Interpretation of Dreams* Freud had been led to infer the existence of unconscious wishes by his discovery of thoughts *transferred* into the preconscious. In this connection, it has always been a case of inferences based on a psychodynamic wish theory; these cannot be confirmed or refuted by assumptions about neurophysiological processes, whether it be those formulated by Freud or their modern equivalents. Instinct, in Freud's metapsychological sense, cannot be declared dead simply because hunger, thirst, and sexuality are regulated by mechanisms other than discharge. Holt's (1976, 1982) evidence is certainly relevant to psychoanalysis, but only provided Freud's metapsychology is assumed to be its basis for scientific explanation. It is precisely this belief which has prevented analysts from recognizing the inadequacy of the dualistic instinct theory pervading all levels of theory and practice.

The explanatory theory of psychoanalysis remained tied to nineteenth century biology, instead of being linked to the experience gathered in the analytic situation. Of course, in the psychoanalytic situation as well as in the metaphoric language of psychoanalytic practice, metapsychology has long since been transfigured, even though its proper burial, and consequently an orderly disposition of the estate, has only recently taken place. For methodological reasons we, in contrast to Rubinstein (1976) and Holt (1976), accept Popper and Eccles' (1977) view of psychophysical interactionism, because theories of identity regularly lead to a monistic materialism, to which Freud had also adhered, despite the emphasis they place on the independence of the psychic and physical levels within the whole. The ubiquitous tendency toward identity theory seems to have its roots in the unconscious. Each of us is identical with his body, but it is also foreign to him because he cannot look into it as an object. Our bodies cause us more puzzlement than external objects, which we can dissect and examine. Finally, we can take up an external position by separating ourselves from the body intellectually. This may be connected with the unconscious yearning for unity which is said to pervade all branches of science; it is the eternal hope that the same set of concepts might one day be valid on some very high level of abstraction. This is an often varied but ever-recurring argument which Adorno (1972 [1955]) criticized with respect to the relationship between sociology and psychology.

We believe that the criticism of instinct energetics has opened new dimensions for scientific depth psychology. One apparent objection to this view is that branches of psychoanalysis deviating from instinct theory often become shallow (Adorno 1952); however, this loss of depth is avoidable. It is probably connected with the fact that many analysts equate the unconscious with instinct or energy. The renunciation of the economic view which results from the rejection of instinct theory inhibits the analyst's fantasizing about his patients' unconscious. After all, the therapeutic process depends on many factors, and our ideas about the motive force have a stimulating effect on the unconscious. Psychoanalytic heuristics will always be oriented on the pleasure principle and on the dynamic of unconscious wishes, even when the economic point of view of instinct theory has been exhausted. The truths that are concealed and expressed metaphorically in Freud's instinct mythology seem to lie in the fact that the id can be understood as an inexhaustible source of human fantasy which points beyond the restricting realities, beyond time and space. In psychoanalysis, libido is considered the "genuine psychic reality," as Adorno (1952, p. 17) demonstrated. To generalize libido into intentionality is to deprive it of its elementary motive force, which one is tempted to describe as being anchored in physical existence. Thus, in criticizing the economic point of view of libido theory, there is good reason to take care not to throw the baby out with the bathwater. Adorno's diagnosis is accurate. Revised and sociologized psychoanalysis tends to fall back into Adlerian superficiality; it replaces Freud's dynamic theory based on the pleasure principle with simple ego psychology (Adorno 1952, p. 2).

The economic principle and the assumptions concerning the regulation of experiences of pleasure and unpleasure by psychic energy have become untenable, both on neurophysiological and clinical psychoanalytic grounds and in view of recent findings on mother-child interaction. The striking, graphic language of Freud's theory suggests similarities between physical and psychic processes which in fact do not exist. If the suggestive power of metaphors leads the analyst to apply them in areas where the comparison is no longer valid, his therapeutic action will also be inappropriate. The crisis of theory cuts deep into psychoanalytic practice.

## 1.4 Metaphors

Freud's background was in late nineteenth century neuroanatomy and neurophysiology, and he employed references to these fields as aids to orientation in the new, unfamiliar territory he was exploring. We should still heed his warning to "resist the temptation to flirt with endocrinology and the autonomic nervous system, when what is needed is *an atmosphere of psychological facts with the help of a framework of psychological concepts*" (1927 a, p. 257, emphasis added). This advice is found in *The Question of Lay Analysis*, at the same point where Freud draws "the true line of division...between *scientific* analysis and its *applications* alike in medical and in nonmedical fields" (p. 257) and makes his famous statement concerning the inseparable bond. It is "not...logical" to distinguish "between medical [i.e., therapeutic] and applied analysis" (p. 257).

Inasmuch as *metaphorical* descriptions rest on *nonpsychological* concepts — as is the case for much of metapsychology — they fail to meet Freud's demands (which, however, he himself disregarded in his pioneer days).

Freud's metaphors — sum of excitation, discharge, cathexis, bond, etc. — came from nineteenth century neurophysiology. There is, of course, nothing to criticize in the use of metaphors as such; they are an integral part of every scientific theory (Grossman and Simon 1969; Wurmser 1977). Metaphors transfer meaning from a primary (familiar) object to a secondary (unfamiliar) object, as shown by Grassi (1979, pp. 51ff.) in his discussion of the historical development of the concept. The comparisons settle nothing by themselves, as Freud once wrote (1933a, p. 72), but they do help to make the analyst feel more at home in the new, unknown territory. Thus it was quite natural for Freud to employ references from neurology, for example in comparing the psychic apparatus to the reflex arc or describing the unconscious, the id, as "a chaos, a cauldron full of seething excitations" (1933a, p. 73), among the many other economic and quantitative metaphors he coined (Rubinstein 1972).

For both practical and theoretical reasons, it is essential to clarify how far the similarity suggested by metaphors extends. It is important to distinguish the common features and differences of the phenomena referred to by metaphors, i.e., to determine the positive and (especially) the *negative* aspects of the analogy (Hesse 1966; Cheshire 1975). An apt comparison reveals the similarity better than an inapt one; however, striking metaphors may only simulate a high explanatory value, in that they lead one to forget to look closely at the dissimilarity — the area of difference. Freud created many metaphors with which psychoanalysts still feel at home today (J. Edelson 1983). While inapt metaphors were abandoned as the theory underwent modification, the area of negative analogy, i.e., the difference, often remained unclarified. It is even probable that many of the metaphors coined by Freud were based on the belief in an isomorphism, i.e., in the equivalence of the items being compared. Otherwise he would not have discussed the possibility — indeed, expressed the hope — that psychoanalytic terminology might one day be replaced by a standardized physiological and chemical terminology following the principles of materialistic monism (1920g, p. 60).

A further complication is that many psychoanalytic metaphors from nineteenth-century neurophysiology are still attributed a scientific validity which they in fact lost long ago in their primary field without ever having been adequately empirically grounded in their secondary field. This old terminology actually deforms psychoanalytic experience and the interpretation of it. The metaphors did once have a useful integrating function, in that they built a bridge from the known to the unknown. Later, the language based on these metaphors played a part in forming the identity of the psychoanalyst within the psychoanalytic movement.

We now come to another language problem. Brandt (1961, 1972, 1977), Bettelheim (1982), and Pines (1985) assert that most of the present problems in psychoanalysis can be traced back to Strachey's alleged substitution of an artificial mechanistic English for Freud's metaphorical and anthropomorphic terminology in order to give the whole a scientific aura. That Strachey's translation displays many weaknesses and downright errors has become apparent to many German-speaking analysts, and there is no doubt that he replaced much of Freud's lucid and vivid terminology with terms which at best mean something to classical scholars. But can this be blamed for the theoretical problems which have such a profound effect on analytic practice? Ornston (1982, 1985 a) has also conjectured that one reason why Freud displayed what Jones (1959, p. 23) called a "cavalier attitude in this matter of translations" was that he positively wanted to retain the richness and variety of associations to everyday language.

Bettelheim's criticism can be illustrated by reference to the translation of *Besetzung* and *besetzen* as "cathexis" and "to cathect." The English words mean nothing to the layman, in contrast to Freud's original terms (*besetzen*: to occupy, fill). But what did Freud himself mean by *Besetzung*? In "Psychoanalysis: Freudian School," his article in the 13th edition of the *Encyclopaedia Britannica*, he wrote:

> From the economic standpoint psycho-analysis supposes that the mental representatives of the instincts have a charge (cathexis) of definite quantities of energy, and that it is the purpose of the mental apparatus to hinder any damming-up of these energies and to keep as low as possible the total amount of the excitations with which it is loaded. The course of mental processes is automatically regulated by the "pleasure-unpleasure principle"; and unpleasure is thus in some way related to an increase of excitation and pleasure to a decrease. (1926f, pp. 265-266)

It is immaterial that Freud himself uses the word "cathexis" here. The important thing is that on the basis of Freud's economic hypothesis — whether expressed in German, English, or any other language — psychoanalysts strove to demonstrate cathexis, using grotesque formulas to depict it (e.g., Bernfeld and Feitelberg 1929, 1930) or describing intricate transformations of the libido (e.g., Hartmann et al. 1949). Even more decisively, analysts often carelessly ascribe an explanatory power to the term "cathexis" because of its seeming quantitative precision. This influences the whole gamut of psychoanalytic practice, for instance the quantitative conception of the mounting tension resulting from silence. Detailed study of the work of Ricoeur (1970) reveals that the quantitative discharge theory permeates even his hermeneutic approach. Disregarding errors in translation, it is precisely the neologisms which have the potential to expose the problems. Freud disliked unnecessarily technical terms, and was dissatisfied when in 1922, for the sake of clarity, Strachey invented the word "cathexis" (from the Greek) as a translation for *Besetzung*. Strachey (see Freud 1923b, p. 63) notes in his introduction to *The Ego and the Id* that Freud may eventually have become reconciled to "cathexis," since he employed the term himself in the German version of the *Encyclopaedia Britannica* article (Freud 1926f, p. 266). Ornston (1985b) has, independently of us, published useful information about the background to Strachey's adoption of this term. The average German reader can guess at the analytic meaning of *besetzen* because he transfers the word's various nonspecialized meanings to the new field, i.e., understands the term metaphorically. In contrast, the neologism "cathexis" can serve as a metaphor only for the classical scholar who knows the meaning of the Greek root.

To restate our point, it is erroneous to claim, as do Bettelheim and Brandt, that Strachey's introduction of neologisms such as "cathexis" or his latinization of the German terms *Ich* and *Über-Ich* to "ego" and "superego" was responsible for creating new problems. On the contrary, Strachey's translations exposed problems which already existed (Ornstein 1982). The issue here is the relationship of explanatory psychoanalytic theory to the patient's subjective experience. Freud set out his policy for proceeding from the described phenomena to the psychoanalytic explanation in the *Introductory Lectures*:

> We seek not merely to describe and to classify phenomena, but to understand them as signs of an interplay of forces in the mind, as a manifestation of purposeful intentions working concurrently or in mutual opposition. We are concerned with a *dynamic view* of mental phenomena. On our view the phenomena that are perceived must yield in importance to trends which are only hypothetical. (Freud 1916/17, p. 67)

From this point of view the use of the Latinate form "ego" (and "superego") rather that an anglicized translation of *Ich* (and *Über-Ich*) is irrelevant, as neither ego nor the analytic use of *Ich* can be equated with the experiencing self (also *Ich* in German). In the introduction to *The Ego and the Id*, Strachey stated, correctly, that Freud's use of the word *Ich* was far from clear:

> The term had of course been in familiar use before the days of Freud; but the precise sense which he himself attached to it in his earlier writings is not unambiguous. It seems possible to detect two main uses: one in which the term distinguishes a person's self as a whole (including, perhaps, his body) from other people, and the other in which it denotes a particular part of the mind characterized by special attributes and functions. (Strachey, in Freud 1923b, pp. 7-8)

Freud was trying to explain an individual's subjective experience by means of the theory of the mind. Therefore no possible improvement in the translation of the German original could help solve problems arising in the theory.

A definite role is played by our understanding of "id" and by whether Hayman's question, "What do we mean by 'Id'" (1969), can be answered in the context of English, French, Spanish, or German society and culture. Yet a substantive it is, and as Breuer stressed in his portion of the joint publication with Freud in 1895, the danger is equally great in all languages:

> One falls only too easily into the mental habit of assuming substance behind a substantive, or of gradually conceiving an object by the term, consciousness. And if one has formed the habit of using such local relationships as "unconscious" metaphorically, he will in time actually build up an idea, in which the metaphor will be forgotten, and which he will manipulate as if it were real. Thus, mythology came into being. (Breuer and Freud 1936, p. 169)

The fact that Breuer's warnings against reification are so little heeded is due to the inadequate consideration of the philosophical aspects highlighted by Dilman (1984, p. 11).

When a German hears the word *Es* he thinks immediately of the impersonal pronoun *es* (it), which in German is used very extensively as the grammatical subject in sentences expressing feelings (e.g., *es tut mir leid*: I am sorry). Kerz (1985) writes that Nietzsche, despite all his criticism of thinking in substances, did not shrink from speaking of will, power, life, force, and so on when attempting to eliminate the constrictions of ego consciousness. In spite of all admonitions, substantives are constantly being reified, and thus the id is also credited with a whole range of human attributes.

Anthropomorphisms are an inevitable part of a use of metaphor in which man unconsciously uses himself as the standard by which all things are measured and accordingly looks for the ego, and in particular for wishes and intentions, in the hidden, still unconscious part of human nature, the id. Despite Freud's physicalistic terminology, he was kept from attributing material substance to the substantivized id by his extensive use of anthropomorphizing metaphors to explain unconscious processes and insofar as he adhered to the psychoanalytic method. Once this line is crossed, however, it is only one short step to diseases of the id and to equation of the id with pathological bodily processes. The understanding of the id in the romantic period and the philosophy of life — Nietzsche's id — becomes Groddeck's psychosomatic id, and the mystical universal science, the target of an insatiable longing, then seems to loom close.

What do we mean by "id"? This question can be answered more satisfactorily when one is familiar with the influence of intellectual history on Freud's decisions, including his following of Nietzsche's usage of the word *Es*. A German speaker familiar with intellectual history will have different associations with *Es* than the English-speaking reader of the Standard Edition will have with "id," but the English, French, and German versions of the psychoanalytic theory of the mind are all equally far removed from the patient attempting to free-associate. Bettelheim (1982) blames the latinization of some basic terms and the relatively low level of education of many of today's patients (who, unlike the educated bourgeoisie of Vienna, are unfamiliar with classical mythology, for instance the legend of Oedipus) for the fact that in his view psychoanalysis has lost Freud's humanity and become abstract.

We regard Bettelheim's arguments as misleading. Freud's theory, like any other, is distinct from subjective experience, and the application of the method in practice has never depended on whether the patient has ever heard of Sophocles' drama. Indeed, the less he knows, the more convincing any therapeutic and scientific discoveries are. Bettelheim's criticism cannot apply to psychoanalytic theory or to the average modern patient, only to the manner in which analysts apply the theory of the id. Certainly theories can be more or less mechanistic, and Freud's theory that displacement, condensation, and plastic representation are the most important unconscious processes is perhaps more mechanistic than Lacan's (1968) thesis that the unconscious is structured in the same way as language. Theoretical propositions about unconscious processes involved in repression have nothing directly to do with the analyst's human responsiveness, but when it comes to the therapeutic application of the psychoanalytic method, human empathy immediately becomes relevant. Professional responsibility then demands that solutions be sought to the problems we summarize at the end of Chap. 10.

Finally, it should be underlined that one reason for the prominence of metaphors in the psychoanalytic dialogue is the fact that they permit the linking of the concrete and the abstract. In addition, the clarification of similarities and differences is a constant factor in therapy (Carveth 1984b). Arlow (1979) called psychoanalysis a metaphoric procedure on the grounds that transference, the typical phenomenon in psychoanalysis, goes back to a metaphoric process, i.e., the carrying over of meaning from one situation to another. We will outline the consequences of this approach for treatment technique in the discussion of transference interpretation in Sect. 8.4.

## 1.5 Training

Psychoanalytic institutions have failed to maintain the inseparable bond between therapy and research. Freud's legacy is passed on principally via the training of therapists, without any appreciable degree of systematic research or treatment in outpatient clinics, as foreseen in Freud's model of how a psychoanalytic institute should function. Stagnation was thus built in, but was initially disguised by the unexpected expansion of psychoanalysis in the U.S.A. after World War II. The social acceptance of psychoanalysis motivated many young doctors to train as analysts. New training centers sprang up. Psychoanalytic concepts formed the basis of dynamic psychotherapy and psychiatry (see Sabshin 1985). But systematic research into the analytic situation, the home ground of psychoanalysis, is just beginning (Schlesinger 1974).

In the U.S.A., apart from a few nonphysicians who are accepted as research candidates on the strength of their talent for interdisciplinary research, only qualified or trainee psychiatrists may train and practice as psychoanalysts. At first glance, therefore, it would seem obvious that the oft-bemoaned stagnation is due to "medical orthodoxy" (Eissler 1965) or to "medicocentric" training (Parin and Parin-Matthèy 1983a). On closer examination, however, this lightning diagnosis turns out to be merely a description of the symptoms, which is, moreover, based on a rather narrow conception of medicocentrism. It is more accurate to say that the goal of training has the same standardizing effect all over the world. Even in countries where training is open to laymen (including nonmedical academics), the institutions turn out psychoanalytic therapists. Specialization in the standard technique equips them to treat patients who are suitable for it.

It is an incontestable fact that almost all nonmedical psychoanalysts give up their previous profession; very few remain active in, or conduct interdisciplinary research from, their original academic discipline. One of the honorable exceptions is the small group of nonmedical psychoanalysts who were qualified scientists before being trained under the auspices of the American Psychoanalytic Association. Favorable external circumstances have assisted most of this group of analysts to work productively in the area of interdisciplinary research and to sustain their competence in their original fields, to the benefit of psychoanalysis. Thus it is the goal of training that imposes restriction and orthodoxy, which is unfairly tagged "medical." In all other areas of medicine, basic research is in fact encouraged, but the emphasis on practice in psychoanalytic training is labeled "medicocentrist."

General and specific scientific questioning, including that in psychoanalytic research, break the chains of every kind of orthodoxy. In psychoanalysis, this leads to cooperation with the *humanities and social sciences.* Freud underlined that alone among the medical disciplines, [psychoanalysis] has the most extensive relations with the mental sciences, and...it is in a position to play a part of the same importance in the studies of religious and cultural history and in the sciences of mythology and literature as it is in psychiatry. This may seem strange when we reflect that originally its only object was the understanding and improvement of neurotic symptoms. But it is easy to indicate the starting-point of the bridge that leads over to the mental sciences. The analysis of dreams gave us an insight into the unconscious processes of the mind and showed us that the mechanisms which produce pathological symptoms are also operative in the normal mind. Thus psycho-analysis became a *depth-psychology* and capable as such of being applied to the mental sciences .... (Freud 1923a, pp. 252-253)

In the endeavor to treat the ill person adequately as a whole, medicine must draw on *all* sciences which could help to investigate, relieve, and cure human suffering. In this sense, the psychoanalytic method is one of many servants, and its master is not a specialist discipline, but rather the patient. More than the established disciplines, psychoanalysis has had (and still has) to fight for its right to determine its scope of activity and research and to work accordingly for the good of patients and society.

Psychoanalysis long remained one of the lesser servants, and Freud had to struggle to prevent it from being subordinated to a master, namely psychiatry. This hampered its practical and scientific development. Eissler (1965) welcomed the separation of psychoanalytic institutions from faculties of medicine and from universities, but in fact this partition was one of the *causes* of the medical orthodoxy he bemoaned. Orthodox attitudes would have had no chance of surviving for long in scientific medicine. Of course, psychoanalysis has for good reason always been medicocentric, in the sense that therapeutic practice is its foundation — and the birthplace of its theory of culture. Scientific investigation, in particular, demonstrates the interdisciplinary position of psychoanalysis and its dependence on exchange with the neighboring sciences. Psychoanalytic approaches can be applied productively in the humanities. However, all interdisciplinary cooperation also leads to relativization of the global claims made on behalf of psychoanalysis, whether as psychology or as theory of culture. In every psychoanalytic institute or university where research groups have been formed in recent decades, ideologies of all sorts have been undermined (Cooper 1984b; Thomä 1983b).

It is not the establishment of separate psychoanalytic institutions as such which has led to rigidity, but rather their one-sided nature, which was bemoaned by no less distinguished an analyst than A. Freud (1971). Kernberg (1985) recently reported that in both structure and function, psychoanalytic institutions are closer to professional schools and theological seminaries than to universities and art schools. This unfavorable state of affairs is met everywhere, i.e., also in apparently liberal centers outside the control of the International Psychoanalytical Association (IPA) which train lay analysts as well as physicians. A. Freud's criticism applies to all places where research is neglected during training and practical experience is limited to a few supervised cases. The increase in the duration of treatment in recent decades and the related intensification of supervision have not relaxed the rigidity to any significant extent.

We cannot go any further into the complex topic of training and supervisory analyses here, but it is revealing that the duration of therapies of patients grows in proportion to the length of training analyses. Training and supervisory analyses thus determine the school-specific features of undiluted, strict, and genuine psychoanalysis. Glover (1955, p. 382) drew attention long ago to the narcissistic components of this unusually high regard for a *quantity*, namely the number of sessions, the duration of analyses in years or decades, and the consequences of these two factors. This problem cannot be left unmentioned in a volume on psychoanalytic therapy, for training and supervisory analyses influence practice and the profession more than all other aspects of training put together. The lengthening of training and supervisory analyses for half a century has created significant problems (A. Freud 1971, 1983; Arlow 1982; Laufer 1982).

A promising sign is that the IPA is now looking at this problem. For example, Kernberg reported his findings at a symposium organized by the IPA, "Changes in Analysts and in Their Training" (Wallerstein 1985). Optimistically, in the long term changes should come about which will allow the realization of Freud's triad of training, patient care, and research. It is plain that evening courses, of the kind held in the traditional psychoanalytic institutions, are inadequate to achieve this goal (A. Freud 1971; Redlich 1968; Holzman 1976).

## 1.6 Directions and Currents

The further psychoanalysis expands, the more difficult it is for the various schools to reach a consensus regarding essential features. The changes heralded in the discussions between Viennese and London psychoanalysts in the 1930s (Riviere 1936; Waelder 1936) took place over the next 25 years.

The result was polarization. On the one hand, according to Rapaport (1967), the psychosocial implications and relationships remained unclarified in the theory of psychoanalytic ego psychology. On the other, the same author described Klein's (1945, 1948) object relationship theory ironically as id mythology. The position of the id in theory and practice is the decisive factor. In Lacan's sphere of influence, ego psychology has been suspected of superficiality, although Freud (1923b) had described the ego as rooted deeply in the id. Thus Pontalis (1968, p. 150) raised the question of whether American ego psychology does not actually destroy fundamental concepts like the unconscious and lead to a psychology of learning.

Klein's theories on early childhood development and her recommendation that deep interpretations be proffered without analyzing resistance led to considerable opposition to ego psychology, represented in A. Freud's *The Ego and the Mechanisms of Defence* (1937). In London, an intermediate group formed between the two poles. North American psychoanalysis followed the ego psychology tradition. The controversy between Kleinians and ego psychologists still continues, but has lost its polemical edge. The majority of psychoanalysts are near the middle of a broad spectrum of views on theory and treatment technique.

A comparative study by Kernberg (1972) presents ego psychologists' criticism of Klein's theory and the Kleinians' response. Klein's influence on psychoanalysis as a whole is considerable: some significant components of her theory have been widely accepted. There is general recognition of the importance of early object relationships for normal and pathological development. The proposition that depressive reactions take place during the first year of life has been accepted even by authors who are not convinced that the depressive position, in the stricter sense, is a normal transitional phase. Ego psychologists who treat borderline cases and psychotic patients orient themselves on the defense constellations which characterize the paranoid-schizoid and depressive positions.

Klein (1935) underlined the importance of the role played by aggression in the early phases of development. Her findings have gained acceptance among analysts who reject specific theses which have their origin in the hypothesis of the death instinct. For example, even Jacobson (1964) also places the early stages of superego formation, and the importance of early superego structures for later psychic development, in the second year of life. Klein's foredating of oedipal conflict to the second and third years of life and her thesis that preoedipal factors and conflicts influence psychosexual development and character formation have also gained broad acceptance.

It seems to be in the nature of things that school-specific one-sidednesses are toned down when they are absorbed into general psychoanalytic theory. Amalgamation of theories inevitably involves mutual influence and permeation. Klein's assumptions on early defense processes have had a productive impact on treatment technique. According to Kernberg, the most important factor here is the interpretation of splitting processes, which clarify the genesis of negative therapeutic reactions as a consequence of unconscious envy, supplementing Freud's understanding of this phenomenon (Sect. 4.4.1).

Klein and the English School also influenced the adherents of object relationship psychology, such as Balint, Fairbairn, Guntrip, and Winnicott. Sutherland (1980), however, stressed the independence of these four analysts from Klein and the English School by calling them the British object relationship theorists. Balint deserves the credit for enabling analysts to employ two- and three-person psychology in treatment technique, having emphasized the importance of the relationship for infantile development as early as 1935. In contrast to Klein, who conceived the object — the maternal person — as being constituted principally by infantile fantasies and their projection, Balint assumed that reciprocity is the basis of object formation.

We prefer Balint's two- and three-person psychology to other theories of interaction for a number of reasons, which we would like to explain by contrasting Balint's understanding with some other approaches which at first glance seem similar. Balint (1935) leaves open what happens between the two people in a relationship. He assumes that some transference and countertransference are personality specific, and that the analyst's own theory influences the analytic situation. Balint's view that adult intrapsychic conflicts are reflected in the relationship distinguishes his two-person psychology from Sullivan's (1953) interpersonal theory, which neglects the patient's subjective experience and instinctual needs. One of the essential differences between Balint's approach and Langs' (1976) bipersonal field is that for Langs it seems to be a given fact that the very existence and the structure of this field are determined especially by the processes of projective and introjective identification. Balint leaves a lot open, whereas Langs and others appear to believe they already know everything that happens in the analytic situation, and, above all, why it happens in the way it does. Naturally, no analyst is free of theoretical conceptions; Balint, however, always stressed that his statements were provisional and emphasized the relevance of the observer's standpoint. This relativization is one of the reasons that Balint opposed dogma and did not found a school. His two-person psychology corresponded to general and specific scientific developments. Erikson extended ego psychology with reference to American philosophers such as James, Cooley, and Mead and their contributions to the development of psychological identity and self-esteem (Cheshire and Thomä 1987).

We come now to another important theme with implications for change in psychoanalytic practice. The advent of object relationship psychology can in part be seen as a sign that patients, because of their growing fundamental insecurity, seek support from the analyst. This should not be regarded solely as repetition of infantile expectations and frustrations. Possibilities are thus opened for expanding the interpretive technique of psychoanalysis to areas which have not been properly explored because insufficient attention has been paid to the here-and-now. In the course of our attempts at integration we have gained a lot from knowing how polarizations have developed, and we would now like to use a few striking examples to show how psychoanalytic technique has ended up in its current position.

The two major international conferences on the theory of treatment, Marienbad in 1936 and Edinburgh in 1961, embrace a period in which much more changed than just treatment technique. Friedman (1978) drew some very revealing comparisons between the two conferences. In Marienbad there was still a great degree of openness, but by 1961 the climate in Edinburgh resembled that of a state of siege:

> The siege atmosphere that hung over this conference distinguished it radically from Freud's writings and from the Marienbad Conference .... The participants at Marienbad gave no sign of struggling to *avoid* a forbidden path; they even felt comfortable referring to unknown influences between patient and therapist. What, then, had happened to make the participants at Edinburgh tread so carefully? Why had interpretation become a battle cry? (Friedman 1978, p. 536)

Like Friedman, we believe that interpretation became a battle cry because the widening scope of psychoanalysis appeared to make it necessary to define the identity of psychoanalysis. Psychoanalysis spread beyond the mainstream. Behavioral therapy and Rogers' client-centered therapy had emerged as rival procedures. The psychotherapy boom started.

The twofold unease led to the establishment of internal and external boundaries, which culminated above all in Eissler's (1953) presentation of the *basic model technique* as the genuine psychoanalytic method. It is interesting that in the Festschrift for Aichhorn, Eissler (1949) had still considered therapy of delinquents to be authentic psychoanalysis. Even in his criticism of Alexander's Chicago School (1950), he declared that psychoanalytic therapy included every technique in which structural change was sought or achieved by psychotherapeutic means, regardless of whether it necessitated daily or irregular sessions and regardless of the use of the couch.

It is plain that the goal was not merely change of any sort, perhaps resulting from suggestion or some other factor. No, Eissler's demand implied that demonstration of the therapeutic efficacy of the method would also show psychoanalytic theory to be accurate, since the theory is oriented on the development of intrapsychic structures. Conclusions about the origin of psychic and psychosomatic illnesses can be drawn from the course of causal psychoanalytic therapy and through the demonstration of change. Thus, despite vehement criticism of Alexander's manipulative use of corrective emotional experience, Eissler was initially in favor of openness, in the spirit of Marienbad. Not until 1953 did he present the basic model technique, whose only tool is interpretation (Eissler 1953, p. 110). The classical psychoanalytic technique is thus "one in which interpretation remains the exclusive or leading or prevailing tool" (Eissler 1958, p. 223). This technique exists nowhere in a pure form.

Boundaries were then drawn which seemed to enable analysts to clearly distinguish the classical technique from the rest of the psychoanalytic and psychotherapeutic world. All the variables in psychoanalytic practice were disregarded: the patient's symptoms and personality structure, the analyst's personal equation, etc. Incidentally, even Eissler believed that such variables could justify variations of technique (1958, p. 222). The basic model technique did more than eliminate all variables except for interpretation; it created a fiction, as Eissler himself admitted in his discussion with Loewenstein: "No patient has ever been analysed with a technique in which interpretations alone have been used" (1958, p. 223). Von Blarer and Brogle (1983) even compared Eissler's theses with the commandments that Moses brought down from the mountain. From the scientific viewpoint, at least, there could be no objection to a purist method such as that demanded in Eissler's basic model technique. However, by and large things went no further than codification, with no thorough investigation of how the commandments work in practice, to what extent they are obeyed, and where they are broken. The only function which the basic model technique fulfilled excellently was that of distinguishing the classical technique from the others, and not even that was supported by empirical studies.

The prevailing mood today is that of a new departure. Sandler, with an unerring sense for the direction the journey is taking, said that "psychoanalysis is what is practiced by psychoanalysts" (1982, p. 44). This pragmatic definition, though strikingly simple, does justice to the diversity of psychoanalytic practice, enjoys wide currency among the general public, and is broadly valid for the individual analysand. We are now talking about practice as it is and also as it is seen from outside, no longer about formal criteria or about ideal demands concerning how practice should be. Sandler supported his thesis by saying that a good analyst modifies his technique from case to case anyway, because what is appropriate varies with the patient. If a patient can only come once or twice a week, the analyst modifies the treatment technique accordingly. The psychoanalytic attitude then becomes the decisive factor, and the perpetually dissatisfying discussions on formal features such as frequency of sessions, duration of therapy, and use of the couch could be discontinued.

Inevitably, we come to the question of what an analyst is and how the psychoanalytic attitude is developed. The problem shifts to training. Sandler believes that instruction in the classical technique creates the best conditions for the development of the analytic attitude, saying that the analyst will not internalize psychoanalysis and find his personal style until he has had many years experience in his own practice. There is certainly no substitute for personal experience, but if flexibility is the criterion of the good analyst, the preparations for practice must be organized accordingly. It can hardly be claimed that the basic model technique — which, for example, forbids the analyst to ask or answer questions — implies a psychoanalytic attitude compatible with Sandler's definition of the good practitioner. It goes without saying that Sandler's emphasis on qualitative aspects does not mean that quantitative aspects are fully immaterial. The time, regularity, duration, and frequency of sessions are important factors on which much depends. Nevertheless, they cannot determine what happens *qualitatively*, and therefore cannot be used as a measure of the difference between psychotherapy and psychoanalysis.

Wyatt (1984) does not regard the psychoanalytic standard technique and analytic psychotherapy as alternatives. If one shares this view, the point which Wyatt raises, at the end of his long study, becomes important: if it is often not possible until late in the course of treatment to judge "whether one is dealing with a *genuine* analysis or a *real* psychotherapy" (p. 96), one would like to know what the difference is between "genuine" and "real." We believe that further clarification of this question will be complicated by the mingling of professional politics and scientific interests. Institutional psychoanalysis tends toward the kind of orthodoxy that thrives on demarcations at the conference table. Empirical studies to improve our knowledge of what constitutes genuine psychoanalysis then seem superfluous.

In practice, the analyst moves along a continuum: no clear demarcations can be drawn. It has never been possible to treat patients with the basic model technique; it is a fiction created for a patient who does not exist. The specific means, led by interpretation of transference and resistance, are embedded in a network of supportive and expressive (i.e., conflict-revealing) techniques, even though particular means are emphasized, as shown by the Menninger study. Kernberg (1984, p. 151) recently suggested differentiating psychoanalysis, conflict-revealing (expressive) psychotherapy, and supportive psychotherapy on the basis of the degree to which the following dimensions are expressed: (1) the principal technical tools such as clarification, interpretation, suggestion, and intervention in the social environment; (2) the intensity of the interpretation of transference; (3) the degree of technical neutrality maintained.

After an analyst has freed himself from drawing sharp boundaries, there is still a wide area in which it is necessary to make *distinctions*. It is a challenge to compare analyses or school-specific techniques with one another and with analytic psychotherapies. We regard such comparative studies as indispensable. If one regards lasting change as the justification for therapeutic action, all methods and techniques lose their self-righteousness; rather, their scientific value becomes relativized by the practical advantage which the patient gains from the therapy. We therefore plead for qualified distinctions, which can but benefit the patient. With the exception of candidates having their training analysis, analysands are not primarily interested in whether they are undergoing analysis or psychotherapy. Patients simply seek the best possible help. The distinctions exist initially in the mind of the analyst. We surmise that frequent good sessions, as defined by Kris (1956a), or frequent mutative interpretations (Sect. 8.4) give the analyst the feeling that he has achieved authentic psychoanalysis. Other features are linked to the intensity of focussing and to the goals which have been set (Chap. 9). The analyst's subjective experience must be checked by means of studies comparing the process and outcome of analysis with the long-term effects. For the time being, we agree with Kernberg (1982, p. 8) that "the strict *separation* of psychoanalysis as a theory and technique from theoretical and technical exploration of psychotherapeutic practice may, for various reasons, damage psychoanalytic work itself."

We localize the damage to two levels: Strict separation, as required most explicitly in the basic model technique, encouraged an orthodox, neoclassical attitude which increasingly restricted the spectrum of indications, and with it the basis for gaining new knowledge. Since the effectiveness of therapy depends by no means only on the analyst's armory of interpretations, limitations also resulted in this area. On the other level, that of analytic psychotherapy, there was much experimentation, variation, and modification, but the relationships of therapeutic variables to psychoanalysis were never made an object of study. At least this is how we understand Kernberg's criticism, although it must be pointed out that numerous studies have been performed precisely in the area of psychodynamic therapies (Luborsky 1984; Strupp and Binder 1984).

## 1.7 Sociocultural Change

The solutions to the current problems of treatment technique cannot be found in imitation of Freud's generous, natural psychoanalytic attitude to his patients, even though such an attitude is a welcome antidote to stereotypes. Freud's solutions to problems of theory and practice can serve as models for the present only inasfar as similarities exist between the situation then and now. The far-reaching changes in our world since the 1930s, including the global insecurity of the nuclear age, affect the individual through the disintegration of social and familial structures. There may be a considerable delay before historical changes influence family life. Generations may pass before historical and psychosocial processes affect family life to such an extent that individuals develop psychic or psychosomatic illnesses. The traditional unconscious attitudes passed on in each individual family may also persist for very long periods, following the rules of a family romance and largely independent of historical and sociocultural change.

The sexual revolution has reduced the repression of sexuality in general, and the contraceptive pill has boosted female emancipation and granted women more sexual self-determination. As predicted by psychoanalytic theory, the incidence of hysterical illnesses has decreased. Conflicts seem nowadays to persist on the oedipal level rather than developing into superego structures (i.e., into the typical Oedipus complex of the fin de siècle).

Since the psychoanalytic method concerns itself principally with the typical familial origin of psychic illnesses, with particular attention paid to childhood, psychosocial influences on adolescents, which offer them a "second chance" (Blos 1985, p. 138), were underestimated until Erikson focussed on them (e.g., Erikson 1959). For many years, the factors through which symptoms are maintained also received insufficient consideration in decisions on treatment technique. This twofold neglect at first had only a few side effects, as the early id analysis and the later ego psychology-oriented analysis of resistance could assume the existence of stable — even rigid — structures acquired at an early stage. The analyst helped the patient to gain greater inner freedom: the strict superego commandments resulting from identification with oppressive patriarchs were exchanged for more human values. Strachey (1934) gave an exemplary account of this therapeutic process.

At about the same time, a theme began to be discussed which has recently moved to the center of attention, namely, the theme of security, which can be seen as a counterpoint to the disintegration of historical and psychosocial structures. It is no coincidence that in the age of narcissism and ideology (Lasch 1979; Bracher 1982), the theme of security has finally come to occupy such an important place in the discussion of psychoanalytic treatment technique, although its origins can easily be traced back to the 1930s and to Freud and Adler. Kohut's innovation probably owes its impact to the fact that patients and analysts are equally dissatisfied with the dissecting nature of conflict psychology and are seeking totality and confirmation — narcissistic security.

Since epidemiologic studies of the incidence of neuroses have only been carried out in recent times (Schepank 1982; Häfner 1985), no exact comparisons can be made with the past. We have to rely on personal impressions, which are doubly unreliable because of the strong element of fashion in diagnostic classification. This having been said, there can be no doubt that today's psychoanalyst is confronted with problems which were not at the focus of attention in Freud's practice (Thomä and Kächele 1976).

Most people in western democracies live in a social system which shields them against strokes of fate, not least against the financial risks of illness. The modern clientele of West German psychoanalysts includes almost no purely self-financing patients. Patients from all strata of society, rich or poor, can now have psychoanalytic treatment at the expense of the insurance system, which in turn is funded by the regular contributions of the insured population. Freud's prediction (1919a) has thus been fulfilled. The therapeutic efficacy of psychoanalysis is today more important than ever. Eissler has also been confirmed in his belief that "socialized medicine will play a great role in [the] future development [of psychoanalysis]. We cannot expect the community to pay the large amounts of money necessary for the analysis of an individual, since symptomatic recoveries are possible in a large number of patients" (Eissler, cited by Miller 1975, p. 151).

We take the view that there is a much closer association than is generally assumed between the scientific grounding of psychoanalysis and its therapeutic efficacy. Social pressure and increasing competition have intensified analysts' efforts to provide a scientific foundation for the effectiveness of what they do.

## 1.8 Convergences

The criticism from inside and outside psychoanalysis has brought about significant changes, including clear trends toward rapprochement and integration of the various currents (Shane and Shane 1980). We believe we are justified in speaking of *convergences* between the different schools within psychoanalysis and also between psychoanalysis and neighboring disciplines. The considerations and the lines of development which we sketch out below plainly show common features, enabling us to erect these two volumes on a firm foundation despite the present anarchorevolutionary situation in psychoanalysis. The following points can be mentioned.

The *object relationship theories* have recognized that the analyst becomes effective as a "new object" (Loewald 1960) and are thus on the way to acknowledging the subject and the intersubjectivity in the analytic situation. Characteristic of this tendency is the discussion on extension of the concept of transference (Sect. 2.5). The psychoanalytic method always had its foundation in the dyadic relationship. Precisely the unconscious elements of object relationships are accessible to the analyst only if he employs an interactional approach. All the indications are that it has now become possible to solve the great therapeutic and theoretical problems of intersubjectivity — of transference and countertransference.

One of the relevant issues in treatment technique is the patient's identification with the analyst's functions (Hoffer 1950). These functions are not perceived as abstract processes; rather, the patient experiences them in the personal context of his therapy. The patient's identifications with the analyst's functions are thus, in the sense described by Loewald, tied to exemplary interactions with the analyst, from which they can be isolated only artificially. The person with whom one identifies is not introjected as an object and stored in intrapsychic isolation. Loewald (1980, p. 48) emphasized that *interactions*, not objects, are introjected.

In fact, the important issue in psychoanalytic descriptions of unconscious elements of object relationships is constituted by aspects of action and their reflection in the (unconscious) world of fantasy. That which is stored as an "internal object" is no isolated item, but a memory image framed in a context of action. It was logical that Schafer (1976) arrived at his action language after Kris (1975) had described action research as the scientific approach appropriate to psychoanalysis. The storage of objects occurs from birth onward within a qualitatively variable context of action. Repeated acts of communication give rise to unconscious schemata which may attain a great degree of stability. Such enduring structures go hand in hand with transference readiness which can be precipitated with varying degrees of speed and ease.

These interactional contexts were implied in psychoanalytic object relationship theories from the very outset. Prominent among the reasons for the great attention paid to them in recent years are the findings on mother-child behavior. The object relationship theories have been enriched by Bowlby's (1969) studies on attachment. Emde (1981) stressed the significance of *social* reciprocity, summarizing research findings as follows:

> The human infant is organized for social interaction from the outset and participates in mutual exchanges with caregivers. We cannot regard individuals in the social surround as static "targets of the drives" and, from this angle, terms like "object relations" are unfortunate in their connotations. (p. 218)

Even the infant constructs his experience in an active way. Affects play a prominent role in these interactional processes.

Libido theory does not cover this process of affective reciprocity. Spitz (1976) demonstrated that Freud viewed the libidinous object principally from the standpoint of the child (and his unconscious wishes), and not against the background of the reciprocal relationship between mother and child. This tradition became so entrenched that Kohut derived self objects from the hypothetical narcissistic way in which the infant sees and experiences things.

Harlow's (1958, 1962) pioneering experiments are instructive in this regard. He raised rhesus monkeys with surrogate mothers made out of wire and terry cloth, i.e., with inanimate objects. These monkeys were unable to play or to develop social relationships. They suffered uncontrollable anxiety and outbursts of rage, hostility, and destructiveness. The adult animals displayed no sexual behavior. Spitz attributed these severe developmental defects to the lack of *mutuality* between surrogate mother and infant monkey. He believes mutuality to be the foundation of the mother-child dialogue. Although he still adheres to the concept of the object relationship (Spitz 1965, pp. 173, 182), it is clear that his descriptions are based on an intersubjective, interactional system.

In the long term, the newer theories of infant development, along with the integration of interdisciplinary theories of communication and action, will probably have considerable consequences on psychoanalysis (Lichtenberg 1983). In all areas, psychoanalysis contributes to the knowledge of the unconscious dimensions of human behavior.

Just as object relationship theories are indispensable for two- and three-person psychology, *ego psychology* would be limited to its very immediate sphere of relevance without "dialogic life" or "you" (Buber 1974). It is of course true that the treatment technique in ego psychology was initially systematized according to the model of intrapsychic conflict, following the example of A. Freud's descriptions in *The Ego and the Mechanisms of Defence* (1937). She presents "considerations bearing upon psycho-analytic therapy" which define the scope of psychoanalytic therapy in terms of *psychic conflict* (pp. 68ff.). At the same time, Hartmann's pioneering study entitled "Ego Psychology and the Problem of Adaption" (1958 [1939]) led to greater exchange with the social sciences, with social psychology playing a mediating role. It has to be said, however, that Carveth's (1984a) critical study highlights the lack of genuine interdisciplinary cooperation.

The criticism of metapsychology and libido theory smoothed the way for the linking of intrapsychic and interpersonal theories of conflict. The interpersonal approach cannot, however, be confined to the concept of "participant observation" (Sullivan 1953). This term, though felicitous, does not make it sufficiently clear that the analyst's participation means intervention from the very beginning of the encounter. (Sect. 2.3). Both his silence and the interpretations he proffers influence his field of observation. He cannot escape the fact that his very participation entails change, even if he deceives himself into thinking he has no specific goals in mind.

The members of an American Psychoanalytic Association discussion group, which met several times between 1977 and 1980 with Lichtenberg as chairman, agreed that "the more we keep values away from being the direct object of our scrutiny, the more they are likely to unwittingly and unconsciously influence our technique and theory" (Lytton 1983, p.576). For practical and scientific reasons, as pointed out by Devereux (1967), nowadays more than ever before the analyst has to accept that he is not just the observer but that he is also observed, i.e., that other psychoanalysts and scientists from neighboring disciplines are investigating what the therapist feels, thinks, and does, and how his thought and action affect the patient. This research into the psychoanalytic situation by third parties has been made possible by the tape recording of analyses. The essential issue is the analyst's contribution to the therapeutic process. In addition, in countries like West Germany, where the costs of treatment are borne by health insurance, society (represented by the scientific community) and the insurers have a right to learn how analysts justify their therapeutic action, with the obvious proviso that the private sphere must be respected.

The dyadic approach to the analytic situation, which is gaining acceptance everywhere, is anything but a carte blanche for subjectivity. On the contrary, precisely because the analyst's competence is such a personal matter, he must accept responsibility for the way in which the theory he prefers affects his countertransference, just as he does for the success of the therapy, or for the lack of it. A growing number of psychoanalysts are therefore calling for practice to be made an object of study (Sandler 1983). It speaks for itself that the congress of the International Psychoanalytical Association in Madrid in 1983 was devoted to "The Psychoanalyst at Work."

The dyadic approach corresponds with the findings of *neonatological research* and the observation of *mother-infant interaction.* Trevarthen (1977) speaks of "primary intersubjectivity." Emde and Robinson (1979), students of Spitz, looked critically at over 300 studies, concluding that they disclosed old prejudices, namely the widespread misconception that the infant is passive and undifferentiated and that his behavior is regulated by instinctual tensions and discharge. The myth of the infant as a passive organism which reacts to stimulation and is attuned primarily to reducing stimulation has become untenable.

The trends which Emde and Robinson detected in research findings have continued. According to Sander (1980) and Peterfreund (1980), the implications of the more recent findings are so great that three myths will have to be laid to rest: the adultomorph (the infant is as I am), the theoreticomorph (the infant is as my theory constructs him), and the pathomorph (the infant feels and thinks like my psychotic patient). Since Freud once called instinct theory "our mythology" (1933a, p. 95), and since myths contain profound truths about man, the process of demythologization is a cause of serious concern among analysts. The psychoanalytic theory of instincts has retained elements of mythology not least because of the connotations of some metaphors — for instance the principle of constancy — which link the human longing for eternity and the mystique of love and death with physical assumptions, thus masquerading as a comprehensive psychobiological explanation.

We are not trying to demonstrate that the intersubjectivity of the therapeutic situation is derived from mother-infant interaction. Our primary concern is the convergence of principles, which shows that the dyadic view of the analytic situation corresponds to human nature as it can be observed from the first moment of life onward. We agree with Wolff (1971), a particularly careful analyst and researcher, when he reminds his colleagues that their most important practical and scientific problems cannot be solved either by observing infants or with the aid of ethology, neurophysiology, or molecular biology. On the other hand, analysts cannot disregard the underlying theories of development when investigating the interpretation rules which they follow when ascribing unconscious meanings to their patients' utterances.

A great role is played by whether or not the treating analyst takes Piaget's work on the development of object constancy into consideration, and by which conceptions of the early mother-child relationship form the basis of his interpretations. Inconsistencies between different theories can be expected because of the complexity of the subject matter and the differences in method. It is thus all the more important for similar results to be acquired by different means or for the implausibility of assumptions such as that of infantile autism to be demonstrated. On the other hand, there are a wealth of studies starting from the factual separateness of mother and child which stress the reciprocity of the interaction (Stern et al. 1977). On the basis of empirical observations, Papoušek and Papoušek (1983) and Papoušek et al. (1984) assume that the infant is *autonomous and has integrative competence.*

Separateness and primary intersubjectivity are the largest and most important common denominators in the results of neonatological research and the recent findings on the therapeutic dyad. We agree with Milton Klein (1981) in regarding birth as the moment of individuation, which implies that each individual newborn begins to *construct* his world actively, creatively, and hungry for stimuli. Brazelton and Als (1979) claim to discern indications of affective and cognitive responses immediately after birth.

However, the precise chronology is not the crucial point. Obviously, the conception that the child actively *constructs* his world does not help us to know how he *experiences* it. Piaget's (1954) theory also assumes that mother-child intersubjectivity is determined by the child's egocentricity, and thus supports the psychoanalytic assumption that the crying child experiences his mother's behavior, whether it be accommodating or rejecting, as though he has caused it. It is of course quite another question whether this egocentricity has the quality of narcissistic omnipotence found in adults.

Emde's (1981) thesis that innate biological schemata regulate the interaction between mother and child is of great importance. On the other hand, the particular features of the schemata constitute individuality: every infant and every mother is as unique alone as they are together in the dyad. Both realize species-specific (general human) mechanisms, i.e., basic biological patterns, in their unmistakable personal way. Mahler's concept of "coenaesthetic empathy" (1971, p. 404), which she uses in reference to common feelings and to shared and deep sensations and perceptions, arose from the observation of mothers and infants. Correspondingly, in therapy it is important to strike a balance between similarity and separateness, between the formation of a we-bond and of the ego.

In the course of the past decade, research into the affective exchange between mother and child has confirmed Winnicott's view: "The infant and the maternal care together form a unit .... I once said: 'There is no such thing as infant'" (1965, p. 39). Winnicott added that he naturally meant that the maternal care is an essential component without which no child could exist, thus distancing himself from Freud's assumptions about primary narcissism and about the transition of the pleasure principle to the reality principle. He also pointed out that Freud himself raised objections to his own thesis:

> It will rightly be objected that an organization which was a slave to the pleasure principle and neglected the reality of the external world could not maintain itself alive for the shortest time, so that it could not have come into existence at all. The employment of a *fiction* like this is, however, justified when one considers that the infant — provided one includes with it *the care it receives from its mother* — does almost realize a psychical system of this kind. (1911 b, p. 220, emphasis added)

If maternal care is included, the fiction collapses and Winnicott's conception of the mother-child unit becomes the point of reference. Of course, there is no doubt that mother and child are different, even though the infant is not yet in a position to delineate himself as an independent person. Hartmann's (1958 [1939]) ego autonomy is biologically rooted, and within the mother-child unit this means that self-perception occurs selectively via the sense organs in exchange with specific other-perceptions. Thus the maternal person is perceived differently by every infant, for two reasons: first, no mother behaves in exactly the same way with each of her children, and second, every child has individual response readinesses which develop within the unit. Otherwise, it would not be possible for Winnicott (1965) to speak of the true and the false self, in addition to emphasizing the mother-child unit. The *true* self refers to the basic feeling of being able to realize one's own potential and free oneself from the restrictions which originated in influence from outside and have found expression in the *false* self.

The empirical findings of research into mother-child interaction can be used to span a divide which has opened up in recent decades in the theory of treatment technique, namely the polarization between the conservative structural theorists and the object relationship theorists. Even an adherent of Balint's (1952) two-person psychology cannot overlook the fact that every patient is unique. The task of the therapeutic dyad, that unit composed of two mutually dependent but independent persons, consists in allowing the patient to establish the greatest possible degree of autonomy.

Our position on two-person psychology must therefore be amended. One-person psychology was constructed according to the model of the natural sciences, and is not appropriate for either the theory or the therapy of psychoanalysis. We agree with Balint's criticism of the theory of psychoanalytic technique and the psychoanalytic theory of development because of their excessive emphasis on intrapsychic processes. Nevertheless, the analyst has the duty to create the optimal conditions for the patient to change on his own, and not to have change forced on him from without. Stress must be laid on one aspect of one-person psychology which represents an obligation for psychoanalysts despite this criticism: The ideal of enlightenment is oriented on the individual, even though self-knowledge, including recognition of unconscious parts of the personality, is tied to two-person psychology.

Remodeling of the psychoanalytic baby along the lines suggested by the results of neonatological research has important consequences for treatment technique (Lebovici and Soule 1970). Every analyst's interpretations, especially his reconstructions of the patient's early childhood, are based on his theory of development. It is for this reason that we speak of the theoretical conception — the model — of the *psychoanalytic baby* or *psychoanalytic infant*, which exists in numerous descriptions of varying precision. This remodeling has only just begun.

These descriptions are constructions created by fathers and mothers such as Freud, Abraham, Klein, Ferenczi, A. and M. Balint, Winnicott, Mahler, and Kohut. Everyone is aware that the various psychoanalytic babies differ greatly. The designers of the models must put up with the fact that their creations are compared.

Kohut's tragic man lies as an infant in the cradle surrounded by an environment (the so-called selfobjects) which only partially reflects his innate narcissism. The fact that Freud's theory of narcissism was the godfather makes the tragedy almost inevitable, but it is nevertheless bathed in a relatively mild light: evil is not a primary force, and oedipal guilt feelings are avoidable, according to Kohut, if the early tragedy is limited and the narcissistic self discovers itself in the mirror of love (Kohut 1984, p. 13). In Kohut's theory, Freud's guilty, oedipal individual and his intrapsychic conflicts are the product of a narcissistic disturbance in early childhood. Without this disturbance, the oedipal conflicts of 3- to 5-year-old children would be principally pleasurable transitional phases, leaving no appreciable guilt feelings as long as a healthy self had already developed. Kohut's theory gives the individual the prospect of a future free of oedipal conflicts. It can be inferred from Kohut's late works that, provided the empathy of the selfobjects is good, the human tragedy also stays within reasonable bounds.

Klein's (1948, 1957) psychoanalytic infant is quite different. This time the godfather was Freud's death instinct, ensuring a malevolence whose early manifestations are unrivalled and which can only be endured by dividing the world into a good breast and a bad breast. The tragedy of the infant's later life is then profound, in contrast to Kohut's mild form, which may find expression in self-ironic humor. Klein's adult was born as Sisyphus, condemned to eternal failure in his attempts to atone for the imaginary wrongs inflicted by hate and envy. Throughout life the processes of projective and introjective identification, and their contents, remain the basic vehicles of interpersonal processes, within families and between groups and whole peoples.

In restricting ourselves to the description of the essential features of two influential models of the psychoanalytic infant, we have highlighted dissimilarities and contradictions. This was our intention. Our current concern is not to advocate pragmatic eclecticism and recommend that the most plausible components be extracted from all the psychoanalytic theories of early childhood and amalgamated with elements of general developmental psychology or parts of Piaget's theory. Rather, we believe that productive eclecticism within psychoanalysis, and within neonatological research into interaction, is only possible if we also examine the aspects which are neglected in the different constructions. It is, after all, disturbing that similar empathic introspective methods — Kohut emphasized his closeness to Klein in this respect — should result in entirely different reconstructions of early childhood.

One possibility, of course, is that contradictory reconstructions originate in the treatment of different illnesses. However, the available literature does not support this hypothesis, which, incidentally, is seldom considered by the fathers and mothers of typical psychoanalytic infants. Sooner or later, the theoreticomorph creation is made the uniform model for explaining the deepest levels of all psychic disturbances: self defects, based on unsuccessful mirroring, and the schizoid-paranoid and depressive positions, founded in innate destructiveness, seem to be the root of all evil.

Instinct mythology is the factor which gives the infants and babies of the different psychoanalytic families their specific narcissistic (Kohut) or destructive (Klein) features. This is why we mentioned the theory of narcissism and the hypothesis of the death instinct, respectively. However, the psychoanalytic babies by no means lose their vitality and their *vis a tergo* if this drive mythology foundation is removed. In common with Freud (1923a, p. 255), we would like to refer to Schiller's lines from *Die Weltweisen* (The World Wise): "For the time being, until philosophy holds the structure of the world together, it [nature] will sustain the gears with hunger and love."

# 2 Transference and Relationship

## 2.1 Transference as Repetition

Transferences arise in all human relationships, and this fact gives Freud's discovery wide significance. Initially, however, he based his definition of transference on observations made in the course of therapy:

They are new editions or facsimiles of the impulses and fantasies which are aroused and made conscious during the progress of the analysis; but they have this peculiarity, which is characteristic for their species, that they replace some earlier person by the person of the physician. To put it another way: a whole series of psychological experiences are revived, not as belonging to the past, but as applying to the person of the physician at the present moment. Some of these transferences have a content which differs from that of their model in no respect whatever except for the substitution. These then — to keep to the same metaphor — are merely new impressions or reprints. Others are more ingeniously constructed; ... by cleverly taking advantage of some real peculiarity in the physician's person or circumstances and attaching themselves to that. These, then, will no longer be new impressions, but revised editions. (Freud 1905e, p. 116)

Later, however, he generalized:

Transference arises *spontaneously* in all human relationships just as it does between the patient and the physician. It is everywhere the true vehicle of therapeutic influence; and the less its presence is suspected, the more powerfully it operates. So psychoanalysis does not create it, but merely reveals it to consciousness and gains control of it in order to guide psychical processes towards the desired goal. (Freud 1910a, p. 51)

Transference is thus a generic term in both senses of the word: First, since a person's past experiences have a fundamental and persistent influence on his present life, transference is universal in *Homo sapiens*. Second, the concept embraces numerous typical phenomena which are expressed individually and uniquely in each one of us. Special forms of transference are found in psychoanalysis, and we will discuss these later. In this chapter we want to demonstrate the dependence of transference phenomena, including resistance, on the analytic situation and its shaping by the analyst — starting with the appearance of his office and continuing with his behavior, his sex, his countertransference, his personal equation, his theory, his image of man, his weltanschauung, etc. Thus, we will be testing the principal thesis of this book on the central core of psychoanalysis — transference and resistance — and investigating the extent of the analyst's influence on the phenomena which are traditionally ascribed solely to the patient. As we are writing for readers whose degree of knowledge varies, we first want to ensure a sound basis for understanding.

Experience has taught that it is not easy to grasp how the view of transference shifted from its being the major obstacle to treatment to the most powerful aid. Of course, the bewildering multiplicity of transference and resistance phenomena had not yet been recognized at the time of the original discovery. Therefore we will start at the beginning of the story. The first discovery was of resistance (association resistance) — to recollection and to the approaching of unconscious conflicts — which owed its strength to the revival of unconscious wishes and their transference to the analyst. Thus the transference actualizes conflicts in the relationship, any obstacle to this being termed transference resistance, though more accurately one should speak of resistance against transference. The psychoanalyst has the greatest difficulty in mastering these transference phenomena, but we must not forget "that it is precisely they that do us the inestimable service of making the patient's hidden and forgotten erotic impulses immediate and manifest. For when all is said and done, it is impossible to destroy anyone in absentia or in effigie." With these famous words, Freud (1912b, p. 108) characterized the here-and-now actuality of transference, which is convincing because of its immediacy and authenticity: nothing can be dealt with successfully "in absentia," i.e., by talking about the past, or "in effigie," by symbolic indirect representation. The development of transference, whether it be positive or negative in nature, is not only opposed step by step by the most varied forms of resistance; the transference can itself become resistance if there is an imbalance between the repetition in present experience and the patient's ability or willingness to replace the transferences with memories, or at least to relativize them. Since the patient "is obliged to repeat the repressed material as a contemporary experience," Freud emphasized in one phase of his thought the necessity "to force as much as possible into the channel of memory and to allow as little as possible to emerge as repetition" (1920g, pp. 18, 19). The analyst should at least not give any occasion for unavoidable repetition, in order to allow the memories to retain their original faithfulness and to avoid their merging with any real impressions: the authenticity of transference in the here-and-now lies ideally in the uninfluenced reproduction of vivid memories actualized as contemporary experience.

The common denominator of all transference phenomena is repetition, which, both in ordinary life and in therapy, apparently arises spontaneously. Freud emphasized the spontaneity of transference to counter the objection that it was *created* by psychoanalysis. In fact, we are all familiar with transference in ourselves and in others. Ms. X or Mr. Y ends up time and again in the same conflict-filled relationships; for example, wishes and expectations are disappointed in the same stereotyped way. New editions and facsimiles seem to be repeated automatically, although at the conscious level the subject makes great efforts to change his behavior.

Freud's purpose was to give psychoanalytic practice a scientific foundation, and therefore he emphasized that transferences are natural phenomena, part of human life, and not artificial products of psychoanalysis. For the same reason, all the relevant rules of treatment are designed to ensure the *spontaneous* occurrence of transference. But what does "spontaneous" mean? From a scientific perspective, we cannot content ourselves with waiting for transferences to occur naturally in analysis as they do in life itself. Looked at more closely, the spontaneity of transferences reveals itself to be conditional on unconscious *inner* expectations and their *external* precipitants. Thus, for *scientific* reasons we must create the most favorable conditions for transferences to happen, and *practical* considerations force us to adjust these conditions according to their therapeutic potential.

Freud's conception of the spontaneity of transference reveals itself as a variable readiness to respond which is released in the interrelationship with objects and the stimuli emanating from them. We can now imagine a kind of autorelease of unconscious responses with no positive external stimulus, as in deprivation of food and drink followed by "hallucinatory gratification of desires" (Freud 1900a). The similarity to the vacuum activities (*Leerlaufaktivitäten*) described by Konrad Lorenz in animals can be mentioned in passing. Creation of the circumstances for such endopsychic autoreleases (apparently independent of external factors) seems scientifically desirable, and not only in order to rebut the accusation of exerting influence. In a deeper sense, it is a matter of the patient's spontaneity in the analysis; he must find himself in the interchange with a "significant other" (Mead 1934). Thus on the one hand, true to the scientific spirit of the time, we have had passed down to us Freud's appeal to get transference phenomena into their purest form, and not to influence them, so that they apparently occur naturally. On the other hand, it is vital for the success of the therapy to create favorable conditions for spontaneity on the part of the patient.

The contradiction between these two aspects was often passed over in such a way that many psychoanalysts believed that by not exerting influence they could promote autorelease just as much as spontaneity in the more profound sense. It was even widely believed that this is a way of combining the demands of theory with therapeutic objectives, although in reality neither is well served. We hope that we can substantiate these claims adequately below.

Theoretical postulates have contributed to the conceptualization of the transference neurosis in the ideal psychoanalytic process as something apparently independent of the participating observer: it develops in the reflection of images by the analyst, who is, ideally, free of all blind spots of countertransference. In the here-and-now the repetition of the genesis of the neurosis is allegedly purer and more complete the less the analyst disturbs these new editions. If some initially unidentified factor X, e.g., the analyst's age, appearance, or behavior, disturbs the ideal course of the therapy, it is a matter not of new editions but rather of revised editions; the patient's memories enable factor X to be traced back to its original meaning in the patient's life history. It seems to have no autonomy. Freud's pioneering observations in the case of Dora (1905e), whose breaking off of treatment was explained by the failure to recognize the factor X in the transference, have led to the neglect of real perceptions in the therapeutic relationship. The ideal model of the psychoanalytic process was elaborated by treatment rules aimed at enabling a pure repetition of the pathogenesis.

Observation of repetition in the most complete transference neurosis possible leads on the one hand — in the search for causes — to reconstruction of the genesis of the illness, and on the other — in the therapy — to emphasis on memory as a curative factor. The transference neurosis is said to be resolved by the patient's realization that his perceptions in the analytic situation are, to a greater or lesser degree, gross distortions. At fault here are projections through which earlier wishes and fears and their repercussions are transported into the present. The model of this analytic process is summarized in Freud's "Remembering, Repeating, and Working-Through" (1914g). This triad came to be regarded as an ideal through its association with Freud's recommendations on treatment technique, although he himself followed them in an assured and flexible fashion rather than dogmatically. In therapy, Freud always attached great importance to the potential influence of suggestion in the context of transferences — though admittedly this cannot be inferred from his technical writings (Thomä 1977; Cremerius 1981b). He considered this influence possible only in the degree to which the patient's experience of dependence on his parents had been good and he was thus capable of so-called *unobjectionable transference.* According to Freud, this is the root of suggestibility, which is used as much by the analyst as by the parents. It can hardly be doubted that suggestibility, in the sense of receptiveness for new experiences, presupposes a certain readiness to trust others that is rooted in the life history. However, trust and suggestibility also have an "actual genesis" (i.e., a basis in the reality of the here-and-now transactions of therapy) which for Freud went without saying. Actual genesis was largely neglected in the theory of treatment technique; for a long time, the genesis of transference relegated the present, including the analyst's situational and actual influence, to the background.

The willingness to neglect the here-and-now — in the sense of new experience as opposed to repetition — becomes more understandable when we consider how the recognition of transference appears to resolve a number of issues:

1. It became possible to reconstruct the origin of psychic and psychosomatic disorders in the interpersonal field of transference.
2. It became possible to diagnose typical neurotic response readinesses and to make so-called dispositional explanations, because internalized conflicts which manifest themselves as thought and behavior patterns in repetitions could be observed in the relationship to the doctor, in transference.
3. Internalized conflict patterns, i.e., conflict patterns which have been absorbed into the structure, can be transformed by transference into object relationships and observed *in statu nascendi.*

The scientific goal was to explore the circumstances of the original development of the neurosis as thoroughly as possible and to create standardized conditions for this process. The view that explanation of the etiology would ideally also resolve the neurosis was in accordance with Freud's causal understanding of therapy, by which past and even obsolete determinants of wishes and anxieties — which, however, still live on in the symptoms — should be repeated in a pure form, i.e., uninfluenced by the analyst. Even this incomplete outline of the solutions reached through the discovery of transference gives an idea of why the actual genesis of the patient's experience and behavior was neglected, and why no commensurate place in the official genealogy of psychoanalytic technique has been accorded to the autonomous here-and-now, the decisive core of therapy. The theoretical and practical solutions provided by the revolutionary paradigm have to be relativized in regard to the influence which the analyst exerts through his individual technique (as determined by his theory), through his personal equation and countertransference, and through his latent image of man.

## 2.2 Suggestion, Suggestibility, and Transference

The relationship between transference and suggestion is two sided. On the one hand, suggestion derives from transference: people are suggestible because they "transfer." Freud traces the suggestibility contingent on transference back to its developmental prototypes and explains it by the child's dependence on its parents. Accordingly, the patient perceives the doctor's suggestion as a derivative of the parental suggestion. On the other hand, suggestion is viewed as an independent tool for steering transference. Trust in the efficacy of this tool is based on experience with hypnotic suggestion. In this respect the double meaning of suggestion originates in the difference between hypnotic and analytic therapy. Freud comments:

> Analytic treatment makes its impact further back towards the roots, where the conflicts are which gave rise to the symptoms, and uses suggestion in order to alter the outcome of those conflicts. Hypnotic treatment leaves the patient inert and unchanged, and for that reason, too, equally unable to resist any fresh occasion for falling ill .... In psychoanalysis we act upon the transference itself, resolve what opposes it, adjust the *instrument* with which we wish to make our impact. Thus it becomes possible for us to derive an entirely fresh advantage from the power of suggestion; we get it into our hands. The patient does not suggest to himself whatever he pleases: we guide his suggestion so far as he is in any way accessible to its influence. (1916/17, pp. 451-452, emphasis added)

The part of this passage which we have emphasized can be interpreted in several ways. One obvious interpretation is to see, in the "instrument" which we "adjust," the transference which would be shaped and instrumentalized accordingly by the psychoanalyst. However, a position outside of transference is needed for the analyst to be able to make transference an instrument. Freud saw in suggestion not only the patient's insight, but also the force which works on transference. Thus suggestion becomes the instrument which "makes an impact" on transference and shapes it.

The two faces of suggestion and the intermixture of suggestion and transference, which have always been obstacles to the understanding of psychoanalytic therapy, have two main causes. First, psychoanalytic suggestion developed from hypnotic suggestion. It was therefore only natural for Freud to stress the new and different form of therapeutic influence by contrasting it with the kind of suggestion practiced previously. Suggestibility was explained in terms of life history and conceived as regression into passive dependence, which naturally means that one is strongly or totally dependent on something from the outside and assimilates what is instilled or suggested. By attributing the effect of suggestion to transference, Freud also threw light on the capriciousness of the successes of hypnosis, since only positive transference produces total trust in the hypnotist and his actions, as if the subject were safe in his mother's bosom. The limits of hypnotizibility and the failure of suggestive therapies have thus become explicable with the help of the psychoanalytic theory of transference (see Thomä 1977).

The second reason, which led to the derivation of the psychoanalyst's influence on the patient from the latter's capacity for transference, has already been hinted at. The genesis of trust/mistrust, affection/aversion, and security/insecurity in the relationships to parents and other close relatives during the preoedipal and oedipal phases and in adolescence establishes the personal response readiness, which can be classified according to typical unconscious dispositions. The effect of these unconscious dispositions is that contemporary experiences are measured against unconscious expectations, i.e., the new material is experienced according to an old, more or less fixed "cliché."

As response readiness, transferences are bound to the past in which they originated. The doctor's suggestion, i.e., the influence exerted by the psychoanalyst, will not be determined by its autonomous, change-oriented function, but will be derived from the patient's life history.

In contrast to suggestive therapies, psychoanalysis calls for the exposition and resolution of transference.[1] The necessary suggestion and suggestibility are derived from transference, which thus seems, as Münchhausen claimed to have done, to be able to pull itself up by its own hair. However, appearances deceive. Münchhausen divided himself by ego splitting, making his hand the center of his self and the rest of his body an object. The fact is, of course, that transference does *not* pull itself up by its own hair. Freud divided transference into two classes. Unobjectionable transference is comparable to Münchhausen's hand; it is credited with possessing the powers which overcome the instinctive *positive* or *negative* transference. Unobjectionable transference is a characteristic and abstract hybrid from the preoedipal, preambivalent period of infantile development in which the basis for trust was formed. In this respect the concept of unobjectionable positive transference is also tied to the past; however, it survives only as response readiness and forms a certain component of that which we term "therapeutic alliance" or "working alliance" (Zetzel 1956; Greenson 1965). These are not fixed quantities, any more than Sterba's (1934) ego splitting, but rather dispositions which can manifest themselves in various ways under situational influences (see Sect. 2.5).

[1] In "An Autobiographical Study" (1925d, p. 27) Freud described his experience of using hypnosis to induce catharsis. He explained his discontinuation of the technique by saying "that even the most brilliant results were liable to be suddenly wiped away if my personal relation with the patient became disturbed. It was true that they would be reestablished if a reconciliation could be effected; but such an occurrence proved that the *personal emotional relation* between doctor and patient was after all stronger than the whole catharsis process, and it was precisely that factor which escaped every effort at control" (emphasis added).

Thus the transference theories simply describe how clichés or, more generally, unconscious response readinesses, are formed. They leave open, however, what the analyst contributes to the particular manifestation of these entities, and above all, Freud's descriptions fail to clarify adequately how to overcome them. With suggestion, derived from transference, one remains rooted in a cycle of events facing backward. To clarify this problem, we point to one of Freud's theses on psychoanalytic therapy which has received little attention: "But, by the help of the doctor's suggestion, the new struggle around this object [i.e., the doctor] is lifted to the highest psychical level: it takes place as a normal mental conflict" (1916/17, p. 454).

Recourse to *doctor's suggestion* does not do justice to the far-reaching, instantaneous, and novel influence exerted by the analyst. The outcome of this struggle differs from that of earlier conflicts in that it is waged by both sides with new weapons which facilitate elevation to "the highest psychical level." We will concern ourselves with this exacting goal in Chap. 8. Strachey's (1934) mutative interpretation is a particularly typical psychoanalytic tool for change in that it is the furthest removed from the conventional form of suggestion.

## 2.3 Dependence of Transference Phenomena on Technique

In contrast to the idealized theory of technique, which attempted to formulate standardized experimental conditions, psychoanalytic practice has from the outset been characterized by a flexibility oriented toward the therapeutic objective, rules being adapted according to the desired change. A questionnaire which Glover (1937, p. 49) first reported at the Marienbad symposium showed that 24 English analysts did indeed differ greatly in their application of important rules of technique. The critical discussion of the effects on transference of applying rules flexibly was interrupted by political events. Not until the years after the war was significantly more light thrown on the decisive part played by the psychoanalyst in the therapeutic paradigm of psychoanalysis. Three pieces of work which all appeared in 1950 (Balint and Tarachow; Heimann; Macalpine) marked a turning point, and from one point of view, Eissler's work published in the same year could also be included (see Chap. 3). In her article "The Development of the Transference," Macalpine reports after a thorough study of the literature that despite fundamental differences of opinion on the nature of transference, there is surprising agreement on its origin: it is assumed that it arises spontaneously in the analysand. Macalpine supports her dissenting view — that transference is induced in a susceptible patient by the particular structure of the therapeutic situation — by listing 15 factors, and describes how typical technical procedures all contribute to the patient's regression, so that his behavior can be viewed as a response to the rigid, infantile setting to which he is exposed. She describes the typical situation as follows:

The patient comes to analysis in the hope and expectation of being helped. He thus expects gratification of some kind, but none of his expectations are fulfilled. He bestows his confidence and gets none in return; he works hard but waits in vain for praise. He confesses his sins, but receives neither absolution nor punishment. He expects analysis to become a partnership, but is left alone (Macalpine 1950, p. 527).

The 15 factors (to which others could be added) yield numerous possible combinations, which lead to a variable picture of how a patient experiences the therapeutic relationship, or how the analyst induces transference through his application of the rules. Macalpine wants to show that transference arises *reactively*. It is thus logical to expect that every variation of the situational precipitants stimulus will lead to different transferences. The field dependence of transference becomes clear when one considers the multitude of possible combinations yielded by selective neglect of one or other of only 15 factors, quite apart from the differences between the various schools in their emphasis on certain aspects of interpretation. Thus it becomes understandable why the patient Mr. Z. had different transferences in his two analyses with Kohut (1979; cf. Cremerius 1982). Macalpine's convincing argumentation gained only little acceptance. Cremerius (1982, p. 22) recently voiced the criticism that many analysts still see transference as an "endopsychic, inevitable process." Apparently, the recognition of the analyst's influence on transference is so unsettling that convincing theoretical argumentation has as little effect as the unequivocal observations which Reich summarized (1933, p. 57) by saying: "Transference is always a faithful mirror of the therapist's behavior and analytic technique."

Eissler is considered one of the most influential exponents of the *basic model technique* (see Thomä 1983 a). His work on modifications of the standard technique and the introduction of the "parameter" (1958) contributed greatly to the formation of the neoclassical style and to psychoanalytic purism. His dispute with Alexander and the Chicago School (1950) delimited the classical technique from its variants, and almost totally overshadowed the fact that this piece of work contains an aspect which concedes the psychoanalyst's influence on transference a greater scope than the basic model technique really permits. What was then at issue? After Freud's death and the consolidation of psychoanalysis after World War II, the question of which variations in technique still lie within a correct understanding of psychoanalysis became prominent in theoretical controversies, although even among orthodox psychoanalysts there is a wide spectrum of practice. On the other hand, by defining rules precisely it is possible to exercise discipline and draw sharp lines. In the 1950s, the unexpected growth of psychoanalysis brought an abundance of problems. The natural reaction to the emergence of numerous forms of psychodynamic *psychotherapy* derived from psychoanalysis was to define the psychoanalytic method strictly and to keep it pure (Blanck and Blanck 1974, p. 1). The simplest way of defining a method is through rules of procedure, as if following them not only protects the psychoanalyst's identity, but also guarantees an optimal, particularly profound analysis.

Thus Eissler's (1950) practically and theoretically productive proposal was almost completely ignored. He defined psychoanalytic method in terms of its goal; vis-à-vis the technical modalities, including the handling of transference, he favored a great degree of openness and goal-oriented flexibility. He stated that any technique can be termed psychoanalytic therapy as long as it strives for or achieves structural personality changes using psychotherapeutic means, regardless of whether sessions are daily or irregular and whether the couch is used or not.

The method can hardly be defined sufficiently in terms of its objective, except under the tacit assumption that only strict psychoanalysis strives for or achieves structural change — which is probably also Eissler's position. Nevertheless, Eissler provided here an early indication — one running counter to his basic model technique — that a more meaningful way of developing an appropriate theory of psychoanalytic technique, and of improving psychoanalytic practice, than censoring the method is to investigate the changes that the treatment strives for and achieves. It is dubious whether the regression produced by the standard technique, with its special transference contents, is the optimal way of changing the structure and therefore the symptoms (see Chap. 8). We cannot shut our eyes to the fact that some therapies do not have a favorable course (Drigalski 1979; Strupp 1982; Strupp et al. 1977; Luborsky and Spence 1978), but to blame this on an inaccurate determination of indications (i.e., to conclude that the patient is not analyzable) is to deceive ourselves. The standard technique has narrowed the definition of analyzability and placed ever-higher demands on the strength of the ego functions of the suitable patient, but there has been insufficient discussion of the problem that complications, right up to so-called transference psychoses, could be due not to the inaccurate determination of indications, but rather to the production of specific regressions displaying excessive sensory deprivation (see Thomä 1983a). Such omissions weigh even more heavily when there is simultaneous failure to prove that certain ways of handling transference do indeed lead to changes in structure and symptoms.

Bachrach's thorough and comprehensive discussion of the concept of "analyzability" (1983, p. 201) is one of the contributions exemplifying the promising developments in the whole field of psychoanalytic theory and practice. Instead of the usual one-sided, and in many respects problematic, question of the patient's suitability, we should now be asking which changes take place in which analysand with which difficulties when the psychoanalytic process is applied in which way by which analyst. The boundaries of transference are being constantly pushed back by self-critical questions, as defined by Bachrach, in spite of simultaneous rigidity. Thus, as shown by Orr's survey as early as 1954, psychoanalysis has long been on the way to a new understanding of transference. Variations of treatment techniques create specific transferences which must be understood operationally.

## 2.4 Transference Neurosis as an Operational Concept

In his introduction to the discussion of the problems of transference at the 1955 IPA Congress, Waelder (1956, p. 367) emphasized the analyst's influence: "As the full development of transference is the consequence of analytic situation and analytic technique, changes of this situation or technique can considerably alter the transference phenomena."

Glover (1955, p. 130) also stressed that "*the transference neurosis in the first instance feeds on transference interpretation*; in other words the transference, starting in a fragmentary form, tends to build itself on the foundations of transference interpretation."

Balint (1957, p. 290) stated even more clearly: "Heaven knows how big a part of what he [the analyst] observes — the transference phenomena happening under his eyes — may have been produced by himself, viz. they may be responses to the analytic situation in general or to its particular variety created by his correct, or not so correct, technique."

The essential findings of the American Psychoanalytic Association symposium "On the Current Concept of Transference Neurosis," with papers by Blum (1971) and Calef (1971), confirm the view emphasized by Waelder and Macalpine. Basically, the introduction of the term transference neurosis expresses Freud's recognition that general human transference is transformed into a systematized relationship under the influence of the analytic situation and in the presence of particular neurotic types of transference readiness (although Freud underestimated this influence or believed he could limit it with standardized conditions). Loewald (1971) underlined the field dependence of transference neurosis by stating that it is not so much a quantity that can be found in patients, but more an operational concept. We agree with Blum (1971, p. 61) that it is still meaningful to talk of transference neurosis if you understand the term to include all transference phenomena against the background of a modern theory of neurosis. In this sense, transient transference phenomena are just as much operational concepts as is symptomatic transference neurosis. We therefore do not differentiate between particular phenomena, e.g., situational transference fantasies, and the transference-neurotic transformation of symptoms of some nosologic class (disease group), including narcissistic neuroses, which Freud equated with psychoses. Transference neurosis is therefore a kind of artificial neurosis. In his *Introductory Lectures* (1916/17, p. 444), Freud writes:

> We must not forget that the patient's illness, which we have undertaken to analyze, is not something which has been rounded off and become rigid but that it is still growing and developing like a living organism .... All the patient's symptoms have abandoned their original meaning and have taken on a *new* sense which lies in a relation to the transference. (Emphasis added)

The context of this quote places strict limitations on the "new sense." Other points in the text, where transference neurosis is spoken of as a "new condition" replacing the "ordinary neurosis" and "giving all the symptoms of the disease a new transference meaning," also restrict the innovative side of real experience to the favorable conditions for the awakening of memories which follows from the repetitive reactions (Freud 1914g, pp. 154-155). Since Freud did not consistently view the growth or development of the transference neurosis, which grows like a living creature, as an interpersonal process within a therapeutic relationship between two individuals, the psychoanalyst's major contribution to this "new, artificial neurosis" (Freud 1916/17, p. 444) remained concealed. The depth of these problems is shown in Freud's rigorous choice of terminology when discussing the overcoming of the transference neurosis (1916/17, p. 443). His words do not reflect the ideal of freedom, but rather betray helplessness: "We overcome the transference by pointing out to the patient that his feelings do not arise from the present situation and do not apply to the person of the doctor, but that they are repeating something that happened to him earlier."

Even more forcibly, he then used a word which did not belong to his usual vocabulary: "In this way we *coerce* him to transform his repetition into a memory" (1916/17, p. 444, emphasis added; Strachey translated *nötigen* as *oblige*).

One further, obsolete meaning of transference neurosis should briefly be mentioned, namely its nosologic use in Freud's sense of the term. This use cannot be supported, as even people undergoing treatment for so-called ego defects or other deficiencies, perversions, borderline states, or psychoses develop transferences. Freud's theoretical assumptions concerning narcissism initially prevented recognition of the peculiar transferences displayed by borderline cases and psychotics, leading to the confusing nosologic differentiation between transference neuroses and narcissistic neuroses. All patients are capable of transference, and it is therefore invalid to define hysterical, phobic, and compulsive neurotic syndromes tautologically as transference neuroses and to contrast them with narcissistic neuroses. The various categories of illness differ in the form and content of transference, but it is never absent.

## 2.5 A Controversial Family of Concepts: Real Relationship, Therapeutic Alliance, Working Alliance, and Transference

We have already met the father of this family of concepts, although he did not identify himself as such. In Freud's work we find him in the person of the doctor to whom the patient attaches himself, as well as in the "real relationship," whose stability is a counterweight to transference. But what would a family be without a mother? We find her in the "unobjectionable transference" which early in the life history begins to build the quiet but solid background of trust. Unobjectionable transference is thus mother of the family of concepts we are now going to discuss. We attribute to real maternal reference persons the greatest influence on the establishment of attitudes of trust toward the environment. If a patient's trust outweighs his mistrust, stable unobjectionable transference (in Freud's terminology) can be expected. Why, then, when the father and mother of the family of concepts already existed, were new terms introduced which differ from one another and, like actual children, sometimes take more after the mother and sometimes more after the father? Sandler et al. (1973) pointed out that until the introduction of the concept of treatment alliance, Freud's inclusion of both unobjectionable and libidinal transference under positive transference was a source of confusion. Their work shows that the treatment alliance is made up of widely differing elements. Indeed, Zetzel's (1956) understanding of the therapeutic alliance is based on the model of the mother-child relationship. In her opinion the early phases of an analysis resemble the child's early phases of development in several ways. The conclusion Zetzel drew for the therapeutic alliance was that especially at the beginning of the treatment, the analyst should model his behavior on that of the good mother. In contrast, Greenson's (1965) working alliance includes above all the real or realistic elements of the relationship which Fenichel (1941) had still called rational transference.

A controversial family: What are the points at issue, and who is involved? At issue are the relationships and hierarchies within the family: the significance of transference compared with the real relationship, and in general the many conscious or unconscious elements in the analytic situation which affect the interaction between patient and analyst and cannot have their origin exclusively in the past.

We hope the reader will indulge us when we talk of the concepts as if they were quarrelsome people in order to shorten and simplify our description. Later we will name a few authors who breathe the fighting spirit into the concepts. Insufficient consideration has been given to the fact that the concepts get along so badly because they belong to different schools of practice. The monadic concepts quarrel with their dyadic brothers and sisters. Transference, like Sterba's ego splitting and Freud's fictive normal ego, is monadic, whereas all relationship concepts are dyadic in design and purpose. Already the quarrel begins: But surely we speak of the transference relationship as an object relationship? Yes, we do, but without thus forsaking one-person psychology, as Klein's theory shows. So, this means we cannot disregard Balint's two- and three-person psychology. Transference resists this, for fear that it, the family's favorite child and the one to whom we owe our professional existence, could suffer just as much as the patient and we ourselves.

We do not need to repeat why Freud conceived transference monadically or why the interactional-dyadic members of the family were long nameless, having an even greater efficacy for being unrecognized and underground. The family of concepts therefore had to be enlarged by the addition of members who had always been there, but had been described in detail only colloquially. We recommend Freud's chapter "Psychotherapy of Hysteria" (1895d, p.282), where there is a wonderful description of how the patient can be won over as a "coworker" for the therapy. All the evidence indicated that Freud continued primarily to attempt to "ally" himself with the patient, to form one party with him. We emphasize that "not every good relation between an analyst and his subject during and after analysis [is] to be regarded as a transference" (Freud 1937c, p.222). But in the meantime, positive transference has become the strongest motive for the analysand to participate in the work (1937c, p.233). The relationship is formalized in a "contract" or "pact"; how "loyalty to the alliance" is cultivated remained unspoken (the words in quotation marks come from Freud's late work, 1937c, 1940a). Particularly instructive is the fact that Freud orients himself in his late work more toward monadically conceived diagnoses, to ego changes, which do not permit adherence to the contract. He continues, though, to emphasize that the analyst "acts as a model...as a teacher" and that "the analytic relationship is based on a love of truth — that is, on a recognition of reality" (1937c, p.248). From the context it is clear that at least the reality of the analyst as a person is also at issue, but how this affects transference is left open.

If treatment strategies had been developed to solve the problem of the recognition of truth, we could spare ourselves the discussion in Sects. 2.7 and 2.8. Instead, there are confrontations, typical of a family feud, between monadic concepts like unobjectionable transference, ego splitting (Sterba 1934), and fictive normal ego (Freud 1937c) and the dyadic concepts which have their colloquial prototypes in Freud's work: induction of the we-bond (Sterba 1940), the therapeutic alliance (Zetzel 1956), and the working alliance (Greenson 1965). Within the family, issues in the dispute include who has a particularly close relationship with whom, and whether all the members are not really descendants of unobjectionable transference, i.e., of the early mother-child relationship. If the controversies are to be understood, it is absolutely essential to appreciate that transference is proud of its subjective, psychic truth, which nonetheless contains distortions. It is said that if negative transferences gain the upper hand, they can completely paralyze the analytic situation. The basic prerequisite for cure, namely the realistic relationship, is then undermined. Here Freud introduced an apparently objective or external truth — patient and analyst are based in the real external world (1940a, p. 173) — which, examined more closely, is in fact no less subjective than the truth which comes from transference. The introduction of the real person, the subject, into the working alliance does not prevent verification of the truth; on the contrary, it makes the subjectivity of our theories manifest. The individual analyst's responsibility is thus all the greater, and he must be expected to subject his practice to scientific examination, beginning with critical reflection on his own thinking and methods, i.e., with *controlled* practice.

We will now look more closely at the genealogical tree of the members of the family. We will start with ego splitting as prototype of the monadic concepts and progress to the we-bond and its derivatives. Freud described "the ideal situation for analysis," the only one in which the effectiveness of analysis can be fully tested, as

> when someone who is otherwise his own master is suffering from an *inner conflict* which he is unable to resolve alone, so that he brings his trouble to the analyst and begs for his help. The physician then works *hand in hand* with one portion of the *pathologically divided* personality, against the other party in the conflict. Any situation which differs from this is to a greater or lesser degree unfavorable for psychoanalysis. (Freud 1920a, p. 150, emphasis added)

Sterba reduced Freud's description to its real, influential essence: Out of the division emerged splitting, and the patient's ability to recognize inner conflicts as determinants of his illness became a particularly important criterion of indication for the technique. Ultimately, it seemed that the only people suitable for psychoanalysis were those whose endopsychic conflicts were on the oedipal level. The fact that Kohut explicitly viewed self psychology and the technique for treating narcissistic personality disturbances as complementing the classic therapy of oedipal conflicts should suffice to illustrate the consequences of ego splitting as a misunderstood catchword. It is certainly simpler if the patient is already conscious of his conflicts, but the analyst must always be willing to help establish a sound therapeutic relationship. In the later reception of ego splitting it was widely forgotten how induction of the we-bond can be promoted by including the elements of the relationship which are not transference determined, although Sterba (1934, 1940) and Bibring (1937) emphasized identification with the analyst, the we-bond, as a basis of therapy.

Because of the one-sided, rather negative conceptualization of psychoanalytic treatment, the genuine and extremely pleasurable experiences of discovering new areas of life through insights and we-bonds are underestimated, being viewed merely as sublimations. If, like Fürstenau (1977), one declares the relationship between analyst and patient to be a "relationship of a nonrelationship," one remains within an understanding of therapy in which the psychoanalyst is assigned a rather negative and paradoxical significance. On the other hand, it is misleading to talk of relationship, partnership, or encounter when it is unclear how these dimensions are shaped therapeutically. Freud taught us the analysis of transference, but relationship was for him self-evident, so that transference and relationship ran through his therapies side by side but unconnected. Today, however, it is important to recognize and interpret the influence of the two phenomena on one another; we therefore regard it as a mistake to employ a negative definition of the analytic situation and the particular interpersonal relationship which constitutes it, whether as relationship of a nonrelationship or as something asymmetrical, as if natural human relationships (e.g., groups that eat, live, and work together) were symmetrical like geometric shapes. The community of interests between analyst and analysand also has its asymmetries, but the starting point is decisive: the dissimilar positions, or the problem itself, which can only be solved by concerted, albeit varying efforts. It is in our view a mistake to make a partnership out of the community of interests, just as it must be antitherapeutic to stress the asymmetry so strongly that identifications are rendered more difficult or even prevented altogether.

However ambiguous the present family of concepts may seem, it became essential for both practical and theoretical reasons to find a concept to complement the equally manifold forms of transference, as the theory of transference attempts to explain the patient's contemporary behavior and his so-called analyzability in terms of the past. Ultimately, the patient's ability to overcome his negative and positive transferences, or resistance to transference, would go back to the mild positive and unobjectionable transference in the early mother-child relationship. One can see that the analyst's influence here would be essentially secondary in nature, i.e., merely derived.

This theory of transference not only failed to match therapeutic experience; on closer inspection, it also becomes clear that psychoanalytic ego psychology, with Sterba's therapeutic splitting of the ego as an early member of the family of concepts, had to lead to the working alliance, in the form of a treatment technique counterpart to the theory of autonomous ego functions. When the patient reflects on his utterances or observes himself, whether independently or assisted by the analyst's interpretations, he does not do this from an empty position. The analyst's ego may, because of its normality, be considered a fiction, but what he thinks and feels about the patient, and how he perceives the patient's transference, is by no means fictive. Just as the patient does not stumble into a no-man's-land when he emerges from his transferences, neither does the analyst fall into a void when he speculates on the patient's unconscious fantasies or attempts to explore his own countertransference. How he approaches the patient is influenced just as much by his views about transference as by his opinions about the patient's realistic perceptions. Knowledge of genesis alone is not sufficient; a position outside this knowledge is necessary to allow us to recognize transference phenomena and call them by their name. The patient is also partially outside the transference; otherwise, he would have no possibility of having the new experiences that the analyst encourages through his innovative approaches. Transference is thus determined by non-transference — and vice versa.

The fact there is something beyond transference, namely identification with the analyst and his functions, is shown by the establishment of a therapeutic relationship which does not end with the discontinuation of treatment. The ideal of the resolution of transference was part of a monadically conceived treatment process, and thus it is no surprise that we do not actually encounter it in reality (see Chap. 8). It is true, of course, that there have always been differences in evaluation: unobjectionable transference was in any case not an object of analysis for Freud and was therefore outside the realm of what was to be resolved.

To facilitate understanding, we repeat that Zetzel explained the patient's ability to form a relationship in terms of the unobjectionable mother transference. Zetzel's therapeutic alliance is therefore derived from, and fits well into, the traditional theory of transference. Over the years, Greenson's working alliance has freed itself the most from the theory of transference. There are practical and theoretical reasons why Greenson's (1967) declarations of independence extended over many years and the links to the father- or motherland — i.e., transference — remained unclear. Thus he spoke of the working alliance as a transference phenomenon (1967, pp. 207, 216) but at the same time stressed that the two were parallel antithetic forces. How can this contradiction be resolved? Insofar as one equates transferences with object relationships (in the analytic sense) in the therapeutic situation, then the working alliance is also an object relationship with unconscious components, and thus requires interpretation.

Over the past decades, the expansion of the family of concepts we have been discussing was accompanied by extension of the concept of transference. The reader will not find it easy to reconcile these two trends, one stressing the non-transference-determined elements (the therapeutic relationship), the other emphasizing transference. The recognition of non-transference-determined elements and the perception of transference as a comprehensive object relationship (transference relationship) arises from separate traditions of psychoanalytic practice which have common roots. Fifty years ago, Sterba (1936, p. 467) stated that transference was essentially an object relationship like any other, although he simultaneously stressed the necessity of differentiation. The essential contribution to the extension of the concept of transference was made by Klein and the "British object relationship theorists," to use a phrase coined by Sutherland (1980) to describe Balint, Fairbairn, Guntrip, and Winnicott and to stress their independence and originality within the English school. The ahistoric, almost unchangeable quality ascribed by Klein to unconscious object-oriented fantasies means that they are always present and extremely effective. Thus, in the here-and-now, deep interpretations of unconscious fantasies can also be made immediately (Heimann 1956; Segal 1982).

Transference was ascribed a unique significance by Klein's school in the context of her special object relationship theory. The rejection of primary narcissism initially had fruitful therapeutic consequences. According to this theory, unconscious transference fantasies focus immediately on the object, the analyst; even more important, they seem to be unconcealed by resistance and thus immediately open to interpretation. In ego psychology, one wrestles with strategies of interpretation typified by catchwords such as surface, depth, positive and negative transference, and interpretation of resistance, but Klein's theory recommends immediately interpreting suspected unconscious fantasies as transferences. Anna Freud related transference interpretations almost exclusively to the past (1937, p. 27), conceding a situational genesis only to resistance. In strict resistance analysis, as propounded by Reich and then by Kaiser (1934) and criticized by Fenichel (1953 [1935a]), the analyst broke his silence only with occasional interpretations of resistance. Klein thus relaxed the rigidity of resistance analysis and replaced silence with a new stereotype: immediate transference interpretation of unconscious, object-oriented fantasies and their typical Kleinian content of the "good" and above all the "bad" breast.

In Klein's theory, the here-and-now is understood exclusively as transference in the sense of ahistorical repetitions (Segal 1982). It is questionable, though, whether one can credit the unconscious parts of experience with a timeless, ahistorical, special existence, however impressive the storage of latent dream thoughts in long-term memory may be. The unconscious has no existence of its own; it is bound to the historicity of human existence. In Klein's view of transference, repetition assumes such great importance that temporality — past, present, and future — seems to be suspended. For this reason the question of change through new experiences was long neglected by the proponents of this theory (Segal 1964). Yet the patient must come to terms with the analyst and the latter's view of the psychic reality of present and past in order to free himself of transference and open himself up for the future. The here-and-now can at the very most only partially also be a then-and-there, otherwise there would be no future — which, revealingly, cannot be localized with such handy adverbs.

Thus the traditional definition of transference limits this concept to that which is not new in the analytic situation, i.e., to the repetitive new editions of intrapsychic conflicts which have their origin in past object relationships and are automatically triggered off in the treatment situation. But since new material emerges in the therapy, it became imperative to accentuate this side of the analysand-analyst relationship by means of the special terms that we have introduced as the dyadic members of the family of concepts associated with the working alliance. At the same time, however, the interpretation technique of ego psychology remained bound up with the past and with the intrapsychic conflict model. Since transference was viewed as a circumscribed distortion of perception, the analyst practicing ego psychology asks himself: What is now being repeated, which unconscious wishes and fears are being enacted, how are they blocked, and — above all — to whom do they relate? What mother or father transference is now being duplicated on me? Obviously these questions refer primarily to the past, which, unnoticed by the patient, is being repeated. Certain rules of treatment behavior allow the repetition to attain full impact and permit it to be convincingly traced back to unconsciously preserved, dynamically active memories. The analyst behaves passively and waits until the mild, positive transference grows into resistance. Finally, he interprets the resistance.

"The here-and-now is primarily important because it leads back to the past where it originates." In our opinion, this statement by Rangell (1984, p. 128) characterizes succinctly an interpretation technique which concerns itself primarily with memories, relegating the contemporary relationship, i.e., the interactional approach, to second place. Exaggerating, one could say that only the transference portions of the dyadic therapeutic process are noted and attention is rapidly turned to the past and to memories. Although Rangell acknowledges the significance of the working relationship when he states that interpretations can be made only after such a relationship has been built up, he emphasizes that the analyst need make no special effort in this direction (1984, p. 126). Sterba's view was entirely different; he encouraged induction of the we-bond:

> From the outset the patient is called upon to 'co-operate' with the analyst against something in himself. Each separate session gives the analyst various opportunities of employing the term 'we', in referring to himself and to the part of the patient's ego which is consonant with reality. (Sterba 1934, p. 121)

The issue is thus one of treatment technique priorities. That transferences are object oriented is undisputed, since the wishes which rise from the unconscious into the preconscious are primarily associated with objects, even though the latter are not mentally represented in the very early stages of life. According to Freud's *topographic* theory of transference as laid out in *The Interpretation of Dreams*, these intrapsychic events form the basis of the clinical transference phenomena. The theoretical assumptions correspond to the experience that transferences — like dream formation "from above" — are triggered by a real day residue. Realistic perceptions, which vary in their course, thus concern the analyst. Neglect of this day residue, and thus of interaction, in interpretation of transference is a serious omission which can have grave consequences. The general neglect of the day residue in transference interpretation is inherent in this theory, and is linked with the avoidance of realistic ties with the person of the analyst, because these run counter to the paradigm of treatment technique based on mirror reflection. Thus, the obvious discrepancy between the consideration of the day residue in the customary interpretation of dreams "from above" and the neglect of it in the interpretation of transference is explained by reference to the past (and prevailing) clinical theory and practice of transference.

It was not only in Klein's school that the extension of the theory of transference led to considerable alterations in treatment technique. We would like to illustrate this by reference to a controversy between Sandler and Rangell. The following passage contains the essential points of Sandler's arguments:

It seems clear that the introduction and description of these object-related processes, particularly the object-related defences, reflected a major new dimension in the analytic work and in the concept of transference. The analysis of the here-and-now of the analytic interaction began to take precedence, in terms of the timing of interpretations, over reconstruction of the infantile past. If the patient used defences within the analytic situation which involved both him and the analyst, this was seen as transference, and increasingly became a primary focus of attention for the analyst. The question "What is going on now?" came to be asked before the question "What does the patient's material reveal about his past?"

In other words, the analytic work became more and more focused, in Britain certainly, on the patient's use of the analyst in his unconscious wishful fantasies and thoughts as they appeared in the present — i.e. in the transference as it is explicitly or implicitly understood by most analysts, in spite of the limited official definition of the term. (Sandler 1983, p. 41)

Rangell's criticism is fundamental. He raises the question: "Is it still resistance and defences first, as it has been with Freud, Anna Freud, Fenichel and others? Or have we moved to what is promulgated by many as transference first, or even transference only?" He says it all boils down to a new polarization: many psychoanalysts everywhere now give the here-and-now precedence over reconstruction and insight. "Ultimately we may have to decide between two different concepts of transference, intrapsychic versus interactional or transactional. The same choice may need to be made between the intrapsychic and interactional models of the therapeutic process" (Rangell 1984, p. 133).

We believe that the decisions have been made and that the controversies are dogmatic in origin. It is in the very nature of the concept of transference that it needs to be supplemented if it is to meet the demands of therapeutic practice and a comprehensive theory of cure. The same goes for the choice between the intrapsychic and interactional models of therapy. After all, it is not a question of either-or, but rather one of not-only-but-also. Should some shabby compromise be made? Not at all. Psychoanalysis as a whole lives from integration, whereas each school attempts to retain its own individuality. This is the root of the continuing controversies which we will now illustrate with some typical examples. In our opinion, recognition of the fact that these controversies are dogmatic in origin must benefit psychoanalytic practice — clarification leads to change, and not only in therapy. Our examples make some problems plain. Rosenfeld's (1972) criticism of Klauber's (1972a) emphasis on the analyst's personal influence reached the level of personal polemic. Eissler (1958), in contrast to Loewenstein (1958), strictly separated interpretation from the person. Brenner (1979a) believed he could show, using some of Zetzel's cases as examples, that the introduction of the therapeutic alliance and other devices would be totally superfluous if only transference were analyzed well — such crutches being necessary only if the analysis of transference is neglected. And indeed, he has no difficulty in demonstrating omissions in Zetzel's analyses. Curtis, in a balanced statement of opinion (1979, p. 190), stresses where the danger lies, namely in seeing the therapeutic alliance and the whole family of concepts as a goal in itself, i.e., in creating a new, corrective object relationship instead of a tool for analysis of resistance and transference. In the light of this argumentation, it becomes clear why Stein (1981) even found fault with Freud's unobjectionable transference — for every type of behavior has unconscious aspects, which sometimes can or even must be interpreted in the here-and-now, even when they are unobjectionable, whatever their origin. In the analytic situation, one factor or another always gets neglected. If, like Gill and Hoffman (1982), one concentrates on the analyst's contribution to the genesis of "resistance to the transference," one can lose sight of the unconscious genesis, as Stone (1981 a) rightly pointed out.

The youngest branch in this family of concepts is Kohut's comprehensive understanding of transference in the framework of his theory of selfobjects. It is comprehensive in the sense that Kohut (1984) considers human relations and the life cycle as the history of unconscious processes of seeking and finding selfobjects. These are archaic object relationships in which self and object, or I and you, are fused. The objects are described as a part of one's self, and the self as a part of the objects. Correspondingly, the special forms of transference described by Kohut, e.g., twinship or fusion transference, are variations within an interactional unit. Kohut's theory can be distinguished from other object relationship theories by the exceptional emphasis on the grandiose exhibitionistic expectations attributed to the infant. According to Kohut, the development of stable self-confidence is dependent on the recognition of and response to these expectations. Kohut's theory of selfobjects thus put disturbances of object relationships in a genetic relationship with disturbances of self-confidence — the eidetic component, the showing of one's self and the reflection in the eye of the maternal reference person, playing a very outstanding role.

Since human dependence on the environment lasts for one's entire life, Kohut's theory of selfobjects has both a general and a specific consequence for treatment technique. All patients depend on recognition, because of their insecurity, and they transfer the corresponding expectations to the analyst. In addition, Kohut described specific selfobject transferences and provided a genetic grounding for their interpretation, i.e., one referring to the origin. According to the summary given by Brandchaft and Stolorow (1984, pp. 108-109):

> These selfobject relationships are necessary in order to maintain the stability and cohesion of the self while the child gradually acquires, bit by bit, the psychological structure it needs to maintain its own self-regulatory capability. The course of selfobject relations reflects the continuity and harmony of the developmental process through its various hierarchically organized stages. In the "omnipotence" which has been described as characteristic of the pathology of archaic object relations (M. Klein, Rosenfeld, Kernberg) we can recognize the persistence of the confident expectation that these selfobject needs will be met. Where archaic selfobject needs persist, the differentiation, integration, and consolidation of self structures and the developmental line of selfobject relationships have been interrupted. Thus archaic, poorly differentiated and integrated selfobjects continue to be needed, expected, and used as substitutes for missing psychological structure.

The relationship to the analyst is thus molded by comprehensive unconscious expectations, which seem to require a completely different kind of reflection than that which Freud introduced with his mirror analogy. Although Kohut (1984, p. 208) emphasizes that he applies the psychoanalytic method in an even stricter sense than that prescribed by Eissler's basic model technique, the interpretations of selfobject transference appear to convey a great deal of recognition. We will discuss this issue in more detail in Chap. 4.

The misgivings expressed in this representative compilation of controversies can all be justified, as it is always easy to show that an analyst has missed opportunities to interpret transference. We believe that these controversies can be raised to a productive level of discussion if their different theoretical assumptions are recognized and if the orthodoxies of the various schools can be overcome.

The followers of Klein, of Eissler's basic model technique, and of Kohut differ in their views of the typical contents of transference. At the same time, followers of these schools cling to their respective purist understandings of transference.

The very fact that each school describes typical transferences speaks for the analyst's influence on the transference contents, but no consequences have been drawn from this fact in the schools themselves. It can hardly be doubted that relativization — toward the analyst's own standpoint — would be inevitable if consequences were actually drawn. The field of transference is pegged out, tilled, and cultivated in different ways by the various theories and their corresponding treatment techniques. Transferences are defined by nontransference and vice versa. It is thus indispensable in theory and in practice that theories of transference oriented toward the past be supplemented. It is as understandable as it is illuminating that the strict schools, in contrast, neglected the transference-independent working alliance, as taking account of it would have meant replacing an intrapsychic model of transference and therapy with an interpersonal conceptualization. In school-independent psychoanalytic practice, decisions along these lines have long since been made. And the controversy between Sandler and Rangell about the here-and-now of transference interpretation concerns far more than priorities of interpretation technique. The analyst's apparently harmless change of approach, now first asking "What's happening now?," has enormous therapeutic and theoretical consequences, which affect, for example, the relative importance placed on construction and reconstruction. If one considers the complete current transference relationship, in its broadest sense, one recognizes the interactional, bipersonal approach, and thus the analyst's influence on transference. It is therefore misleading to speak only of an extension of the concept of transference. What we have here is a changed perspective, which long ago began to develop unobtrusively in psychoanalytic practice. The relationship between here-and-now and then-and-there has always been seen as important, although only more recently have we fully realized how strongly "what's happening now" is influenced by us.

Neurotic, psychotic, and psychosomatic symptoms have their roots in the patient's life history, and the observation of repetitions and conflicting reinforcements yields vital insights into psychogenetic and psychodynamic connections. Therapeutically, it is decisive how long and with what degree of attentiveness the analyst wears his retrospective glasses, when he puts on his reading glasses to improve his close vision, and where his glance rests longer. The relationship between the different perspectives largely determines what is viewed as transference. Finally, what about the comprehensive understanding of transference, in which the relationship to the analyst is central?

Interpretations of transference can be made on various preconscious or unconscious levels of this object relationship. The patient's perspective is deepened and extended by his confrontation with the analyst's opinions. Although the ideal is mutual communication, the analyst's influence can become particularly great if he takes the extended, comprehensive view of transference (transference relationship). Thus Balint criticized the stereotypic interpretations of transference, which make the psychoanalyst all-powerful and the patient extremely dependent. The target of his criticism was Klein's technique, in which the transference relationship is viewed exclusively as repetition. The more interpretations of transference are made, the more important it is to heed the real precipitating stimulus in the here-and-now and not to lose sight of the patient's external reality.

We hope we have shown that it is necessary to recognize the working alliance (Freud's real relationship) as a therapeutically essential component of the analytic situation, and always to take it into account. Otherwise we get stuck in Münchhausen's paradox, and transference must pull itself out of the swamp by its own hair. Schimek (1983, p. 439) spoke of a clinical paradox whereby transference is resolved by the force of the transference. Ferenczi and Rank had already drawn attention to this in their book *Development Goals of Psychoanalysis* (1924, p. 20): it would be a *contradictio in adjecto*, an impossibility, to use the patient's love of the doctor to help him do without this love.

Finally, we would like to emphasize that we are not dealing with constant personality traits when it comes to the patient's ability to establish a working alliance. The analyst's contribution to the therapeutic dyad can positively reinforce or negatively weaken the alliance. E. and G. Ticho (1969), in particular, pointed out the interrelationship between the working alliance and the transference neurosis. Luborsky (1984) has since provided empirical evidence that the working alliance has a decisive influence on the course and outcome of treatment. The proof of the change, which Freud (1909 b) called for on practical and theoretical grounds, justifies and limits both the scope of the psychoanalytic method and the influence exerted by the psychoanalyst through his handling of transference, a vital part of the analytic process.

## 2.6 The New Object as Subject: From Object Relationship Theory to Two-Person Psychology

Freud spoke of the "new object" and of the "new struggle" which he said leads out of transference: the first phase of therapeutic work is the genesis of transference through the liberation of the libido from the symptoms, the second phase is the struggle for the new object, the analyst (1916/17, p. 455). It is clear that the innovative side of the struggle consists in the new object, whose qualities were especially elaborated by Loewald (1960). It speaks for the productive psychoanalytic zeitgeist that Stone's (1961) influential book on the psychoanalytic situation appeared almost at the same time. We believe that the path from the new object must inevitably lead to recognition that the subject is the participant observer and interpreter guided by his subjective feelings and theory. The weight of the therapeutic work is borne not by the new object, but by the person, the psychoanalyst. Through his interpretations, the analyst shows the patient step by step how he sees him, enabling him to see himself differently, gain new insights, and change his behavior. The new subject has an innovative effect on the patient. How could suggestion, as part of the transference to be eliminated, possibly bring about change? Repetitions are not suspended by the patient being talked out of them in sublime, interpretative suggestion. But this is how the therapeutic changes would have to be explained if the psychoanalyst's influence were included in the analogy of transference and suggestion.

Freud drew such analogies, thus contributing to distortions which delayed deeper understanding of the therapeutic function of the new subject.[2] The subject is of course also used as object, as Winnicott (1971) noted. The transferences take place on the object. The therapeutic problem is to end the repetition, to interrupt the neurotic, self-reinforcing vicious circle. Now there are two people who can act self-critically. If the vicious circle of compulsive repetition is to be broken, it is essential that the patient can discover new material in the object, as Loewald (1960) put it. The analyst as person fails largely or completely to meet the patient's expectations in certain areas — particularly the area of his symptoms or special difficulties in his life — which have previously always been fulfilled by virtue of unconscious steering mechanisms.[3]

Because the psychoanalytic theory of instincts speaks of the object, and this usage has also been adopted in object relationship psychology, the fact is easily overlooked that we are dealing with living beings, with people who are affected by one another. The psychoanalyst offers at least implicit solutions to problems, even unspoken, when he believes he is discussing nothing more than transference. Today, thanks to the many painstaking studies of Freud's technique, which Cremerius (1981 b) critically examined and interpreted, we know that the founder of psychoanalysis had a comprehensive, pluralistic concept of treatment and used a wide range of therapeutic devices. The revolutionary significance of the introduction of the subject in observation and therapy remained concealed, however, because the associated severe problems were a heavy burden on psychoanalytic theory and practice. Only in recent decades has it become possible to solve these problems (see, e.g., Polanyi 1958).[4] Freud

---

[2] The "person of the doctor," with which the patient has a "proper rapport" in an "effective transference," is in Freud's theory of technique only "one of the imagoes of the people by whom he was accustomed to be treated with affection" (1913 c, pp. 139–140).

[3] Freud regularly explains the "new" in terms of biographical patterns — the child's "faith." The following is one example: "This personal influence is our most powerful dynamic weapon. It is the *new* element which we introduce into the situation and by means of which we make it fluid .... The neurotic sets to work because he has *faith* in the analyst .... *Children*, too, only believe people they are *attached* to." (Freud 1926 e, pp. 224-225, emphasis added)

[4] Weizsäcker's explicit "Introduction of the Subject into Medicine" lacked the methodology which could have cracked the therapeutic and theoretical problems of the special interpersonal encounter in psychotherapy.

tried to reeliminate the subject immediately and shift it outside the realm of "psychoanalytic technology" (Wisdom 1956; see Chap. 9). The subject surfaces again in the discussion of treatment technique, this time reduced to countertransference, which should be kept to a minimum for the sake of objectivity. Freud left the subject in the extratechnical area, where the analyst as real "person" remained until very recently, if only in the theory of technique. Now transformations are taking place, however, which change Freud's therapeutic and theoretical paradigm. Gill broke new ground with his "The Point of View of Psychoanalysis: Energy Discharge or Person?" (1983), in which he pleaded convincingly for the integration of interpersonal and intrapsychic interaction and for the synthesis of instinct theory and the object relationship theories. Simply the fact that an author who three decades ago, together with Rapaport (1959), extended the metapsychologic points of view now sees the person as more central than energy discharge, and everything else as subordinate, should provide food for thought. More important, of course, is that and how psychoanalytic observations change under the primacy of the person, or more correctly, from the point of view of Gill's conception of interaction between persons.

The cornerstones of psychoanalysis — transference and resistance — were laid on the foundation of an idealized scientific detachment (Polanyi 1958, p. VII), and elimination of the resulting construction faults can only increase their load-carrying capacity.

As we know from Lampl-de Groot (1976), Freud worked on two therapeutic levels — sometimes relationship, sometimes transference. Lampl-de Groot says it was clear when Freud was speaking to her as a real person and when as a transference object. The differentiation between these two aspects must have been very marked, as relationship and transference are not only complex systems in themselves, but are also closely entwined. This raised many theoretical and practical problems, for which Freud found a monadic solution in the ideal therapy model and a dyadic solution in practice.

Anchoring the pluralistic view in the theoretical paradigm, and not just practicing it, meant investigating the implications of all the psychoanalyst's influences on the patient (and vice versa). No model for this was created. In recent years it has become public knowledge how Freud practiced psychoanalysis. The model handed down was the monadic one, which Freud's successors refined with the aim of achieving the purest form of transference. In fact, in the whole of Freud's work there is no detailed discussion of the actual "real relationship." The analyst's influence is traced back to his predecessors in the patient's life history, i.e., the parents, and termed unobjectionable transference. This was bound to lead to confusion (Sandler et al. 1973). The real relationship seems to be in opposition to transference and threatened by it: intensive transference can allegedly wrench the patient out of the real relationship with the doctor (Freud 1912b, p. 105; 1916/17, p. 443). And there — with such global descriptions or negative characterizations (distortion of the real relationship by transference) — the matter remains. Thus Freud later adds that every good (therapeutic) relationship is to be viewed as transference; it could also be founded in reality (Freud 1937c, p. 221). We have no words to describe anything new, including the innovative components of problem-solving strategies.

A. Freud (1937) points out that we describe everything in the analytic situation which is *not* new as transference. Therefore the spontaneity of the transference neurosis, which according to her is not created by the doctor, is emphasized time and again. "Abolition" or "destruction" (Freud 1905e, p. 117) of the transference neurosis will, indeed must, lead to elimination of the symptoms, since, as Freud said later (1916/17, p.453), when transference has been "dissected" or "cleared away," those internal changes which make success inevitable have, according to theory, then been achieved. Only rarely in Freud's work is there any intimation of how much the psychoanalyst contributes to the patient's problem solving and thus to his new potentials, his freedom of decision.

## 2.7 The Recognition of Actual Truths

The fundamental uneasiness which gripped Freud the human being, Freud the doctor, and Freud the scientist on the discovery of transference did not fade away. After making the discovery (1895), Freud emphasized the vital therapeutic significance of transference in the postscript to "Dora," whose treatment ended in December 1900 and was written up as a case history in January 1901. The idea that we "destroy" transference by bringing it into the realm of the conscious originated in this "Fragment of an Analysis of a Case of Hysteria" (Freud 1905e). Later, in the *Introductory Lectures* (1916/17), Freud wrote that we must "compel" the patient to make the shift from repetition to recollection.

That is one of the signs showing that Freud's uneasiness persisted. The problem had resisted solution by the treatment rules which had in the meantime been formalized, although one of their principal goals had been to facilitate the handling of transference. The aggressiveness of Freud's metaphors (dissection, destruction) may show that he too was painfully touched by the actual, situational truth, i.e., by the realistic component of every transference. There are many ways of rejecting the patient's realistic observations, and paradoxical though it sounds, one widespread interpretation of transference is one of them. The interpretation we mean is offered when the patient has made relevant observations which are realistic, and thus in principle potentially accurate. Instead of accepting a perception as plausible, or contemplating the effects of a realistic observation on the unconscious and on its enactment in transference, the analyst often offers interpretations which take into account only the distortion of perception: "You think I would withdraw from you like your mother—I could get angry like your father." It is true that shifting an impulse to the past can have a relieving effect, because the patient is thus freed from an ego-dystonic impulse in the present, as A. Freud described (1937). However, the form taken by the interpretation of transference is vital. If it is constructed as though the patient is just imagining everything in the here-and-now, the situational truth in the patient's perception is ignored, often leading to grave rejections and irritations which result in aggression. If these are then interpreted as reprints or new editions of old clichés (Freud 1912b, p.99), then we have the situation that A. Freud discussed. She pointed out the fact that "analyst and patient are also two real people, of equal adult status, in real personal relationship to each other," and wondered "whether our — at times complete — neglect of this side of the matter is not responsible for some of the hostile reactions which we get from our patients and which we are apt to ascribe to 'true transference' only" (1954a, pp. 618-619). Balint's (1968) descriptions of artifacts, in the sense of reactively reinforced repetitions, also prevent us from contenting ourselves today with the careful raising of questions. Not only the consequences of the real personal relationship on the treatment process are important, but also the recognition of the analyst's enormous influence on transference. We can no longer ignore the fact that the "hypocrisy of professional practice" — drawn to our attention by Ferenczi (1955 [1933]) — can even produce transference-neurotic deformations. Freud (1937 d) assumed that "historical [life-historical] truths" even lay behind psychotic misperceptions of reality.

The life-historical relevance of these historical truths can at best be reconstructed. The actual truths, however, can be demonstrated *ad oculos*, and with their recognition the component of transference affected or triggered by the analyst becomes all the clearer. The fear that acceptance of the patient's realistic perceptions could pollute the transference beyond recognition is unfounded. On the contrary, through the patient's contributions, deeper truths can be broached. If the realistic, situational truths are accepted as such, i.e., integrated into the interpretation technique as initially autonomous elements, the procedure is no different than when one starts from the day residues and takes them seriously. The analyst reveals no details of his private life, makes no confessions (cf. Heimann 1970, 1978; Thomä 1981, p. 68). The atmosphere changes radically with the admission, as a matter of course, that the patient's observations in the here-and-now and in the analyst's office could be absolutely accurate. According to Gill it is essential, in cases of doubt, to assume at least the plausibility of the patient's observations, for the following reasons. No one is in a position to sound himself out with full self-knowledge, or to control the impact of his unconscious. One should, therefore, be open to the possibility of patients noticing things which have escaped one's own attention. Any argument over who is right will probably end up with the patient withdrawing, due to his dependence, and noting the experience that his remarks *ad personam* are not welcome. In this situation the analyst will have given no good example of composure and shown no willingness to take someone else's critical opinion as a starting point for self-critical reflections. Gill and Hoffman (1982) showed that systematic investigation of the analyst's influence on the form taken by transference is possible.

The ideal of pure mirror reflection must be abandoned not only because it is unattainable and can, from the epistomological viewpoint, lead only to confusion; from the psychoanalytic viewpoint, it must even be therapeutically harmful to strive after this fata morgana, because the patient can experience pure mirror reflection of his questions as rejection. Sometimes it is not just the patient's imagination that his observations or questions are at least irksome (see Sect. 7.4). The mirror reflection of questions is experienced as evasion;

actual truths are bypassed. Patients who are so disposed undergo malignant regressions, in the course of which the historical truths also become deformed, because the contemporary realistic perceptions are obstructed. Although it seems that the patient is saying everything that occurs to him, he has preconsciously registered the analyst's sensitive points and unconsciously avoids them. It is often no illusion or transferred feeling; the patient does not only *feel* that this or that question or observation might be unwelcome — his critical and realistic observations often *are* unwelcome. One cannot deal properly with these problems if one's own narcissism prevents recognition of the plausibility of realistic observations. If, on the other hand, one strives to base one's interpretation technique on the situational realities and their consequences for transference, essential changes occur. These changes not only affect the climate, they also facilitate the establishment of a therapeutically effective relationship, as new experiences are made in the here-and-now which contrast with the transference expectations. It now seems a natural step to place a particular construction on Freud's statement, quoted above, that conflicts are raised to the highest psychic level and thus abolished: the analyst's recognition of his realistic perceptions enables the patient to complete psychic acts and reach the agreement with the subject/object which is one of the most important preconditions for the formation of object constancy and self-finding. The ability to complete psychic acts in this way characterizes the genuine, therapeutically effective experiences in the psychoanalytic situation.

However, there are unfavorable consequences for the new "artificial neurosis," as Freud also called the transference neurosis, if the psychoanalyst's interpretations bypass contemporary realistic perceptions or attribute them to distortions. What we are confronted with here is nothing less than a violation of the love of truth which Freud (1937c, p.248) wanted to practice through the recognition of reality. However, the very problem of how the analyst recognizes realistic perceptions has still not been cracked by any development in treatment technique. Just as denied historical truths lie at the root of psychotic processes, chaotic transference neuroses or even transference psychoses can be created by failure to recognize actual truths. According to psychoanalytic theory, the summation of an infinite number of unconsciously registered rejections of realistic perceptions can result in a partial loss of reality. It can thus hardly be doubted that the analyst's shaping of the transference neurosis also has a bearing on the outcome of the treatment and the more or less problematic resolution of transference. The fundamental difficulties in resolving transference, which go beyond the individual case, are probably linked with the great underestimation of the effects of the therapeutic one-to-one relationship on the course of treatment.

## 2.8 The Here-and-Now in a New Perspective

We have tried to show that the analytic situation involves complex processes influencing both parties. Systematic investigations are thus methodologically difficult and demanding. How a real analyst's personal equation, countertransference, theories, and latent anthropology act on the patient cannot be grasped in its entirety, either clinically or theoretically. The typical dilemma therefore arises time and again: the complex real person cannot be used as a tool in treatment technique, but on the other hand, investigation of one section of the here-and-now does no justice to the complexity of the situation. Difficult situations are the true test of the master! Gill and Hoffman's qualitative and quantitative studies (1982) are centered on the theme of resistance to transference, including the analyst's contribution to its genesis and to its alteration in the here-and-now. Both aspects of this resistance must be emphasized. The here-and-now is self-evident, as the therapeutic change can only take place at the current moment — in the present. Of course, Gill and Hoffman's theory also assumes that resistance (and transference) originates partially in the past, but they stress the situational, actual aspects of the genesis of resistance. Their reasons for placing less importance on the reconstructive explanation are as follows: In psychoanalytic technique the analyst's contribution to transference and resistance was neglected. The reconstruction of the genesis of transference must also start in the here-and-now. In our opinion, one can arrive at the earlier determinants of neurotic, psychosomatic, and psychotic states in a therapeutically effective and theoretically convincing manner only if one always, even when making causal connections, starts with the factors that maintain the state in the here-and-now. Exactly this is the central point of Gill and Hoffman's theory. It is a remarkable fact that the here-and-now, the essential pivot of therapy, has only recently laid full claim to its deservedly prominent position. The simultaneous extension of the concept of transference, which is now understood by many analysts as the entirety of the patient's object relationship to the analyst, has already been described in Sect. 2.5 above as a sign of a radical transformation. Retrospection and the reanimation of memories has always served to resolve them in order to widen the perspective for the future. Although repetition has dominated the traditional understanding of transference, we would like to quote two striking passages from Freud; their therapeutic and theoretical potential is, in our opinion, only now being fully realized. In "Remembering, Repeating and Working-Through" (1914g, p. 154), he states:

> The transference thus creates an intermediate region between illness and real life through which the transition from the one to the other is made. The new condition has taken over all the features of the illness; but it represents an artificial illness which is at every point accessible to our intervention.

And in the *Introductory Lectures* (1916/17, p. 444) we read:

> The beginning of the treatment does not put an end to this development; when, however, the treatment has obtained mastery over the patient, what happens is that the whole of his illness's new production is concentrated upon a single point — his relation to the doctor. Thus the transference may be compared to the cambium layer in a tree between the wood and the bark, from which the new formation of tissue and the increase in the girth of the trunk derive. When the transference has risen to this significance, work upon the patient's memories retreats far into the background. Thereafter it is not incorrect to say that we are no longer concerned with the patient's earlier illness but with a newly created and transformed neurosis which has taken the former's place.

It is no wonder that the enormous implications of these comparisons have remained disconcerting for the psychoanalyst. If one translates these metaphors into practice, and sees transference as the cambium, a plant tissue capable of lifelong division, then the growth and proliferation of transference in all its forms and contents becomes a quantity which is also dependent on the analyst's influences. Indeed, in therapeutic practice all analysts start from the present, the here-and-now. They construct or reconstruct, interpret the past in light of insights gained in the present. We reconstruct the portion of transference whose genesis we suspect is in the past by starting from the here-and-now.

Since human beings are environment-oriented from infancy onwards, and since psychoanalytically we find objects even in narcissistic fantasies — even if they are Kohut's selfobjects on a totally unconscious level — transference can also be nothing other than an object relationship. There never used to be a fuss made about such truisms (see Sterba 1936, and Sect. 2.5). Even Nunberg, who viewed the analytic setting as closely analogous to the hypnotic attachment of the patient to the doctor, credited transference with an autonomous object reference:

Insofar ... as in transference the wishes and drives are directed towards the objects of the external world, ... transference is independent of the repetition compulsion. Repetition compulsion points to the past, transference to actuality (reality) and thus, in a sense, to the future. (Nunberg 1951, p. 5)

The analyst's contribution to transference gives it a process-like quality. Both in the genesis and in the passing of transference, the precipitating and innovative circumstances of the analytic situation are to be taken even more seriously than the past and its partial repetition, because the opportunity for change, and thus for the future development of the patient and his illness, exists only in the present. Central in the expansion of the model of the therapeutic process over the past decades has been the solution of a problem which was described by Gill (1982, p. 106) as follows:

Important though the recognition of the distinction between the technical and personal roles of the analyst is, I believe the current tendency to dissolve this distinction completely is a sign of a more basic problem — the failure to recognize the importance of the analyst's real behavior and the patient's realistic attitudes and how they must be taken into account in technique.

The reconstruction now becomes what it in practice always was: a means to an end. The adaptation of the handling of transference to the goal of the psychoanalytic process — structural change and the logically dependent change in symptoms — is a sine qua non of this argumentation. The influencing of the patient casts doubt on the objectivity of our findings [following Freud (1916/17, p. 452)], but this doubt can be lifted. Freud interpreted the evidence of therapeutic efficacy as proof of the validity of his theoretical assumptions. When resistances are successfully overcome, change (in symptoms) is the necessary and empirically verifiable result, going beyond the evidential feelings of the purely subjective truth-finding of the two participants in the psychoanalytic process. The psychoanalytic influence is vindicated by the evidence of change which can be explained theoretically, especially when the influence itself is made an object of reflection and interpretation. In the intersubjective process of interpretation, which relates to those conscious and unconscious "expectations" (Freud 1916/17, p. 452) on the part of the patient which the analyst suspects on the basis of indications, this influence cannot, as a matter of principle, be ignored. As a goal-oriented intention, it forms part of every therapeutic intervention. If from the very outset the analyst makes his contribution to transference in the full knowledge of his function as new subject-object, there emerges a significant intensification and extension of the therapeutic paradigm of psychoanalysis which is currently in full swing. The discussion between Grünbaum (1982) and M. Edelson (1983) shows that there are considerable theoretical problems to be solved.

To do full justice to the role of intersubjectivity or two-person psychology in the *psychoanalytic technique* it is necessary to go beyond both the traditional object relationship theories and the model of drive discharge. All the objects essential to man are constituted from the very beginning in an intersubjective space which is vitiated by vital pleasures (G. Klein 1969), yet it is not possible to link them closely to the drive discharge model. In their excellent study, Greenberg and Mitchell (1983) showed that the drive/structure model and the relational/structure model are not compatible; it therefore seems logical to seek ways toward an integration at a new level.

In Chap. 4 we will employ the fundamental approaches discussed here in the presentation of typical forms of transference and resistance, including fea ures specific to the various schools, and we will use them to help us to understand the psychoanalytic process (Chap. 9) and the interpretation of transference (Sect. 8.4). It can be deduced from purely theoretical considerations that at least the so-called unobjectionable transference cannot be resolved, but only recently has research also shown empirically how decisively the outcome is affected from the very beginning by the handling of transference.

# 3 Countertransference

## 3.1 Countertransference: The Cinderella in Psychoanalysis

Freud viewed countertransference, even when he first discovered it (1910d), as connected with the patient's transference in a dynamic way. It "arises in him [the physician] as a result of the patient's influence on his unconscious feelings" (Freud 1910d, p. 144). Freud emphasizes that "no psychoanalyst goes further than his own complexes and internal resistances permit" (1910d, p. 145). Thus it is necessary for the analyst to undergo a training analysis in order to be freed of his "blind spots."

Because Freud's recommendations about treatment techniques — expressed in striking metaphors such as to reflect like a "mirror" and to act like an "emotionless surgeon" — were taken literally, countertransference retained a negative meaning for decades. Freud had to place great value on "psychoanalytic purification" (1912e, p. 116) both because of his concern about the dangers that misuse might pose to the psychoanalytic method, and for scientific reasons. The fact that the analyst's "personal equation" (Freud 1926e, p. 220) would still remain even after the influence of countertransference had been mastered (i.e., ideally, eliminated) was regretfully accepted as inevitable. Freud was able to comfort himself with the fact that the personal equation[1] cannot be eliminated from observations even in astronomy, where it was discovered. However, he hoped that training analysis would lead to such a far-reaching balancing of the personal equation that satisfactory agreement would one day be achieved among analysts (Freud 1926e, p. 220).

These reasons were decisive factors in the very different histories of the concepts of transference and countertransference. It was not until much later that their separate paths merged in the realization that "we are dealing with a

[1] Freud knew of the concept's origin in astronomy. The famous case that led to the discovery of personal equation concerned the astronomers Maskelyne and Kinnebrook. Maskelyne, the director of an observatory, dismissed his assistant in 1796 because the latter always observed the passage of stars more than half a second later than he did. He could not imagine that an equally attentive observer using the same method would register systematically different times. It was not until 26 years later that Bessel recognized this possibility, thus solving the discrepancy and leading to Kinnebrook's later rehabilitation. As Russell et al. wrote in 1945, "This personal equation is an extremely troublesome error, because it varies with the observer's physical condition and also with the nature and brightness of the object."

system of relations in which each factor is a function of the other" (Loch 1965a, p. 15). Neyraut came to a similar conclusion in his study *Le transfert* (1974). Kemper (1969) spoke of transference and countertransference being a "functional unity." Earlier, Fliess (1953) had gone as far as to view some transference phenomena as reactions to the analyst's countertransference. Their interaction was also emphasized by Moeller (1977).

While transference changed within a short time from a major obstacle to the most powerful resource in treatment, countertransference retained its negative image for almost 40 years. It contradicted the time-honored scientific ideal which Freud was committed to and which was important to him both out of personal conviction and for the sake of his controversial method's reputation. In the history of science the analogy with the mirror can be found as early as Sir Francis Bacon's theory of idols (1960 [1620]), where it also was associated with the notion of objectivity, namely that true nature becomes apparent after cleaning the observing, reflecting mirror and eliminating all subjective elements. This led to the demand that countertransference, i.e., the mirror's blind spots and other blemishes, be eliminated. The demand that neurotic conflicts, and especially their manifestations toward the patient in countertransference, be overcome developed into a downright phobic attitude on the part of analysts toward their own feelings.

Freud addresses his recommendations in particular to the young and ambitious psychoanalyst who starts off to cure with true psychoanalysis and not with treatment by suggestion. He also warns him against employing too much of his own individuality although the temptation is certainly great.

It might be expected that it would be quite allowable and indeed useful, with a view to overcoming the patient's existing resistances, for the doctor to afford him a glimpse of his own mental defects and conflicts and, by giving him intimate information about his own life, enable him to put himself on an equal footing. One confidence deserves another, and anyone who demands intimacy from someone else must be prepared to give it in return.

But in psychoanalytic relations things often happen differently from what the psychology of consciousness might lead us to expect. Experience does not speak in favor of an affective technique of this kind. Nor is it hard to see that it involves a departure from psychoanalytic principles and verges upon treatment by suggestion. It may induce the patient to bring forward sooner and with less difficulty things he already knows but would otherwise have kept back for a time through conventional resistances. But this technique achieves nothing towards the uncovering of what is unconscious to the patient. It makes him even more incapable of overcoming his deeper resistances and in severer cases it invariably fails by encouraging the patient to be insatiable: he would like to reverse the situation, and finds the analysis of the doctor more interesting than his own. The resolution of the transference, too — one of the main tasks of the treatment — is made more difficult by an intimate attitude on the doctor's part, so that any gain there may be at the beginning is more than outweighed at the end. I have no hesitation, therefore, in condemning this kind of technique as incorrect. The doctor should be opaque to his patients and, like a mirror, should show them nothing but what is shown to him. In practice, it is true, there is nothing to be said against a psychotherapist combining a certain amount of analysis with some suggestive influence in order to achieve a perceptible result in a shorter time — as is necessary, for instance, in institutions. But one has a right to insist that he himself should be in no doubt about what he is doing and should know that his method is not that of true psychoanalysis. (Freud 1912e, pp. 117-118)

The difference between what the psychotherapist and the psychoanalyst may do, or between psychotherapy and psychoanalysis, is as relevant today as it has ever been, and differences can be most easily clarified by using rules. The entire complex surrounding influence became associated with countertransference, creating a formidable practical and theoretical problem. The fear of countertransference is thus not only a personal matter; the analyst's professional responsibility requires him to avoid the unfavorable influences which countertransference came to embody. Countertransference was the Cinderella of psychoanalytic technique, and its other qualities did not become apparent until it too had become a princess. To be sure, there was a preconscious premonition of its hidden qualities long before it gained official recognition, but the whispers could not make themselves heard. Thus the transformation seemed to take place overnight. The admiration now paid to the "new" countertransference creates the impression that many psychoanalysts immediately felt liberated, just as they did after Kohut's brilliant rehabilitation of narcissism. The strength of the phobic avoidance can be recognized in the fact that it was not until 30-40 years after Freud's discovery of countertransference (1910d, p. 144) that the subject was put in a new perspective in publications by A. and M. Balint (1939), Berman (1949), Winnicott (1949), A. Reich (1951), Cohen (1952), Gitelson (1952), and Little (1951). In hindsight, Heimann's original contribution on the subject (1950) was later seen as marking a turning point; we will discuss this publication in detail below.

The history of this concept (Orr 1954; Tower 1956) shows that there were a few forerunners to the above-mentioned publications from the 1950s. The obscurity of the positive aspects of countertransference can be demonstrated by referring to an article by Deutsch, missing from Orr's otherwise comprehensive study. Deutsch published her influential considerations on the relationship between countertransference and empathy in 1926; this line of work was continued by Racker in 1968. The title of Deutsch's article was "Occult Phenomena in Psychoanalysis" — no wonder these ideas remained in obscurity! The publications by Ferenczi (1950 [1919]), Stern (1924), Ferenczi and Rank (1924), W. Reich (1933), and A. Balint (1936) also did not have any significant influence.

Fenichel (1941) recognized relatively early that the fear of countertransference could bring the analyst to suppress every natural human emotion in his reactions toward the patient. Patients who had previously been in treatment with another analyst had often expressed surprise at his (Fenichel's) freedom and naturalness. They had believed that an analyst was somebody special and that he was not permitted to be human, although just the opposite impression should be dominant. The patient should always be able to depend on his analyst's humanity (Fenichel 1941, p. 74). Berman (1949) also emphasizes that the negative evaluation of countertransference had led to rigid, antitherapeutic attitudes. The optimal emotional climate is described, for him, by clinical anecdotes which demonstrate the great therapeutic importance of an analyst's caring and genuine, sincere interest; however, this side of the psychoanalytic process, to which the examples of many reputable analysts have contributed, is handed down primarily in a personal and informal way.

This verbally transmitted wealth of experience did not bear fruit because Freud's rules were ritualized. Yet since the burdens particular to our profession do not change from generation to generation, it is not surprising that this has been a prominent topic in the history of psychoanalysis and has been discussed at all the important symposia held by the International Psychoanalytical Association on psychoanalytic technique for the past half century. The disputes about Freud's suggestions on technique, impressively exemplified by the mirror analogy, emotional coldness, neutrality, and incognito, are repeated regularly because every psychoanalyst is exposed over and over again to the diverse disturbances of a complex situation. Thus a high value is placed on all solutions which promise to be reliable and easy to use. Understandable as it is, however, that novices in particular follow Freud word for word, this should not be viewed as an inevitable repetition compulsion confronting every generation of psychoanalysts in the recourse to the literal meaning of his words instead of to their historical meaning.

The further clarification of the foundations of therapy contributed to putting countertransference in a new light. The fact that numerous authors worked in the same direction simultaneously but independently demonstrates that the time was ripe for fundamental changes.

M. Balint and Tarachow (1950) reported that psychoanalytic technique was entering a new phase of development. The main concern had previously been the analysis of transference, i.e., the patient's contribution to the analytic process. In the phase beginning at that time the analyst's role, especially with regard to his countertransference, moved to the center of practical interest.

For the following reasons we will treat the articles by Heimann (1950, 1960) as exemplary in this connection.

1. Her initial presentation (1950) marks the turning point to a *comprehensive* understanding of countertransference as encompassing *all* the analyst's feelings toward the patient.
2. Heimann emphasized more than any other author the positive value of countertransference as an essential diagnostic aid and even as an instrument for psychoanalytic research. She also attributed the creation of countertransference to the *patient.*
3. Thus the countertransference feelings were in a certain sense depersonalized. Admittedly, they originate within the analyst, but as *products of the patient.* The more completely the analyst opens himself to countertransference, the more useful it is as a diagnostic aid. Heimann traced the *origin* of countertransference back to the patient and initially explained it as projective identification in the Kleinian sense.
4. Heimann initiated the comprehensive conception of countertransference, but after 1950 made numerous critical comments on "misunderstandings." She was stimulated to further clarify her position in discussions which took place in Heidelberg and Frankfurt within the framework of the studies on the interpretive process initiated by Thomä (1967b); this led to her publications on the analyst's cognitive process (Heimann 1969, 1977). Although she finally so distanced herself from the thesis that countertransference is the patient's creation that she expressed amazement at having ever made such an assertion (in a private conversation with B. and H. Thomä on August 3, 1980), this idea had long taken on a life of its own.

We believe it correct to mention such personal recollections here, because most analysts go through a learning process which is full of conflicts and which becomes more and more difficult with the increasing duration of training analyses. Heimann is a typical example. It was not until one of her last publications that she argued for the therapeutic use of countertransference without appealing to projective identification and independently of Klein's theories.

Special maieutic skill was required to free this Cinderella of the negative connotations Freud attached to it from the very beginning. Conceptual changes lead to profound professional and personal conflicts among analysts, which can be lessened if an interpretive connection to Freud can be made plausible. Heimann had good reason to handle countertransference with kid gloves. Today we know (King 1983) that she was urgently advised by Hoffer and Klein not to present her paper "On Countertransference" (1950) at the International Psychoanalytic Congress in Zurich. It is understandable that she used the usual ploy, saying in effect, "Actually, Freud also viewed the matter in a similar way or always acted in this way in his practice; he was simply misunderstood." In this way she diplomatically pointed to "misreadings" which Freud's views on countertransference and his mirror and surgeon analogies had led to. Nerenz (1983) has recently gone even further and asserted that Freud has been misunderstood because of a "legend" in which his comprehensive understanding of countertransference has been reinterpreted and assigned its generally accepted negative connotation.

Yet, of course, even Ferenczi, back in 1918, had spoken of the analyst's resistance to countertransference. Ferenczi described three phases of countertransference. In the first phase the analyst succeeds in gaining "control of everything in his actions and speech, and also in his feelings, that might give occasion for any complications." In the second phase he then sinks into "resistance against the countertransference" and is in danger of becoming far too harsh and rejecting; this would postpone the establishment of transference or even make it completely impossible to achieve. "It is only after overcoming this stage that one perhaps reaches the third, namely, that of the control of the countertransference" (Ferenczi 1950 [1919], p. 188). In the same publication Ferenczi accurately described the optimal attitude of the analyst as "constant oscillation between the free play of fantasy and critical scrutiny" (p. 189). The reader will be surprised to find that Ferenczi, of all people, after acknowledging the role of intuition, continued: "On the other hand, the doctor must subject the material submitted by himself and the patient to a logical scrutiny, and in his dealings and commmunications may only let himself be guided exclusively by the result of this mental effort" (p. 189).

With hindsight it is understandable that even Ferenczi's descriptions of the three phases of mastering countertransference failed to decrease the excessive anxiety which he described as the incorrect attitude. The analyst's acquired ability to control his own feelings and the exaggeration of this ability in resistance to countertransference cannot be altered by the vague observation that this is not the correct attitude. That is to say, if a strict control of feelings is introduced as the first learning experience, then it should come as no surprise that the result is "excessive anxiety" which is retained even when it should be discarded. In any case, Ferenczi's description of countertransference has had only minimal positive influence on its use. Psychoanalysts followed Freud's suggestions about technique very literally.

## 3.2 Countertransference in Its New Guise

There is no better description of the transformation of Cinderella into a radiant beauty than Heimann's following sentence, with its profound implications and consequences: "The analyst's countertransference is not only part and parcel of the analytic relationship, but it is the patient's *creation*, it is part of the patient's personality" (1950, p. 83). If countertransference had until then been regarded as a (more or less) strong neurotic reaction by the analyst to the patient's transference neurosis that was to be avoided as far as possible, now it became part and parcel of the analytic relationship and, later, "comprehensive" countertransference (Kernberg 1965). For Heimann, countertransference includes all the feelings the analyst experiences toward the patient. Her thesis is that

> the analyst's emotional response to his patient within the analytic situation represents one of the most important tools for his work. The analyst's countertransference is an instrument of research into the patient's unconscious .... It has not been sufficiently stressed that it is a relationship between two persons. What distinguishes this relationship from others is not the presence of feelings in one partner, the patient, and their absence in the other, the analyst, but above all the degree of the feelings experienced and the use made of them, these factors being interdependent. (Heimann 1950, p. 81)

It is essential that the analyst, in contrast to the patient, does not abreact the feelings released in him. They are subordinated to the task of analysis, in which the analyst functions as a mirror for the patient.

> The analyst along with this freely working attention needs a freely roused emotional sensibility so as to follow the patient's emotional movements and unconscious fantasies. Our basic assumption is that the analyst's unconscious understands that of his patient. This rapport on the deep level comes to the surface in the form of feelings which the analyst notices in response to his patient, in his "countertransference." This is the most dynamic way in which his patient's voice reaches him. In the comparison of feelings roused in himself with his patient's associations and behavior, the analyst possesses a most valuable means of checking whether he has understood or failed to understand his patient. (Heimann 1950, p. 82)

Since Heimann herself later considerably narrowed her conception of countertransference and wanted to have its area of applicability tested by reliable criteria, we can conclude our discussion of this theme. In psychoanalysis theories not only serve to solve substantive problems, but are embedded in a genealogy or tradition. With the new theory of countertransference, Heimann was very probably attempting to reconcile the conflicting positions of her teachers Reik and Klein. Through his countertransference the analyst hears with Reik's "third ear," and the patient's creation allegedly reaches him via the mechanisms described by Klein.

In the theory espoused by Klein and her school, the analyst's capacity for empathy is dependent on his recognition of the projective and introjective identification processes which underly the psychopathology and which proceed unconsciously in the patient. The following reasons are given for this.

Paranoid-schizoid and depressive positions are viewed as necessary dispositions of general and, under additional conditions, specific psychopathology. The transitions from "normal" to "pathologic" are gradual and smooth. Because of the assumed innate polarity of instincts and the secondary significance of experience, everyone is subject to the development of both positions (as unconscious "psychotic core") and to their effects on projective and introjective identifications.

The fixation point of the psychotic illnesses lies in the paranoid-schizoid position and at the beginning of the depressive position .... If the depressive position has been reached and at least partially worked through, the difficulties encountered in the later development of the individual are not of a psychotic, but of a neurotic nature. (Segal 1964, p.61)

Since the depressive position is unconsciously retained, the neurosis inevitably becomes a universal phenomenon. Because of the general presence of these positions, the psychoanalytic process proceeds evenly according to the dominance of one or the other position insofar as the analyst acts as a *perfect mirror* and promotes the development of the transference neurosis in the sense of the unfolding of projective and introjective identification. These two processes determine the kind of object relationship to internal and external objects, for both patient and analyst.

The analyst's capacity for empathy is explained formally and substantively by the two aspects of identification (Segal 1964). Empathy in its metaphoric representation as a receiver is equated with countertransference (Rosenfeld 1955, p.193). Through self-perception the analyst becomes able to trace a certain feeling back to the patient's projection. Thus Bion concludes the presentation of one vignette with the following words: "It will be noted that my interpretation depends on the use of Melanie Klein's theory of projective identification, first to illuminate my countertransference, and then to frame the interpretation which I gave the patient" (Bion 1955, p.224). Money-Kyrle described the smooth, "normal course" of transference and countertransference as a fairly rapid oscillation between introjection and projection:

As the patient speaks, the analyst will, as it were, become introjectively identified with him, and having understood him inside, will reproject him and interpret. But what I think the analyst is most aware of is the projective phase — that is to say, the phase in which the patient is the representative of a former immature or ill part of himself, including his damaged objects, which he can now understand and therefore treat by interpretation, in the external world. (Money-Kyrle 1956, p.361)

Grinberg (1979) describes the analyst's unconscious answers to the patient's projections as "projective counteridentification."

The substantive and formal connection of empathy to the processes of projective and introjective identification renders only those analysts who have "worked through" the paranoid-schizoid and the depressive positions personally and psychoanalytically fully capable of cognition. In the Kleinian theory of object relationships, unconscious fantasies — as products of instincts — are neglected relative to real persons from one's environment with regard to the constitution of the object in both its form and content (see Guntrip 1961, p. 230; 1968, p. 415; 1971, pp. 54–66). According to this, the analyst fulfills his task best when he acts as an impersonal mirror or neutral interpreter (Segal 1964). The Kleinian psychoanalyst ties his purely interpretive technique to a position of maximum neutrality. In terms of the metaphor, the mirror does not have any more blind spots insofar as the analyst has achieved the most profound insights into his own projective and introjective identifications. The Kleinian school can legitimately continue to claim to be able to employ a purely psychoanalytic technique even for patients other psychoanalysts view as requiring variations or modifications of technique.

From a scientific point of view it is distressing that the familiy ties within psychoanalysis lead to the development of new ideas only by means of a process of bracketing out well-justified criticism. For example, Heimann had neglected Grotjahn's (1950) criticism of Reik's ideas as well as Bibring's (1947) and Glover's (1945) criticism of Klein's teachings. Nevertheless, the liberating effect generated by the decisiveness with which Heimann described countertransference as the patient's creation cannot be valued highly enough. Ten years later Heimann had to straighten out some misunderstandings; "some" trainees had begun to make interpretations according to "feeling," quoting her article in support. When Heimann expressed criticism, the trainees claimed to be following her new conceptualization of countertransference and did not appear inclined to test interpretations on the actual events in the analysis (Heimann 1960). While Heimann had achieved her "main objective...to lay the ghost of the 'unfeeling,' inhuman analyst, and to show the operational significance of the countertransference" (Heimann 1960, p. 10), it is nonetheless necessary for this banishment to be repeated in every generation since the ghost reappears again. Without a doubt this is easier today because a distinguished analyst has set a precedent. Yet other questions remain to be answered, questions which were not posed in Freud's theory of countertransference because they seemed inapplicable in his approach.

## 3.3 Consequences and Problems of the Comprehensive Conception

The road to the integration of countertransference seems to be paved with misunderstandings which not only arise in trainees and which are not only caused by the failure to test interpretations based on countertransference in the analytic situation, as criticized by Heimann. The new understanding of countertransference had implications for basic problems of psychoanalytic technique and consequently led to various attempts to develop answers. At question is nothing less than the analyst's own cognitive process, i.e., the complex in which his therapeutic actions and especially his particular interpretations originate and are founded. The implication of appealing to interpretations based on feeling (as described above) without being concerned about their verification in the analytic situation and about real events is that their justification, i.e., their validity, is eo ipso presumed from the beginning. If countertransference is accorded the status of the central perceptive function, there is more than a remote danger that a reliable power of judgement will be attributed to it.

The concept of countertransference as transformed by Heimann seems to have entered into a close relationship with "evenly suspended attention" (see Sect. 7.3). Yet how can we go from unprejudiced listening to reliable knowledge that our own physical sensations, feelings, fantasies, and rational considerations correspond to the patient's unconscious processes, whether through reciprocity or through complementarity? The fact that Heimann raised countertransference to the level of a research instrument provided support for the naive idea that clarifying the origin of the analyst's fantasies would in itself ensure reliable and valid conclusions with regard to the patient's unconscious processes. However, how does it happen that Heimann's "countertransference" and Kohut's "empathy," closely related tools which cannot conceal their descent from Reik's third ear, arrive at completely different statements about a patient's unconscious? We will concern ourselves with the origin and foundation of interpretations, a topic largely neglected in psychoanalysis, in Chap. 10. Reiss (1983) has presented a thorough study of the problems which have to be solved in an attempt to grasp the interactional origin of empathy.

The huge difference between, on the one hand, the assertion that countertransference is the core of the analytic relationship and the patient's creation and, on the other, the proof of this assertion has hardly been tackled. Heimann's thesis, which goes far beyond merely laying the ghost and far beyond rehabilitating countertransference (including its hypothetical explanatory basis in projective identification), is instead treated as if it were already well founded, especially with regard to very specific thoughts and fantasies which the analyst has in individual cases. We summarize our own investigations of the *genesis* of analysts' fantasies and of their *foundation* in the transformation into interpretations, including the controls in the analytic situation demanded by Heimann, in Sect. 3.5. If countertransference is used as an instrument of perception, we are dealing in part with the solution to the problem Heimann referred to as "control" in the therapeutic situation. This control, in the sense of checking, is all the more necessary because it is easy for the analyst to "fall into the temptation of projecting outwards some of the peculiarities of his own personality, which he has dimly perceived, into the field of science, as a theory having universal validity" (Freud 1912e, p. 117) or to attribute these peculiarities to the patient instead of to himself. Exactly because psychoanalysis attempts to make full use of subjectivity, as Loch (1965a) rightly emphasized, it is essential for analysts to be conscious of subjectivity in order to be able to discuss a personal theory intersubjectively. This requires that countertransference be distinguished from the analyst's personal theory; discussion can clarify which theoretical assumptions actually influence treatment.

The comprehensive concept of countertransference appears to have especially the following theoretical and practical consequences. Without disturbing the still valid demand that the blind spots of countertransference in Freud's sense be overcome, the comprehensive concept led to the creation of links to Freud's receiver model of psychoanalytic perception (see Sect. 7.3). The comprehensive concept revived a tradition Reik had especially fostered. A secondary aspect of this tradition is the related idea that empathic perception from unconscious to unconscious does not recognize any further foundation, whereby a particularly "psychoanalytic" understanding of truth is claimed. It should be noted that cultivation of this tradition in psychoanalysis is not limited to any particular school.

The attempt by psychoanalysts of the Kleinian school to reduce the psychoanalyst's patient-related fantasies to a few typical mechanisms and thus to provide an explanation for his empathy can also be viewed as another consequence of the comprehensive view of countertransference.

Heimann believed that the patient's unconscious partially expresses itself in countertransference. This view remained for her tied to the one-to-one relationship in analysis. The idea that one's own sensations might correspond to and be initiated by the other person's was soon transported into the field of applied psychoanalysis. There it spread like wildfire, because applied psychoanalysis makes it very difficult to exercise the controls demanded by Heimann. Today it is especially popular to view the fantasies of participants at technical seminars as reflections of a patient's unconscious. The more ideas the participants have and the more convincing the moderator is in discerning a common theme in the multitude of perspectives, the more productive these seminars are. They familiarize the participants with fantasies and unconscious wishes hidden behind the manifest phenomena. The joint fantasizing about a patient thus fulfills a primary didactic function, which somehow can also provide benefits for treatment. This "somehow" is of course the crux of the problem, because testable theses are posed only very rarely and because there is usually no feedback on the further development of the case being discussed. More exact clinical verification is probably completely impossible because an infinite number of variations of the themes can be imagined.

Thus we are faced with a dilemma. On the one hand it is instructive when there is much speculating and fantasizing at casuistic seminars, on the other it is often at an immense distance from the absent patient's problems and their unconscious motivation. Opinions differ on this dilemma. It is only possible to take unadulterated pleasure in fantasizing until the question is raised as to the nature of the relationship of the participants' associations to the absent patient's unconscious thoughts. We have stressed the patient's absence as a reminder that the seminar participants have only secondhand information available about him and that this information includes only what the treating analyst has reported. They look through a telescope whose lens system has produced numerous refractions of the characteristics of the object. Our analogy makes it clear that it is impossible to trace the path of the light without exact knowledge of the individual systems. In order at least to learn as much as possible about the treating analyst's approach, the custom of taking protocols of treatment sessions was initiated at the psychosomatic clinic at the University of Heidelberg in the 1960s; this permitted good insight into verbal exchanges (Thomä and Houben 1967; Thomä 1967). Klüwer also bases his investigations into the relationship between transference and countertransference in seminar discussions on detailed treatment protocols. The primary topics discussed in treatment influence the participants' dispositions and judgements. Sessions which are depressive stimulate different reactions than those in which the patient lets the analyst participate in his successes and seeks his approval. To this extent the seminar group is a sounding board. Yet how far is this analogy valid? Klüwer asserts that in seminar groups "phenomena of the transference-countertransference relationship extend into the group via the protocols and direct statements in the discussion; there they can be grasped by the groups more quickly than by the attending analyst" (Klüwer 1983, p. 134). This assertion is supported by an assumption which itself first has to be proved, in other words, a *petitio principii.* Klüwer in addition states "that as a matter of principle all the phenomena considered are interpreted strictly on the *patient* and not on the attending analyst" (Klüwer 1983, p. 134). This procedure certainly ensures harmony in the seminar and relieves the reporting therapist, who apparently does not speak on his own behalf. The patient's voice is heard through that of the analyst.

The critical comment of a seminar participant might, for example, be traced back to the patient who had first put his aggression into the analyst. The patient's aggression reaches the seminar by means of the analyst's unnoticed countertransference, where it can be grasped after being amplified by the sounding board. This schematic description makes it clear that perceptiveness bordering on telepathy would be necessary in order to leap over the many unclarified transformations and get back to the origin of the phenomena of transference and countertransference. Yet the sounding board can do just that! Every instrument of the polyphonous orchestra has its own resonance. Every seminar participant in his own way amplifies the patient's tone. It somehow happens that one resonance appears to have more to do with the patient than the others, and there are always some so far from him that they have practically nothing to do with him. Thus there are some things which have nothing to do with the patient. Yet who in the group knows this? Either the conductor, first violinist, or a distinguished soloist ensures that the resonance is somehow harmonious. Specific group dynamic processes take place which are very distant from the patient. It is not uncommon for the theory of projective identification to give ideas produced by resonance the semblance of scientific validity, where in fact only telepathic powers would suffice to bridge the many gaps in information. These critical comments restrict the didactic value of this seminar style considerably because such seminars promote belief in authority rather than scientific thinking.

The idea that the seminar is a sounding board has spread, especially in Germany, via Balint groups. While Balint himself also related the ideas of the members to the patients for didactic reasons when leading a case seminar, as a conductor he intervened in the resonance in an unobtrusive manner and adopted what appeared practicable to him. Countertransference mysticism held no fascination for him; it thrives above all in Germany and is just as foreign to the pragmatic "English" school as it is to the "British" object relations theorists (Sutherland 1980). The use of countertransference by de M'Uzan (1977, pp. 164–181) is also bound strictly to the analytic situation and to whether the patient can link the analyst's interpretations to his own experience. According to de M'Uzan, intensifying the analyst's sensitiveness for the analysand's unconscious processes sometimes makes the following process possible: In an altered state of consciousness, comparable with slight depersonalization but paradoxically also with increased attentiveness, and without a rationally recognizable connection to the material being studied, the analyst perceives in words and images fragments of the analysand's thoughts which had never been conscious or which had been repressed. After an interpretation has been made, these contents are supplemented, and thus confirmed, by the analysand in the same session or later with associations or dreams.

The analyst must, of course, distinguish the conflicts triggered in him by the patient from his own unconscious conflicts. According to de M'Uzan one indication that conscious contents have been triggered by the patient is that the analyst registers unusual phenomena in subsequent self-observation, including stronger object devotion to the analysand together with a disturbance of his own sense of identity. Exact descriptions of this process in which the patient's association as it were confirms the countertransference — or not — could contribute to demystifying the concept. This psychic activity, which is not peculiar to either being awake, dreaming, or sleeping, is called "paradoxical thinking" (*pensée paradoxale*) by de M'Uzan (1977). It occurs in an instant when the psychic state of the analyst has become largely identical to that of the analysand. This paradoxical thinking is considered to originate in the zone between the unconscious and the preconscious because of the patient's partly incomprehensible and fragmentary speech.

The comprehensive concept of countertransference finally became so broad that it encompassed everything; it became identical with the analyst's entire psychic reality. McLaughlin (1981) therefore suggested abandoning the concept after it had become so inflated as to merge into psychic reality. However, it is just as impossible to eliminate established speech habits, whose meanings are obvious to every analyst, as it is to abolish the phenomena to which they refer. For this reason McLaughlin's suggestion will not find any resonance, although it should be taken seriously at a deeper level. In pychoanalysis concepts not only take on expanded meanings, they are also redefined. Numerous and contradictory definitions are formulated, leading inevitably to confusion. For example, Heimann had to add that there are of course also habitual blind spots not caused by the patient, which thus would not be termed countertransference according to the new nomenclature. Heimann now called this habitual countertransference the analyst's transference. After the redefinition of countertransference, it was not clarified which of the many thoughts and fantasies which constitute the analyst's evenly suspended attention were imposed upon — or, as it is called in jargon, invested in — him by the patient.

Heimann not only laid a ghost and extended or redefined a concept, she created a special new theory (initially in association with Klein's mechanisms of projective and introjective identification); it was not generally recognized, however, that this theory had not yet passed the tests of scientific validity. That countertransference is the patient's creation was presented as a fact. Heimann had thus not been misunderstood at all by trainee psychoanalysts faithful to her theories. It was not until 10 years later that her statement was reclassified as a hypothesis inasmuch as clinical *control* was now urgently advised. During this period Heimann became critical of Klein's theories; her understanding of countertransference also changed accordingly because her belief in the explanatory power of projective identification had begun to waver. For example, she (Heimann 1956, p. 304) long continued to believe in the death instinct and derived disavowal and other resistance mechanisms from it. Those who presume the theory of projective identification to be valid still maintain that all countertransference anwers are determined by the patient. Such assertions must, in accordance with Sandler (1976, p. 46), be strictly rejected, because they make further clarification apparently superfluous and present a hypothesis as self-evident.

We hope we have clarified why the struggle for better definitions alone cannot resolve the confusion and why the suggestion that a concept be removed from circulation is not very productive. Concepts as such have a subordinate significance, essentially fulfilling a function within a theory and within a school of thought. Shane (1980) showed that the unwitting acceptance of rules of behavior from training and supervisory analysts can function as school-specific countertransference. Freud's and Heimann's definitions of countertransference fulfilled functions in different theories of therapeutic interaction and of the analytic processes dependent on it. Everything indicates that the phobic avoidance of feelings suggested by Freud's theory had unfortunate consequences, except in Freud's own treatments – Freud applied his rules flexibly (Cremerius 1981 b; Kanzer and Glenn 1980). It is just as certain that Heimann's innovations in treatment technique changed and reappraised more than a concept. "Making use of our subjectivity means to make it conscious." We agree completely with this demand by Loch (1965 a, p. 18), which he supported with the following famous sentence from Freud's letter to Binswanger (1962, p. 65): "A person is not free until he recognizes and overcomes each manifestation of his countertransference."

## 3.4 Concordance and Complementarity of Countertransference

We shall now consider a few attempts to describe typical examples of countertransference. Within the framework of Klein's theory, Racker (1957) distinguished among an analyst's countertransference reactions according to two forms of identification, calling them concordant and complementary. In concordant identification the analyst identifies himself with the corresponding part of the patient's psychic apparatus, ego with ego, superego with superego, and id with id. The analyst thus experiences the feeling in himself in the same way the patient does. The expression "complementary identification," which goes back to Deutsch (1926), describes the analyst's identification with the patient's objects of transference. The analyst then experiences feelings in the same way as the patient's mother or father, while the patient reexperiences feelings like those he had earlier with regard to his parental imagoes. Deutsch spoke out very early in favor of using countertransference:

I call this procedure the "complementary position" in contrast to identification with the infantile patient. Only together do they form the essence of unconscious countertransference, the *utilization* and purposive mastering of which belong to the most important tasks of the analyst. This unconscious countertransference is not to be confused with the course-affective conscious relationship to the patient. (Deutsch 1926, p. 423, emphasis added)

Sandler added a role-theoretical supplement to the complementary position by tracing the interaction between patient and analyst back to the intrapsychic role relationship that each tries to impose on the other. "What I want to emphasize is that the role-relationship of the patient ... consists of a role in which he casts himself, and a *complementary* role in which he casts the analyst at that particular time" (Sandler 1976, p. 44). Although it is difficult to expand role theory to include intrapsychic and unconscious processes, complementarity comes close to observation and experience according to this view. The analyst deals in a reflective manner with the roles unconsciously attributed to or imposed on him, reaches an understanding about it with the patient, and thus makes it possible for the patient to achieve an altered enactment. The therapeutic process could be described in role theory as a path leading more and more to the actual role that the patient not only plays but would like to be. The roles which are tailor-made for the patient are the ones which come closest to him (to his "true" self). The analyst's complementary function is essential; the reenactment would be more difficult if he refused the complementary role.

With the help of complementarity as a fundamental principle of social interaction, we are now also able to grasp why Ferenczi was able to make the observation reported above as early as 1919 (1950). Namely, the analyst's resistance to countertransference makes it more difficult for transference to be achieved, because an object that acts in a completely impersonal way tends to be repulsive. Equally, it would be a mistake to believe that such an object is especially appropriate to help old imagoes become faithful reflections of reality, and thus to secure their intellectual reconstruction. In role theory and from symbolic interactionism we are also able to derive why the consequences are bound to be similarly fatal if the comprehensive conception of countertransference explains the analyst's experience as a projection of inner objects. For how is someone to find and change himself through communication with some significant other if the analyst claims to be nothing more than what the patient is? This is exactly the case, however, in the strict Kleinian interpretation technique based on the theory of projection and introjection. That such interpretations could nonetheless be therapeutically effective is on an entirely different level. This could, for example, be associated with the fact that speaking about shifting good and bad elements back and forth facilitates identification with human nature in general and with one's own unconscious fantasies in particular.

Melanie Klein and her school deserve our praise for having extended the perceptive capacity of analysts for their countertransference and deepened their insights into the nature of evil in man. However much the patient contributes to the enactment of countertransference, this phenomenon arises in the analyst and he is responsible for it.

In our opinion the therapeutic turning point occurs precisely at the point of reflection on role enactment and role responsiveness. Building role theory into a stage model which goes back to Mead (1913) makes it possible to say that the psychoanalytic situation permits continuous trial action to take place so that both participants can move from the stage to the auditorium quickly and easily and can thus observe themselves.

Both are virtually on the stage and in the audience at the same time. The patient's self-representation contains expressions of his favored leading role and enigmatic supporting role whose latent meanings are especially important to the analyst. Also in their roles as observers, the patient and the analyst do not remain on the same seats: the scene being enacted on the stage changes with the perspective. The analyst's interpretations contribute to the change in perspective, interrupt the patient's talking or silence, and contain metacommunications, i.e., information about the exchange taking place. Overemphasizing the metacommunicative aspect of the interpretation means failing to recognize that interpretations have the same effect on actors' portrayals as a director's instructions. That the director himself is also on the stage is demonstrated especially by the transference interpretations that add dramatic depth to the dialogue.

There are several objections to this stage model of the psychoanalytic dialogue, as we have extended it following Habermas (1971) and Loewald (1975). In fact, no analogy expresses the psychoanalytic situation properly; all comparisons are flawed. Yet the weaknesses of our analogy do not lie where the reader who takes exception to role theory or to the comparison of treatment for severe mental illnesses with a stage play might suppose. The tears wept there are no less authentic and real than those shed in real life. The transference and countertransference feelings are also authentic. With reference to Freud's profound remarks on the authenticity of transference (1915a, especially pp. 166-170), we would like to emphasize the responsibility of the analyst, who, as the director, is also responsible for his own countertransference. The comprehensive concept makes a virtue out of necessity, i.e., the inevitability of countertransference: the more, the better! In end effect this would mean, for example, the more countertransference, the better. This is an absurd consequence of the countertransference euphoria which in some places has now replaced the earlier evasion of it! Eissler has made the following ironic comment on these excesses:

> Countertransference was clearly defined by Freud as a psychic process in the analyst that is detrimental to the psychoanalytic process. It amounts to no less than a perversion of theory and practice when it is heralded as highly effective in bringing about the patient's cure. Jokingly, I might say that we seem to be not far from the point when candidates will be advised to resume their training analyses, because they do not form countertransferences to their patients. (1963a, p. 457)

In the sense of the enlarged stage model we maintain that while the analyst is greatly affected by the patient, he can only fulfill his professional task when, as director and observer in one, he remains conscious of the great effect of his thoughts and actions in the analytic situation. Since, as Freud (1915a, p. 169) emphasized, the analyst also "evokes this love," he is partially responsible for the ideas which the patient forms about authenticity and reality in general and in particular. In terms of the stage model we reach the result that the analytic situation offers the patient a greater degree of freedom than real life does. Freud took the opposite view; he believed that the dependence of transference on infantile experience and the latter's inevitable repetition limit one's freedom. Although this statement is partially valid, it does not take the fact into account that reenactment and role responsiveness in the analytic situation enlarge the realm of freedom because the possible forms of action enable restrictive templates to be resolved.

Reenactment permits the analyst to exert influence from the outset, which makes it easier for the patient, through therapy, "to acquire the extra piece of mental freedom" which for Freud was the goal of "a strictly regular, undiluted pychoanalysis" (Freud 1915a, pp. 170, 171).

The stage analogy thus does not founder on authenticity. On the contrary, it is possible to speculate that things on the stage or in a dream are even more authentic because we know that we will escape again. Of course, we also know that pleasure seeks to achieve not only eternity but also reality.

It is precisely the restrictions of the psychoanalytic situation which create a secure realm for the patient to discover the roles that he had previously not been able to *occupy* or *cathect* adequately. The two meanings of the German *besetzen* are both important. The theory of cathexis concerns the unconscious inner world and its energetic regulation, which is far from being enacted, far from the level of expression. The analogy reaches its limit here, just as in the fact that in psychoanalysis formation and movement are largely restricted to verbal action. The animation of images evoked through countertransference is part of the analyst's cognitive process. Part of the patient's unconscious instinctual desire can be an inner image that an object stimulus fits, in harmony, like a key fits a lock. Supplement, correspondence, and agreement characterize certain aspects of an interactional event. Whether the inner stimulus, the instinct, creates the image or the outer object provokes the endopsychic stimulus — we will pass over this age-old problem, to which Kunz (1946a) dedicated a two-volume study. As Freud showed, the "loose connection" of the instinct with the object constitutes human development.

## 3.5 Should the Analyst Admit Countertransference?

We will now draw consequences which open new perspectives and bring the difficult problems of handling countertransference closer to a solution. We are referring to the controversial question of whether the analyst should admit his countertransference to the patient. Most analysts reject this proposition, referring to Freud's experiences and the incognito rule he derived from them. However, Winnicott (1949), Little (1951), and Searles (1965, pp. 192–215), in particular, gave examples to justify exceptions. Heimann warned for decades against confirming the patient's realistic perceptions, discovering only late that the analyst's admission of a feeling relating to a patient does not amount to a personal confession and does not burden the patient with the analyst's own personal problems. Upon closer examination it is clear that Freud's recommendations referred to not letting the patient participate in the analyst's personal conflicts, even with well-meaning intentions, because it confuses or burdens the patient and can keep him from finding his own life style. Heimann also argued in this way until a late study with the pungent title "On the Necessity for the Analyst To Be Natural with His Patient." In a certain therapeutic situation Heimann not only let herself be led by a feeling, but even communicated it. She commented on this as follows:

> The communication of my feelings in violation of the rules appeared to me as something natural. I was somewhat surprised myself and thought more about it later. The description of one's self in another person is a well-known strategy of our patients, a compromise between the desire for frankness and resistance to it, and it is usual to tell this to our patients. I could have done this without mentioning my feelings. Thus I later tried to find formulations omitting my feelings, but I did not like any of the interpretations; they all seemed a little cramped. My self-supervision did not produce anything better. As detailed elsewhere (Heimann 1964), I am against an analyst communicating his feelings to his patient and giving him an insight into the analyst's private life, because this burdens the patient and distracts from his own problems. While I did not find a better interpretation than that my patient had given, I recognized that the statement that I shudder at a 15-year-old having the mental caliber of a 70-year-old in reality does not disclose anything about my private life, just as my assertion does not that the female patient identified with the girl. (Heimann 1978, pp. 225-226)

It is essential that the communication of a feeling be considered in the sense of complementarity. This is the reason that Heimann can say that she has not revealed anything about her private life. We are concerned with a feeling tied to a situation; this feeling is, so to speak, part of an interaction and makes it clear to the patient what effect he has on the "object." We would like to discuss this aspect on a general level because we are convinced that still another way can then be found to employ countertransference profitably.

All patients find it incomprehensible that analysts apparently cannot be irritated by any affect and that they react to hopelessness with the same equanimity as to contempt and hate. Analysts also appear to maintain their neutrality when confronted with intense transference love. Yet appearances are deceptive, as we knew even before the comprehensive concept of countertransference was formulated. What must the effect be, however, if the analyst indirectly ruins his credibility by putting himself beyond good and evil and indicating to the patient what the patient, based on his unconscious wishes, intends to do with the analyst as the transference object? Part of the usual interpretation strategy is also the intention to show the patient that he really means another object, such as his father, mother, or sibling. Thus the analyst cannot be personally affected! Escaping from this theoretically and therapeutically regrettable situation requires conceding, at least in principle, that the analyst can be affected and moved. Neutrality in the sense of reflective restraint begins after countertransference has been experienced, and makes our professional task possible by creating a distance to the natural physical-sensual complementary reactions which can be triggered by the patient's sexual and aggressive impulses. We therefore consider it vital to let the patient participate in the analyst's reflections, including those about the context and background of interpretations, in order to facilitate his identifications. This permits us to regulate the relationship of closeness and distance to the analyst as the "object." Heimann described this process; we have tried to describe its fundamental significance.

# 4 Resistance

## 4.1 General Factors

The vocabulary employed to deal with the patient's resistance is confusing and rich in metaphors whose primary meaning is based on man's struggle for existence, or even on war. In fact, it contradicts common sense that a patient seeking help because of emotional or psychosomatic suffering should also display forms of behavior that Freud summarized by the term "resistance." Yet most important is that we emphasize that at the same time patients *primarily* seek special help in the relationship to their doctor and the transference relationship to the psychotherapist. The appearance of resistance phenomena is *secondary*; they are the consequence of disturbances which lead inevitably to resistance in one form or another. Such *disturbances* in the therapeutic relationship provided the occasion for the original observation of resistance. Thus we can still say with Freud (1900a, p. 517), "Whatever interrupts the progress of analytic work is a resistance." Analytic work is performed in the therapeutic relationship. Thus the basic pattern exhibited by resistance is directed *against* the transference relationship which is being sought (see Chap. 2).

The patient seeking help comes to realize, just like his therapist, that the process of change itself is unsettling because the balance that the patient has attained, even at the cost of serious restrictions of his internal and external freedom of movement, guarantees a certain degree of security and stability. On the basis of this balance, events are unconsciously expected and imagined, even though they may be unpleasant in nature. Although the patient consciously desires a change, a self-perpetuating circle is created, maintained, and reinforced because the balance, however pathological its consequences may be, contributes decisively toward reducing anxiety and insecurity. The many forms that resistance takes have the function of maintaining the balance which has been achieved. This reveals different aspects of resistance:

1. Resistance is related to the change which is consciously desired but unconsciously feared.
2. The observation of resistance is tied to the therapeutic relationship, whereas parapraxes and other unconsciously motivated phenomena can also be observed outside therapy. Resistance is part of the therapeutic process.
3. Since the continuation of the analytic work can be disturbed in a multitude of ways, there are no forms of behavior that cannot be employed as resistance once they have attained a certain strength. The cooperation between

therapist and patient suffers if the resistance surpasses a certain level of intensity, which can be detected on a wide range of phenomena. An increase in transference to the level of blind infatuation can become resistance in the same way as excessive reporting of dreams or overly rational reflection on them.

4. *Qualitative* and *quantitative* criteria are thus used in the evaluation of resistance. For example, positive and negative transference become resistance if they reach an intensity which inhibits or prohibits reflective cooperation.

Glover (1955) distinguishes between obvious, crude forms of resistance and unobtrusive forms. The crude forms include arriving late, missing sessions, talking too much or not at all, automatically rejecting or misunderstanding all the analyst's utterances, playing ignorant, constantly being absentminded, falling asleep, and, finally, terminating the treatment prematurely.

These crude disturbances create the impression of conscious and intentional sabotage and touch the analyst at an especially sensitive spot. Some of the forms of behavior mentioned above, such as arriving late and missing sessions, undermine the analytic work and suggest global interpretations that can at best be considered educational measures or at worst lead to power struggles. Such complications can develop with particular rapidity at precisely the beginning of therapy. It is therefore essential to remember that the patient is primarily seeking a supportive relationship. As long as the analyst does not let himself become entangled in a power struggle, signs of positive transference can be recognized in subtle forms of evasiveness during the session, and also interpreted, even as early as the beginning of therapy. Then the power struggle that might result from the challenge which the attacks on the existential conditions of therapy would logically constitute does not necessarily take place.

Resistance to work has become "resistance to the psychoanalytic process" (Stone 1973). Many individual and typical resistance phenomena have been described since 1900. These can be classified — although with the inevitable loss of vividness — according to general qualitative and quantitative points of view and according to the genesis of the resistance. Since resistance to the psychoanalytic process is observed as transference resistance, this form of resistance has always been at the center of attention. It is therefore appropriate first to clarify how and why transference resistance appears.

### *4.1.1 Classification of the Forms of Resistance*

Freud first discovered transference as resistance, as the *main obstacle*. Patients — women in particular, which is significant — did not keep to the prescribed patient-doctor stereotype with regard to their rules and relationships, but incorporated the therapist into their own personal fantasy worlds. As a doctor, Freud was irritated by this observation. Because of their bad consciences and their shame at having thus mentally violated a convention, patients concealed their fantasies and developed a *resistance* to the sexual feelings and desires they transferred to Freud. Since Freud had not provided any real cause for the actual genesis of these desires, i.e., for the situation precipitating them, it seemed appropriate to examine the prehistory of unconscious patterns of expectations more closely. The study of transference as a "false connection" led into the past world of unconscious desires and fantasies and finally to the discovery of the Oedipus complex and the incest taboo. When it became possible to derive the doctor's influence from the parents' (and from the patient's *unobjectable* relationship to them), analysts' understanding of transference shifted from that of it being the main obstacle to therapy to it being the most powerful therapeutic tool, as long as it does not turn into negative or overly positive erotized transference.

The relationship between transference and resistance (in the concept of transference resistance) can be described schematically as follows: After overcoming the resistance to transference becoming conscious, therapy in Freud's theory is based on mild, unobjectable transference, which thus becomes desirable and the analyst's most powerful tool. Positive transference — in the sense of a relationship sui generis — forms the foundation of therapy (see Chap. 2).

This working relationship, as we would call it today, is endangered if positive transference is intensified and if polarizations — called transference love or negative (aggressive) transference — are created. Transference thus again becomes resistance if the patient's attitude to the analyst is erotized (transference love) or turns into hate (negative transference). According to Freud, these two forms of transference become resistance if they prevent *remembering.*

Finally, in the resistance to the *resolution* of transference we find a third aspect. United in the concept of transference resistance are resistance to transference becoming conscious, resistance in the form of transference love or negative transference, and resistance to the resolution of transference.

The concrete forms taken by the different elements of transference resistance are dependent on how the therapeutic situation is structured by rules and interpretations. For example, resistance to transference becoming conscious is a regular component of the introductory phase. The later ups and downs of this form of resistance reflect dyad-specific fluctuations. A paranoid patient rapidly develops a negative transference, just as a nymphomaniac quickly develops erotized transference. It is the intensity of these transferences which makes them resistance. A wide spectrum separates these extremes, and within it the analyst decides which forms of behavior to interpret as resistance. Freud's later classification (1926d) provides diagnostic criteria in this regard, listing superego resistance, id resistance, and resistance based on the secondary gain from illness in addition to repression resistance and transference resistance.

Thus the modern classification into two forms of ego resistance (repression resistance and transference resistance), superego resistance, and id resistance goes back to Freud's revision of his theory in the 1920s. Since transference resistance retained its central role, in structural theory the two basic patterns of transference resistance (the overly positive, erotized transference and the negative, aggressive transference) remained the focus of therapeutic interest. This is the reason that we have further differentiated the concept of transference resistance.

In our discussion of the theory of transference (see Chap. 2), we do not deal with the complications arising from the fact that both basic patterns of transference resistance can make the cure more difficult. With negative transferences, the aggressive rejection can gain the upper hand, and therapy can reach a stalemate or be terminated (Freud 1912b, 1937c, p. 239).

It is noteworthy that Freud retained the polar classification of resistance into negative (aggressive) and overly positive (erotized) forms although between 1912 and 1937 the modification of instinct theory and especially the introduction of structural theory had led to the classification of resistance into five forms. This element of conservativism in Freud's thought is probably related to the fact that in his treatments he continued to adhere to the conception of the polarization of love and hate in the oedipal phase of conflict and its transference, as pointed out by Schafer (1973) and others. This, as well as universal human ambivalence, leads inevitably to positive and negative transferences.

Yet what occurs with the intensification of transference to the point where it becomes resistance, whether as transference love or as insurmountable hate? Without wanting to minimize the human potential for hate and destructiveness, there can be no doubt that the role treatment technique plays in precipitating resistance in the form of negative transference has long been neglected (Thomä 1981). A. Freud (1954a, p. 618) finally raised the question of whether the occasionally complete neglect of the fact that analyst and patient are both adults in a real, personal relationship to each other might be responsible for some of the aggressive reactions that we trigger in our patients and that we possibly only consider as transference.

The same is true of transference love, especially inasfar as erotized transference dooms analysis to failure or seems to render any attempt at analysis pointless. Naturally, we also know of other cases of transference love, such as those described by Nunberg (1951), Rappaport (1956), Saul (1962), and Blum (1973). It is clear that erotized transferences can become resistance. Yet we would like to point to the fact that the influence of the analyst and his treatment technique on the development of negative and erotized transferences is often mentioned only in passing, even in the most recent publications. This occurs despite the general recognition of how strongly negative transferences — and the same is true for erotized transferences — are dependent on countertransference, treatment technique, and the analyst's theoretical position.

In our analytic work we ask, as Schafer (1973, p. 281) does:

> How are we to understand his or her living in just this way, producing just these symptoms, suffering in just this way, effecting just these relationships, experiencing just these feelings, interfering with further understanding in just this way and at just this time? What wish or set of wishes is being fulfilled to the extent possible? Is it in this sense that clinical analysis eventuates in investigation of affirmations ("wish-fulfillments")? This is what is meant finally by analysis of resistance and defence. What are they *for*? What is this person *for*?

Schafer was correct in putting the question as to the function of resistance and defense at the end. Habitual self-defense against unconsciously imagined dangers is the consequence of a life-long process of failing to find security and satisfaction in interpersonal relationships. In the next section we will therefore deal with the function resistance has in regulating a relationship.

### *4.1.2 Function of Resistance in Regulating Relationships*

Emphasizing the function that resistance has in regulating relationships makes it necessary for us to pay special attention to the relationship between resistance and transference. Specifically, in transference resistance the intrapsychic model of conflict (repression resistance) is linked with object relationship psychologies and with the interpersonal model of conflict. Freud established this connection in the transformation of his theory of anxiety in "Inhibitions, Symptoms and Anxiety" (1926d); the appendix to this paper contains the above-mentioned classification of resistance into five forms. It should be remembered that Freud traced *all* neurotic anxieties back to real dangers (i.e., to threats) from without.

Castration anxiety and anxiety regarding the loss of an object or of love are thus products whose genesis requires two or three persons. Nevertheless, the internal emotional processes received one-sided emphasis in the psychoanalytic model of conflict. On the one hand, discharge theory suggests that precisely severe annihilation anxieties should be derived from quantitative factors. On the other hand, the situational influence on the genesis of anxieties, in the sense of a real danger, was neglected. And with regard to indications, the cases considered especially suited for psychoanalysis are those which exhibit stable structures, i.e., internalized conflicts. The question then is what disturbs the homeostasis, the internal balance.

Analysts orienting themselves on the intrapsychic model of conflict have to respond as Brenner (1979b, p. 558) does: "Whatever mental activity serves the purpose of avoiding unpleasure aroused by an instinctual derivative is a defense. There is no other valid way of defining defense."

Analysts putting more emphasis on object relationships as a part of theory take a point of view of which Brierley (1937, p. 262) was a very early advocate:

> The child is first concerned with objects only in relation to its own feelings and sensations but, as soon as feelings are firmly linked to objects, the process of instinct-defence becomes a process of defence against objects. The infant then tries to master its feelings by manipulating their object-carriers.

### *4.1.3 Resistance and Defense*

We consider it especially important to clarify the interrelationship between resistance and defense. These two terms are often used synonymously. However, resistance phenomena can be observed, while defense processes must be inferred. In Freud's (1916/17, p. 294) words, "We have proposed to give the pathogenic process which is demonstrated by the resistance the name of *repression*."

Synonymous use of the terms "resistance" and "defense" can easily give rise to the misunderstanding that the description itself provides an explanation for the function of resistance. In clinical jargon, psychodynamic connections are thus often given a global description: Negative transference serves as a defense against positive feelings; self-defects and early abandonment anxieties are warded off by means of hysterical flirting; and so on.

Yet the important task consists in recognizing the individual instances of such psychodynamic connections, i.e., the specific psychic acts, and in rendering them therapeutically useful. Freud proceeded in this way when he constructed the prototype of all defense mechanisms — repression resistance — and related it to the patient's manner of experiencing and to symptoms. In this description, a form of resistance is linked with the prototype of all defense mechanisms.

It should be emphasized that the concept of resistance belongs to the theory of treatment technique, while the concept of defense is related to the structural model of the psychic apparatus (Leeuw 1965).

Typical forms of defense, such as identification with the aggressor, imply complex and multistage defense processes (repression, projection, splitting, etc.). These unconsious processes form the foundation for a multitude of resistance phenomena (Ehlers 1983).

The further development of the theory of defense mechanisms thus made the so-called defense resistances beyond the prototypical form (repression resistance) more accessible to therapy. It is possible to describe repression resistance using Nietzsche's famous phrase in *Beyond Good and Evil*: "'I did it,' says my memory. 'I cannot have done it,' says my pride and remains adamant. Finally, my memory complies." For psychoanalysis, of course, the *unconscious* processes of self-deception are the focus of interest (Fingarette 1977).

The most important practical consequence of structural theory is the application of the typology described by A. Freud (1937) to clinical resistance phenomena. The "transference of defense," for example, proves to be "resistance to transference" in the sense described above. The fact that resistance is spoken of in some cases and defense in others results in part from the similar meaning of the words. Another reason is that clinical experience of typical forms of resistance has for decades been described in the terminology of defense processes. Finally there is a linguistic relation between a person's unconscious defense processes and his actions: The patient disavows, makes good, turns against his self, splits, tries to undo something, regresses.

The preference for defense terminology probably expresses a tendency which led to Schafer's *action language* (1976). Close examination of typical forms of defense leads beyond the theory of defense mechanisms and makes it necessary, for example, to look at the complex phenomena of acting out, repetition compulsion, and id resistance. These mechanisms serve in different ways to maintain a balance and cause the specific resistance to changes. Thus psychoanalytic terminology refers for the sake of brevity to resistance, e.g., by means of regression, projection, or disavowal. Since the process of inferring the unconscious defense mechanisms starts from resistance, i.e., they cannot be immediately experienced or directly observed, the relationship between resistance and defense revolves around complicated problems of construct validation. We hope that we have demonstrated convincingly that the use of "resistance" and "defense" as synonymous and global terms is objectionable.

The general points of view mentioned so far concern topics that we will deal with in more detail in the following sections of this chapter. Emphasis will be placed on the following points: Since Freud attributed resistance, from its discovery onwards, a function in regulating relationships, we will devote Sect. 4.2 to its protective function in relation to anxiety. In this regard it proves essential that other affect signals also be considered. We have already given transference resistance a special place in these introductory remarks because of its great significance, and will return to it in connection with repression in Sect. 4.3.

Prompted by Freud's classification, we present superego and id resistances in Sect. 4.4. These forms of resistance owe their names to Freud's far-reaching revision of his theories in the 1920s. The reorganization of instinct theory and the substitution of structural theory (id, ego, and superego) for the topographical model (with the layers unconscious, preconscious, and conscious) went back to, among other things, Freud's experiences in the analytic situation. The discovery of unconscious feelings of guilt in so-called negative therapeutic reactions led to the assumption that significant portions of the ego and the superego are unconscious. At the same time, Freud was deeply impressed by repetition compulsion, which he attempted to explain by means of the conservative nature of the instincts attributed to the id. Thus the powers of the id also seemed to explain the steadfast nature of the erotized and the negative, aggressive forms of transference and the superego resistance. The critical discussion of superego and id resistances has had theoretical and practical consequences, which we will describe in Sect. 4.4.1 using the example of the present-day understanding of negative therapeutic reaction.

In Sect. 4.4.2 we discuss recent developments in theories of human aggression. A short discussion (Sect. 4.5) is devoted to secondary gain from illness, listed in Freud's classification under ego resistance. This unusually important form of resistance is discussed in detail in Chap. 8 in the context of the factors working to maintain the symptoms. In our opinion, secondary gain from illness has received far too little attention in the psychoanalytic technique.

Finally, in Sect. 4.6 we turn to identity resistance as described by Erikson. This form of resistance is the prototype of a group of resistance phenomena which are of crucial clinical and theoretical significance. As such, the phenomena described as identity resistance are not new. Erikson's innovation is the theoretical reorientation by which he links the function of resistance (and also the unconscious defense processes) to the maintenance of the feeling of identity or self, which is psychosocial in origin. This introduces a superior regulatory principle. The separation of the pleasure-unpleasure principle from the economic principle and discharge theory by no means has to lead to a neglect of Freud's discoveries concerning man's unconscious world of desires. On the contrary, along with G. Klein and many other contemporary analysts we believe that the psychoanalytic theory of motivation gains in plausibility and therapeutic utility if the instinctive search for oedipal and pregenital gratifications is understood as an essential component in developing a *feeling of self*. The assumption that there is an interdependence between a regulation of self-feeling (as ego or self-identity) and the gratification of desires originates in the experience acquired in psychoanalytic practice. It also leads us out of the dilemma that Kohut ended up in as a result of his two-track theory of development, with independent processes of (narcissistic) self formation and (libidinal) object formation. It is easy to show the absurdity of separating (narcissistic) self formation from (instinctive) object relationship: There are no disturbances of object relationships without disturbances of self, and vice versa.

## 4.2 Anxiety and the Protective Function of Resistance

Freud encountered resistance in hysterical patients in his therapeutic attempts to revive their forgotten memories. As Freud turned to hypnosis and the pressure procedure in his preanalytic period, everything in a patient which opposed the doctor's attempts to influence the patient was considered resistance. These powers, which were directed outward, i.e., against the doctor's attempts to influence the patient, were for Freud a mirror image of those internal powers which had led to and maintained dissociation during the genesis of the symptoms.

> Thus a psychical force, aversion on the part of the ego, had originally driven the pathogenic idea out of association [and thus led to dissociation] and was now opposing its return to memory. The hysterical patient's "not knowing" was in fact a "not wanting to know" — a not wanting which might be to a greater or less extent conscious. The task of the therapist, therefore, lies in overcoming by his psychical work this resistance to association. (Freud 1895d, pp. 269-270)

From the very beginning, therapeutic observation was linked with a psychodynamic explanatory model, according to which the strength of the resistance indicated the degree to which associations and symptoms were distorted (Freud 1904a). The discovery of unconscious instinctual impulses and oedipal wishes and anxieties added to the knowledge on the motives of resistance and strengthened their key role in treatment technique. Sandler et al. summarize:

> The entry of psychoanalysis into what has been described as its second phase and the recognition of the importance of inner impulses and wishes (in contrast to painful real experiences) in causing conflict and motivating defense did not bring about any fundamental change in the concept of resistance. Nevertheless resistance was now seen as being directed not only against the recall of distressing memories but also against the awareness of unacceptable impulses. (1973, p. 72)

The starting point was "not wanting to know." What now required explanation were not being able to know, the self-deceptions, and the unconscious processes which led to the distorted reproduction of instinctual wishes.

The descriptive recording of resistance phenomena has meanwhile been completed. Less than a hundred years after Freud's discovery there is probably hardly a human impulse which has not yet been described in the literature with regard to its relationship to a specific resistance. It will not be difficult for the reader to acquaint himself with the feeling of resistance if he imagines communicating absolutely everything that passes through his mind to a fictive listener.

A function of resistance in the therapeutic dialogue is to regulate the relationship. Freud therefore viewed it from the very beginning in the context of the patient's relationship to the doctor; he understood it as being connected with transference. As we have already mentioned, the relationship-regulating (border guard) function of resistance was later neglected as a result of the restrictive model of conflict and structure. The context of the discovery of resistance remained decisive, however, for all later explanatory attempts: Why do resistance phenomena appear in the therapeutic relationship and what purpose do they serve? Freud (1926 d) later answered this question in a global way: All resistance phenomena are correlates of anxiety defense. He classified anxiety, an unpleasurable affect, with the prototype of the defense mechanisms, repression. In Freud's generalizing manner of expression, anxiety stands for, as it were, shame, sadness, guilt, weakness — ultimately all unpleasurable affect signals.

As a result anxiety became the most important affect in the psychoanalytic theory of defense. Freud (1929 d) was then able to say that anxiety, the escape and attack reactions belonging to it, and their counterparts in the emotional sphere constitute the core problem of neuroses. The unconscious defense processes are thus biologically anchored. Yet the emphasis put on anxiety as the motor of mental and psychosomatic illnesses also led to a situation in which other independent affect signals received too little attention. Today affect signals must be viewed in a more differentiated way for both theoretical and therapeutic reasons. Not going beyond the historical prototype, i.e., anxiety and the defense against it, means not doing justice to the wide spectrum of disturbing affects. An analyst ignores the patient's own feelings and experience if he makes anxiety interpretations while the patient is warding off a qualitatively different emotion. It is one thing that many phenomena culminate in anxiety, which is the reason we can speak of shame anxiety, separation anxiety, and castration anxiety. It is quite another thing that extensive parts of the hierarchy of affects contain independent elements whose phenomenology has not been the subject of growing interest among psychoanalysts until recent decades.

There are several reasons for this. Rapaport (1953) was probably the first to draw widespread attention to the fact that there is no systematic psychoanalytic theory of affects. The derivation of affects from instincts and Freud's view that affects represent instinctual energy were factors unfavorable for a subtle phenomenological description of qualitatively different affective conditions. As a result of the revision of anxiety theory, signal anxiety became the prototype of affective conditions. Freud did separate signal anxiety to a large degree from the economic process of discharge (1926 d, p. 139); he described typical danger situations and distinguished between different affective conditions, one example being the pain affect. Yet the anxiety affect was given an exclusive role in psychoanalysis, not the least important reason being that many affects do indeed have an anxiety component (Dahl 1978).

We now want to illustrate a differentiated consideration of an affect and its relation to anxiety, using the example of shame and basing our description on the studies by Wurmser (1981). A person suffering from *shame anxiety* is afraid of being exposed — and thus humiliated. According to Wurmser, a complex shame affect is arranged around a depressive core: I have exposed myself and feel humiliated; I would like to disappear; I don't want to exist any more as a creature that exposes itself in such a way. The contempt can only be erased by eliminating the exposure — by hiding, by disappearing, and if necessary by being obliterated.

Shame still exists as a means of protection, as preventive self-concealment, as a *reaction formation*. It is obvious that the protective function of resistance is particularly related to feelings of unbearable shame. According to Wurmser, all three forms of shame — shame anxiety, depressive shame, and shame as a reaction formation — have a subject pole and an object pole. A person is ashamed *of something* and with reference *to someone*. A subtle phenomenological analysis of different affective conditions is significant for treatment technique, especially because it makes it possible to make a psychoanalytic statement of what would be *tactful* at that moment. A tactful procedure for dealing with resistance analysis is then not only a result of sympathy and intuition. We see, in today's emphasis on countertransference, a sign that the manifold forms of emotions and affects are attracting increased interest.

The protective function of resistance can also be described for other affects. Krause (1983, 1985) and Moser (1978) have demonstrated that aggressive emotions such as vexation, anger, rage, and hate are employed as inner signals in the same way as anxiety and can trigger defense processes. It is certainly also possible for aggressive emotions to accumulate to the point where they constitute an anxiety signal, and anxiety theory is therefore so elegant, concise, and encompassing. Freud's genius worked like Occam's razor, subordinating a few at least partially independent affective signal systems to the prototype, as if they were vassals.

It is therapeutically inadvisable to pay special attention to the anxiety signal. Moser used the following argument to support the technical rule that the independence of other affect signals should be accepted.

> These affects [vexation, anger, rage, hate, etc.] are employed as internal signals in the same way as anxiety, given that affective experience has at all reached the developmental level of an internal reporting system (signal system). In many neurotic developments (e.g., in neurotic depressions, compulsion neuroses, neurotic character disturbances) the aggressive signal system is completely stunted or poorly developed. These are patients who do not notice their aggressive impulses, consequently do not recognize them, and cannot classify them in a situational context. Such patients either demonstrate aggressive behavior without noticing it (and are also unable to recognize it as such afterwards) or react to environmental stimuli precipitating aggression with emotional activation, analyze the stimuli in a different way, and interpret them as, for instance, anxiety signals. In this case a shifting takes place from the aggressive to the anxiety signal system .... In the theory of neurosis these substitution processes have been described as typical affective defense mechanisms, using the terms "aggression as anxiety defense" and "anxiety as aggressive defense." Thus there are good reasons to devise an "aggression signal theory" in addition to anxiety signal theory. (Moser 1978, p. 236-237)

Waelder described the development of psychoanalytic technique by using a series of questions which the analyst asks himself. First "the question [was] constantly in his mind: *What are the patient's desires?* What does the patient (unconsciously) want?" After the revision of anxiety theory, "the old question about his desires had to be supplemented by a second question also continuously in the analyst's mind: *And of what is he afraid?*' Finally, the insights into unconscious defense and resistance processes led to the third question: "*And when he is afraid, what does he do?*' (Waelder 1960, pp. 182-183). Waelder stated that no further aspects had yet been added to help orient the analyst in his examination of the patient.

Today it is advisable to pose a series of further questions, such as: What does the patient do when he is ashamed, when he is pleased, when he is surprised, when he feels grief, fright, disgust, or rage? The manner in which emotions are expressed varies widely, and may be preceded by unspecific arousal stages. Emotions and affects — we use the two terms synonymously — can therefore be interrupted in the undifferentiated prestage (at the root, so to speak), but they can also accumulate to form anxiety. The wide range of affects should be kept in mind with regard to technique because the designation of qualitatively different emotions can facilitate integration or make the accumulation of affects either more or less difficult.

Naturally there have always been a number of other questions which did not concern Waelder at this point. From therapeutic and dyadic points of view — we must be careful not to lose sight of these — the analyst asks himself many questions having a common denominator, such as: What am I doing that causes the patient to have this anxiety and that provokes this resistance? And above all: What do I contribute to overcoming them? In discussing these diagnostic considerations it is necessary to distinguish the different affect signals from one another. Today even an analyst as conservative as Brenner (1982) acknowledges that depressive affects and unpleasurable anxiety affects are factors of equal significance in the precipitation of conflicts. The fact that it is dubious to attribute autonomy to precisely the complex depressive affects in the signal system is not important for our discussion. The decisive point is to have a comprehensive grasp of pleasure-unpleasure regulation and conflict genesis, and not to limit oneself to anxiety, however important this prototypical affect signal may be.

The communicative character of affects must be given special consideration in the theory of defense processes (and of resistance), as Krause (1983) has emphasized. Freud had adopted the importance he attached to emotional expressive behavior in his early writings from Darwin (1872). In his later instinct theory, affects were treated increasingly as products of discharge and cathexis. The instinct finds a representative in the idea and the affect, and it discharges internally: "Affectivity manifests itself essentially in motor (secretory and vasomotor) discharge resulting in an (internal) alteration of the subject's own body without reference to the external world; motility, in actions designed to effect changes in the external world" (Freud 1915e, p. 179). In this statement Freud described the relationship of instinct and affect in a one-sided manner: Affects have become instinctual derivatives, and their communicative character seems to have been lost. As can be seen in Krause's comprehensive overview, the instinct-affect interaction is in fact complex and does not proceed in only one direction (from instinct to affect). We will deal with this complicated problem here only inasfar as our understanding of resistance is concerned.

There are lasting consequences for the therapeutic attitude, of course, if anxiety, rage, disgust, and shame—to name a few affect conditions—are traced back to changes in the body's balance in a one-sided manner. It leads to a neglect of the interactional genesis of anxiety, rage, disgust, and shame and their signal function. Yet it is precisely these communicative processes which make comprehensible the infectious nature of affects observed by Freud in group processes. The interrelatedness which characterizes the precipitation of affects in others, either amplifying or weakening the circular process, forms the foundation of empathy. Thus, in therapy the analyst can also feel that emotions have a communicative character as a result of his empathic understanding of the affective condition.

Basing feelings and affects on dualistic instinct theory has led to a confusion of instinct with affect, of libido with love, and of aggression with hostility, as especially Blanck and Blanck (1979) have pointed out. If this confusion is carried over to signal anxiety, the capacity for perceiving other affect systems is limited. The fact that different affects and their dyadic functions should be taken into consideration in communication is gaining in importance in psychoanalytic object relationship theories. We would like to describe the relationship-regulating function of affective communication and the defense function of resistance associated with it by referring to a passage from Krause. After describing the complicated blend of affects and instinctual acts in sexual interaction, he concludes:

> Before a terminal act of sexual nature can take place between two persons, they have to ensure that they get together at all, i.e., the distance between the partners must be reduced and finally eliminated. This can only happen if the anxiety affect generally accompanying such processes is outweighed by the antagonistic affects of joy, curiosity, interest, and security. This takes place by means of the mutual induction of positive affects. (Krause 1983, p. 1033)

Krause refers to a mutual induction of positive affects and to the reduction in an anxiety affect. It is beyond doubt that in the case of impotence the terminal physiological act can be disturbed by the unconscious castration anxiety or that frigidity can develop as a result of an unconscious shame anxiety. At issue here is the interplay of emotional components such as security, trust, curiosity, and joy with lust, that is with sexual excitement and acts in a strict sense. This meshwork of purposive wishes striving for the climax of desire, positively coupled with emotions, is generally abridged in psychoanalysis to the scheme of oedipal and pregenital instinctual gratifications and object relationships. In doing this, analysts easily lose sight of the wide range of qualitatively different emotions. Balint (1935) was one of the first to discuss this problem, using the example of tenderness. Object relationships and countertransference probably play such a dominant role in current discussions because they are related to genuine and qualitatively distinct emotional experiences which are not simply a function of the phases of libidinal development.

Everyday psychoanalytic experience shows that a patient can relinquish resistant behavior if he feels secure and has gained trust. Such experience agrees with the results of psychoanalytic studies of mother-child interaction. We would like to mention Bowlby's (1969) findings on attachment and the significance of the child's affective exchange with its mother, because Harlow's

(1958) deprivation experiments with young monkeys suggest a convergent interpretation.

While the gratification of hunger, the oral component instinct according to psychoanalysis, is the necessary precondition for survival, the emotional object relationship is the prerequisite for sexual maturation. Monkeys who when young are deprived of contact with their mothers for a sufficient period of time and have only wire puppets or fur substitutes — i.e., monkeys deprived of the object which makes an emotional tie possible and, to use an anthropomorphizing expression, offers security — are not able to perform sexual acts. Krause offers the explanation that the deprivation makes it impossible for a monkey to experience in the presence of another the affects (security, trust, curiosity, and joy) which are necessary to perform sexual acts. According to Spitz's (1965) interpretation of these findings mutuality and dialogue are missing.

On the other hand, affective security can be sought in addictive instinctual gratification in the form of overeating or excessive masturbation. The interplay of instinctual processes and affective signals can lead to reversion processes. This is the reason that one speaks in terms of warding off anxiety by means of sexualization or of regression to oral patterns of gratification; it is widely accepted that this occurs in many illnesses.

Especially impressive, for example, is a manifestation of virtually addictive transference love without the recognition of any diagnostic factors indicating the existence of an addictive structure. The question is then whether and to what extent the patient seeks support from excessive masturbation, and whether the patient is not able to find this support in the analytic situation because the analyst does not provide affective resonance. Psychoanalysts commonly impose an inordinant amount of restraint on themselves because they associate affect signals with anxiety and trace this anxiety back to anxiety over the intensity of an instinct. The analyst's capacity for resonance can develop more freely if affects are viewed as the carriers of meaning (Modell 1984a, p. 234; Green 1977) instead of as instinct derivatives, because response is not equated with gratification.

The division of instinct theory into affective and cognitive aspects was based in part on the fact that therapeutic experience had shown that "recollection without affect almost invariably produces no result. The psychical process which originally took place must be repeated as vividly as possible; it must be brought back to its *status nascendi* and then given verbal utterance" (Freud 1895d, p. 6). The consequence of this observation for the theory of resistance and defense processes was the assumption of a division between affects and ideas. We think that the significance of the splitting processes is not that the instinct is represented twice, both as idea and as affect, as if it were naturally split. On the contrary, the interactive affective processes are actually also cognitive in nature; it is thus possible to say that expressive behavior is linked to the understanding of affects. It is true that this unity of affect and cognition, of feeling and idea, can be lost. Yet regardless of which affects are involved in conflict genesis and in the disturbance of the feelings of security and self, a balance has in any case been established in the sphere of symptoms and is further stabilized by repetitions.

Everyone knows how difficult it is to change habits that have become second nature. Although patients seek a change in regard to their suffering, they would like to leave the related interpersonal conflicts untouched. The relationship conflicts constituting the various forms of transference resistance are thus the objects of such intense struggles because the compromises which they involve, though associated with significant disadvantages, provide a certain degree of security. Caruso's (1972) suggestion that we speak of exchange mechanisms instead of defense mechansisms in the interpersonal sphere is therefore just as convincing as Mentzos' (1976) interactional interpretation of defense processes.

The defense processes restrict or interrupt the affective-cognitive exchange. The consequences of the defense process of disavowal are by definition more external and those of repression are more internal. Yet these are differences of degree: where there is disavowal and denial, repression or its manifestations can also be detected. We emphasize the adaptive function of resistance especially because the patient's strong reluctance to cooperate with the treatment is often viewed as negative. If analysts assume that patients, with the help of their resistance, have reached the best possible solutions to their own conflicts and thus maintain an equilibrium, then they will be better able to confront the task of creating the best conditions to eliminate the resistances.

A patient cannot admit his feelings toward the analyst to himself, whether because of his self-respect or his fear of the analyst. The everyday psychological meaning of this narcissistic protection is shown clearly by Stendhal: "You must be careful not to allow free rein to hope before you are sure that admiration exists. Otherwise you would achieve only an insipid flatness quite incompatible with love, or at least whose only cure would be in a challenge to your self-esteem" (1975, p. 58).

When can a patient be sure that he has gained "admiration"? How can he determine that he has not created "an insipid flatness quite incompatible with love?" The analyst must be able to answer these questions if he wants to be able to handle transference resistance in a productive manner. Yet Stendhal's words also refer to the important function of nonverbal communication (more closely associated with the preconscious) with regard to the genesis of feelings indicative of a relationship, whether they be love or resistance. It is instructive in this regard that Erikson's description of identity resistance, to which all unalloyed forms of resistance can be subsumed, has found little resonance in psychoanalysis. This probably has to do with Erikson's strong psychosocial orientation, because the link binding resistance to the feeling of security (Sandler 1960; Weiss 1971) or to the feeling of self (Kohut 1971) in order to avoid injuries is not very different from identity resistance.

## 4.3 Repression and Transference Resistance

Prototypical for Freud's understanding of the effects of inferred defense mechanisms was his description of repression resistance. Repression resistance has remained the prime manifestation of defense mechanisms, even after A.

Freud's systematization of the theory of defense mechanisms. We agree with the description by Sandler et al. of the function of the forms of resistance originating in defense mechanisms. According to them, repression resistance occurs when the patient defends "himself against impulses, memories and feelings which, were they to emerge into consciousness, would bring about a painful state, or would threaten to cause such a state." They continue:

The repression-resistance can also be seen as a reflection of the so-called "primary gain" from the neurotic illness, inasmuch as neurotic symptoms can be regarded as being last-resort formations aimed at protecting the individual from conscious awareness of distressing and painful mental content. The process of free association during psychoanalysis creates a constant potential danger-situation for the patient, because of the invitation offered to the repressed by the process of free association, and this in turn promotes the repression-resistance. The closer the repressed material comes to consciousness, the greater the resistance, and it is the analyst's task to facilitate, through his interpretations, the emergence of such content into consciousness in a form which can be tolerated by the patient. (Sandler et al. 1973, p. 74)

With reference to this passage, we would like to emphasize once more that observations of visible feelings and behavior suggest the assumption that unconscious or preconscious defense processes are active. The nature of the self-deception, the distortion, the reversal — in short, the transformation and the interruption — becomes increasingly evident the closer the patient gets to the origin of his feelings within the protection of the analytic situation. This is linked to authenticity of feelings and experience, and therefore the surface of one's character is often called a facade or even character armor (Reich 1933). This negative evaluation of the surface can unfortunately strengthen the self-assertion, i.e., raise the resistance, of those patients who initially cannot accept this assessment. This is an unfavorable side effect of the character analysis introduced by Reich.

Reich's systematization, which thematizes the form-content problem, should of course not be measured by its abuses. Reich's (1933, p. 65) discovery that "character resistance expresses itself not in the *content* of the material, but in the *formal* aspects of the general behavior, the manner of talking, of the gait, facial expression and typical attitudes" (emphasis added) is independent of the libido-economic explanation of character armor. Reich gave a very astute description of indirect affective expressive behavior, which manages to manifest itself somewhere despite the resistance.

The affect appears in bodily and especially in facial expression, and its cognitive or fantasy components change in size according to whether they are temporarily separated or repressed. We refer to these processes as isolation or splitting. Reich showed that defense processes uncouple the affect from its cognitive representative and modify it in various ways. Krause correctly points out that Reich's point of view has not been further developed theoretically, and continues:

This marked the disappearance of the influence of Darwin's affect theory on psychoanalysis. It was based on the fact that Freud, because of his background in neurology, was only able to view affect as a motor discharge leading to an internal change in one's own body, and ignored the social and expressive portion of the affect and the link between it and idiosyncratic action. As a consequence, the fact was overlooked that affect socialization takes place in part by means of an automatic and constant control exercised by the motoric-expressive system, that this is the only way to prevent the initial development of the affect, and that this can often be successfully accomplished without the development of an unconscious fantasy. (Krause 1985, pp. 281-282)

The great growth of clinical knowledge by the 1930s made a systematization possible and even necessary. In 1926 Freud (1926d) was still able to restrict himself to referring to the prototype, namely repression resistance. Yet, based on A. Freud's list of defense mechanisms, it was imperative after 1936 to speak of regression, isolation, projection, and introjection resistance and of resistance by undoing, by turning against oneself, by reversal into the opposite, by sublimation, and by reaction formation. Reich, in fact, oriented his theory of character analysis primarily around resistance in the form of reaction formations. The diagnosis of reaction formation is a valuable aid in the evaluation of resistance in the therapeutic situation, as shown in Hoffmann's (1979) critical analysis of psychoanalytic characterology. We would like to remind readers of the forms of resistance corresponding to the reaction formations in oral, anal, and phallic characters.

According to the definition given by Sandler et al. (1973, pp. 74-75) for transference resistance,

although essentially similar to the repression-resistance, [transference resistance] has the special quality that it both expresses, and reflects the struggle against, infantile impulses which have emerged, in direct or modified form, in relation to the person of the analyst. The analytic situation has reanimated, in the form of a current distortion of reality, material which had been repressed or had been dealt with in some other way (e.g. by its canalization into the neurotic symptom itself). This revival of the past in the psychoanalytic relationship leads to the transference-resistance.

The history of Freud's discovery of transference resistance in the course of his attempts to promote free association is still instructive (Freud 1900a, p. 532; 1905e, p. 118; 1912b, pp. 101ff.). It is the story of a disturbance in association which occurs when the patient is dominated by an association relating to the person of the doctor. The more intensively the patient is concerned with the person of the doctor — which naturally also depends on the amount of time the doctor spends with the patient — the more his unconscious expectations are revived. The hope for a cure links with yearnings for wish fulfillment which do not conform to an objective doctor-patient relationship. If the patient transfers to the analyst unconscious desires which are already repressed in his relationships to significant others, then the strongest resistance to further communication can be evoked and can find expression in concealments or silence.

We would like to emphasize that transference resistance was discovered in the form of resistance *against* transference, and as such it can be observed over and over again by every analyst, even in initial interviews. A legitimate question, however, is why we make such a fuss about an everyday event, by emphasizing that the primary phenomena are to be understood as resistance to transference.

The technical rule that the analyst should begin at the surface and work down toward the "depths" simply means that the analyst should interpret the resistance to transference *before* the transferred ideas and affects and their earlier forms in childhood. Glover (1955, p. 121) especially warned against every rigid and absolute application of the rule, and emphasized that we *usually* are concerned first with resistance to transference. Together with Stone (1973) and Gill (1979), we place great value on terminologically distinguishing resistance to transference, and especially to the patient becoming aware of transference, from the phenomenology of transference in general. We hope to be able to demonstrate the advantages offered by the unwieldy phrase "resistance to awareness of the transference" by adopting the distinction which Stone (1973, p. 63) made between "three broad aspects of the relationship between resistance and transference":

> Assuming technical adequacy, the proportional importance of each one [of these aspects] will vary with the individual patient, especially with the depth of psychopathology. First, the resistance to awareness of the transference, and its subjective elaboration in the transference neurosis. Second, the resistance to the dynamic and genetic reductions of the transference neurosis, and ultimately the transference attachment itself, once established in awareness. Third, the transference presentation of the analyst to the "experiencing" portion of the patient's ego, as id object and as externalized superego simultaneously. (Stone 1973, p. 63)

Out of the multitude of meanings given to the concept of resistance, we consider it very important technically to emphasize resistance to the establishment of awareness of the transference. This lends expression to the fact that transferences in the widest sense of the word are the primary realities. This must be the case since man is born a social animal. Resistance can only be directed against something extant, e.g., against the relationship. Clearly, we are referring to a comprehensive understanding of transference as relationship. Differentiations are introduced when the analyst shows the patient here and there that an act of avoidance, hesitation, or forgetting is directed at a — deeper — relationship.

Keeping sight of the adaptive function reduces the danger that resistance interpretations might be taken as criticism. It is therefore advisable for the analyst to conjecture about the object of resistance and about how reflex-like adjustments are achieved even in the initial phase of therapy. According to the steps outlined by Stone, an essential factor is the speed with which the analysis proceeds from the here-and-now to the then-and-there, from the present into the past. Of course, the handling of repression resistance occurs in the present. The therapeutic potential is rooted both in the multiple comparisons between the patient's retrospection and the way the analyst sees things, and in the discovery that the patient draws conclusions by analogy in the therapeutic situation. The patient wants to create a perceptual identity where something new could be perceived; peculiarly, the patient's appropriation of unconscious memories goes hand in hand with an increased distance to the past.

Merely by being different from the other people, the analyst contributes to this far-reaching affective and cognitive process of differentiation. The numerous similarities to other people that the analyst also exhibits can be strengthened in the analytic situation by countertransference. The analyst stimulates the patient's capacity to differentiate by calling feelings and perceptions by their right name. To recapitulate for the sake of clarity, resistance to transference is not referred to or defined as such; on the contrary, we recommend avoiding all words also used in the language of psychoanalytic theory. The important point is to speak with the patient in his own language, in order to gain access to his world.

Nonetheless, the analyst provides the feelings of hate and love with, for instance, an oedipal meaning by referring to them in this context. This is also true for all the other forms and contents of resistance and transference. Which transferences and resistances originate in the here-and-now depends very largely on the way the analyst conducts the treatment (see the reasons given in Chap. 2). Whether the patient's initial resistance to becoming consciously aware of transference develops into a transference resistance, in the sense that the patient only wants to repeat something in his relation to the doctor rather than remembering and working through, and whether this transference resistance develops into transference love and erotized transference, only to change into an alternation of such phases or even finally into a negative transference — these fates of transference resistance are dyadic in nature, however great the contribution of the patient's psychopathology may have been. We hope that the fact that we have begun with resistance to conscious awareness of transference proves to be advantageous with regard to the discussion of the other transference resistances. This form of resistance accompanies the entire course of treatment, because the handling of every conflict or problem in the therapeutic situation can lead to a resistance.

In Chap. 2 we have discussed the most important conditions that must be satisfied in order to affirm Freud's statement that transference becomes "the most powerful therapeutic instrument" in the hands of the physician (1923 a, p. 247). With regard to transference resistances, we can paraphrase Freud to the effect that the importance for the dynamic of cure that the analyst's influence has in the genesis and course of the three typical transference resistances can hardly be overestimated. To recapitulate, these three resistances are resistance against transference, transference love, and the transformations of the latter to either its more intense form, erotized transference, or its reversion to the opposite extreme, i.e., to negative (or aggressive) transference.

## 4.4 Id and Superego Resistance

In the introduction to this chapter (Sect. 4.1) we describe the typology of five forms of resistance which Freud devised in the wake of his revision of anxiety theory and in the context of his structural theory. The observation of masochistic phenomena and the interpretation of acts of severe self-punishment led Freud to assume the existence of unconscious parts of the ego. The conception of superego resistance was thus a significant enrichment of the analytic understanding of unconscious feelings of guilt and negative therapeutic reactions. Superego resistance becomes psychologically comprehensible in the context of the psychosexual and psychosocial genesis of the superego and of ideals and in light of the description of identification processes in the life of an individual and in groups, as described by Freud in *The Ego and the Id* (1923 b) and *Group Psychology and the Analysis of the Ego* (1921 c). In recent decades a large number of unconscious motives for negative therapeutic reactions have been revealed by psychoanalytic studies. The negative therapeutic reaction will be discussed in a section of its own due to the significance of these discoveries for treatment technique. First, however, we will try to provide a description of Freud's theoretical explanations of id and superego resistance.

The clinical phenomena leading to id resistance have already been mentioned. They are the negative and the erotized forms of transference inasfar as these become an unresolvable resistance. Freud traced the fact that some patients are not willing or able to give up their hate or transference love back to certain features of the id which are also present in the superego. Yet, id resistance and superego resistance have one clinical feature in common: they make the cure more difficult or prevent it completely. Freud had noticed that these hardly comprehensible forms of resistance occurred in addition to the protective measures of ego resistance, i.e., in addition to repression resistance and resistance based on secondary gain (Sect. 4.5). He then traced erotized transference and negative therapeutic reaction back to resistance against the separation of the instincts from their previous objects and paths of libido discharge. We will turn now to the explanations Freud gave for apparently refractory erotized transference infatuations and incorrectible negative transferences.

The reader may be surprised that id and superego resistances are discussed in the same section. Yet while the id and the superego are located at opposite poles of Freud's structural theory, these poles are linked by the instinctual nature of man that Freud hypothesized. Because of this link, Freud traced the very different phenomena of id and superego resistance back to the same roots. Freud viewed negative therapeutic reaction and insurmountable transference love ultimately as the result of biological powers which manifest themselves as repetition compulsion in analysis and in the individual's life.

As therapist, Freud nonetheless continued the search for the psychic causes of malignant transferences and regressions. In his late study *Analysis Terminable and Interminable* (1937c), he discusses the problems involved in gaining access to latent conflicts which have remained undisturbed throughout a patient's life until therapy begins. He also deals briefly with the influence that the analyst's personality can have on the analytic situation and on the treatment process. Yet the psychological explanation of successes and failures, i.e., the classification of the factors contributing to a cure and of the way they can become effective in the analytic situation, was no longer one of his central interests. Freud's speculations (derived from a philosophy of nature) about the economic basis of id and superego resistance grew out of his observation of the apparently inevitable repetition of love and hate, of erotized transference and negative transference.

The obscure id and superego resistances seemed to evade explanation in terms of depth psychology. This obscurity was partially illuminated, but simultaneously sealed, for Freud by his fascination with the assumption of repetition compulsion, whose basis he sought in the conservative nature of the instincts. His assumption that the death instinct is the condition for repetition compulsion obscured the significance of the discovery of superego resistance. Similarly, id resistance seemed irresolvable because of the conservative nature of the instincts.

We have mentioned that different kinds of phenomena are covered by id and superego resistances, and we are aware that Freud attributed different economic bases to them. Freud saw a greater chance of achieving modification of id resistance in *working through* (see Chap. 8) than of obtaining modification of superego resistance. According to Freud, in the one case we are dealing more with the termination of libidinal attachments, which is frustrated by the inertia of the libido, in the other with the struggle against the consequences of the death instinct. Freud sought and believed he had found the common denominator of these two forms of resistance in the conservative nature of instincts: in the "adhesiveness" (1916/17, p. 348), the "inertia" (1918b, p. 115), or the "sluggishness" (1940a, p. 181) of the libido. In Freud's view, the patient seeks repetition because of the adhesiveness of the libido instead of foregoing the gratification of erotic transference and relying on remembering and the reality principle. Hate — negative transference — then results from the disappointment.

The patient thus puts himself into situations in which he repeats previous experiences without being able to remember the libidinal objects which serve as models for his love and hate. Indeed, he insists that everything happening is occurring in the present and is not the result of his love/hate of his father/mother. In fact, however, the analyst is the object of the love and hate previously directed at the mother and father. These recurrences do not violate the pleasure principle; fundamental is disappointed love. In repetition compulsion in the sense of superego resistance, another, negative power is at work: the aggression derived from the death instinct.

To help the reader grasp these complicated problems, we will now describe how repetition compulsion was discovered, basing our account on Cremerius (1978). We will then discuss, using the example of the so-called negative therapeutic reaction, the immense expansion of our genuinely analytic understanding of this phenomenon, and of repetition compulsion as a whole, when freed from Freud's metapsychological speculations.

The phenomenon of repetition compulsion gives ample evidence that people get themselves into similar unpleasant situations again and again with fateful inevitability. In *Beyond the Pleasure Principle* Freud described the power of repetition compulsion, using the examples of fate neurosis and traumatic neurosis. For Freud the shared feature of these two forms of neurosis is the fact that states of suffering apparently occur inevitably in people's lives. It is possible for traumatic experiences, even those belonging to the past, to dominate a person's thinking and feeling for years. Painful constellations of typical disappointments and catastrophes in personal relations then result apparently through no fault of the patient's and recur in an apparently inevitable manner.

Precisely because of the recurrence of traumatic events in dreams, Freud now presented a very plausible psychological theory oriented around problem-solving. The treatment of patients with traumatic neuroses also shows how repetition is employed by the ego, as it were, to master the traumatic experience of loss of control. In therapy the patient actualizes this traumatic experience, with the goal of ridding himself of the accompanying painful affects and the hope that the analyst can master them for him. Repetition compulsion can thus be understood as an attempt to tie the traumatic experience into an interpersonal context, and thus to integrate it psychically. We will go into this in more detail in the discussion of dreams (Chap. 5). In the Introduction (Chap. 1), we have already drawn attention to the fundamental significance of problem-solving as a framework for treatment technique. Nothing is more natural than to view the apparently incomprehensible and inevitable fate neuroses as manifestations of unconscious, i.e., psychic, patterns of behavior.

Yet Freud's psychoanalytic studies did not seem at this point to lead any further. The negative therapeutic reaction became the decisive piece of circumstantial evidence in favor of the hypothesis of a superego resistance derived ultimately from the death instinct. For the sake of brevity, we have skipped a few steps of the argument, but Freud reached this conclusion and accepted it to the end. In the posthumously published *An Outline of Psychoanalysis* (1940a, p. 149), he wrote: "There can be no question of restricting one or the other of the basic instincts to one of the provinces of the mind. They must necessarily be met with everywhere." Freud repeats in this statement his earlier assumption that when the life and death instincts are disentangled, the superego is the pure form of the latter (1923b, p. 53).

We are now in a position to state the following: Freud's discovery of unconscious guilt feelings, of the negative therapeutic reaction, and of superego resistance as a whole stood at the beginning of his revision of his theory. Since significant portions of the ego are unconscious, it was only natural for him to replace the topographic division (unconscious, preconscious, and conscious) by structural theory. At approximately the same time, the dualism of life and death instincts was given new meaning. The causes of repetition compulsion were seen (and sought) in the conservative nature of the instincts, whether in the inertia of the libido or in the death instinct with its yearning to return to an inanimate state. Freud's linkage of this new, dualistic theory of instincts with structural theory seemed to explain why attempts at psychoanalytic therapy are frustrated by id resistance, irresolvable erotized transference, and by superego resistance — because of the cathexis of the unconscious areas of the superego with destructive instinctual elements.

In hindsight it is impossible to disagree with the view that precisely the instinctual explanations of id and superego resistances caused a delay in the therapeutic application and *depth-psychological* understanding of the unconscious guilt feeling and of the negative therapeutic reaction. Overcoming these forms of resistance is definitely no simple matter, but exactly Freud's speculations on natural philosophy constitute the factor making the analyst into a Don Quixote, mistaking windmills for giants and battling them in vain. There is also no need for us to feel like Sisyphus; Lichtenstein's (1935) little known phenomenological and psychoanalytic interpretation of the myth of Sisyphus, which was not translated into English until 1974, can also lead out of the dead end of pseudobiological assumptions on repetition compulsion.

### *4.4.1 The Negative Therapeutic Reaction*

In his report on the case of the Wolf Man (1918b, p.69), Freud described his patient's "transitory 'negative reactions'":

> Every time something had been conclusively cleared up, he attempted to contradict the effect for a short while by an aggravation of the symptom which had been cleared up. It is quite the rule, as we know, for children to treat prohibitions in the same kind of way. When they have been rebuked for something (for instance, because they are making an unbearable din), they repeat it once more after the prohibition before stopping it. In this way they gain the point of apparently stopping of their own accord and of disobeying the prohibition.

In analogy to raising children, Freud speaks here of prohibitions that children disobey. It seems significant that there is a worsening of the symptom concerned after a conclusive clearing up and that Freud considers the disobedient and negating behavior to be an expression of *independence.* Problem solving is done jointly, whereas stopping voluntarily is an expression of assertion and independence. Freud also put the therapeutic relationship at the focus of attention in the later, comprehensive definition of negative therapeutic reaction. He observed:

> There are certain people who behave in a quite peculiar fashion during the work of analysis. When one speaks hopefully to them or expresses satisfaction with the progress of the treatment, they show signs of discontent and their condition invariably becomes worse. One begins by regarding this as defiance and as an attempt to prove their superiority to the physician, but later one comes to take a deeper and juster view. One becomes convinced, not only that such people cannot endure any praise or appreciation, but that they react inversely to the progress of the treatment. Every partial solution that ought to result, and in other people does result, in an improvement or a temporary suspension of symptoms produces in them for the time being an exacerbation of their illness; they get worse during the treatment instead of getting better. They exhibit what is known as a "negative therapeutic reaction". (Freud 1923b, p.49)

Although the situation Freud described here was extreme, the description might nonetheless still apply to some extent to very many, and perhaps even to all, difficult cases of neurosis (Freud 1923b, p.51).

In view of the obeservation that very many patients react negatively precisely when the analyst expresses satisfaction with the progress of treatment and especially to accurate interpretations, it is surprising that Freud finally let himself be led instead by the model of intrapsychic conflict and by the conception of superego resistance. From the negative therapeutic reaction he concluded that there is an unconscious sense of guilt "which is finding its satisfaction in the illness and refuses to give up the punishment of suffering" (1923b, p.49). Freud later repeated this explanation in a slightly modified form:

> People in whom this unconscious sense of guilt is excessively strong betray themselves in analytic treatment by the negative therapeutic reaction which is so disagreeable from the prognostic point of view. When one has given them the solution of a symptom, which should normally be followed by at least its temporary disappearance, what they produce instead is a momentary exacerbation of the symptom and of the illness. It is often enough to praise them for their behaviour in the treatment or to say a few hopeful words about the progress of the analysis in order to bring about an unmistakable worsening of their condition. A non-analyst

would say that the "will to recovery" was absent. If you follow the analytic way of thinking, you will see in this behaviour a manifestation of the unconscious sense of guilt, for which being ill, with its sufferings and impediments, is just what is wanted. (Freud 1933a, pp. 109-110)

Finally, Freud traced the unconscious masochistic tendency — the motive of the negative therapeutic reaction — back to the aggressive and destructive instinct, i.e., the death instinct. The latter, together with the conservative nature of the instincts based on it, is also the reason for the failure of the interminable analysis, as we can read in Freud's late study *Analysis Terminable and Interminable* (1937c, pp. 242-243):

One portion of this force has been recognized by us, undoubtedly with justice, as the sense of guilt and need for punishment, and has been localized by us in the ego's relation to the super-ego. But this is only the portion of it which is, as it were, psychically bound by the super-ego and thus becomes recognizable; other quotas of the same force, whether bound or free, may be at work in other, unspecified places. If we take into consideration the total picture made up of the phenomena of masochism immanent in so many people, the negative therapeutic reaction and the sense of guilt found in so many neurotics, we shall no longer be able to adhere to the belief that mental events are exclusively governed by the desire for pleasure. These phenomena are unmistakable indications of the presence of a power in mental life which we call the instinct of aggression or of destruction according to its aims, and which we trace back to the original death instinct of living matter.

When we nowadays rediscover the negative therapeutic reaction and unconscious guilt feelings (in the form of superego resistance) during treatment, we are in a more favorable position than Freud was. In the meantime many analysts have pursued the question of why precisely the intensification of the relationship between patient and analyst, which is associated with an accurate interpretation and an increase in hope, can lead to the feeling "But I don't deserve this." Many patients quickly realize this tendency in themselves, and their accounts often contain components of what Deutsch (1930) misleadingly termed fate neurosis. In the statement "I don't deserve better," for example, the sense of guilt as such is not unconscious. On the contrary, the object-related pleasurable and aggressive wishes, which push into the foreground at precisely the moment transference is strengthened, i.e., upon rediscovery of the object, want to enter into the realm of experience.

There is therefore hardly anything in the psychoanalytic treatment technique better suited than the negative therapeutic reaction to demonstrate the unfavorable consequences of the doctrinaire assumptions of instinct theory and structural theory. In fact, the resolution of superego resistance leads away from Freud's metapsychological assumptions and toward a comprehensive interactional theory of conflict capable of providing an understanding of superego formation and thus of superego resistance. The internalization of prohibitions, i.e., superego formation, is tied in Freud's theory to oedipal conflicts. The object relationship psychologies provide more significant information on why it is particularly the analyst's expressions of optimism which lead to disturbances in the transference relationship. A wealth of emotions are contained in self-punishment and masochistic tendencies. It is therefore not surprising that many observations published in the last few decades significantly facilitate the resolution of superego resistance. It would be gratifying if the individual results could be reduced to a common denominator.

Grunert (1979) has argued that the numerous forms taken by the negative therapeutic reaction should be conceived as a recurrence of the process of detachment and individuation, in Mahler's (1969) sense, and that the unconscious motivations of the negative therapeutic reaction should be sought there. Using the passages from Freud that we have quoted above and referring especially to Spitz (1957), Grunert demonstrates convincingly that this defiant behavior can also be understood positively, as negation serving the striving for autonomy. Considering that the process of detachment and individuation also includes the later rapprochement, i.e., encompasses practically everything that takes place between mother and child, then it is not surprising that Grunert views this phase and its revival as the common denominator for the typical constellations of transference and countertransference. A more exact examination of unconscious guilt feelings leads beyond oedipal rivalry. Superego resistance proves to be only the tip of a pyramid anchored deep in the world of unconscious wishes. The child's development inevitably leads out of the symbiosis. The child is inquisitive, curious, and eager for new experiences. In the therapeutic regression, rapproachement to unconscious fusion wishes also strengthens the tendencies toward differentiation (Olinick 1964, 1970).

The contribution the analyst makes toward the new discoveries is therefore decisive. Asch (1976) and Tower (see Olinick 1970, pp. 658ff.) have recognized different aspects of this negativism in the context of symbiosis or primary identification. Grunert uses one patient's meaningful, transference neurotic utterances to describe different facets of the process of detachment and individuation. As an example of separation guilt he gives the statement: "The separation will destroy either you or me." The following sentences illustrate the striving for autarky with simultaneous deprivation anxiety: "I want to control what is happening here, so that you lose in value." "If I show how well I am, I have to go." The passive struggle with the father was manifested, for example, in the following statement: "As a failure, I'll force him/you to accept my conditions." Grunert, like Rosenfeld (1971, 1975) and Kernberg (1975), views envy of the analyst as a particularly powerful motive behind the negative therapeutic reaction.

Even Freud's early descriptions disclose that a worsening occurs exactly when the analyst could expect gratitude. Klein's (1957) ideas on envy and gratitude are therefore especially relevant for a deeper understanding of the negative therapeutic reaction. Characteristically, the increase in dependence goes hand in hand with a growth in their denial by means of aggressive ideas of omnipotence. These are, admittedly, process-related quantities which are correlated with technique.

The negative therapeutic reaction is, however, also the response to an object felt to be pathogenic, as the character anaylsis of masochistics shows. These patients had to submit in childhood to a parental figure who they felt did not love them but despised them. To protect itself against the consequences of this perception, the child begins to idealize its parents and their rigid demands. It attempts to meet these demands and condemns and devalues itself in order to be able to maintain the illusion of being loved by its parents. When this form of relationship is relived in transference, the patient *must* respond to the analyst's interpretations with a negative therapeutic reaction. The patient turns the tables, so to speak, by taking the position of the mother who had mocked his opinions and by putting the analyst into the position of the child who is constantly unjustly treated but still desparately strives for love. Parkin (1980) calls this a situation of "masochistic enthralment" between subject and object.

Awareness of these unconscious motivations behind the negative therapeutic reaction has contributed to a positive modification of psychoanalytic technique. Our survey makes it clear that the common denominator that Grunert found in Mahler's process of detachment and individuation proves to be a good classifying principle. In our opinion, however, the question of whether disturbances of this phase, comprising the period from the 5th to the 36th month of life, have special relevance for the negative therapeutic reaction cannot yet be answered. In any case, we believe it is important to pay attention to what the analyst contributes to the therapeutic regression and to his interpretation of it based on his countertransference and his theoretical approach (Limentani 1981).

### *4.4.2 Aggression and Destructiveness: Beyond the Mythology of Instinct*

Since Freud's derivations of the superego and id resistances are incorrect, the limits of the applicability of the psychoanalytic method do not lie where he had thought. The hereditary and constitutional factors which contribute so decisively to molding every individual's potential for growth and development are not to be found where Freud's definition of instincts localized them. Neither id resistance (as erotized transference) nor superego resistance (as masochistic repetition) derives its quality from the conservative nature of the instincts which Freud felt compelled to assume on the basis of his metapsychological speculations on the death instinct. The introduction of an independent aggressive or destructive instinct and its derivation from the death instinct, which reached its culmination in Freud's *Civilization and Its Discontents* (1930a), had positive and negative consequences for treatment technique. In *Beyond the Pleasure Principle* (1920g), Freud had described repetition compulsion and the conservative character of instinctual life. Ten years later he was amazed at "how we can have overlooked the ubiquity of non-erotic aggressivity and destructiveness and can have failed to give it its due place in our interpretation of life ... I remember my own defensive attitude when the idea of an instinct of destruction first emerged in psycho-analytic literature, and how long it took before I became receptive to it" (Freud 1930a, p. 120).

Adler had in fact allotted the aggressive instinct a special and independent place in his theory of neurosis. Freud (1909d) had described the role of hate merely casuistically, for example as a feature of compulsion neurosis, but derived the phenomena of aggression from the sexual and self-preservative instincts. Waelder summarizes the theoretical revision of the 1920s in the following way:

While they had previously been thought of as explainable in terms of sexual and self-preservative drives — the dichotomy of the early psychoanalytic instinct theory — and in terms of the ego, they now came to be seen as manifestations of a destructive drive. (Waelder 1960, p. 131)

Despite the mixed reception given to Freud's new instinctual dualism, as the publications by Bibring (1936), Bernfeld (1935), Fenichel (1953 [1935b]), Loewenstein (1940), and Federn (1930) show, the indirect consequences it had on treatment technique were substantial even where the theory as such was met with skepticism or rejection. According to Waelder's description (1960, p. 133), even analysts who did not believe in the existence of a death instinct, i.e., understood the aggressive instinct on the basis of the clinical psychological and not the metapsychological theory of psychoanalysis, "were quick to accept the new theory on impressionistic grounds." Waelder, referring to Bernfeld (1935), traces this back to the following circumstance:

The old theories could *not* be *directly* applied to the phenomena; the latter had first to be analyzed, i.e., their unconscious meaning had to be investigated .... But classifications such as "erotic" or "destructive" could be applied directly to the raw material of observation, without any previous analytic work of distilling and refining (or with a bare minimum of it) .... It is easy to say that a patient is hostile, much easier than, e.g., the reconstruction of an unconscious fantasy from transference behavior. Could some of the popularity of the concept be due to the deceptive ease of its application (or misapplication)? (Waelder 1960, pp. 133-134)

Waelder invites theoretical comparison by compiling a list of the explanatory modalities of the older psychoanalytic theory of aggression. In his opinion, it is possible to provide a good explanation for aggressive and destructive phenomena using the older theory, i.e., without recourse to the assumption of an independent aggressive instinct:

A destructive attitude, action or impulse may be

1. the reaction to (a) a threat to self-preservation or, more generally, to purposes usually attributed to the ego; or the reaction to (b) the frustration, or threatened frustration, of a libidinal drive. Or
2. it may be a by-product of an ego activity such as (a) the mastery of the outside world, or (b) the control of one's own body or mind. Or
3. it may be a part or aspect of libidinal urge which in some way implies aggressiveness against the object, such as, e.g., incorporation or penetration.

In the first case, we may feel hostile to those who threaten our lives or thwart our ego ambitions (1a), or to those who compete with us for the same love object (1b). In the second sense, the normal attempt of the growing organism to acquire mastery of the outside world implies a measure of destructiveness as far as inanimate objects are concerned, and a measure of aggression with regard to man or animal (2a). Or it may manifest itself as a by-product of the control, gradually required, of one's body or as a by-product of our struggle to acquire control over our mind (2b), related to the fear of being overwhelmed by the strength of the id. Finally, it may be part and parcel of a libidinal urge, or an aspect of it, such as in oral biting, oral incorporation, anal sadism, phallic penetration, or vaginal retentiveness (3). In all these instances aggression appears, sometimes a very dangerous aggression; but there is no compelling need to postulate an inborn drive to destroy. (Waelder 1960, pp. 139-140)

Implicit in Waelder's classification are two aspects of principle which deserve special emphasis. We can consider this behavior from the points of view of spontaneity and reactivity. The spontaneous and reactive portions of human action and feeling have been mixed from the very beginning. Nutritional, oral, and sexual activity each have a relatively high level of spontaneity. The preponderance of the influence of rhythmic physical and endopsychic processes over that of precipitating stimuli is one of the defining features of instinctual behavior. Waelder, in contrast, emphasizes the reactive nature of aggressiveness. Aggressiveness would be impossible, of course, without the spontaneous activity which characterizes man just as it does other living things. In this sense Kunz (1946b, p. 23) said that "spontaneity constitutes the foundation which makes reactivity possible."

Since Freud described the development of human spontaneity in terms of libido theory — and hunger and sexuality do indeed have all the features of an instinct — it was a natural step to grasp the likewise ubiquitous aggressiveness as a primary instinct. A factor which has probably contributed to this right up to the present day is the idea that we can only do justice to the social significance of aggressiveness if we concede it a primary position next to sexuality.

The assumption that aggressiveness is reactive in origin seems to make it into a secondary phenomenon, even to minimize its importance. This is by no means our intention, and we would like to point out that the noninstinctual origin of aggressiveness — we will justify this assumption in detail later — is precisely what constitutes its evil nature. To introduce this line of argument, it is advantageous to distinguish between aggressive and destructive actions and their unconscious and conscious antecedents. Given a gradual transition from aggression to destruction, it is impossible to clearly define destructiveness as referring to devastation and extermination, ultimately as the killing of a fellow human being. In contrast, expansive and aggressive activities are not necessarily painful, but may in some situations even be pleasurable.

Reconsidering Waelder's list, it is apparent that he views the manifestations of aggressiveness as reactions to frustration or danger, as by-products of self-preservation, or as phenomena accompanying the sexual instinct. What then remains for Waelder is the particularly malignant "essential destructiveness" which eludes our understanding. He used this phrase to refer to

> manifestations of aggression which cannot be seen as reactive to provocation because they are so vast in intensity or duration that it would be difficult to fit them into any scheme of stimulus and reaction; which cannot be seen as by-products of ego activities because they neither are accompaniments of present ego activities nor seem explainable as derivatives of former by-products of ego activities; and, finally, cannot be seen as part of sexual drives because no sexual pleasure of any kind appears to be attached to them. (Waelder 1960, p. 142)

As an example of essential destructiveness, Waelder referred to the most monstrous case in history: Hitler's insatiable hatred of the Jews. He added, "It is difficult to see how it could be explained on a reactive basis because of its limitlessness and inexhaustibility" (Waelder 1960, p. 144).

We fully agree with Waelder that the limitlessness and inexhaustibility of this hatred and similar forms of destructivenss are not adequately explained by the stimulus-reaction scheme. Of course, Freud's discovery of unconscious response readiness had made it possible to grasp precisely those actions which had eluded understanding, i.e., those which have no recognizable cause or are completely out of proportion to the cause. This disproportion between cause and reaction characterizes unconsciously directed trains of thought and action, especially delusional ones. The inexhaustible and insatiable will for destruction that took hold of large portions of the German people under Hitler is something far beyond what we usually characterize as instinctual phenomena.

We mention this most monstrous of cases of destructiveness here because we believe that the holocaust is an extreme experience which has contributed to the revision of the psychoanalytic theory of aggression. The events of recent history have, however, also revived the belief in a death instinct; consequently, the far-reaching revisions initiated at the beginning of the 1970s have remained largely unnoticed. Whichever events of persecution, whichever apocalyptic threats, and whichever independent developments within psychoanalysis may have contributed to it, in recent years there has been a fundamental revision of the psychoanalytic instinctual theory which has hardly been recognized.

On the basis of subtle psychoanalytic and phenomenological analyses of aggressive and destructive phenomena, Stone (1971), A. Freud (1972), Gillespie (1971), Rochlin (1973), and Basch (1984) all independently reached the conclusion that malicious human destructiveness in particular lacks the features which customarily characterize instincts, such as sexuality and hunger, both within psychoanalysis and outside it. It is true that A. Freud, with reference to Eissler (1971), made a vain attempt to rescue the theory of the death instinct. Yet her clear line of argument, to the effect that the features of an instinct such as source and special energy are absent from aggression, leaves no room for the death instinct. That birth and death are the most significant events in a human life, and that any psychology worthy of the name has to assign death an important role in its system, as A. Freud emphasizes with reference to Schopenhauer, Freud, and Eissler, are not indications of the existence of a death instinct, but of a psychology of death (Richter 1984).

The clinical observations of children and adults in analyses as well as the direct observations of children that A. Freud mentions are all included in the territory marked out by Waelder. The fact that the criticism of the instinctual theory of aggression has so far had few consequences is surely related to our continued use of the wonted vocabulary. A. Freud continued to base her descriptions of clinical observations on instinctual theory even after the instinctual character of aggression had been refuted, as shown by her observation that:

> Children in analysis may be angry, destructive, insulting, rejecting, attacking for a wide variety of reasons, only one of them being the *direct discharge of genuine aggressive fantasies or impulses.* The rest is aggressive behaviour in the service of the ego, i.e., for the purpose of defence: as a reaction to anxiety and effective cover for it; as an ego resistance against lowering defences; as a resistance against the verbalization of preconscious and unconscious material; as a superego reaction against the conscious acknowledgement of id derivatives, sexual or aggressive; as a denial of any positive, libidinal tie to the analyst; as a defence against passive-feminine strivings ("impotent rage"). (A. Freud 1972, p. 169, emphasis added)

Yet what is the situation with regard to the reasons for the discharge of genuine aggressive fantasies? After A. Freud had denied that aggression has an energy of its own, it obviously became impossible to assert that such energy can be discharged. Her use of the compact expression "genuine aggressive fantasies or impulses" also requires comment. It is most probable that diffuse, undirected explosions or those involving an object which is only accidentally present — the famous fly on the wall — occur reactively, as the result of previous injuries coupled with an incapacity to defend oneself which may have internal or external reasons. The gratification of aggression is not comparable with the satisfaction of hunger or with the pleasure of the orgasm. After verbal disputes one has the feeling, "At last I've told him what I think of him." The gratification of aggressive destructive impulses thus serves to reconstitute a damaged sense of one's worth. The fact that a person feels better after an emotional outburst than before is clearly also associated with the release of tension, but this tension also arises reactively and is based on fantasies in the widest sense of the word.

The conception that human aggressiveness and destructiveness lack the features of an instinct by no means minimizes their importance. On the contrary, it is precisely the especially malicious, timeless, and insatiable form of hate, which erupts unpredictably and without apparent reason, which now becomes accessible to psychoanalytic explanation.

In her criticism of the aggressive instinct, A. Freud reaches the same conclusions as Kunz, a constructive, even endearing critic of psychoanalysis; we will refer to the results of his studies. The fact that Kunz's phenomenological analyses have been forgotten is, incidentally, one of the many signs of the insufficient communication between disciplines. Forty years ago Kunz wrote that

> there is no aggressive "instinct" in the sense in which we acknowledge the instinctual nature of sexuality and hunger .... We therefore do not argue about the word "instinct," because we can of course impute "instincts" or "an instinct" to all living behavior and even to cosmic events .... The question is rather: given that we have decided, for example, to give the name "instinctual acts" to the actions serving to gratify sexual desire and hunger, and to presume that they are at least partially determined by the dynamic mechanisms we term "instincts," is it appropriate also to describe acts of aggression and destruction as "instinctual" and call the imputed moving factor the "aggressive instinct"? ... Or are the differences between the two complexes of phenomena so pronounced that using the same terminology for both of them is inevitably misleading and a barrier to cognition? This is indeed our opinion. The aggressive, destructive movements differ in essence from actions due to sexual excitement and hunger, despite the many similarities. (Kunz 1946b, pp. 33-34, 41-42)

A. Freud concludes that human aggression lacks everything specific: the organ, the energy, and the object. Kunz emphasized that aggression

> *altogether lacks the specificity, both in feeling and in the forms of its manifestations* .... The correctness of the hypothesis about the nonspecific nature of aggression is supported, for one thing, by the absence of an organ or field of expression primarily serving aggression. We have been able to determine that there are preferences for certain zones of the body, changing in the course of life, and have to admit the possibility that such links can also form and harden secondarily. Yet there is no original — albeit nonexclusive — organ serving aggression which corresponds to the digestive tract for hunger or the genital zone for sexuality. (Kunz 1946b, p. 32)

Kunz provides further support for his assumption that aggression is nonspecific by referrring to the absence of an object reserved for it.

Spontaneous activity, as the basis of the object relations, is the precondition for the reactivity Kunz discusses here. We therefore agree with Kunz when he emphasizes that the *enormous effect* and the *constant readiness* of aggression and destructiveness can only be comprehended properly if assumed to be reactive in nature.

If aggressions were based on a specific aggressive instinct, it would presumably fit, just as the other needs rooted in instincts do, into the more or less pronounced and never completely absent rhythm of tension and relaxation, unrest and rest, deprivation and fulfillment. Certainly, there is also a saturation of aggressive impulses, both when the gratification immediately follows the origin of the impulse and after a long-deferred discharge. Yet it does not obey an autonomous phasic alternation, but is connected to the appearance and diminution of those tendencies whose nongratification remains associated with the actualization of the aggressions. An apparent exception is the accumulated aggressiveness which results from the earlier inhibition of numerous impulses, becomes a kind of permanent character trait, and discharges from time to time for no (apparent) reason. (Kunz 1946b, pp. 48-49)

Turning to the theoretical and practical consequences of this criticism, the nonspecificity of the alleged instinctual nature of human aggressiveness makes a differentiated consideration necessary. Such consideration has led to a division of the complex field and to the formation of partial theories. Their empirical validity is accordingly limited. Merely a partial aspect is explained by time-honored theories such as the frustration-aggression theory, on which, for example, Dollard et al. (1967 [1939]) tested empirically based psychoanalytic assumptions regarding the sudden change of positive transference into hatred (see Angst 1980). From psychoanalytic points of view it must be emphasized that even in experimental research on aggression the degree to which an individual is *affected* by an event previously characterized by individual concepts such as "frustration, attack, and arbitrariness" (Michaelis 1976, p. 34) proves to be a decisive influence for his aggressive behavior.

Interestingly, Michaelis arrives at a process model of aggression. He states: "The decisive factors are not acts of frustration, attacks, or arbitrary acts, but rather the *direction* of the event and thus the degree to which an individual is affected" (Michaelis 1976, p. 31). We believe that the technical knowledge which makes it possible for us to discover the factors precipitating aggressive impulses, fantasies, or acts is oriented around the degree to which one is affected or feels injured. A treatment technique situated *beyond* the mythology of instinct has to undertake a differentiated phenomenological and psychoanalytic analysis of the situational origin of aggressive impulses and fantasies as recommended by Waelder.

The loose attachment of the instinct to its object, as described by Freud, distinguishes human instincts significantly from animal instincts and their regulation by innate stimulus mechanisms. This difference is the basis of the *plasticity* of human object choice. It is fairly safe to say that this loose association is the expression of an evolutionary jump which characterizes the process of man's development. Lorenz (1973) uses the term "fulguration" to describe the situation. The metaphor of the sudden brightness emanating from a flash of lightning accurately expresses the transformation of unconscious life to a state of conscious awareness. Let there be light — with reference to the biblical story of creation, one could say that with lightning speed the fulguration created light, throwing shadows and making it possible to distinguish light and dark, good and evil. And what about the thunder which usually follows the lightning? Its strongly amplified echo reaches us today in the knowledge that the fulguration, as the evolutionary jump, brings with it the capacity to form symbols and thus the potential to employ destructiveness in the service of grandiose fantasies.

The destructive goals of human aggression such as the annihilation of fellow humans or even entire groups of people — such as the attempted genocide of the Jewish people in the Holocaust — is beyond biological explanation. Nobody would ever consider minimizing these forms of aggression by explaining them as manifestations of so-called evil. It is illuminating that a biologist, von Bertalanffy (1958), was the one to remind psychoanalysts of the significance of symbol formation for the theory of human aggression.

The capacity to use symbols not only makes possible man's cultural evolution; it also enables an individual to distinguish himself from others and allows barriers to communication to be established between groups. These processes can contribute to conflicts being so waged "as if they were conflicts *between different species*, the aim of which even in the animal kingdom is generally the destruction of the opponent" (Eibl-Eibesfeldt 1980, p. 28). At this point it is necessary to distinguish between intra- and interspecies aggression. A typical feature of the destructiveness directed at fellow men is that the targets are discriminated against and declared to be subhuman. In intergroup aggression, alternating mutual disparagement has always played a significant role. As a result of the development of the mass media, the influence of propaganda has grown beyond all bounds in our lifetime — for good as well as for evil. In his famous letter to Einstein, Freud contrasted human aggressiveness and its destructive degenerate form particularly to emotional attachment by means of identification: "Whatever leads men to share important interests produces this community of feeling, these identifications. And the structure of human society is to a large extent based on them" (1933 b, p. 212). Such processes of identification are also the basis of the therapeutic relationship, and thus negative, aggressive transference is a variable which depends on many factors.

In contrast to the processes just described, aggressive animalistic behavior is endogenously controlled by rhythmic processes. In behavior research, Lorenz has described object discharges which consume the instinct and could be called aggressive. There appear to be analogies between substitute activities and aggression discharged onto the object of displacement, between vacuum activities and blind, seemingly objectless actions (Thomä 1967 a). The therapeutic recommendations that Lorenz (1963) makes in his well-known book, entitled in German *Das sogenannte Böse* (literally, the so-called evil), are, accordingly, at the level of time-honored catharsis and affective abreaction. Lorenz basically says that there should be a psychohygienic reduction in the accumulated potential for aggression that could mean the end for mankind, and advises that this be achieved by means of more harmless forms of instinctual discharge, such as sports. Discharge theory and catharsis were influential in the formulation of these recommendations. Some instances of harmless negative transference become comprehensible in this way. The aggressiveness reactively produced by frustration is part of the negative transference.

Following A. Freud's argumentation, however, all simple patterns of explanation and analogies become dubious, since human aggression has no energy reservoir or object of its own. While interspecies animal aggression consists only of the finding and killing of prey, human destructiveness is insatiable. Fantasy activities are not bound by the constraints of space and time, and this seems to have led to boundaries not being reliably established and maintained by ritual as they are in the animal kingdom (Wisdom 1984). Aggressive behavior between members of the same animal species, whether between sexual rivals or for seniority or territory, ceases when the weaker animal acknowledges defeat by means of a submissive posture or flight (Eibl-Eibesfeldt 1970). In the animal kingdom, distance can end the rivalry; in contrast, distance is a precondition for human destructiveness: the image of the enemy is distorted beyond recognition.

As already mentioned, von Bertalanffy traced human destructiveness back to man's capacity to form symbols and distinguished it from instinctual aggressiveness as seen in animal behavior. The factor that gives human aggressiveness its evil quality and makes it so insatiable is its tie to conscious and unconscious fanatasy systems, which apparently are generated out of nothing and degenerate to evil. Man's capacity to form symbols is in itself beyond good and evil.

An analyst cannot, of course, be satisfied with the view that omnipotence fantasies and destructive aims arise out of nothing, as it were. We know that injuries that appear completely banal can precipitate greatly exaggerated aggressive reactions in sensitive people and especially in psychopathologic borderline cases. Destructive processes are set in motion because unconscious fantasies give the harmless external stimuli the appearance of a serious threat. Psychoanalytic investigation of this connection regularly leads to the recognition that the extent of the injury from without is in direct proportion to the amount of aggression that the subject has relieved himself of by means of projection. Klein (1946) earned the honor of describing this process as an object relationship within the framework of the theory of projective and introjective identification.

Yet the question as to which childhood experiences are instrumental in the formation of grandiose and destructive fantasies (and their projection with subsequent control of the object) has remained unanswered. It is a part of every mother's experience that strong aggressive reactions appear especially with frustration in small children, just as it is part of everyday knowledge that the tolerance of frustration is lowered by continued pampering. Freud therefore described both excessive denial and pampering as undesirable in child raising.

If the history of the development of fantasy systems with grandiose ideational contents is traced back, one finally arrives at the question of how firmly the assumption of archaic unconscious ideas of omnipotence and impotence is founded. The theory of narcissism provides a clear answer to these questions: Kohut's inborn grandiose self reacts to every injury with narcissistic rage. Awareness of the phenomenology of increased sensitivity to injury and narcissistic rage — here we prefer to speak of destructiveness — is obviously one of the older and least controversial facts of psychoanalysis. In view of the criticism directed at metapsychology, the important thing now is to provide an unprejudiced clarification of the role of man's capacity to form smybols in the origin of human destructiveness.

If one considers self-preservation to be a biopsychological regulatory principle that can be disturbed both from within and from without, one reaches a perspective from which it is possible to attribute to self-preservation the ability both to attain a reflective, oral mastery of the object and to establish a sophisticated delusional system of destruction subserving grandiose ideas. The fantasy associated with symbolization processes, in the widest sense of the concept, is ever-present. Since fantasy is linked to the capacity to form internal ideational representations, infantile aggression can hardly have the archaic significance assigned to it by the assumption, from instinctual theory, that the narcissistic libido is expressed in the infantile omnipotence. The grandiose fantasies lead us to conscious and unconscious wishes, which are inexhaustible because of their loose connection and plasticity.

It is significant that oral and sexual desires are satiable, whereas instrumentalized aggressiveness is ever-present. Aggressiveness subserves a self-preservation primarily determined by psychic contents. We thus take up Freud's old classification and endow it with a psychosocial meaning. Freud initially attributed aggression to the instinct for self-preservation, which he also called the ego instinct, and contrasted this instinct to the sexual one responsible for species preservation. According to this classification, included in the ego instincts is the mastery of the object with a view to self-preservation. By means of an immense extension of what Freud termed self-preservation, it is possible to view human destructiveness as a correlate of self-preservation. Thus, neither human destructiveness nor species preservation can now be conceived as purely biological regulatory principles. They nonetheless remain related to each other because the intensity and extent of the destructiveness are interdependent with grandiose fantasies and their fulfillment.

This assumption contains a reactive element inasmuch as the increase in fantasies of grandeur is accompanied by an increase in the danger posed by imagined enemies. A *circulus vitiosus* thus develops that finds more and more realistic occasions to transform the imagined enemies into real opponents fighting for survival. Such self-preservation is no longer grounded in biology. The struggle is not one for animalistic survival, which may well be guaranteed and as a rule is. It is even possible to say that the *Homo symbolicus* cannot fully develop and put his inventions at the disposal of aggression until a sufficient margin of security has been achieved, i.e., until the loose connection between the nurturing instinct and the object has been stabilized to the extent that the struggle for the daily bread is no longer man's sole or primary preoccupation (Freud 1933a, p.177). Why do social revolutionaries, such as Michael Kohlhaas (to mention a figure from German history, immortalized by a novel by H.

Kleist), fight? The primary reason was certainly not to obtain compensation for the material injustice inflicted on Kohlhaas when the nobleman robbed him of his horses.

Since self-preservation, in its narrow and comprehensive sense, is tied to the gratification of vital needs, the problem of the connection between deprivation and the compensatory increase in envy, greed, revenge, or power fantasies is still of great practical importance. Yet Freud demonstrated, using the example of the consequences of childhood pampering, that aggressiveness is not only compenstory in origin. Pampering creates an aggressive potential in adults in that a moderate demand is later experienced as unbearable: aggressive means are employed for self-preservation, i.e., to preserve the pampered state of the status quo.

The consequences which the revision of the theory of aggression has on treatment technique affect both superego resistance, i.e., the negative therapeutic reaction, and negative transference. The greater the insecurity in the analytic situation, i.e., the more serious the threat to self-preservation, the stronger aggressive transference has to be. Moser stressed what consequences the analytic situation can have, especially if the aggressive signals are not recognized at an early stage:

> If attention is not paid to the aggressive signals (anger, rage) and if they do not lead to any behavior activities to change the precipitating situation, the emotional activation progresses. (This corresponds to Freud's thesis of signal summation.) The overactivation finally shows itself in a state of anger or rage in which plainly only uncontrolled aggressive behavior is possible .... The analytic situation forestalls motoric aggression through systematic conditioning which, coupled with insight, operantly reinforces the nonaction. There is therefore an inclination to somatisize affective outbursts inasmuch as they cannot be headed off interactively by the analyst's interpretation. (Moser 1978, p. 236)

One possible disadvantage of premature interpretations of negative transference was pointed out by Balint:

> In this latter case the patient may be prevented from feeling full-blooded hatred or hostility because consistent interpretations offer him facilities for discharging his emotions in small quantities, which may not amount to more than a feeling of some kind of irritation or of being annoyed. The analyst, interpreting negative transference consistently too early — in the same way as his patient — need not to get to grips with high intensity emotions either; the whole analytic work may be done on "symbols" of hatred, hostility, etc. (Balint 1954, p. 160)

Kohut grasps negative transference as the patient's reaction to the psychoanalyst's actions; this led him to criticize the conception that human aggressiveness is rooted in man's instinctual nature, and to interpret destructiveness in the framework of a theory of the self.

Kohut drew consequences from the untenability of the view that human destructiveness is a primary instinct which deepen our understanding of aggressive transference. Although we do not share his opinion that destructiveness represents a primitive disintegration product (Kohut 1977, p. 119; 1984, p. 137), without a doubt narcissistic rage belongs to the processes maintaining the delusion-like self and identity systems being discussed here. Examples of these systems can be found especially in personal and collective ideologies. The difference between aggression and destructiveness is considerable. Pure aggression, directed at the persons or objects standing in the way of gratification, disappears quickly after the goal has been reached. In contrast, the narcissistic rage is insatiable. The conscious and unconscious fantasies have then become independent of the events precipitating the aggressive rivalry and operate as insatiable forces of cold-blooded destruction.

For the treatment technique it is essential that the numerous injuries be identified that the patient *actually* experiences in the analytic situation, rather than perceives through the magnifying glass in exaggerated form. The childish powerlessness which is revived by the regression in the analytic situation reactively leads to ideas of omnipotence, which can take the place of direct controversies if the realistic precipitating factors in the here-and-now are not taken seriously. Narcissistic patients refuse to become involved in everyday aggressive conflicts because for them it immediately becomes a question of all or nothing. Because of their heightened sensitivity to injury, these patients are trapped within a vicious circle of unconscious fantasies of revenge. In the case of personal or collective ideologies, an enemy is created whose qualities facilitate projections. It can thus be observed with great regularity that narcissistic rage is transformed into everyday, relatively harmless aggressive rivalry if it has been possible in the analytic situation to trace the offenses back to their roots.

We quoted from Freud's letter to Einstein partly for technical reasons. Negative, aggressive transferences must be viewed in the context of whether it is possible to create significant common ground in the sense of Sterba's (1934, 1940) we-bond (see Chap. 2). Negative, aggressive transference also has a function with regard to regulating distance, since identifications arise by means of imitation and appropriation and this interpersonal exchange is inevitably connected with disturbances. Finding the optimal distance is crucial particularly for at-risk patients, who at first sight appear to require a special degree of support and empathy. A correctly understood professional neutrality, which has nothing to do with anonymity, contributes to this (T. Shapiro 1984).

The technical consequences we can draw from these considerations correspond to a certain extent to Kohut's recommendations. It is essential that the real stimulus in the here-and-now be linked to its incontestable meaning. This real stimulus can possibly even lie in the fact that the patient turns to the analyst for help. The question of how rapidly the analyst can move from the here-and-now of the injury to the then-and-there of the origin of increased sensitivity is a topic we will discuss against the background of case studies in volume two.

## 4.5 Secondary Gain from Illness

One of Freud's five forms of resistance was ego resistance, which "proceeds from the 'gain from illness' and is based upon an assimilation of the symptoms into the ego" (1926d, p. 160). In evaluating the external forces which codetermine and sustain the psychic illness, it is useful to bear in mind the distinction between primary and secondary gain from illness that Freud made in 1923 in a footnote to his account of the Dora case (1905e). Between 1905 and 1923 the ego was assigned a much greater significance in theory and technique with regard to the origin of symptoms, specifically relating to defense processes. According to the 1923 footnote: "The statement that the motives of illness are not present at the beginning of the illness, but only appear secondarily to it, cannot be maintained" (Freud 1905e, p.43). And in *Inhibitions, Symptoms and Anxiety* (1926d, p.98) Freud wrote, "But usually the outcome is different. The initial act of repression is followed by a tedious or interminable sequel in which the struggle against the instinctual impulse is prolonged into a struggle against the symptom."

Precisely a case exhibiting a stable structuring of symptoms is characterized by a course in which the primary conditions are so mixed with the secondary motives that they can hardly be distinguished.

In obsessional neurosis and paranoia the forms which the symptoms assume become very valuable to the ego because they obtain for it, not certain advantages, but a narcissistic satisfaction which it would otherwise be without. The systems which the obsessional neurotic constructs flatter his self-love by making him feel that he is better than other people because he is specially cleanly or specially conscientious. The delusional constructions of the paranoic offer to his acute perceptive and imaginative powers a field of activity which he could not easily find elsewhere.

All of this results in what is familiar to us as the "(secondary) gain from illness" which follows a neurosis. This gain comes to the assistance of the ego in its endeavor to incorporate the symptom and increases the symptom's fixation. When the analyst tries subsequently to help the ego in its struggle against the symptom, he finds that these conciliatory bonds between ego and symptom operate on the side of the resistances and that they are not easy to loosen. (Freud 1926d, pp.99-100)

Freud also comments on this topic in his *Introductory Lectures*:

This motive ["a self-interested motive on the part of the ego, seeking for protection and advantage"] tries to preserve the ego from the dangers the threat of which was the preciptitating cause of the illness and it will not allow recovery to occur until a repetition of these dangers seems no longer possible .... I have already shown that symptoms are supported by the ego, too, because they have a side with which they offer satisfaction to the repressing purpose of the ego .... You will easily realize that everything that contributes to the gain from illness will intensify the resistance due to repression and will increase the therapeutic difficulties .... When a psychical organization like an illness has lasted for some time, it behaves eventually like an independent organism .... (Freud 1916/17, pp.382, 384)

The secondary gain from illness amplifies the *circulus vitiosus*. The analyst should therefore pay special attention to the situative factors in and outside the analytic situation which maintain the symptoms. We attribute very great significance to secondary gain from illness, understood in a comprehensive sense, and deal with it in the sections on working through and restructuring in Chap. 8.

## 4.6 Identity Resistance and the Safety Principle

The reader will not have overlooked the fact that we have often referred to a uniform functional principle in addition to the numerous different resistance phenomena. We would now like to discuss this principle. In addition to the great differences between these phenomena, not amazing considering the complexity of the phenomena, there are also very revealing similarities. Independently of one another, analysts from different schools attribute to resistance and defense processes a function oriented on self-regulation and the safety principle. In Kohut's self psychology, instinctual gratification is subordinate to the self-feeling. Sandler (1960) subordinated the pleasure-unpleasure principle to the safety principle. In Erikson's *identity resistance*, the most important regulator is identity, which viewed phenomenologically is the Siamese twin of the self. Erikson provides the following description of identity resistance:

> We see here the most extreme form of what may be called *identity resistance* which, as such, far from being restricted to the patients described here, is a universal form of resistance regularly experienced but often unrecognized in the course of some analyses. Identity resistance is, in its milder and more usual forms, the patient's fear that the analyst, because of his particular personality, background, or philosophy, may carelessly or deliberately destroy the weak core of the patient's identity and impose instead his own. I would not hesitate to say that some of the much-discussed unsolved transference neuroses in patients, as well as in candidates in training, is the direct result of the fact that identity resistance often is, at best, analyzed only quite unsystematically. In such cases the analysand may resist throughout the analysis any possible inroad on his identity of the analyst's values while surrendering on all other points; or the patient may absorb more of the analyst's identity than is manageable within his own means; or he may leave the analysis with a lifelong sense of not having been provided with something essential owed him by the analyst.
>
> In cases of acute identity confusion, this identity resistance becomes the core problem of the therapeutic encounter. Variations of psychoanalytic technique have this one problem in common: the dominant resistance must be accepted as the main guide to technique, and interpretation must be fitted to the patient's ability to utilize it. In these cases the patient sabotages communication until he has settled some basic—if contradictory—issues. The patient insists that the therapist accept his negative identity as real and necessary—which it is, or rather was—without concluding that this negative identity is "all there is to him." If the therapist is able to fulfill both these demands, he must prove patiently through many severe crises that he can maintain understanding and affection for the patient without either devouring him or offering himself for a totem meal. Only then can better-known forms of transference, if ever so reluctantly, emerge. (Erikson 1968, pp. 214-215)

We do not disregard the differences between these conceptions. Kohut derives self-feeling and its regulation from narcissistic selfobjects, while Erikson's identity feeling and the identity resistance associated with it have a more psychosocial founding. While it is true that self-feeling and identity can hardly be differentiated phenomenologically, Kohut's and Erikson's different derivations have consequences for treatment technique. The same applies to the safety principle, which Henseler (1974, p. 75) linked closely to the theory of narcissism. The *safeguarding aspects* of the neurotic *life style* occupy much of Adler's theory. Freud (1914d, p. 53) considered Adler's word "safeguarding" to be better than his own term "protective measure."

We can again refer back to Freud's concept of self-preservation as "the highest good" and find there the best common denominator for resistance and defense. Who would doubt that self-preservation occupies an especially high, if not the highest, rank among the regulating factors, or "governors," as Quint (1984) recently documented using case studies. Self-preservation in the psychological sense is effective as a regulating factor by means of the unconscious and conscious contents which have been integrated in an individual's life to constitute the personal identity. The interpersonally developed sense of self, the self security, the self confidence etc. are themselves dependent on the satisfaction of certain internal and external conditions.

Many of these interdependences are in fact conceptually included in the structural theory of psychoanalysis. As soon as we discuss the concepts of superego and ego-ideal in clinical terms we tend to transform them into substances and call them internal objects, even though they are characterized by their motivational strength. This usage goes back to Freud's discovery that in the case of depressive self-accusations "the shadow of the object fell upon the ego" (1917e, p. 249).

As a result of the very expressive metaphor in Freud's description of internal objects it can be easily overlooked that these objects are in a context of action: a person does not identify himself with an isolated object, but with interactions (Loewald 1980, p. 48). That intrapsychic conflicts can arise through such identifications as a result of the incompatibility of some ideas and affects is one of the oldest items of knowledge in psychoanalysis. When Freud (1895d, p. 269) spoke of incompatible ideas against which the ego defends itself, the word "ego" was still colloquially used and equated with person and self. The obvious question is then why so much discussion is being devoted nowadays to self-regulation or the safety principle if they have always had a place in theory and technique and if the understanding of resistance and defense has been oriented on their safeguard, which also forms the background to structural theory. The limitation of ego psychology to intrapsychic conflicts and their derivation from the pleasure principle in the sense of the *instinctual discharge model* have proven to be a Procrustean bed too narrow for interpersonal oedipal conflicts — at any rate when the aim is to gain a comprehensive understanding of these conflicts. The rediscovery of holistic references and regulatory principles within two-person psychology — such as security, self-confidence, and object constancy — indirectly makes apparent what had been lost as a result of disorientation and fragmentation. Not that narcissistic pleasure had ever been forgotten in psychoanalysis, but by raising the pleasure gained in self-fulfillment to a principle Kohut not only rediscovered something old, but gave narcissism a new meaning.

Yet the numerous types of interdependence of self feeling can easily be overlooked if self feeling is made the primary regulatory principle. The patient's resistance is then quite logically understood as a protective measure against injuries and finally against the danger of self-disintegration. Kohut not only discarded the instinctual discharge model, but also neglected the dependence of self-confidence on psychosexual satisfaction. The effects of these new forms of one-sidedness are, however, in many cases favorable. This is not surprising considering that the self-psychological treatment technique conveys much confirmation and acknowledgement. In addition, the analyst's thematization of injuries as a result of a lack of empathy and his admission of this situation create an atmosphere favorable to therapy; they promote self-assertion, thus indirectly reducing many anxieties. So far, so good.

The problem consists in the fact that the patient's resistance is now understood as a protective measure against injuries and ultimately against the danger of self-disintegration, as if self-disintegration no longer required explanation. Self-disintegration is ontologized instead of psychoanalytic research being conducted into the extent to which, for example, unconscious aggressions assume the form of anxiety concerning the loss of structure (whether in the form of the end of the world or of one's own person). The sociologist Carveth (1984a, p. 79) has pointed to the consequences of the ontologization of fantasies: "It would seem that psychoanalysis (like social analysis) is perpetually in danger of conflating phenomenology (or psychology) with ontology, the description of what people imagine to be the case with statements of what is in fact the case." After describing Freud's understanding of women's lack of a penis as such a conflation, Carveth continues:

> Similarly, Kohut observed that many analysands suffering from narcissistic problems think of their "selves" as prone to fragmentation, disintegration, or enfeeblement under certain circumstances. It is one thing to describe such fragmentation fantasies; it is quite another to evolve a psychology of the self in which "the self" is actually thought of as some "thing" that can either cohere or fragment. (Carveth 1984a, p. 79)

In support of his criticism Carveth cites Slap and Levine (1978) and Schafer (1981), who represent similar points of view.

Kohut places special emphasis on the relationship-regulating function of selfobject transferences, and above all on everything that the patient seeks in the analyst, whether it be in the idealizing selfobject transference, in the twinship transference, or in the mirror transference. These signals emitted by the patient serve, in Kohuts opinion, to compensate for empathy deficiencies. Patients unconsciously seek to compensate defects, and the resistance has a protective function, i.e., to ward off new injuries. The grandiose or idealizing transferences are taken by the analyst as signs of early disturbances. These disturbances are not primarily frustrated gratifications of instincts but rather deficiencies in the confirmation which the child's self-feeling is dependent on.

Despite our criticism of Kohut's theory, we attach great value to his technical innovations. Yet at first glance it is surprising that in some cases the anxiety over structural disintegration can improve even though the unconscious aggressions in the transference relationship referred to above have not been worked through. This is probably associated with the fact that the promotion of self-assertion in Kohut's technique both indirectly actualizes the aggressive portions of personality and reduces the frustration aggression.

To what extent Kohut's transference interpretations have a specific effectiveness cannot in our opinion be answered. The regulation of self-feeling and the analyst's therapeutic contribution toward it have a special significance, regardless of the validity of individual aspects of interpretations. We would like to illustrate the advance in treatment technique attained by Kohut's ideas by referring to a self-psychological interpretation of narcissistic resistance, described by Abraham in 1919, which was at that time irresolvable.

Abraham (1953 [1919], p. 306) described a form of resistance for narcissistic and thus easily injured patients with labile ego feeling who identify with the doctor and behave like superanalysts instead of personally coming closer to him in the transference. Abraham's patient saw himself, so to speak, through the eyes of his analyst and made the interpretations he thought were accurate for himself. The author did not consider the possibility that such identifications may be indirect attempts to come closer. This is all the more surprising since it is Abraham to whom we thank the description of oral incorporation and the identification associated with it. Abraham was apparently not yet able to fruitfully apply the knowledge that primary identifications can be the earliest form of emotional attachment to an object (Freud 1921c, pp. 106-107; 1923b, pp. 29-30). Strachey (1934) later described the identification with the analyst as object relationship. More recently, Kohut has brought us closer to understanding the primary identifications in the different selfobject transferences and the technical ways of dealing with them. It is true, however, that Kohut on the other hand seems to neglect the fact that identifications have a defensive function and thus can subserve the resistance to independence.

# 5 Interpretation of Dreams

## 5.1 Dreams and Sleep

Ever since Freud's seminal study, the interpretation of dreams has been the most popular area of psychoanalytic theory and technique. The analyst's interpretations of dreams are as dependent on his conception of the function of dreaming as they are on his theory of the genesis of the dream and on the modification of the dream up to the moment of the manifest dream report. What dreams a patient remembers, the way in which he relates them, and the point at which he relates them in the particular session and in the framework of the analysis as a whole are all factors contributing to the interpretation. Not least, both the interest in dreams and the (sometimes more, sometimes less productive) way they are dealt with during treatment are critical for the interpretation of the dreams themselves and for the conduct of treatment in general.

In this introductory section we must briefly outline the most important findings of experimental dream research, even though doing so makes interpreting dreams appear more problematic than before. Freud's view that dreams are the guardian of sleep must now be regarded as disproved; on the contrary, sleep is the guardian of dreams (Wolman 1979, p. VII). This is one of the fundamental conclusions which must be drawn from the many psychobiological investigations of dream and sleep. The nature of the REM phases of sleep and their specific biological and psychological functions are nevertheless still a source of scientific controversy. H. Gill's (1982) description of REM phases as a third form of mental existence underlines once more the importance of Freud's basic approach, i.e., that dreams should be seen as a *via regia* to hidden aspects of human existence.

Two questions are central to current empirical dream research: one concerns the psychic function of dreams, the other, the affective cognitive processes of dream genesis (Strauch 1981). After the discovery of REM sleep, dream research aimed at establishing relationships between dreaming and physiological processes (Fisher 1965). More recently, though, disenchantment with this correlative research has been registered. Strauch (1981), for instance, urges a return to genuinely psychological types of problems. The goal is to reestablish the significance of dreaming as a psychological phenomenon. Freud travelled a similar path to reach his *Interpretation of Dreams* (1900a). His route has been traced by Schott (1981) in a comparative study of the development of Freud's theories. Even though we have not reached the same point of departure — some important postulates of Freud's dream theory (though not those of interpretation) have been refuted — it remains clear that physiological conditions and psychological meanings belong to completely different dimensions.

Even in the future, it can hardly be expected that the established methods of dream interpretation as practiced by the various schools of psychotherapy will be influenced by the results of dream research. Dreaming has a value of its own in the therapeutic process, even if the underlying dream theories have to be modified. (Strauch 1981, p. 43)

Research into sleep and dreaming over the past 30 years has already done much to modify our conception of dreaming. The future will show whether and how this influences the practice of dream interpretation.

## 5.2 Dream Thinking

One of the thorny theoretical problems regarding dreams and dreaming is that of reaching an appropriate understanding of the relationship between image and thought. Freud himself addresses this problem in a footnote added in 1925 to *The Interpretation of Dreams*:

I used at one time to find it extraordinarily difficult to accustom readers to the distinction between the manifest content of dreams and the latent dream-thoughts. Again and again arguments and objections would be brought up based upon some uninterpreted dream in the form in which it had been retained in the memory, and the need to interpret it would be ignored. But now that analysts at least have become reconciled to replacing the manifest dream by the meaning revealed by its interpretation, many of them have become guilty of falling into another confusion which they cling to with equal obstinacy. They seek to find the essence of dreams in their latent content and in so doing they overlook the distinction between the latent dream-thoughts and the dream-work. At bottom, dreams are nothing other than a particular *form* of thinking, made possible by the conditions of the state of sleep. It is the *dream-work* which creates that form, and it alone is the essence of dreaming — the explanation of its peculiar nature. I say this in order to make it possible to assess the value of the notorious "prospective purpose" of dreams. The fact that dreams concern themselves with attempts at solving the problems by which our mental life is faced is no more strange than that our conscious waking life should do so; beyond this it merely tells us that that activity can also be carried on in the preconscious — and this we already knew. (1900 a, pp. 506-507)

The immediate characteristics of dreams are, according to Freud (1933 a, p. 19), manifestations of the phylogenetically more ancient modes of operation of the mental apparatus which can come to the fore during regression in the sleeping state. Thus, he described dream language in the 13th of the *Introductory Lectures on Psycho-Analysis* (1916/17) as being characterized by archaic traits. Dream language, which predates our development of thought language, is a picture language rich in symbolic relationships. Accordingly, man's use of symbols transcends the limits of the respective language communities (1923 a, p. 242). Condensation, displacement, and plastic representation are the processes which determine form. In contrast to the waking state, in which thinking proceeds in gradations and differentiations and is oriented around logical distinctions in space and time, in sleep there is regression, with boundaries becoming blurred. This blurring of boundaries can be felt when falling asleep. Freud described the wish to sleep as a motif for the induction of this regression.

The formal elements of dream language are termed "dream work," which Freud summarized as follows: "The achievements I have enumerated exhaust its activity; it can do no more than condense, displace, represent in plastic form and subject the whole to a secondary revision" (1916/17, p. 182). The dreamer represents the world, including his self, differently than in his waking thinking and in his everyday language. Thus the problem is not just to describe the formal characteristics of dream language; the difficulty lies in their translation. Thoughts are transformed into images, and images are described in words (Spence 1982a). The direction in which the translation is made, i.e., whether from thought language into dream language or vice versa, is by no means a matter of indifference. On the contrary, keeping this in mind makes it possible to understand some of the contradictions which affect the relationship of images to latent dream thoughts and have also determined the rules of translation relevant to the psychoanalytic interpretation of dreams. The inner perceptions which are still possible under the conditions of sleep probably have to be interpreted as visual metaphors; a decisive determinant of this is the neurological process of distribution of the stimuli in the brain.

These translation rules concern the relationships between dream elements and the latent meaning elements they represent, which Freud, with strange vagueness, called "the 'genuine' thing" (1916/17, p. 151). In the *Introductory Lectures*, he initially distinguished "three such relationships — those of a part to a whole, of allusion and of plastic portrayal." The fourth is the symbolic relationship (1916/17, pp. 151, 170). According to Freud, the relationship between symbol and dream element is constant, and this facilitates translation:

> Since symbols are stable translations, they realize to some extent the ideal of the ancient as well as of the popular interpretation of dreams, from which, with our technique, we had departed widely. They allow us in certain circumstances to interpret a dream without questioning the dreamer, who indeed would in any case have nothing to tell us about the symbol. If we are acquainted with the ordinary dream-symbols, and in addition with the dreamer's personality, the circumstances in which he lives and the impressions which preceded the occurrence of the dream, we are often in a position to interpret a dream straightaway — to translate it at sight, as it were. (1916/17, p. 151)

This view is based on the assumption that the dreamer himself is incapable of associations endowing the symbol with meaning, because his regression in the therapeutic situation is insufficient to allow him direct access to the picture language.

What we are now concerned with is the nature of the relationship between the manifest and the latent dream element, or, as Freud put it, the relationship between dream elements and their "'genuine' thing." From the very outset there are great difficulties in understanding this relationship, as Freud himself makes clear: the manifest dream element is not so much a distortion of the latent as "a representation of it, a plastic, concrete portrayal of it, taking its start from the wording. But precisely on that account it is once more a distortion, for we have long since forgotten from what concrete image the word originated and consequently fail to recognize it when it is replaced by the image" (1916/17, p. 121). Our attention is drawn here to the basic problem of the relationship of word and image. Dream language expresses itself predominantly in visual images, and the task of therapeutic translation consists of transforming images into words and thoughts. Although thoughts must be viewed as secondary in regard to the original representation, they are of primary importance for therapy because thoughts expressed in words make the therapeutic dialogue possible. We hope we can now make it clear why the concept of latent dream thought underwent a profound change of meaning in Freud's writings: initially identical with the day residue, it eventually becomes "the 'genuine' thing" of the dream, transformed by the dream work into the manifest dream and now translated back, so to speak, by the interpretive work — *the dream work is retransformed by the interpretive work.* In contradiction to the primacy of picture language, in a certain sense the latent dream thought now takes its place on the deepest level, where it in turn fuses with the wish requiring translation.

We can now illustrate this argument by describing the transformation in meaning undergone by the latent dream thought. Freud started from the concept of interpretive work, and it was natural at the outset for him to equate the day residues (the dream motif) with the latent dream thoughts (1916/17, p. 199). In the theory of dream work, i.e., of dream genesis, the latent dream thoughts are transposed under the influence of dream censorship into a different mode of expression, which "harks back to states of our intellectual development which have long since been superseded — to picture-language, to symbolic connections, to conditions, perhaps, which existed before our thought-language had developed. We have on that account described the mode of expression of the dream-work as *archaic* or *regressive*" (1916/17, p. 199). Today we would say rather that the work on the dream is carried out with regressive methods. With the definitive change in meaning, "everything we learn in interpreting the dream" is termed latent dream thoughts (1916/17, p. 226). The great predominance of the interpretive work over the theory of dream genesis is clear from the identification of the dream censor with the resistance to the uncovering of the latent dream thoughts, which in turn represent, above all, wishes repressed to different levels. This predominance of wishes among the latent dream thoughts is explained on the one hand by the universal significance of the world of wishes, and on the other by the special attention paid by psychoanalysts from the very outset to the wishful aspect of dreams. Freud's general point of view — i.e., that dreams are in essence nothing else than a special form of our thinking (1900 a, p. 506) — was neglected until Erikson published "The Dream Specimen of Psychoanalysis" (1954).

Systematic studies have now made it possible to ascertain whether dream thinking is complementary to waking thinking or whether the one blends into the other. Some findings indicate that there is a correspondence between daydreaming and night dreaming, and it can be shown that distortion and expression of affect increase progressively from daydreams through fantasies to night dreams. It has also been shown that it is possible to identify sex-specific differences for certain needs (Strauch 1981, p. 27). Generally, it is now thought that the configuration of the dream contents reflects the principal personality traits of the dreamer (Cohen 1976, p. 334).

This perspective has also gained support from the results of broad-based investigations carried out by Foulkes in the field of developmental psychology (1977, 1979, 1982). Foulkes pointed out the parallelism in cognitive and emotional development between the waking state and the dream report. Giora (1981, p. 305) also underlines the danger of taking only the clinical material into consideration and neglecting the existence of other types of dreams, e.g., logical and problem-solving dreams, when discussing the theory of dreams. We now know that dreams in REM sleep tend to be irrational and those in non-REM sleep rational, which suggests that the primary-process mechanisms of dream work are linked to specific physiological conditions. Ferenczi (1955 [1912]) was already thinking along these lines when he reported on "dirigible" dreams. These dreams are deliberately shaped by the dreamer, who rejects unsatisfactory versions. We can sum up by saying that currently many authors reject theories which accord dream thinking a special status, preferring instead to integrate dream thinking into the general principles of psychic function.

Based on EEG examinations, pharmacological experiments, and theoretical considerations, Koukkou and Lehmann (1980, 1983) formulated a "state fluctuation model" which centers on the idea that the brain shifts between different functional states, each of which has its own selectively accessible memory stores. According to this model, the formal characteristics of dreams (i.e., the product of the primary process and the dream work) result from:

1. Recall during sleep of memory material (actual events, thought strategies, symbols, and fantasies) which was stored during development and which in the adult waking state either cannot be read completely or has been so heavily adapted to the here-and-now by the waking thought strategies that it is no longer recognizable. Also recall of new (recent) memory material and its reinterpretation according to the thought strategies of the functional states during sleep.
2. Fluctuations of the functional state in various stages of sleep (much more narrowly defined and much shorter than the four classical EEG stages) which occur spontaneously or as a response to new stimuli or signalling stimuli during sleep. This results in the transformation of contents in the course of shifting between memory stores (functional states) and leads to
3. The formation of new associations, which, in the absence of an alteration of functional state to the waking state, cannot be adapted to current reality, as the sleeper employs the thought strategies of the functional state (developmental level) he is in (Koukkou and Lehmann 1980, p. 340).

## 5.3 Day Residue and Infantile Wish

There is hardly a step in Freud's theory of dreams bolder than the one linking the attempt at wish fulfillment with the postulate that this must be an infantile wish, i.e., "the discovery that in point of fact *all* dreams are children's dreams, that they work with the same infantile material, with the mental impulses and mechanisms of childhood" (1916/17, p. 213). In *The Interpretation of Dreams*, Freud gives, in contrast to the infantile wish, an impressive wealth of evidence for the operational effectiveness of wishes which originate in the present, and for motives which Kanzer (1955) termed the "communicative function" of dreams. In addition, we must remember Freud's distinction between dream source and dream motor; the selection of material "from any part of the dreamer's life" (Freud 1900a, p. 169) and the introduction of this material as causal moment of the dream are two quite separate things.

We believe that Freud retained the concept of the primacy of the infantile wish for heuristic reasons and on grounds of treatment technique. We will not go into the question of how often interpretation has succeeded in convincingly tracing dream genesis back from the day residues (the immediate precipitating factors) to infantile wishes, and showing the latter to be the deeper, more essential causes. Freud illustrated the relationship between the day residues and the (infantile) unconscious wish by comparing it to a commercial enterprise, which always needs a capitalist to provide the financing and an entrepreneur with an idea and the vision to carry it through. The capitalist is the unconscious wish, supplying the psychic energy for dream formation, the entrepreneur is the day residue. However, the capitalist could also have the idea, or the entrepreneur the capital. Thus the metaphor remains open: this simplifies the situation in practice, but impedes the attempt to understand it theoretically (Freud 1916/17, p. 226).

Later, Freud (1933a) transformed this metaphor into the theory of dream genesis from above (from the day residue) and from below (from the unconscious wish). The fact that the capitalist is equated in the original metaphor with the psychic energy which he provides reflects Freud's assumption concerning energy economy, in which psychic energy is seen as the basic force behind the stimulus, the force which creates the wish and presses for its fulfillment — even if only through a kind of abreaction in the form of hallucinatory gratification. (One can also borrow a term from ethology and call such abreactions vacuum activities in the absence of the instinct-gratifying object.)

One consequence of this theoretical assumption is that, strictly speaking, discovery of the infantile wish by interpretation must involve the rediscovery and reproduction of the original situation in which a wish, a need, or an instinctual stimulus arose but was not gratified, and therefore no genuine abreaction to the object could take place. It was against this hypothetical background that Freud voiced the expectation, even to patients themselves — as we know from the case of the Wolf Man — that penetration of the screen memory would reveal the original situation of wish and frustration (the primal scene). According to the Wolf Man, Freud's expectation was not met, i.e., the screen memory was not penetrated and the Wolf Man did not remember the primal scene. The Wolf Man's later life is well documented (Gardiner 1971), and the conclusion can be drawn that his relapses — indeed the very fact that his illness became chronic — were due far less to inadequate illumination of infantile, incestuous temptation and frustration situations than to his idealization of Freud (and psychoanalysis) as a defense against a recent negative transference.

Implicit in this assumption that infantile wishes are the dream motor is a theory of the storage of memories. This theory was conceived by Freud in *The Interpretation of Dreams* (1900a, Chap. 7) and had considerable consequences on the structuring of psychoanalytic treatment in that it laid the emphasis on remembering and on discharge of excitation. Although it is only rarely possible for the infantile wish and its environment to be reconstructed or affectively and cognitively revived with any confidence, the illumination of childhood amnesia is the ideal, particularly for more orthodox psychoanalysts. This is especially true for the time from which, for psychobiological reasons, there can probably be only sensorimotor memories. The plausibility of such reconstructions is one thing, but their therapeutic effectiveness is another, as Freud indicated clearly enough when he said: "Quite often we do not succeed in bringing the patient to recollect what has been repressed. Instead of that, if the analysis is carried out correctly, we produce in him an assured conviction of the truth of their construction which achieves the same therapeutic result as a recaptured memory" (1937d, pp. 265-266). Occasionally, subsequent questioning of the patient's mother provides support for the plausibility of reconstructions, by yielding final confirmation of events which had been assumed from the outset and apparently already verified during analysis (e.g., Segal 1982). What value such data have in connection with the subjective truth of the fantasy life and with the alteration of the latter under the influence of treatment is a problem which we cannot go into here (see Spence 1982a).

As we have seen, there are many aspects to the demonstration of the existence of the unconscious, infantile dream wish, and we can only touch on its clinical relevance. We can summarize by saying that there are gaps in the theory of wish fulfillment with regard to demonstrating the unconscious, infantile wish element, and that this leads to other problems, e.g., how to reconcile stereotypical anxiety dreams with the theory.

The day residue functions as an affective bridge between thinking in the waking state and dream thinking. The identification of the day residue, by reference to the patient's associations, usually leads to a first, immediate understanding of the dream. This bridge function can be seen particularly clearly in experimental dream research, when subjects are woken in the night and questioned about their dreams. Greenberg and Pearlman (1975, p. 447) observed this process from the perspective of the psychoanalytic situation, and underlined the relatively undistorted incorporation of affect-charged events into the manifest dream.

However, referring to Schur's (1966) supplementary comments on Freud's Irma dream, we emphasize that a restricted conception of "day residue" obscures any links there might be with events lying somewhat further in the past. Freud's own associations to the Irma dream soon led him back to the covert criticism made by his friend Otto, who the previous evening had informed him of Irma's not altogether satisfactory condition. Freud did not mention, in *The Interpretation of Dreams*, the extremely critical situation with regard to the patient Emma a few months after she had been operated on by his friend Fliess. For Freud, the day residue stands at the intersection of two associative lines, one of which leads to the infantile wish, the other to the present wish: "From every element in a dream's content associative threads branch out in two or more directions" (1901a, p.648). If we free ourselves from the dichotomy of current and infantile wish sources and adopt instead the concept of the associative network according to which past and present become entwined in many temporal stratifications (Palombo 1973), we gain access to the thesis that the main function of dreaming is the development, maintenance (regulation) and, when necessary, the restoration of psychic processes, structures, and organization (Fosshage 1983, p.657).

We know very little about whether the control of these assimilative and adaptive processes in the psychic *milieu interne* always requires recourse to infantile, repressed wishes, or whether this is necessary only in selected cases, i.e., when a recent conflict begins to resonate with an unsolved infantile conflict situation. Speculative, but nevertheless highly interesting, is Koukkou and Lehmann's (1980, 1983) neurophysiological thesis that the variation in EEG patterns in the REM phases strongly suggests that the doorway to early memories might be open several times each night, in which case exchange processes between present and past may well take place.

Freud's idea that the infantile wish is the motor of dream formation has not been confirmed, and in light of the findings of modern research must be rejected as superfluous. He formulated this hypothesis before it became known that dreaming is a biologically based activity that is controlled by an internal clock and needs no foundation in the psychic economy. We must ask which of the dreams recalled and recorded by means of the REM technique in dream research would actually be remembered in psychoanalysis, and which would have fulfilled their psychological function by being dreamed and *not* remembered. Nevertheless, it is clinically relevant which dreams are remembered and to whom they are told. The communicative function of dreaming (Kanzer 1955) remains a purely psychological-psychoanalytic question which has a different relevance for each of the three areas which are considered important: problem solving, information processing, and ego consolidation. These perspectives are not mutually exclusive, as Dallet (1973) rightly pointed out, and the empirical support for them differs greatly. As we saw above in the discussion of dream thinking (Sect. 5.2), over the years the hypothesis that the function of dreaming is mainly to help deal with reality has lost ground to the view that it is important for the dreamer's intrapsychic equilibrium and for the maintenance of his psychic functions. We will now present some of the important contributions to the development of the theory of dreams.

### *5.3.1 Wish Fulfillment Theory: A Unifying Principle of Explanation*

Freud clearly felt it important to have a uniform principle of explanation and to stick to it, despite all the theoretical and practical difficulties he encountered, which we will elaborate on below. He sought to solve these difficulties by equipping the wish, in its capacity as the motive force of dream genesis, with theoretical powers comprising many elements from various sources. Freud preferred this move toward uniformity to other approaches as early as 1905, though without providing a convincing justification.

I argued in my book, *The Interpretation of Dreams* (1900a), that every dream is a wish which is represented as fulfilled, that the representation acts as a disguise if the wish is a repressed one, belonging to the unconscious, and that except in the case of children's dreams only an unconscious wish or one which reaches down into the unconscious has the force necessary for the formation of a dream. I fancy my theory would have been more certain of general acceptance if I had contented myself with maintaining that every dream had a meaning, which could be discovered by means of a certain process of interpretation; and that when the interpretation had been completed the dream could be replaced by thoughts which would fall into place at an easily recognizable point in the waking mental life of the dreamer. I might then have gone on to say that the meaning of a dream turned out to be of as many different sorts as the processes of waking thought; that in one case it would be a fulfilled wish, an another a realized fear, or again a reflection persisting on into sleep, or an intention (as in the instance of Dora's dream), or a piece of creative thought during sleep, and so on. Such a theory would no doubt have proved attractive from its very simplicity, and it might have been supported by a great many examples of dreams that had been satisfactorily interpreted, as for instance by the one which has been analyzed in these pages.

But instead of this I formulated a generalization according to which the meaning of dreams is limited to a single form, to the representation of *wishes*, and by so doing I aroused a universal inclination to dissent. I must, however, observe that I did not consider it either my right or my duty to simplify a psychological process so as to make it more acceptable to my readers, when my researches had shown me that it presented a complication which could not be reduced to uniformity until the inquiry had been carried into another field. It is therefore of special importance to me to show that apparent exceptions — such as this dream of Dora's, which has shown itself in the first instance to be the continuation into sleep of an intention formed during the day — nevertheless lend fresh support to the rule which is in dispute. (Freud 1905e, pp. 67-68)

In order to be able to adhere to the uniform principle of explanation, Freud had to undertake great theoretical and conceptual efforts, which we will now briefly summarize. The genesis, nature, and function of the dream are founded in the attempt to eliminate psychic stimuli by means of hallucinatory gratification (Freud 1916/17, p. 136). One component of this teleological functional theory is the thesis that the dream, or the dream compromise, is the guardian of sleep, helping to fulfill the desire to remain in the sleeping state (Freud 1933a, p. 19).

Expansion of the concepts of wish and gratification allowed even those dreams which appeared to contradict wish fulfillment theory — so-called punishment dreams — to be integrated into it. The understanding of the dream as a compromise between various tendencies made it possible for the essential motivation for the form taken by the manifest dream to be attributed sometimes to the wish for sleep, and sometimes to the need for self-punishment, interpreted as a wish and located in the superego.

It was also possible to incorporate into the traditional teleological functional theory the fact that people sometimes wake up during anxiety dreams. This was accomplished by means of the supplementary hypothesis that in nightmares, the guardian of sleep reverses its normal role and interrupts the sleep to stop the dream from becoming even more frightening. Many attempts to mitigate the anxiety can then theoretically be accommodated around this emergency function, e.g., the sleeper's simultaneous awareness that "it's only a dream." This interpretation of anxiety dreams is based on the hypothesis of protection against stimuli, and more broadly on Freud's economic hypothesis, which is of course also embodied in the idea that the dream constitutes an attempt to eliminate psychic stimuli by means of hallucinatory gratification.

The contradictions and inconsistancies in the explanations of dreaming based on wish fulfillment theory cannot simply be eliminated. The fact that Freud nonetheless always considered the wish to be the motive force in dreaming is presumably connected with *psychoanalytic heuristics*. In Sect. 3.1 we have emphasized that there were good reasons for the fact that psychoanalytic heuristics is oriented on the pleasure principle, i.e., on the dynamic of unconscious desires (see also Sects. 8.2 and 10.2). It is important, however, to distinguish between the *discovery* of unconscious desires, that the psychoanalytic method can disclose, and the *explanation* of dreaming and dream work as the expression of desires (see Sect. 10.2). Wishes and longings will influence human life day and night even after metapsychology and its fundamental principle (drive economy) are dead, that is, can no longer be viewed as the foundation of wish fulfillment theory.

### *5.3.2 Self-Representation and Problem Solving*

We now want to deal with the reasons why, with regard to ego formation, so much more emphasis was placed on wish theory than on the significance of identification, which can also be recognized in many dreams. Already in Freud's *Project for a Scientific Psychology* (1950 a), we find the noteworthy sentence: "The aim and end of all thought processes is thus to bring about a *state of identity*" (p. 332). In some ways, this idea in this context addresses for the first time a problem that goes far beyond the realm of dream language and was later discussed in connection with Romain Rolland's "oceanic feeling" of man's community with space (see Freud 1930 a, pp. 64-66).

Let us suppose that the object which furnishes the perception resembles the subject — a *fellow human-being*. If so, the theoretical interest [taken in it] is also explained by the fact that an object *like this* was simultaneously the [subject's] first satisfying object and further his first hostile object, as well as his sole helping power. For this reason it is in relation to a fellow human-being that a human-being learns to cognize. Then the perceptual complexes proceeding from this fellow human-being will in part be new and non-comparable — his *features*, for instance, in the visual sphere; but other visual perceptions — e.g. those of the movements of his hands — will coincide in the subject with memories of quite similar visual impressions of his own, of his own body, [memories] which are associated with memories of movements experienced by himself. Other perceptions of the object too — if, for instance, he screams — will awaken the memory of his own experiences of pain. (Freud 1950 a, p. 331).

We refer back to this passage from the *Project for a Scientific Psychology* because here visual and motor perception of one's self and the other are linked with gratification through the object. In the wish fulfillment theory of dreams, gratification has become separated from the cognitive visual processes. Since we would like to stress the major and long underestimated importance of these processes for an empirically founded self psychology, this passage, which gives Freud a place in the genealogy of symbolic interactionism, is particularly opportune. Consider Cooley's neat rhyme: "Each to each a looking-glass reflects the other that doth pass" (1964 [1902], p. 184). We will deal with the consequences of incorporating these processes into the theory and practice of dream interpretation in the following, but can say already that doing so relativizes wish fulfillment theory without robbing it of its heuristic and therapeutic significance. Wish fulfillment theory had to be furnished with more and more supplementary hypotheses, diminishing rather than increasing the importance of the wish in the sense of instinctual wish; in addition, there was the problem of the theory's power to explain the polymorphic phenomenology of dreaming (Siebenthal 1953; Snyder 1970).

In contrast to wish fulfillment theory, whose inner contradictions led him to make repeated additions and amendments, Freud never had to revise his statement in *The Interpretation of Dreams*: "It is my experience, and one to which I have found no exception, that every dream deals with the dreamer himself" (1900a, p.322). We would like to quote fully his elaboration of this statement, which was repeated almost word for word in his later work:

> Dreams are completely egoistic. Whenever my own ego does not appear in the content of the dream, but only some extraneous person, I may safely assume that my own ego lies concealed, by identification, behind this other person; I can insert my ego into the context. On other occasions, when my own ego *does* appear in the dream, the situation in which it occurs may teach me that some other person lies concealed, by identification, behind my ego. In that case the dream should warn me to transfer on to myself, when I am interpreting the dream, the concealed common element attached to this other person. There are also dreams in which my ego appears along with other people who, when the identification is resolved, are revealed once again as my ego. These identifications should then make it possible for me to bring into contact with my ego certain ideas whose acceptance has been forbidden by the censorship. Thus my ego may be represented in a dream several times over, now directly and now through identification with extraneous persons. By means of a number of such identifications it becomes possible to condense an extraordinary amount of thought-material. The fact that the dreamer's own ego appears several times, or in several forms, in a dream is at bottom no more remarkable than that the ego should be contained in a conscious thought several times or in different places or connections — e.g. in the sentence "when *I* think what a healthy child *I* was". (1900a, pp.322-323)

In a footnote, Freud gives a rule to follow when in doubt regarding which of the figures appearing in the dream conceals the ego: "the person who in the dream feels an emotion which I myself experience in my sleep is the one who conceals my ego."

In Freud's later observations that the figure who plays the leading role in the dream is always oneself (1916/17, p.142; 1917d, p.223), this fact is again attributed to the narcissism of the sleeping state and to the loss of interest in the entire external world, narcissism here being equated with egoism. Incidentally, it is also possible to establish a link to wish fulfillment theory, since self-representation always includes wishes. Thus the dreamer always has unfulfilled wishes, be they ungratified instinctual needs or products of man's unique creative fantasy.

The narcissism of the sleeping state and the regressive form of thinking in dreams may correspond to a loss of interest in the external world if "interest" and "external world" are understood in the way that the distinction between subject and object seems to decree; we believe, however, that the interest is linked with the external world in a deeper sense, eliminating the subject-object,

I-you differentiation in order to achieve identity via identifications. Rereading the passage quoted above particularly attentively, it becomes even clearer that Freud is talking about *self-representation* through *identification*, i.e., about the establishment of commonality. However, the dreamer is egoistic inasmuch as he can give his thoughts and wishes free rein, without any regard for the animate or inanimate object referred to (the same goes for daydreams). From the developmental standpoint, the fact that self-representation in dreams can make use of the other persons and of animals and inanimate objects can be attributed to the primary lack of separation. This is the origin of the magic of thoughts, as well as that of gestures and actions.

To date, psychoanalysis has accorded greater therapeutic and theoretical significance to wish fulfillment via the object and to the role of the object relationship in dreams than to Freud's basic thesis that the dreamer always dreams about himself (often represented by others). In addition to the factors already mentioned, we believe that other reasons for this can be found in the history of psychoanalysis. Wish fulfillment theory, together with the instinct theories which substantiate it, served to distinguish psychoanalysis from Jung's theory of dreams. Jung first introduced the self as the subjective element, contrasting his "constructive" understanding to the reductive analytical one. Later he expanded his "constructive method" considerably, altering his terminology somewhat in the process:

> I call every interpretation which equates the dream images with real objects an interpretation on the objective level. In contrast to this is the interpretation which refers every part of the dream and all the actors in it back to the dreamer himself. This I call interpretation on the subjective level. Interpretation on the objective level is analytic, because it breaks down the dream content into complexes of memory that refer to external situations. Interpretation on the subjective level is synthetic, because it detaches the underlying complexes of memory from their external causes, regards them as tendencies or components of the subject, and reunites them with that subject. (In any experience I experience not merely the object but first and foremost myself, provided of course that I render myself an account of the experience.) In this case, therefore, all the contents of the dream are treated as symbols for subjective contents.
>
> Thus the synthetic or constructive process of interpretation is interpretation on the subjective level. (Jung 1972 [1912], p. 83)

The use of the subject level becomes Jung's most important heuristic principle, and he states that the relationships initially understood as being at the object level should also be raised to the subject level (1972 [1912], pp. 94-95). At the same time, the subject level disregards not only the personal ego and the representation of subjective attributes through other figures in the dream, but also the biographical background of such representations. Everything personal is embedded in archetypes, the interpretation of which also gives the objects a deeper meaning. Other figures in the dream are viewed not as substitutes for the dreamer's own ego, but as exponents of archetypal patterns, i.e., schemata which govern life and determine the form taken by intrapersonal affective cognitive processes as well as interpersonal experience and action. In Jung's image of man, the life cycle is understood as an assimilation of unconscious archetypal images. At the center of this assimilation is the self:

> The beginnings of our whole psychic life seem to be inextricably rooted in this point [the self], and all our highest and ultimate purposes seem to be striving towards it .... I hope it has become sufficiently clear to the attentive reader that the self has as much to do with the ego as the sun with the earth. (Jung 1972 [1928], p. 236)

Jung's theory of archetypes and Freud's theory of symbols meet at the point where Freud assumes the existence of general supraindividual structures of meaning. Since the configuration of these structures depends on individual and socioculturally imparted experience, the Freudian psychoanalytic interpretation of dreams cannot look on self-representations as manifestations of archetypal contents. Some analysts, though, are of the opinion that self-images do have archaic contents, and this can be illustrated using the example of Kohut's perception of the self-state dream.

In addition to the normal, well-known type of dream, whose latent contents (such as instinctual wishes, conflicts, and attempts to solve problems) can, in principle, be verbalized, Kohut believes he has discovered a second type, which he calls the "self-state dream." With these dreams, free association leads not to deeper understanding, but at best to images which remain on the same level as the manifest content of the dream. Investigation of the manifest content and the associative enrichment indicates that the healthy elements of the patient react with anxiety to the unsettling changes in the state of the self, e.g., its threatened disintegration. As a whole, then, dreams of this second type are to be comprehended as plastic representations of a menacing disintegration of the self.

Kohut explained this using the example of dreams of flying. In particular, we refer the reader to three dreams which he first mentioned in 1971 (pp. 4, 149) and to which he drew attention again in 1977 (p. 109). Briefly, Kohut views dreams of flying as highly threatening representations of the grandiose self, the danger being the disintegration which he equates with the appearance of a psychosis. This is the source of the interpretation — which Kohut does not want confused with a supportive maneuver — according to which various events in the patient's life, including the interruption of the analysis, revive old grandiose delusions. The patient fears that they will reappear, but even his dreams clearly show that he can overcome the problem with humor (Kohut 1977, p. 109). Kohut sees in humor a kind of sublimation and conquest of narcissistic delusions of grandeur, i.e., a kind of distancing (see also French and Fromm's [1964] concept of "deanimation" as a defense and a means of facilitating problem solving).

Nothing is more natural than to see dreams of flying as self-representations and wish dreams. For people today, unlike Icarus, flying is a realistic experience. We believe that the consequences which developments in technology have for the formation of unconscious schemata should be investigated in more detail before venturing anything so definite as Kohut's statement that dreams of flying are particularly alarming representations of the grandiose self. And beyond the practical questions of treatment technique, such interpretations show what consequences theoretical assumptions can have if they are taken as proved. Kohut requires no associations to interpret these dreams, because they are allegedly at an archaic level of function. However, we regard this — like the general question of the interpretation of symbols — as an unclarified problem in the psychoanalytic theory of the interpretation of dreams.

Lüders (1982) distinguishes between self dreams and object relationship dreams, but seems to accept that dreams featuring interacting figures can also be interpreted from the point of view of the self. He emphasizes that dreams are interpretations, though without the regulation and the control which in waking consciousness both indicate and betray the activity of the ego. In his view it is the contradiction between the self-concept and the real self, the imagined and the actual capacity to act, which determines the shape that dreams take. Either the self-concept has been modified without this affecting the real self, or the actual capacity to act has undergone an unsymbolized modification. The changes which have expanded or restricted the capacity to act can be positive or negative; in either case the dreamer learns, through the interpretation, what condition his real self is in and what potential he has for recognition and action at the time of the dream, how he really feels, and what sort of mood he is in. Whether the dreams are of flying or falling, dying or being born, about the dreamer's mother or the analyst, each dream individually translates the unperceived, unsymbolized alteration in the dreamer's capacity to act, and every interpretation of a dream clarifies and differentiates the self-image he has constructed.

With this conception of the self aspect of dreams, Lüders underlines their problem-solving function, seeing each manifest dream as an interpretation of the dreamer's unconscious state of mind and assigning central importance to the integrative function of the analyst's interpretation (as French [1952, p. 71] had done; see also French and Fromm [1964]). We also particularly share Lüders' categorical opinion that "every scene and person is a metaphor which illustates the invisible and unarticulated dynamic and whose meaning can only be ascertained with the help of the dreamer's associations and memories. The language of the dream is private, not universal" (1982, p. 828).

Since Freud, an increasing number of functions have been ascribed to dreaming, that is to say, wish fulfillment theory has been enriched. One important extension of Freud's theory is French's (1952) suggestion that dreams should be viewed as attempts at problem solving and that consideration be given not only to the wish itself but also to the obstacles standing in the way of the wish, of its fulfillment, and of conscious awareness of it. In their further elaboration of this idea, French and Fromm (1964) see two major differences between Freud's theory of dreams and their own. The first is Freud's one-sided theoretical interest in the infantile wish, which he sees as the essential motor of the dream work. The second lies in the fact that Freud's technique of reconstructing the dream work is essentially limited to following up chains of associations. French and Fromm, in contrast, do not consider thought processes to be a chain-like succession of separate items, but rather view thinking as something which proceeds in "Gestalten" (p. 89).

The "problem solving" spotlighted by French and Fromm (1964) does not remain general, as it is a personal, ubiquitous, and never-completed task for every individual. At various points French and Fromm limit the term to social adaptation, thus giving problem solving a more specific meaning with emphasis on relationship conflicts.

The relationship between a dream and an attempt at problem solving comes up in Freud's work after 1905, in the *Introductory Lectures* (1916/17, p. 222):

For it is quite correct to say that a dream can represent and be replaced by everything you have just enumerated — an intention, a warning, a reflection, a preparation, an attempt at solving a problem, and so on. But if you look properly, you will see that all this only applies to the latent dream-thoughts, which have been transformed into the dream. You learn from interpretations of dreams that people's unconscious thinking is concerned with these intentions, preparations, reflections, and so on, out of which the dream-work then makes the dreams.

Freud went on to clarify some concepts and then to ask (p. 223): "The latent dream-thoughts are the material which the dream-work transforms into the manifest dream. Why should you want to confuse the material with the activity which forms it?" In the ensuing reflections Freud underlined once more the function of the dream as wish fulfillment.

The theory of dreams was considerably influenced by philosophical speculation concerning compulsive repetition. The alternative, psychologically more plausible explanation — which Freud had contemplated for recurring anxiety dreams, and from which, in contrast to the death instinct hypothesis, useful therapeutic measures can be derived — was relegated to the sidelines. This leads us to plead even more strongly that the motivational interpretation of anxiety dreams be treated as an attempt to master difficult traumatic situations.

In practice, the introduction of the concept of the death instinct affected only those analysts who incorporated it, as a latent image of the world or of man, into the clinical theory of psychoanalysis. Most analysts followed Freud's therapeutically very fruitful and theoretically plausible alternative interpretation of recurring anxiety dreams, which regards them as a form of deferred mastering and thus, in a broad sense, as problem solving. Kafka (1979), in his overview of examination dreams, speaks of their reassuring function, and clarifies them as a transitional form between traumatic dreams and anxiety dreams.

Similarly to the way in which punishment dreams were incorporated into wish fulfillment theory by expanding the concept of the wish and localizing the wish in the superego, recurring anxiety dreams could also have been included in the expanded theory by ascribing the ego a wishlike need for mastery (Weiss and Sampson 1985). Although envisaged by Freud, this alternative was not theoretically developed, which is all the more astounding considering that it was used intuitively by many analysts and that it can be validated clinically with no great difficulty. Experience shows that if old determinants of anxiety are worked through while self-confidence (ego feeling etc.) increases, then stereotypic recurring anxiety dreams about traumatic situations will subside. The symptoms may also improve inasmuch as they are rooted in the dreams and can be reviewed as manifestations of these specific unconscious determinants (see Kafka 1979).

Thus although Freud had not hesitated in the context of a psychological interpretation of punishment dreams to view the wish and its gratification as arising in psychic areas other than that of instinctual life, he now shied back from extending wish fulfillment theory any further. He had been able to accommodate punishment dreams in the superego without abandoning his system, but to assign a wishlike character to problem solving itself would have destroyed the system. Problem solving would then have become a paramount principle, and instinctual wishes, as parts of the integral self-representation, would have had to be subordinated to it.

What could have led Freud not to view anxiety dreams as attempts at wish fulfillment in the sense of mastering, i.e., stemming from the ego, even though he had not hesitated to attribute punishment dreams to motives in the superego? We suspect that so many problems were created by the reorganization of the dualistic theory and by the conversion of the first topography to the second, structural topography that the theory of dreams has still not been completely integrated into structural theory (Rapaport 1967) despite the attempts which have been made (Arlow and Brenner 1964). For example, on the basis of structural theory, it would have been very natural to consider the ego as having an anxiety-mastering function in dreams too, and to view the recurrences as attempts at problem solving. Freud had already given a convincing example of problem solving in a dream which he interpreted in *Fragment of an Analysis of a Case of Hysteria* (1905 e), and in very positive terms described problem solving in dreams as a continuation of waking thinking at a preconscious level (in notes to the 1914 and 1925 editions of *The Interpretation of Dreams* [1900 a, p. 579 and p. 506 respectively] and in the *Introductory Lectures* [1916/17, p. 236]).

Yet Freud also remained skeptical toward attempts to ascribe a creative character to dream work (1923 a, p. 242). We attribute the fact that he nevertheless adhered to the idea of reducing the meaning of dreams to one single type of thought (namely the attempt at wish fulfillment) to a basic principle immanent in his system and rooted in his latent anthropology, i.e., his image of man and the world. We are referring to his attempt to attribute psychic phenomena, and thus the genesis, meaning, and nature of dreams, ultimately to physiologic processes. Needs and wishes are undoubtedly closely connected with instinct in its capacity as a borderline concept between the psychic and the physiologic, which is why dreaming was considered as the discharge of internal stimuli. Freud's confirmation of his latent image of man in practice, i.e., in dream interpretation, cannot, however, be dismissed as finding the Easter eggs that he himself had hidden, or, in other words, as a confirmation of bias and presuppositions. Even if wish fulfillment theory cannot be upheld in the sense of instinct discharge, it remains a primary heuristic principle that all psychic phenomena, including dreams, be viewed as expressions of wishes and needs. An essential element is lost whenever this regulatory principle is ignored.

## 5.4 Self-Representation Theory and Its Consequences

We would like to summarize Freud's thesis that every dream represents the dreamer himself, and to draw some conclusions which extend his thesis. The contradictions in the psychoanalytic theory of dreams (dream work) arise from the fact that therapeutic translation (interpretation work) does not yield the meaning behind the manifest dream content without encountering resistance by the dreamer. One problem which arises in the interpretation work is that of determining the relationship between the latent dream thoughts uncovered by interpretation and the manifest dream content (i.e., between the latent and the manifest dream).

Inconsistencies arise in attempts at translation, because Freud now assumed a kind of genetic relationship, in which the thought — the later phenomenon from the point of view of developmental psychology — was subordinated to the archaic symbolic mode of expression in the shape of a simultaneously operative latent wish. The following statement is characteristic: "You will see, too, that in this way it becomes possible in regard to a large number of *abstract* thoughts to create pictures to act as substitutes for them in the manifest dream while at the same time serving the purpose of concealment" (Freud 1916/17, p. 121, emphasis added).

It is quite clear that Freud is concerned here — as indeed in all his work — with the relationship of preliminary stages to the final form, i.e., with the theme of transformation and with the problem of the divergence and development of psychic constellations. The above-mentioned contradictions are also ultimately related to the great difficulty in comprehending transformation rules and their determinants when wish, image, and thought, or affect and perception, have been separated from each other even though they comprise a unit of experience. Think, for example, of the transformation of the wish into "hallucinatory wish fulfillment." Since a primary infantile wish was subordinated to the latent thought in the chain of events assumed by the theory, this may also be viewed as a kind of transformation problem, which might explain the contradictory statements concerning "manifest" and "latent." If one adopts the abbreviated term *latent dream* to describe the meaning of the *manifest dream* revealed by interpretation, without localizing the meaning itself to a seemingly real preliminary stage, one need not concern oneself with theoretically inadequate attempts at problem solving, but can regain an openness oriented on the special form of thinking in dreams.

We have already indicated which processes of psychological development create the basis for the appearance of the person of the dreamer in every dream. Yet questions of detail remain open if we choose the formulation that the dream is a self-representation in which the dreamer is involved at least insofar as he expresses his subjective view of a part of his world in picture language. His subjective view of himself and of the part of his life represented in the dream is — even independently of the regression — ego-oriented. The other dramatis personae, their words, and their actions are invented and staged by the playwright, at least inasmuch as they cannot effectively contradict the dream author's characterizations and settings.

The author, however, does not have complete freedom of choice concerning material and means of representation, which are in fact to a large degree predetermined by the following restrictions: As long as there are no thoughts which force themselves on us irresistibly in the waking state or in neurotic or psychotic illnesses, we feel that we are masters in our own house, with sufficient freedom of choice between various possible courses of action. Even when the scope for choice is actually very limited by external or internal factors, and when, from the motivational point of view, our freedom of will seems to dissolve into dependence, we still lay claim, at least subjectively, to the possibility of choosing to do one thing and not another. If it were otherwise, we would not be able to achieve the ideal aim of psychoanalysis, which is, by means of insight into the determinants of thought and action, to enlarge an individual's realm of freedom and his capacity for responsibility for himself and those around him, i.e., to free him from the inevitable consequences of unconscious processes. In dreams, the subjective feeling of being master in one's own house, and at least potentially free, is lost. We experience this loss particularly strongly when we fight our way out of sleep during anxiety dreams, against which we are totally helpless, and overcome the loss of freedom by reasserting the ascendancy of the ego. The lessening of the resistance to repression, together with the processes molding dream formation (dream work) described by Freud, allows unconscious areas of psychic life to emerge which the ego would prefer not to acknowledge and against which barriers are erected. It is one of the established general principles of psychoanalysis that these unconscious strivings nevertheless produce symptoms, precisely because they return through the back door and deprive the master of the house of his power and his freedom. The relevance of this general principle for human life is controversial in some specific contexts in individual psychopathology and in the history of collectives.

From the dynamic point of view, it would seem natural to look particularly closely at what effects the lessening of repression resistance during sleep has on the dreamer's world of wishes. Since wishes are by their very nature directed at objects and strive for gratification, and since there are no limits to human imagination — i.e., it goes far beyond the immediate gratification of vital needs — frustrations inevitably emerge. In view of the basic significance of wishes, and the fact that even in paradise wish fulfillment would probably never catch up with human fantasy — to say nothing of real failures or of the incest taboo, which is probably the only taboo to transcend almost all sociocultural boundaries and have universal validity (Hall and Lindzey 1968) — it is no wonder that Freud restricted the practical therapeutic consideration of the meaning of dreams to the representation of wishes. On the one hand the world of wishes is inexhaustible, and on the other there are always restrictions, prohibitions, and taboos which prevent wishes from being fulfilled. Thus, wishes involve so many imagined or genuine mortifications, which can be nourished endlessly from the individual's surplus fantasy, that a particularly strong resistance is built up to acknowledging and consciously recognizing them. Freud therefore attributed to the dream censor a masking and encoding function which permits only the *attempt* to fulfill wishes.

There can be no wish or instinct divorced from the subject, and even where the subject does not yet experience itself with an ego feeling or sense of identity, i.e., in infancy, it is treated as a hungry entity and called by its own name. In a sense, expressing hunger by crying is the self-representation appropriate to the subject's age. The infant itself does not understand it as such, but those around it do. Although adults can gain insight into the way children experience the world, our theories of how they see and feel things are always products of the adult mind. Because they concern the preverbal phase of developement, constructions and reconstructions of a child's internal world cannot be based on verbal information. They thus pose particular problems of scientific verification, which, however, we cannot go into more deeply here.

We mention this potential — and frequent — "confusion of tongues between adults and the child" (Ferenczi 1955 [1933]) because we now want to go into the relationship between the child's way of seeing things and adult thinking, using the example of the translation of the child's dream language into the language of waking thinking. By the way, we are still dealing with translation from one language to another even when the special form of thinking in dreams is not characterized as strongly by infantilisms and peculiarly colored memory elements as Freud assumed it to be. From time immemorial, the fact that people live in two worlds, that of normal language during the day and that of dream language at night, has been a source of uneasiness. An important aspect of the art of the dream-reader was the interpreting of the strange language and world of dreams in such a way that their content could be harmonized with the dreamer's conscious desires and intentions. During the siege of Tyre, Alexander the Great dreamed of a dancing satyr, which the dream-reader Aristandros interpreted as *sa Tyros*, "thine is Tyre" (Freud 1916/17, p. 236). It can hardly be disputed that Aristandros achieved some insight into Alexander's world of wishes, and he probably already intuitively understood something of the self-fulfilling function of prophesies. Perhaps the prophesy brought luck by strengthening Alexander's resolve!

Approaching the night side of our thinking can also be disturbing for the patient when his associations revolve around the manifest dream content, the search for meaning is left entirely to him, and his reading is left unchallenged. Even patients who are strongly motivated by curiosity or who are, on the basis of previous experience, inclined to grant that dreaming has a creative function are disturbed by the sinister nature of some dreams. It is often possible to understand this apprehensiveness in the context of resistance in one form or another, and thus to be able to offer means of overcoming it. Because it occurs so commonly and so regularly, and is by no means always confined to the initial phase of treatment, we would like to describe it using the more general term "identity resistance" (Chap. 4), that is to say, resistance rooted in the patient's adherence to his conscious image of himself and the world, i.e., to his previous identity.

Identity resistance is directed not only outward, against the opinions and influences of others — specifically the analyst — but also inward, particularly against the different representation of the self and the world in dreams. This internal aspect is what Erikson means when he speaks of identity resistance and the fear of changes in the identity feeling (1968, pp. 214-215). He described identity resistance particularly in the context of the phenomenology of identity confusion in puberty and early adulthood. The motivation for the identity resistance displayed by analysands who adhere rigidly to their conscious view of things, and thus have considerable reservations concerning the self-representation in their dreams, is quite different. It seems obvious that these two psychopathologically very different groups, which vary both in age and in symptoms, require different treatment. Plain common sense tells us we should behave differently when we want to stabilize identity distinctions which are blurred and confused than when — at the other extreme — we want to break down barriers which have become rigid and almost insurmountable. This differentiation in treatment can be substantiated theoretically.

There can be no doubt that greater therapeutic and theoretical significance has been attached to wish fulfillment via the object and to the object relationship in dreams than to Freud's basic thesis that the dreamer always represents himself, often in the guise of other figures.

The above thoughts on identity and identity resistance make it necessary for us now to consider the concept of identification in the sense of "just as." Freud (1900 a, p. 320) states that a figure in a dream can be made up of parts of a number of different people, and says that this "construction of a composite person" (p. 321) cannot be differentiated clearly from identification. When construction of a composite person is not completely successful, another figure appears in the dream.

We have traced Freud's assumption (1923 c, p. 120) that the dreamer's ego can appear more than once in the same dream — in person and concealed behind other figures — back to the dream language's direct conversion of common features or similarities into visual images. Instead of giving verbal expression to thoughts such as "I am similar to..." or "I wish I was like...," the dreamer portrays the person with whose beauty, strength, aggression, sexual potency, intelligence, sophistication, etc. he would like to identify. This substantively multifaceted process makes it possible for human development to take place and for the individual to learn from a model. One could say that while the gratification of instincts ensures animal survival, identification is necessary to guarantee the ontogenesis of a person in the given sociocultural context. We thus support Freud's thesis that primary identification is a direct or original form of the association of feelings with an object, occurring earlier than any object relationship, and thus has basic constitutive significance for human development (Freud 1921 c, pp. 106-107; 1923 b, p. 31).

The effortlessness with which the dreamer distributes his own opinions, intentions, or actions between several figures is linked with the probably irreducible nature of the formal structure of this special language, a structure which resembles the composition of picture puzzles. These, by the way, were very popular in 19th-century Vienna, which may explain why Freud chose them as a metaphor for the structure of dreams — a metaphor of which even Wittgenstein approved in spite of his general hostility to psychoanalysis.

It seems a natural step to describe representation of the dreamer by another person as projection, but the depth of self-representation through others would be limited if it were to be attributed to projection in general and defense in particular. Nevertheless, it is not uncommon for dreamers to have trouble recognizing themselves in others, or to see the mote in another's eye without noticing the beam in their own. The primitive level of psychological development to which dreamers can regress enables subject and objects to be interchanged. The differentiation of ego and not ego, of subject and object, is not yet complete in this phase (and is fortunately never absolute, even in the healthy adult, otherwise there would be no such thing as mutual and shared happiness, let alone the "oceanic feeling"; see Thomä 1981, pp. 99-100).

In this context we would like to refer again to the painstaking investigations by Foulkes (1982), which showed that the dream reports of 3- to 4-year-old children describe actions carried out by other people. At the dream level, children of this age thus live principally from identification, not from projection.

In contrast to his faithfulness to the assumption that the function of dreaming is the representation of wishes, Freud later (1923c, pp. 120-121) repudiated as speculation the proposition that *all* figures appearing in dreams are fragmentations or representations of the dreamer's own ego. But who had upheld this proposition? It is our view that Freud's criticism might have been directed against Jung's interpretation at the subjective level. Alternatively, it is conceivable that this opinion was held by other psychotherapists or that it had just emerged within psychoanalysis. Finally, it is possible that Freud wanted to warn in advance against regarding this point of view as absolute. Consistently throughout his whole work, he adheres to the view that the dreamer can appear more than once in a dream and be concealed behind others. An absolutist conception would have breached the all-embracing heuristic principle of finding the infantile root of the motivating dream wish whenever possible.

An absolutist theory of self-representation would thus have come to rival wish fulfillment theory as the primary concept of psychoanalytic dream interpretation. In fact, though, practical therapeutic dream interpretation was as far from realizing this at the beginning of the 1920s as it had been when Freud wrote *The Interpretation of Dreams*, in which all those factors were already covered which had also proven their worth in the understanding of Dora's dreams. In other words, in the process of looking for latent wishes, including *the* infantile dream wish, other aspects of dreams and their meaning were constantly being discovered, including the problem-solving and conflict-mastering functions. There was always a great variety of approaches to dream interpretation, but never any tendency to replace wish fulfillment theory with an equally comprehensive theory of self-representation.

It is important not to forget Freud's view that it is the regression in sleep that makes it possible for the dreamer to represent himself through several dream figures. This facilitates the cross-border traffic between "I" and "you," between subject and object, and makes them interchangeable in the sense of reciprocal identification in the dream drama. The emergence of magic wishes allows objects in dreams, as in fairy tales, to be transformed ad libitum. Being and having, identification and wishes, are no longer opposites but two aspects of the dream process.

In view of all this, it seems natural to seek the target of Freud's criticism outside the Freudian schools of psychoanalysis and to find it in Jung's interpretation of dreams at the subjective level. Even if we should be mistaken in this assumption, we hope at least that our error is productive for the pursual of our topic. For historical and practical reasons, any discussion of self-representation in dreams must include both interpretation at the subjective level, which is intimately related to Jung's self concept, and Kohut's narcissistic, self psychological interpretation.

## 5.5 Technique

With the conception of the dream as a means of self-representation, we would like to pave the way for an expanded understanding of dreaming which will lead us out of the irresolvable contradiction inherent in wish theory. In latent dream thoughts and wishes we see unconscious self elements which have a considerable share in the conflict and which also contain a description of the problem, perhaps even an attempt at problem solving in the dream. We also see the dreamer's ideas about himself, his body, his behavior patterns, etc. The relationship between problem solving in the present and that earlier in the life history not only reveals repressed wishes and conflicts, but also displays rehearsals of future actions. When the dream is understood as self-representation in all its conceivable aspects, the analyst will be receptive to what is most important to the dreamer and will measure the success of his interpretations not only by how much they contribute to the understanding of how the patient currently functions, but also, and most importantly, by how far they help the patient to attain new and better ways of seeing things and to produce improved patterns of behavior. Vitally important though the dreamer's past is, with all its obstacles to his development, his life takes place in the here-and-now and is oriented toward the future. Dream interpretation can contribute considerably to altering an individual's present and future.

Before we turn to dream interpretation in the stricter sense, we would like to raise a few questions relating to the remembering of dreams and to the patient's dream reports. The therapeutic usefulness of dreams is not, however, restricted solely to their interpretation with the aid of associations, i.e., the revelation of the latent dream thought. Monchaux (1978) regarded the function of dreaming and the reporting of dreams (in the sense of unconscious wish and defense in the transference relationship) as just as important for the dreamer as the actual dream itself.

Let us begin with a practical question: Should we encourage patients to write out their dreams, for instance directly upon waking? Freud (1911 e) came out clearly against this proposal, in the belief that dreams are not forgotten when the basic unconscious content becomes capable of being worked on. Abraham (1953 [1913]) shared this view, supporting it with an at times amusing case history. Slap (1976) reports briefly how he requested a patient to record in writing a part of one dream which she found very difficult to describe orally, and relates that this course of action helped in understanding the dream.

The fact (which has sometimes been critically noted) that a patient's dream reports bear or acquire a distinct resemblance to his analyst's theoretical orientation is not evidence for the analyst's theory, but for the fact that patient and analyst influence each other. No one should be astonished if the two parties are brought closer together by the reporting, common exploration, and eventual comprehension of dreams. The productivity of a patient with regard to his dream reports is naturally also determined largely by the way in which the analyst reacts to the reports and by whether he gets the feeling that the analyst is interested in them. Thomä (1977) has shown clearly that this rapprochement is not a result of therapeutic suggestion. In order for a patient to be able to report a dream, he must feel sufficiently secure in the therapeutic relationship. Hohage and Thomä (1982) give a brief account of the interplay between the transference constellation and the patient's potential for concerning himself with dreams.

Grunert (1982, p. 206) argues against the restrictions inherent in Freud's suggestion that consideration of the manifest dream content alone, without including the dreamer's associations, may be of no use in interpretation. She writes: "Contrary to Freud's practice, the analyst should not be afraid to give serious consideration to the manifest imagery and events in the dream and the accompanying or symbolized emotions and affects." It follows that he should interpret accordingly.

### *5.5.1 Freud's Recommendations and Later Extensions*

After the numerous formulations of his advice on interpretation technique scattered throughout *The Interpretation of Dreams* (1900 a), Freud summarized his recommendations in various publications. In *Remarks on the Theory and Practice of Dream-Interpretation* (1923 c, p. 109) he wrote:

> In interpreting a dream during analysis a choice lies open to one between several technical procedures.
>
> One can (*a*) proceed chronologically and get the dreamer to bring up his associations to the elements of the dream in the order in which those elements occurred in his account of the dream. This is the original, classical method, which I still regard as the best if one is analysing one's own dreams.
>
> Or one can (*b*) start the work of interpretation from some one particular element of the dream which one picks out from the middle of it. For instance, one can choose the most striking piece of it, or the piece which shows the greatest clarity or sensory intensity; or, again, one can start off from some spoken words in the dream, in the expectation that they will lead to the recollection of some spoken words in waking life.
>
> Or one can (*c*) begin by entirely disregarding the manifest content and instead ask the dreamer what events of the previous day are associated in his mind with the dream he has just described.
>
> Finally, one can (*d*), if the dreamer is already familiar with the technique of interpretation, avoid giving him any instructions and leave it to him to decide with which associations to the dream he shall begin.
>
> I cannot lay it down that one or the other of these techniques is preferable or in general yields better results.

These recommendations include all the essential elements of dream interpretation, although the analyst has a great deal of latitude concerning relative importance and sequence of application. The recommendations given 10 years later (1933 a) are similar, but attach a new importance to the day residue.

The analyst now has the material with which he can work. But how? Although the literature on dreams has meanwhile grown to almost unmanageable proportions, elaborate recommendations on interpretative technique have remained rather rare.

In light of their view of dreaming as problem solving, French and Fromm list three conditions which interpretations must fulfill:

1. The various meanings of the dream must fit together.
2. They must fit the dreamer's emotional situation at the moment of dreaming.
3. It must be possible to reconstruct the thought processes in a way which is free of contradictions.

French and Fromm (1964, p. 66) describe these factors as the "cognitive structure" of the dream, constituting the decisive test of the validity of the reconstruction and thus of the interpretation. They emphasize that the ego in dreams not only has the task of solving problems, but must also avoid too great an involvement in the focal conflict, which would make problem solving more difficult. This avoidance should really be termed "distancing." One well-established means of distancing is what French and Fromm call "deanimation": a conflict with other people is de-emotionalized or technicized, to make it easier to find solutions for the problem which now has the appearance of a merely technical obstacle. "Cognitive structure of the dream" is the expression French and Fromm use to describe the "constellation of intimately related problems" (p. 94), by which they mean the dreamer's current relationships in everyday life, that to the analyst, and the connection between the two.

Dream interpretation, in common with other forms of interpretation, must comprise three components: the transference relationship, the current external relationship, and the historical dimension. This is necessary because the problem — it is a neurotic one — apparently cannot be solved by the patient in all three of these areas. French and Fromm are very rigorous in their endeavor to come up with a recognizable, meaningful connection ("evidence") to the material from the same (and previous) sessions. Any gaps and contradictions are useful indicators that other, perhaps better hypotheses should be tested. Although they are by no means opponents of intuition, they mistrust intuitive dream interpretation since it mostly covers only one aspect of the dream and leads the analyst into the trap of the "Procrustean bed" technique (1964, p. 24), i.e., the temptation to fit the material to the hypothesis, and not vice versa. The consideration of isolated aspects is in their view the most common reason for differences of opinion in dream interpretation. Their call for the analysis of several dreams in order to achieve historical interpretations (p. 195) is interesting. Other authors have also urged investigation of series of dreams (e.g., Greenberg and Pearlman 1975; Cohen 1976; Greene 1979; Geist and Kächele 1979).

To ensure complete clarity we would like to list again the requirements which French and Fromm believe dream interpretation should fulfill:

1. The various meanings of a dream must fit together.
2. They must fit the dreamer's emotional situation "at the moment of dreaming."
3. Beware of taking a part for the whole.
4. Beware of the Procrustean bed technique.

5. Two steps:
   a) current problem
   b) similar historical problem (remember the transference aspect).
6. Testability: reconstruction of the cognitive structure of the dream, contradictions as important indicators for new ideas (analogy: puzzles).
7. Several dreams are necessary for historical interpretations.

Lowy (1967) draws attention to one restriction on interpretation activity: he does not interpret aspects which would be helpful and supportive for the dreamer. This corresponds roughly to the technique of not interpreting mild, positive transference before it turns into resistance. He warns urgently against making over-hasty interpretations: "the suppressing capacity of unconsidered interpretations is real, and this may result in depriving the subject of needed explicit experiencing of certain self-created figures and scenes" (p. 524).

A frequent subject of discussion is symbol interpretation, which occupies a special position because of the general validity of symbols. However, this position is relativized by Holt's illuminating definition of symbols as a special form of displacement. According to him, symbols are to be treated as displacements of another kind:

> I propose, therefore, that we consider symbolism a special case of displacement, with the following characteristics: a symbol is a socially shared and structuralized displacement-substitute. The first characteristic, its being used by a large number of people, implies the second one and helps explain it: if any particular displacement-substitute were a purely *ad hoc*, transitory phenomenon, one would indeed have to assume some kind of "racial unconscious" or other type of pre-established harmony to account for the fact that many people arrive at the same displacement. (Holt 1967, p. 358)

Associations are the prerequisite and the basis for the analyst's interpretations. They are the bricks which he employs to build his understanding of the dream and of the problem and to construct his alternative solutions for the dreamer, and which constitute an important part of what is termed the "context" of the dream. Sand (in an unpublished manuscript entitled "A Systematic Error in the Use of Free Association," 1984) has discussed the significance of the "context" from the scientific point of view. Reis (1970) investigated the forms taken by free association regarding dreams and used an actual case to illustrate the specific problem that patients are sometimes unable to associate to dreams in particular.

Freud (1916/17, pp. 116-117) postulates a quantitative relationship between resistance and the requirement for associations necessary to understand a dream element:

> Sometimes it requires only a single response, or no more than a few, to lead us from a dream-element to the unconscious material behind it, while on other occasions long chains of associations and the overcoming of many critical objections are required for bringing this about. We shall conclude that these differences relate to the changing magnitude of the resistance, and we shall probably turn out to be right. If the resistance is small, the substitute cannot be far distant from the unconscious material; but a greater resistance means that the unconscious material will be greatly distorted and that the path will be a long one from the substitute back to the unconscious material.

It is in the field of dream interpretations that the technique of free association was particularly consolidated and refined (see Sect. 7.2). At the same time, the technique obtained its theoretical foundation from the assumed inverse symmetry between the dream work and the genesis of free associations. Thus, Freud (1900a, p. 102) defines free association as "involuntary ideas." The dream is perceived as the product of a regressive process through which the dream thought is transformed into a visual image.

Freud assumed that a patient who free-associates on the couch is in a regression similar to that of the dreamer. The patient is thus in a particularly favorable positon to describe the dream images and also interpret them. Through the process of association, one by one the components of the dream become intelligible in the waking state; that is, the patient is in the position to dismantle that which was assembled in the dream (Freud 1901a, pp. 636-642).

Since the method of free association can today no longer be regarded as a simple inversion of dream work, it is advisable to adopt a pragmatic attitude to free association and not to overlook the meaningful role which the analyst plays — merely by actively listening — in creating the connections he interprets. We have already shown clearly, using the example of Kohut's dream interpretations, how much influence theoretical assumptions can exert.

We use the expression "theme-centered association" to describe the associations which the dreamer, prompted by the analyst, has concerning the individual elements of the dream; these are the associations which characterize classical dream interpretation. Although theme-centered association is still employed occasionally, with positive consequences for the interpretative work, the literature contains few such analyses of dreams. We are not ashamed to be old-fashioned in this respect, and do not believe that the patient's freedom is restricted by the focused dream interpretation derived from theme-centered association. Naturally, in theme-centered association too, the question soon arises as to which of the patient's associations are still connected with the manifest dream, and, most importantly, which are linked with his latent thoughts and his specific unconscious wishes. However, the association resistance, albeit circumscribed, gives some indication of the path to pursue in the context of the dream.

At this juncture we would like to mention just one further point, namely that the technique of dream interpretation described by Freud as "classical" (1923c, p. 109; see above) has almost fallen into oblivion. Kris does not give a single example of this technique. He has a comprehensive understanding of the method and the process of free association: it is a common process whereby the dreamer attempts to express all his thoughts and feelings in words, and the analyst, prompted by his own associations, helps him to fulfill this task (Kris 1982, pp. 3, 22).

The patient's ability to associate freely, or more freely, can be regarded as an expression of inner freedom, and thus as a desirable goal of treatment. However, it is not the analyst's own associations, or his evenly suspended attention as such, which help the patient to open up; the essential factor is how the analyst arrives at useful interpretations and what effect these have on the patient. Directly after every intervention — every interruption of the patient's flow of words — the session becomes centered on this one theme. Even total absence of response to an interpretation is a reaction which the analyst will note. The analyst's evenly suspended attention then operates in a theme-centered fashion to the same degree as the patient centers on one theme, i.e., reacts to his interventions rather than ignores them. How the analyst derives his interpretations from the patient's associations, how he finds the right words — in a nutshell, psychoanalytic heuristics — is not the subject of this section (see Chap. 8). The more varied the patient's associations are, and the more he goes into detail, the more difficulty the analyst has in making his selection and also in justifying it on the basis of patterns or configuration in the material. It is therefore expedient on the one hand to consider what the patient is saying from the point of view of continuity — which of the last session's themes is being continued today? — and on the other hand to regard the current session as a unit — which problem is the patient trying to solve?

Spence (1981) proposes dividing associations into "primary" and "secondary" in order to arrive at the "transformation rules" he wants to establish. The basis for the use of association is the "correspondence postulate" which we mentioned above (Spence 1981, p.387): the associations correspond to the dream thoughts because the regression during association corresponds to the state of "benign regression" during sleep or when in love. Primary associations are those which are causally linked to the dream; they lead to the details of the dream. Secondary associations are those prompted by the dream itself; they lead away from the dream. Because of the significance of this differentiation, and in order to show his argument more clearly, we would like to quote Spence at some length:

1. We must partition the dreamer's associations into a primary set (the presumed causes of the dream) and a secondary set (triggered by the dream as dreamt but having no significant relationship to the creation of the dream). The primary associations should all come from about the same time period in the patient's life — as a working hypothesis, let us take the twenty-four hours preceding the dream. The more restricted this time period, the more confidence we can have that we have identified truly primary associations. If, on the other hand, we significantly increase the size of our search space (to include, for example, the patient's total life), we thereby reduce the chances of finding anything significantly related to the *cause* of the dream and increase the chances of capturing only secondary associations.
2. We need to rewrite the primary associations as a minimum set of propositions. The purpose of this step is to represent each association in some standard canonical form, making it easier for us to discover the underlying similarity of the set and paving the way for a discovery of the rules of transformation.
3. We have to reduce the causative propositions to a restricted set of one or more transformation rules. Each rule (or rules), applied to the canonical proposition, should generate one or more of the details of the actual dream; the complete set of rules, together with the full set of propositions, should account for *all* details in the dream. Thus, at the end of this procedure, we will have reduced the manifest dream to (a) a set of underlying propositons, and (b) a set of one or more transforming rules. The transforming rules might share some of the same primary-process mechanisms. (1981, p.391)

Spence's essential concern is to reduce the multiplicity of meanings which led Specht (1981) to ask how interpretation of dreams differs first from astrology and the interpretation of oracles, and second from the schematic interpretation of symbols on which popular books on dream interpretation are based.

Let us address first the criticism of arbitrariness, which appears to receive support even from within our own ranks. Waelder (1936), discussing theories of neurosis, writes:

If one were to unearth such possible theories — theories which view the neurosis as the simultaneous solution of three or more problems — and in addition to consider the possibility of subordinating one problem to the other, the number of such theories of the neurosis would reach many tens of thousands. (1936, p. 55)

A little later, he continues:

Finally, we may look for the operation of this principle even in dream life; the dream is the sphere wherein over-determination was originally discovered. Nevertheless, the general character of dreams remains the reduction of the psychic experience as well in relation to its content (receding of the superego and of the active problems of the ego) as in relation to the way of working (substitution of the manner of working of the unconscious for the manner of working of the conscious in *attempted solutions*) and finally in the chronological sense (receding of the actual in favor of the past). In consideration of all these reduction or regression developments which mean a change in the problems and a reversion in the specific methods of solution from the manner of working of the conscious to the manner of working of the unconscious, the dream phenomena can also be explained through the principle of multiple function. Every occurrence in the dream appears then likewise in eightfold function or clearly in eight groups of meaning. The distinction of the dream is characterized only through the change or the shifting of the problems and through the relapse in the manner of working. (1936, pp. 58-59, emphasis added)

Implicit in this is that if several factors are taken into account, the number of possible interpretations of a dream runs, as a matter of principle, into the "tens of thousands." The dream is thus a "concentration" of many different endeavors and has an infinite number of potential meanings. According to Specht (1981), however, the possible tentative interpretations of a dream are not unlimited. Specht formulates and tests a theory of dream interpretation, referring to the "indistinct horizon" of psychoanalytic concepts and interpretation rules (p. 776). He proposes, in conformity with similar problems of scientific theory, that "dream interpretations should also be comprehended as recommendations and not as descriptive statements" (p. 783). He proposes understanding the dream in the sense of the assumed wish, even if the dreamer is not aware of the wish. Specht defines a wish as "a tendency, founded in the concrete life situation, which the dreamer has not yet been able to accept" (p. 784). He works with the concept of "antecedent constellation" (p. 765), by which he means "the psychic situation preceding the dream." Following Roland (1971), he emphasizes — like Sand (see above) but independently — the decisive importance of the "relevant context." Both concepts — rightly, we believe — leave the temporal dimension entirely open, so that both the day residue and traumas occurring decades earlier can be included. Specht comes to the conclusion that the possibilities for dream interpretation are limited by (1) the rules of interpretation, (2) the dreamer's free associations, and (3) the number of wishes which are anchored in the antecedent constellation and which are prevented (by countermotives, which remain to be specified) from attaining the level of conscious awareness. If in the majority of the dreams no correspondence can be determined between the possible tentative interpretations for a dream and the wishes anchored in the antecedent constellation, Specht would reject the theory as false. "The theory of dreams is thus in principle falsifiable, in sharp contrast to the interpretation of oracles" (p. 775).

He lays down the following criteria for scientific dream interpretation:

1. Description of the antecedent constellation
2. Application of the rules of interpretation
3. Reporting of the patient's free associations
4. Description of the countermotives (with psychogenesis?)
5. Consideration of various dream wishes
6. Justification of the choice of the "right" interpretation
7. Elaboration into interpretations
8. Their effect (taking account of the criteria for the "right interpretation" — among others, the emergence of new material)

In disputes over scientific theory, we should not allow ourselves to forget that dream interpretation has a practical origin in the patient's wish for such interpretation (Bartels 1979): he wants to close the breach between his dreams and his conscious life, in order to preserve his identity, as Erikson (1954) pointed out in his interpretation of "the dream specimen of psychoanalysis" — Freud's Irma dream.

# 6 The Initial Interview and the Latent Presence of Third Parties

## 6.1 The Problem

Patient and analyst usually meet for the first time in the waiting room, but each has already formed some kind of image of the other. Consider a patient who has arranged his appointment on the telephone or in writing. He has outlined his problems in brief or has written a detailed account of his life and current situation to emphasize the urgent need for a consultation. He may also have expressed his doubts and his hopes that this analyst, whom he has heard of through the grapevine, will take him on as a patient and that his long-postponed decision to undergo analysis will now lead swiftly to successful treatment of his chronic symptoms. For his part, the analyst has already learned or inferred much about the patient's life and current situation from the way in which the patient has come or been referred to him and from the content and form of the letter or telephone call. Thus even before the first encounter, processes of transference, countertransference, and resistance have been set in motion. In anticipation of the first meeting our imaginary patient may even have dreamed of a house whose similarity to the building where the analyst's office is located was obvious to him on waking. For his part, the analyst may have noticed in himself signs of positive countertransference in the more comprehensive sense of this term. Since the patient has described his work situation in a way which permits the analyst to assume that he has considerable flexibility with regard to appointments, the analyst has checked his appointments schedule to see what he can offer.

Two things can be gathered from this brief account of an imaginary typical case. First, transference, countertransference, and resistance begin before the first encounter between patient and analyst. Second, the patient's hopes also start to affect his dream thinking before the initial interview. It is for these reasons that this chapter comes after the chapters dealing with those aspects. With regard to transference, countertransference, and resistance, we would like to underline the vital importance of the analyst's attitude for the first meeting and all subsequent encounters. We emphasize this particularly for those who have chosen to read this chapter first because it offers an introduction to psychoanalytic practice. The somewhat more experienced reader will see from our outline of the preliminaries that the outcome of the initial interview with this imaginary model patient can be predicted with some certainty even on the basis of this small amount of information. In such cases no great diagnostic acuity is needed, and the decision to commence an analysis has almost been made before the analyst has racked his brain over specific indications. In a few cases an initial interview or a lengthy phase of clarification can be dispensed with. It is then clear to both participants — patient and analyst alike — that the initial interview may mark the commencement of treatment. Every analyst is familiar with such swift decision-making processes which have nothing to do with the fascinations of mutual attraction; quite the opposite, they lead so smoothly to four or five sessions of treatment per week because the expectations on each side complement each other well. Everything fits, so to speak: age, level of education, severity of symptoms, a successful professional career which gives the patient financial independence and flexibility with regard to appointments.

It comes as no surprise that the psychoanalytic literature contains many more discussions of the opening phase of treatment than of the initial interview. We would also prefer to skip discussion of the initial interview and proceed directly to treatment rules and the commencement of treatment itself. However, we cannot act as though we deal principally with ideal patients, whose motivation for seeking treatment is good and who are aware of the connection between their symptoms and the problems and conflicts in their lives, i.e., who already have the psychoanalytically desirable insight into their illness. Such patients do exist, but are few and far between; in reality things are quite different. As soon as an analyst's patients have a wide range of psychic and physical problems (i.e., cover a broad nosologic spectrum) and are not all financially independent and well-educated, the initial interview assumes decisive importance. Once the initial interview is no longer ascribed the dubious alibi function of allegedly identifying the patient who is suitable for psychoanalysis, it is possible to share Freud's pioneer spirit and the pleasure he took in experimentation.

We regard the initial interview as the first opportunity for the psychoanalytic method to be adapted to the particular circumstances of the individual patient. The first encounters carry a heavy burden of responsibility. The information which must be gained in just a few meetings will be incomplete and unreliable. On principle, only in absolutely clear-cut cases may it be stated with certainty that a given patient *cannot* be helped by psychoanalysis, as the psychoanalytic method is based on the establishment by the analyst of a special interpersonal relationship with the patient as an individual in order to be able to exercise a beneficial therapeutic influence on disturbances, symptoms, and illnesses which are partly or wholly *psychic* in origin. Thus we employ a somewhat pretentious word and speak of an *encounter* in which all technical rules and specialized terms are embodied.

Plainly one must go beyond mere generalization. The further therapeutic methods and techniques are developed and refined, the more clearly they are related to the theory of the origin of the given illness and the more precisely their efficiency can be predicted. And the better the circumstances surrounding the origin of the condition are known and the more exactly the mechanisms of the remedy have been clarified, the greater is the accuracy of prognostic statements. Thus, in medicine, standardization and generalizability of a technique — its applicability to the typical case, but with the flexibility to allow for adaptation to the individual patient — represents the scientific and practical ideal. In this way, errors in treatment technique can be described as deviations from an established norm. The full relevance of this emerges in the identification of instances of malpractice.

Can this ideal be applied to psychoanalysis, and can we expect the initial interview to yield the information we need to establish a positive indication for treatment? This would mean that indication and prognosis are interrelated, as is plain in the questions every patient asks: "What are my chances of improvement or cure from analysis? Is the treatment less likely to be successful if I can only come twice a week?" Such questions are awkward for every analyst. This is the reason that we have openly admitted that we too are happy to work under standardized conditions, under the proviso that the diagnosis implies a clear psychogenesis, so that indication and prognosis can be grounded.

If the selection of patients suitable for the standard psychoanalytic technique were the only issue of importance in the initial interview, it might seem that we could proceed directly to therapy, i.e., to the psychoanalytic process, the course of which determines the prognosis. But appearances are deceiving; the technical standards designed for the so-called suitable case are formal criteria, and as such remain outside the essence and substance of the process and possibly even interfere with it. It is for this reason that we must take so many different factors into account in talking about the initial interview, and this multiplicity must be viewed in the context of the comprehensive tasks that have to be achieved. By tracing a few lines of development, we would like to widen the perspective and use the psychoanalytic attitude to shed light on the initial interview from various angles. We emphasize the importance of the analyst's *attitude*, for example in the attention he pays to transference, countertransference, and resistance. Frequently the psychoanalytic tools, in the strict sense, cannot be utilized, so that the analyst's attitude and the way he handles the patient's communications are essential. Thus a specific psychoanalytic interview technique was late to develop, although psychoanalysis soon influenced the psychiatric interview in the USA and history-taking in German psychosomatic medicine.

Our aim in this chapter is to do justice to both the general requirements of interviewing and the special characteristics of the psychoanalytic interview. We therefore have to familiarize the reader with a broad range of views, because although the medical model for the establishment of positive indications was adopted in the standard technique of psychoanalysis, hardly any analyst — except in the rare clear-cut cases mentioned above — is in the position to form a definite opinion on the basis of just a few meetings with the patient.

It is not surprising that in those cases in which it seems to the analyst that the very first meeting can be conducted in a way approximating the basic model technique, the patients turn to be suitable for an analysis under standard conditions. It is indeed important how, for example, the patient reacts to trial interpretations, since for obvious reasons this may provide useful pointers to his capacity for insight and awareness of conflicts. Even more important is the experience that patients' reactions to trial interpretations and to other special tools of psychoanalytic technique depend on a multitude of determinants, for example timing. Many factors are involved in determining how long a patient needs to become so familiar with the psychoanalytic dialogue as conducted by the individual analyst — and the spectrum is wide — that he can grasp the meaning of trial interpretations. All things being equal, the same holds true for all criteria. Finally, our conviction that the form taken by the initial interview should be adapted to the particular circumstances of the individual patient influences our description.

## 6.2 Diagnosis

Freud's diagnostic explorations served to exclude somatic illness or psychosis. The limitations of the psychoanalytic method seemed to be defined much more by the constraints of outpatient as opposed to inpatient treatment than by restrictions of technique. Freud, who in any case never hesitated to take on seriously ill patients, saw temporary inpatient treatment in emergencies as a means of considerably extending the applicability of the psychoanalytic method (Freud 1905 a). As soon as the elementary preconditions had been satisfied and questions of payment and appointments settled, the fundamental rule was explained and the analysis began. Then as now, general psychosocial factors such as education, age, and motivation were highly relevant. Freud did not take a detailed history until the first phase of treatment; his preliminary interview was brief, as can be seen in the case of the Rat Man (1909 d, p. 158).

Freud's patients were all "in analysis"; after he had discontinued hypnosis he made no distinction between various forms of psychoanalytic therapy — there was just his psychoanalytic method. He principally treated serious cases, patients who could not cope with life, i.e., those with whom and for whom psychoanalytic therapy was developed (Freud 1905 a, p. 263).

The problem of selection first arose when demand began to outstrip supply, as Fenichel reported about the clinic of the Berlin Institute:

> The difference between the total number of consultations and the number of analyses it was possible to undertake necessitated a disagreeable sifting-out process. It goes without saying that the primary criteria were those of indication for analysis, but in addition the Institute imposed two conditions for the acceptance of a patient for psychoanalytic treatment: the case had to lend itself to scientific research and to teaching. (Fenichel 1930, p. 13)

The ratio of consultations to treatments initiated was at that time about 2.5:1. The prevailing climate at the Berlin Institute with regard to initiating psychoanalytic treatment was one of enthusiasm for experimentation, and this is underlined by the high proportion of analyses (241 of 721) which were broken off:

> The breaking off of a relatively large number of analyses after only a short time can be explained. In most of these cases, the patients' accessibility to analysis was doubtful from the outset but they nevertheless underwent a "trial analysis," at the end of which the analyst had to recommend termination. (Fenichel 1930, p. 14)

Trial analysis served to establish indications more definitely, and was plagued from the outset by the patient asking: "If it turns out at the end of the trial analysis that I'm not suitable for psychoanalysis, what kind of treatment am I suitable for?" This obvious question rocks the very foundations of the patient's existence. It would seem that the problem could be avoided by not expressly agreeing on a trial analysis, i.e., the analyst could decide on a trial period without telling the patient, but this would be irreconcilable with the psychoanalytic attitude. Moreover, the trial analysis can only be valid as a test of suitability in the context of a standardized technique which the same analyst would also use later. The patient's behavior during the trial analysis would thus be seen from the viewpoint of one particular understanding of the rule. Not many of the patients now seeking consultations at psychoanalytic outpatient clinics would be judged suitable in a trial analysis conducted according to the basic model technique. It is plain why the trial analysis was dropped; the rejection at the end can be very painful for the patient if he is simply branded "unsuitable for psychoanalysis" and not given any suggestions as to alternative treatment.

Of course, dropping the trial analysis did not solve the problem, but just shifted it to the initial interview. As we will show later, this burden will not be reduced to a level which is bearable for both participants, or constructively soluble, until an adaptive establishment of indications has become a fundamental aspect of diagnosis and therapy. First, however, we would like to stress that the problems which had to be solved in the initial interview in the clinic of the old Berlin Psychoanalytic Institute are still encountered in all large clinics; private practice is not affected as strongly. For this reason, most publications on the subject of the initial interview stem from experience authors have gathered in institutions. In addition, few psychoanalytic training centers expressly teach interview technique. The following major lines of development can be discerned: In general diagnostics, psychoanalysis has over the years adopted the nosologic system from psychiatry. The diagnostic models of psychosomatic medicine were and are oriented around physical symptomatology. The psychoanalytic initial interview is a relatively late achievement and was developed in large outpatient clinics.

The psychoanalytic attitude and psychoanalytic thinking exerted a great influence on psychiatric exploration technique. Here, as anywhere in history, there may be asynchronous phases lasting decades, and interdisciplinary influence may long go unrecognized, but there can be no doubt that psychiatric diagnostics underwent a change with Bleuler's (1910) assimilation of psychoanalytic thinking. Brill, Putnam, and other psychiatrists acquainted themselves with the psychoanalytic technique through Bleuler's Burghölzli school and helped to diffuse it among psychiatrists in the USA, where the way had already been paved by Meyer's ideas on social hygiene and psychotherapy. The influences of psychodynamic thinking were perceptible as early as the 1930s. The individual steps have been traced by Gill et al. (1954), whose important contribution is the definition of the psychodynamic interview technique. They contrast the traditional psychiatric exploration with the "dynamic interview," which has three aims:

The first aim is to establish *rapport* between two strangers, a professional person and a human being who suffers psychologically and often makes others suffer. A serious attempt to understand the patient, a warm human contact and some mutual appreciation have to be established regardless of who therapist and patient are. All writers on interviewing have stressed this and we are in basic agreement on this point. The second aim is *appraisal* of the patient's psychological status. The third aim is *reinforcement* of the patient's wish to continue with therapy whenever this is indicated, and to plan with him the next step in this direction. (Gill et al. 1954, pp. 87-88)

The psychiatric diagnosis is rooted in the appraisal of the total situation and corresponds to Balint's concept of total diagnosis. Gill et al.'s inclusion of the development and support of a patient among the tasks of the initial interview marks in our opinion a significant step away from the purely diagnostic interview in the direction of therapeutic action.

Sullivan's "interpersonal theory of psychiatry" (1953) put great emphasis on the relationship aspect. Unresolved is whether Sullivan really founded a truly interpersonal psychotherapy, as Greenberg and Mitchell (1983) claim, or returned to a largely intrapsychically oriented approach (Wachtel 1982). The clarification of this issue depends on how the analyst's role as participant observer is realized in practice.

In the course of the 1950s, numerous different psychodynamically oriented interview strategies were developed by psychoanalysts working within dynamic psychiatry. It was during this period that Deutsch described the "associative anamnesis" in the context of his teaching activities:

The method called "associative anamnesis" consists in recording not only what the patient said, but also how he gave the information. It is of consequence not only that the patient tells his complaints, but also in what phase of the interview, and in which connection he introduces his ideas, complaints and recollections of his somatic and emotional disturbances. (Deutsch and Murphy 1955, vol. 1, p. 19)

An approach centered on exploration and description of the psychopathology was replaced by observation of the dynamic of what takes place, without putting too much stress on the relationship component, but rather using it to create a situation conducive to investigation. It is rewarding to look at this integration of psychiatry and psychoanalysis — as sought, for example, by Redlich and Freedman (1966) — from the point of view of the various blends of descriptive psychopathology and recognition of the relationship which have emerged.

Kernberg's "structural interview" (1977, 1981) is a good example of the second generation of psychoanalytically oriented psychiatric initial interviews following in the tradition of the dynamic interview. He attempts to relate the history of the patient's personal illness and his general psychic functioning directly to his interaction with the diagnostician. Kernberg's technical guidelines recommend a circular process. On the one hand, returning continually to the patient's problems and symptoms defines the psychopathological status; on the other, attention is focussed on the interaction between patient and therapist in the psychoanalytic sense, and interpretations, including interpretations of transference, are given in the here-and-now. The main goal is clarification of the integration of ego identity or identity diffusion, the quality of the defense mechanisms, and the presence or absence of the capacity for reality testing. This permits the differentiation of personality structure into neuroses, borderline personalities, functional (endogenous) psychoses, and organically determined psychoses. The interviewer mobilizes clarification, confrontation, and interpretation in the effort to gather material which will yield important prognostic and therapeutic information. He is particularly concerned to appraise the patient's motivation, his capacity for introspection, his ability to work together with the therapist, his potential for acting out, and the danger of psychotic decompensation. Occasionally, unconscious connections are offered as interpretations to a neurotic patient, or a borderline patient is told about splits in his self-representations. From the patient's reactions, conclusions can be drawn which help the therapist decide on further diagnostic and therapeutic measures.

The structured classification of differential diagnosis follows the nosologic system of psychiatry in the division into three main categories — endogenous and exogenous psychoses and neuroses. Kernberg adds borderline disturbances as a fourth category. Despite the circular form of the dialogue, the main theme of Kernberg's interview, which he makes more concrete by means of particular questions in the beginning, middle, and end phases, follows the psychiatric phenomenological concept of looking first for psychoses resulting from cerebral disorders, next for functional psychoses, and only then for borderline disturbances and neuroses. Through his use of terms like "diagnostics," "exploration," and "cardinal symptoms," Kernberg shows that he stands with one foot planted firmly in descriptive psychiatry. The interviewer's structuring activity naturally affects the interaction. A certain restriction of freedom in the way the relationship between patient and therapist begins to form is accepted in order to gain the information necessary for differential diagnosis. The structural interview is nevertheless a balanced blend of psychopathologic description and relationship analysis, and meets the diagnostic, therapeutic, and prognostic demands placed on the initial consultation. It also covers a broad spectrum of illnesses which are only encountered, whether in private practice or in institutions, in the absence of restrictive preselection processes ensuring that the analyst almost exclusively treats neuroses. In our opinion, Kernberg has achieved a good synthesis of the various functions of the first meeting. If one considers that almost all American psychoanalysts have had psychiatric training, it becomes more comprehensible why no great emphasis is placed on the initial interview in the curricula of American psychoanalytic institutions (Redlich and Freedman 1966).

Greatly simplified, one could say that the psychoanalytic attitude and psychoanalytic thinking influenced the psychodynamic interview technique and that this in turn affected psychoanalytic practice. In the framework of these reciprocal influences there are particular nodal points which characterize the main tasks of the initial interview. In the following description, we are aware that our emphasis on certain aspects exaggerates the differences.

First we will deal with biographical anamnesis, because the question of the connection between the patient's life history and his current symptoms comes up in every initial interview. If one is to proceed from the precipitating situation—in psychoanalytic terms, from the situation of temptation and frustration—to explanation of the psychogenesis in the sense of Freud's complementary series, it is indispensable to learn something about the patient's childhood. In order to grasp the potential emotional relevance of this information, however, it is essential to incorporate it into the psychopathology of the conflict, and thus in the wider sense into a theory of personality. It must therefore be noted even at this juncture that the psychoanalytic initial interview is rooted partly in the attempts made in the 1920s and 1930s to systematize the theory of therapy. Finally, we come to the interactional interview model which Balint developed at the Tavistock Clinic, influenced by object relationship psychology and the significance of the interchange between doctor and patient in the here-and-now.

The beginnings of psychosomatic medicine in Heidelberg after the war were strongly influenced by von Weizsäcker's (1943) question: "Why does a disease appear *now*, and why does it appear precisely *here* in this organ or system?" The development of the associated interview technique of "biographical anamnesis," and its evolution into "systematic history-taking" have been described by Thomä:

> The central aim of "biographical anamnesis" (see Ruffler 1957) is to use questions to throw light on the patient's life situation at the time of the onset of the symptoms and then to describe this situation precisely .... Biographical anamnesis was not primarily concerned with a psychotherapeutic goal, i.e., with achieving change, but with the diagnosis of the past. No special consideration was given to the doctor-patient relationship or to its specific expression in transference and countertransference. (Thomä 1978, p. 254)

The temporal associations between the patient's current situation, previous events in his life, the origin of his symptoms, and their variable intensity naturally form the starting point for many more or less systematized interview techniques. The triad of "object loss, hopelessness, and helplessness" (Engel and Schmale 1967), which can be observed in many different illnesses, forms the theoretical background for the mode of dialogue recommended by Engel (1962). Adler (1979, p. 329) describes Engel's method as a technique of history-taking which puts the doctor in a position, by virtue of his knowledge of developmental psychology and the theory of neurosis, to integrate psychic, social, and somatic data and recognize their significance.

It is generally true that the therapeutic appropriateness of these information-seeking and insight-providing techniques for structuring interviews is largely determined by the way they are applied. If the analyst succeeds in using typical conflicts in the patient's life to show him *ad oculos* something of the latent dynamics and the connections, this method facilitates access particularly to those patients who would otherwise have no direct, unhindered insight into the psychogenesis of their symptoms.

In this technique, diagnosis drew on a more or less well consolidated theory of neurosis, and the conducting of the dialogue in practice was oriented on the psychoanalytic treatment technique as systematized in the 1920s and 1930s. Experience gained in psychoanalytic outpatient clinics was decisive in this respect. Particularly great emphasis was placed on diagnostic ability at the outpatient clinic of the old Berlin Psychoanalytic Institute, and it became necessary to make the findings comparable. Teaching and research thus promoted systematization. Alexander's early work provides an excellent example; his later research on specificity in psychosomatic medicine, at the Chicago Psychoanalytic Institute, would not have been possible without a diagnostic interview model (Alexander 1950).

Schultz-Hencke's (1951) "goal-directed anamnesis," which served the purpose of diagnosing the symptom-precipitating situations of temptation and frustration, neglected the relationship and transference aspect of the initial interview. Schultz-Hencke related these situations, which Freud had introduced into psychoanalytic terminology and practice, to his own theory of conflict and structure. The later extension of this interview technique was termed "biographical anamnesis" and described in detail by Dührssen (1972, 1981).

In recent years, the expectation has decreased that we will be able to identify typical, highly characteristic constellations of conflicts as discussed by Alexander and French (1946) under the heading of specific hypotheses. The variability of psychodynamic conflict patterns, and their no more than loose connection to the clinical picture, i.e., their "nonspecificity" (Thomä 1980), has relativized the diagnostic component of the initial interview.

The Tavistock model, which is closely associated with Balint's work, stresses the therapeutic relationship in the here-and-now, i.e., the functional unit of transference and countertransference. In the late 1950s, Mitscherlich introduced this model in the Psychosomatic Clinic of the University of Heidelberg, where it proved extremely productive in that from the very beginning of the dialogue it drew the analyst's attention to the current processes of exchange between him and the patient (Künzler and Zimmermann 1965). Some important points which invite special consideration when making a written summary of the dialogue are as follows:

*Development of the Doctor-Patient Relationship*

1. How does the patient treat the doctor? Are there any changes in this respect? Does this point to habits of behavior or to his relationship to the illness?
2. How does the doctor treat the patient? Are there any changes in the course of the interview?
   a) Was the doctor interested in the patient's problems?
   b) Did he have the feeling he could do something for him?
   c) Did he notice any human qualities on the part of the patient which he liked in spite of all the patient's faults?

*Important Moments in the Interview*

The focus of attention here is the development of events within the interview, i.e., the results of transference and countertransference.

1. Surprising statements or expressions of emotion by the patient, parapraxes etc., obvious exclusion of specific periods of his life or particular people in his environment, and so on.

2. What interpretations were offered in the course of the interview, and what were the patient's reactions?

*Findings and Assessment*

1. How is the disturbance expressed in the patient's life (listing of the symptoms revealed in the interview, including those the analyst vaguely suspects at this juncture)?
2. Presumed significance of the disturbance, expressed in psychodynamic terms.
3. Choice of therapy:
   a) Suitability for a short therapy (focal psychotherapy); reasons
   b) Potential arguments against
   c) Suitability for psychoanalysis; reason
   d) Refusal of any form of psychotherapy; reasons
   e) Other possibly suitable forms of treatment
4. Next goals: What does the doctor consider the essential symptom, the one he wants to tackle first? How might the treatment of this symptom affect other symptoms? Thoughts on the frequency and duration of treatment.

In the next section it will be made even clearer how the spirit of Balint's model influenced the understanding of the therapeutic aspects of the initial interview. Although many are unaware of its origin, this model — whether in its original form (Balint and Balint 1961, pp. 69-70; Balint et al. 1972, pp. 19-20) or modified — has in many places become a guide for the therapeutic conception of the initial interview.

## 6.3 Therapeutic Aspects

The introduction of the Tavistock model changed the conception of the initial interview: psychoanalysis was incorporated into the interview as a therapeutic method, and diagnosis was subordinated to therapy. Or perhaps we should be more cautious and say that the diagnostic and therapeutic functions of the first consultation were now seen as equal in importance. We base our discussion of this qualitative change on Balint's work. Although many other analysts have of course contributed to the therapeutic function of the initial interview being given its rightful place in the first encounter between analyst and patient, we have good reason to concentrate on Balint, as it is precisely with regard to the structure of the interview that his influence on German psychoanalysts is particularly strong. The emphasis put on the therapeutic task creates just that flexibility which we consider essential if one is to achieve an adaptive assessment of indications. The fact that this interview style was originally developed for a special form of therapy, i.e., focal therapy, does not reduce its utility for psychoanalysis in general. On the contrary, obtaining genuine solutions to problems in such a short time is the strongest indication that broader and deeper conflicts might also be reached in a therapeutically useful manner in the course of a longer analysis.

Indeed, hardly any other factor has had as great an influence on the way the analytic dialogue is conducted as the interview technique developed within the framework of focal therapy. Balint's considerations often apply in the same way to the physician and to the psychoanalyst. This emphasizes the wide-reaching interactional nature of the interview; it can be extended to cover many different situations. Central, however, is the observation of the bipersonal process, which Balint stressed as important for the comprehension of the patient's life history. The conception of two-person psychology means that the analyst creates a relationship between what the patient says and how he behaves in the analytic situation, and then uses this relationship diagnostically and therapeutically. Accordingly, the result of the investigation depends on how the analyst behaves in this professional relationship and what he learns from it. Ultimately only what the patient contributes can be used in diagnosis, but his contributions must be understood as "the sum total of the patient's reactions to a particular doctor, at a particular moment, in a particular setting" (Balint and Balint 1961, p. 167). This puts the doctor or psychoanalyst in a situation which is theoretically interesting, but in practice hard to solve. The differentiation of function and tasks leads to this one-sided version of interaction. As regards treatment technique, the object relationship which develops is considered to be determined principally by the patient's inner need for such a relationship (see Beckmann 1974).

The general message that psychoanalysts have also received from Balint's writings for physicians in general is that the attempt should be made to use "the patient's potentiality for developing and maintaining human relationships" (Balint and Balint 1961, p. 183) as a criterion for decisions. The acceptance of Balint's ideas enabled the initial interview to be varied widely within psychoanalysis and applied in many different fields (Junker and Waßner 1984). The renewed reflection on the parameters of the interview which is necessary in each individual case simultaneously permitted innovations that played a part in the development of various types and configurations of the initial meeting (home visit, consultation with family doctor, psychoanalytic counseling, etc.). Interviews without previous appointment, as introduced at the Sigmund Freud Institute originally for purely practical reasons, create unforeseen new forms which demonstrate just how much the content of an interview is determined by the conditions under which it takes place (Argelander et al. 1973). This kind of interview meets the expectations of a patient in acute distress. The analyst, for his part, sees the patient at a time of crisis in which the therapeutic possibilities are circumscribed and limited. Unaccustomed for the analyst, but perhaps therefore important, is the opportunity — analogous to the general practitioner — to lend immediate short-term therapeutic support and thereby possibly create an atmosphere of trust conducive to a subsequent analysis. Wherever analysts reserve time for consultations at short notice — whether in their own practices or, as is more usually the case, in institutions — a wealth of new possibilities emerge. The patients who avail themselves of this opportunity are mostly those who do not fit into the rigid framework of analytic practice and thus enrich the analyst's store of experience.

The longer patients must wait for the psychoanalytic initial interview, the greater the selection among the patients the analyst eventually sees. There are two psychodynamic factors at work here. On the one hand, the patient who has taken the step of making an appointment is already in a therapeutic situation. In conscious and unconscious fantasies, he is trying out preexisting patterns of transference to the analyst, although they have not yet met. On the other hand, his unconscious resistance is inevitably reinforced by the frustration of waiting.

Questionnaires and tests before the initial interview place the patient under stress and also, understandably, awake expectations in him. He is then tense when the interview comes and often expects more than the analyst is in a position to give. The different expectations aroused by the differing settings in institutions and in private analysts' offices must be made a topic of discussion at an early stage.

Additional differences in the expectations toward the initial interview arise from the range of treatment available, which differs from place to place and is usually not completely familiar to the patient. To avoid disappointments, suitable preparation concerning the goals of the interview is an important first step in the introductory phase (*recommendation 1*). The interview is an unaccustomed situation for patients, and most errors in the consequences drawn from their behavior stem from inadequate preparation. Cremerius gives one clear example of this in his criticism of the situational structure of the interview technique employed by the French psychosomatic-psychoanalytic school (Cremerius 1977a).

Educated and uneducated patients vary so widely in their prior knowledge of psychoanalysis (Cremerius 1977a) that the way the dialogue is conducted must be adjusted accordingly. A striking example of the patient's prior understanding and the analyst's erroneous interpretations of it is provided — probably unintentionally — by Schröter (1980) in his essay on specific reactions to the treatment process and the social distance to the therapist: "It nevertheless seems that lower-class patients are typically irritated to a greater degree than others by the special features of the psychoanalytic dialogue" (p. 60).

It irritates us that a sociologically trained author here postulates a form of the psychoanalytic dialogue which seems to make no allowances for variation in the conditions under which the patient's everyday communication takes place. We cannot let this rigidity — as though the unconscious were accessible only via a form of psychoanalytic dialogue oriented toward an upper middle class standard — go uncriticized, particularly since we have good models for conducting the interview according to the patient's potentialities (Deutsch and Murphy 1955).

It would seem more profitable to study the Balints' recommendations concerning the necessary conditions for a successful interview (Balint and Balint 1961, pp. 187-188), which we would now like to summarize. *Recommendation 1* (see above) stresses the importance of proper and adequate introduction to the encounter — particularly relevant with regard to the social component of the differences in patients' expectations. *Recommendation 2* is the creation and maintenance of an appropriate atmosphere, in which the patient can open up enough for the therapist to be able to understand him. This is a test of the interviewer's capacity for active empathy, and thus of his ability to adjust himself to every new patient. Difficulties are inevitable here as well, necessitating continuous examination of the analyst's contribution to the dialogue. The Balints emphasize this by pointing out that a doctor who always reassures the patient as soon as he notices the latter is under stress will gain material different in nature to that gathered by a doctor who only listens passively and lets the patient "stew" or steer the interview himself.

Statements about a patient should therefore always include information on the situational parameters created by the interviewer which have acted as "stimuli" — in the Balints' sense of the word — on the patient (*recommendation 3*).

It is very important that the psychoanalyst have some idea of the future direction of the relationship before he begins to mold it in the interview. The concrete interview plan (*recommendation 4*) depends on whether the analyst can anticipate that the interview relationship will develop into a therapeutic relationship, or whether it is certain from the outset that the relationship will end at least provisionally after this one encounter because the patient will be either placed on the waiting list or referred to a colleague.

The duration of the interview is another of the parameters determined both by practical external considerations and by the complexities of the interaction. On the one hand the therapist is emotionally and scientifically curious, on the other his need for security leads to great differences in the form the interview takes.

One practical problem which is often overlooked is the patient's lack of information as to the duration of the interview. After all, the initial interview frequently follows a series of mostly disappointing and often short consultations with doctors. How should the patient know that he can now count on a duration of at least 45 minutes and on the security which this gives? Another matter which must be considered is the question of whether the patient should be informed of the possibility of a second meeting directly at the beginning of the interview, or whether this should be decided at the end on the basis of what the interview has revealed.

Conversely, we believe it is vital that novice analysts, in particular, set themselves a definite framework for the configuration of the initial interview, but avoid having an unlimited number of sessions depending on their own personal degree of insecurity (*recommendation 5*).

These passionately debated details of technique all belong to the area which the Balints seek to embrace in the concept of *elastic interview technique*. The analyst must react differently to different patients and not allow himself to be restricted by stereotypes such as the traditional understanding of countertransference (*recommendation 6*). We can speak of a capacity for countertransference when the analyst recognizes countertransference and can use it to good diagnostic effect (see Dantlgraber 1982). The decisive question is: In which respect does this flexibility have to prove its value? Here too, the Balints go straight to the problems for which there are no universally applicable answers, but which must be solved on an individual basis: "Is it advisable or desirable that a consultation should amount to nothing more than a diagnostic examination, or should it include some sort of therapy, e.g. some highly mitigated form of psycho-analysis?" (Balint and Balint 1961, p. 195). We are of the opinion that the patient should experience in the initial interview what the treatment can mean for him; this is therapeutic in itself. But viewing the initial interview as a model of therapy raises a demand which cannot be satisfied. The interview should be conducted in a manner that gives the patient a basis on which to decide for himself whether he wants to undergo psychotherapeutic treatment and is capable of tackling the problems inevitably associated with its realization. This approach releases the patient from his passive role. Although a certain amount of exploratory diagnostic work is essential and should not be phobically avoided, the goal of the psychoanalytic interview is to find what is going on or has gone on within the patient and how he himself has contributed to his fate. This goal can be reached by means of an appropriate technique, as described clearly and empathically by Rosenkötter:

> When a patient visits a psychotherapist on account of neurotic symptoms or other problems of psychic origin, the first contact between the two is in principle no different from that in other medical consultations. The patient reports his problems, and the therapist tries to find out as much as possible about their occurrence and history and about the life history of the patient in general, in order to gain material on which to base a verdict as to indication and prognosis. An important role is played by the therapist's experience and gift for empathy. The therapist must allow sufficient time to enable the patient to enter the dialogue spontaneously and of his own free will; any questions he needs to ask should accompany and supplement the patient's report in a cautious manner, and he should take care to maintain a beneficent, neutral, reserved attitude. He should avoid specific questioning, definitive statements, and instructions, which tend to lead patients in general to adopt an attitude of passive, magic expectation toward doctors. (1973, p. 989)

The Balints' comments on the initial interview, which are relevant for the analyst as well as for psychotherapy in medical practice, were taken up by Argelander, who in a series of publications (Argelander 1966, 1967, 1970; Argelander et al. 1973) devoted himself to the interaction between patient and investigator:

> For the experienced psychotherapist, Balint's statement says that every interview is also grasped as an analytic situation and features specific moments of transference to the given interviewer and the given surroundings at the given time. The patient's very varied communications — verbal information, proffered behavior, ideas induced in the interviewer, and so on — are grouped or, more accurately, crystallized around this interpersonal relationship, the heart of the examination as Balint called it. They receive from this action center a directive which leads to the patient's problems unfolding in characteristic fashion before the eyes of the given examiner. (1966, p. 40)

Argelander varies and elaborates these themes in the later publications. Taking Balint's theses to their conclusion, he describes the interview as "an analytic situation in which we use our psychoanalytic instrument also for diagnostic purposes" (1966, p. 42). Even though it is taken for granted that the analyst adapts the psychoanalytic instrument to the special external structure of this initially restricted analytic situation — it must remain in harmony with the current reality and the ego-related process — this interview technique often demands more than analyst and patient are in a position to deliver. Argelander

(1966, 1967) distinguishes between two areas of experience which he tries to relate in the interview: the registering of objective facts and the development of subjective experiencing.

The fusion of these two areas of experience (with the objective subordinated to the subjective) constitutes the specific psychoanalytic access. In this concept, the three essential working steps are characterized by observation of behavior, questioning for "objective" information, and a specific kind of perception which takes the form of empathic understanding of the unconscious object relationship. This third function is precisely that understanding of process activity which occurs in long analyses:

We know from psychoanalytic experience that in an object relationship internal psychic processes are projected externally and can be perceived and experienced subjectively. For this reason we give the patient the chance to initiate an object relationship in the initial interview, leaving the form, content, and dynamic of the relationship to be determined by his own individual personality. His spontaneity is fully safeguarded. Our appearance, age, sex, character, temperament, etc. are concrete situational factors which stimulate the examinee to transfer preexisting inner feelings, expectations, conflicts, ideas, and fantasies to the examiner. (Argelander 1967, p. 431)

This "transference theory" of the initial interview owes its indisputable attractiveness to the fact that the painstaking, slowly developing processes of mutual understanding and communication in the psychoanalytic process are apparently comprehended at the very first attempt, during the first encounter.

In his further elaboration of this position (1970), Argelander separated the three sources of information, which he termed objective, subjective, and scenic. This is somewhat arbitrary, as he himself says, but useful in practice. "Scenic information is dominated by the experiencing of the situation, with all its emotional stimuli and ideational processes" (1970, p. 14). The specific understanding achieved in scenic cognition was developed and structured in Balint group work and in case discussions (Argelander et al. 1973). The accumulated experience of Argelander and his colleagues underlines the fact that in an interview material is usually gathered relatively rapidly "in order to put analytic perception and thinking on an operational basis" (Argelander et al. 1973, p. 1004). The Balint group experience was confirmed in this setting, which (although different) shared a similar structure by virtue of the brevity of the interviews. Despite the very positive response among German-speaking analysts to Argelander's model of the initial interview, his own admonitions and self-critical comments have not received corresponding attention: "The exercises in scenic understanding should thus serve to accentuate the preconscious perception and thought processes more strongly and in this way mobilize the analyst's natural creative potential" (Argelander et al. 1973, p. 1009). The capacity to perceive preconscious processes can be improved through training.

Without this training nothing more than extravagant fantasies and wild speculation can be expected .... This fact cannot be stated often enough, as our specialty is particularly guilty of ignoring it. The failures are then swiftly blamed on the hopelessly overstressed subjective factor, and eventually the whole method is discredited. (Argelander et al. 1973, p. 1010)

Our assessment of this interview style can be related to Argelander's own reservations. It is one thing for a group led by a specially gifted psychoanalyst to dedicate itself to developing a highly differentiated interview style, but quite another to evaluate how well such a procedure can be taught and learned. In addition, we doubt whether this method, when applied in too purist a fashion, achieves the special results it was designed to achieve, i.e., to enable the selection of a specific therapeutic procedure "oriented toward the patient's present inner conflict situation (e.g., short therapy) or his current transference disposition and its needs, conflicts, and forms of expression (e.g., group therapy)" (Argelander 1966, p. 41). Indications for particular treatment procedures cannot be established entirely from the diagnosis of unconscious conflict constellations, as the following discussion of the problems regarding indications will show.

In recent years it has become increasingly clear that although the initial interview is adequate for a subjective appraisal (Dantlgraber 1982), a more differentiated establishment of indications requires consideration of additional factors. The purely subjective impression of a patient's suitability for analysis is not sufficient.

## 6.4 Decision Process

So far we have concentrated on a critical account of past and present conceptions of the initial interview as an event which is simultaneously diagnostic and therapeutic. At the end of the last section we were confronted with the question of what conclusions regarding indications can be drawn from any one technique. As we will now show, the misgivings we mentioned are borne out by the almost complete lack of substance displayed by the results in the copious clinical literature.

Freud's indication criteria were essentially criteria of exclusion: to be excluded are those who do not have a certain degree of education and a fairly reliable character, and also those who themselves feel no necessity to undergo treatment for their problems but are pressured into doing so by their families. "To be quite safe, one should limit one's choice of patients to those who possess a normal mental condition, since in the psycho-analytic method this is used as a foothold from which to obtain control of the morbid manifestations" (1905a, p. 264). Further restrictive criteria which Freud applied were age and the necessity for swift elimination of threatening symptoms, for example in anorexia nervosa.

We attach greater importance to Freud's positive criterion of indication, which is much less widely known: "Psycho-analytic therapy was created through and *for* the treatment of patients permanently unfit for existence" (1905a, p. 263, emphasis added). With the proviso of the existence of a "normal mental condition" as described above, Freud attaches no restrictive significance to the severity of an illness. This viewpoint differs radically from the conclusion reached in numerous round table discussions of analyzability (e.g., Waldhorn 1960); the description of the suitable patient can be summed up as "sick enough to need it and healthy enough to stand it." This shows how far the neoclassical style of treatment technique has departed from Freud's original conception.

We must today still proceed from the assumption that the indication for psychoanalysis can only rarely, if ever, be derived from the nature of the illness. Although a distinction was long made between transference neuroses — considered treatable — and narcissistic neuroses, the fact could not be disguised that the diagnosis of a transference neurosis actually says relatively little about treatability. Before we continue the tangled story of the development of indication criteria, characterized over the decades by the introduction of various terms such as suitability, accessibility, and analyzability, we would like to point out that in doing so we are describing a line of thought which did not originate in Freud's practice.

We believe that to discuss the problem complex from the perspective outlined by Tyson and Sandler (1971) — that of the problems involved in selection of patients *for* analysis — is to start from a false position, one which originated in a legitimate central idea but has become a dance around the golden calf of the basic model technique (see Chap. 1).

The nucleus of many discussions concerning the selection of patients for psychoanalytic treatment is represented by the high demands in terms of personal commitment, money, and time which an intensive analysis places on both patient and analyst. Not for nothing has psychoanalysis been compared to an expedition whose members must be chosen with care. It thus seems that the method may in fact not be successful in all the "patients permanently unfit for existence" for whom Freud originally said psychoanalysis was created, and therefore it is in the interests of both doctor and patient to appraise its applicability in advance in each individual case. This must be borne in mind in reading the following discussion of the problematic nature of indications for psychoanalysis in the standard technique with its high frequency of sessions.

Freud enthusiastically regarded patients with all variants of severe and complex neuroses who could not be treated by more convenient methods (1905a, p. 262) as potential candidates for his new method. Jones (1920), however, introduced the connection between diagnosis and prognosis. His catalogue of indications includes the following diagnoses: (1) hysteria, (2) anxiety hysteria, (3) compulsion neurosis, (4) hypochondria, (5) fixation hysteria. Groups 4 and 5 were considered to have worse prognoses.

Fenichel (1945) took up the idea of connecting the prognosis to the severity of the neurosis:

> In general, therefore, the difficulty of an analysis corresponds to the depth of the pathogenic regression. Thus using analytic knowledge about the depth of the decisive fixation points in the respective neuroses, the neuroses may generally be classified, according to their accessibility to analysis ... (p. 574)

The method, by this time established, is embodied in the words "accessibility to analysis." Fenichel stresses, however, that:

> Many other circumstances must be considered in making the prognosis: the general dynamic relationship between resistances and the wish for recovery, the secondary gains, the general flexibility of the person. (p. 575)

Glover (1955) takes up the concept of responsiveness and assigns diagnoses to one of three categories, "accessible," "moderately accessible," and "intractable."

Tyson and Sandler (1971) state that the symposium "The Widening Scope of Psychoanalysis" shifted the emphasis from diagnostic criteria to criteria of suitability. As A. Freud (1954b) commented, there is no guarantee that two people with the same symptoms will react identically to the same technical intervention. This fact cuts the ground from under the feet of any nosologically oriented discussion of indications. Yet it took a long time before the knowledge that it is impossible to predict the result of treatment for a given patient led to the conclusion that analysts should seek those factors which have a positive effect on the development of a psychoanalytic process. The problem continued to be reduced to the familiar formula "insight into the structure of the neurosis." Freud's (1913c) concept of a trial analysis was elaborated by Fenichel (1945) but has never really been widely adopted. Instead, the initial interview increasingly contains elements of the trial analysis, the intention being to test the patient's ability to handle interpretations (Alexander and French 1946, p. 98). Although the results are sometimes impressive, the fear remains that this situation could create excessive stress, with potentially negative consequences on the decision regarding indication.

Mitscherlich (1967) formulated a minimal requirement which ought to give a greater number of patients access to psychoanalytic treatment: "The ability [of the patient] to react affectively to an understanding offer seems to us the most certain prognostic indicator that ... the symptom does not represent the best outcome which the patient could achieve" (p. 149). Also implied here is the "ability" of the therapist to make an "understanding offer." The problem of the initial interview and the associated problems of indication is complicated by the technical issue of how we can convince patients to cooperate with our "direction of questioning" (Mitscherlich 1967, p. 141). However, since we do not want our portrayal of the problems to end up following the traditional dichotomy between the standard technique and analytically oriented psychotherapies, the simple statement that the patient's cooperation in the initial interview should be won by means of an understanding offer does not suffice. For which goals should it be won? In this light we can now examine more closely the criteria of suitability put forward by Tyson and Sandler (1971), which in our opinion imply processes to reach consensus on goals.

We suggest speaking in terms of a wide range of treatment goals. Psychoanalysis can only fully live up to its ambitious claim of being a path to improved self-knowledge if the self-knowledge which is gained results in a decrease of anxiety and thus in a change in viewpoint and a modification of behavior toward a freer choice of goals. Freud's statement (1909b, p. 121) that "therapeutic success, however, is not our primary aim; we endeavour rather to enable the patient to obtain a conscious grasp of his unconscious wishes" implies a postulate of change that can only be artificially distinguished from narrowly defined medical criteria of success. Psychoanalytic theory postulates that the elimination of repression and the conscious recognition of previously unconscious wishes necessarily bring about a change in psychic processes. The discussion of indications for various forms of psychoanalytic treatment is thus actually a discussion of various goals. The decision to suggest that a patient have several sessions of analysis a week implies the assumption that he can in all probability achieve profound changes in his psychic processes which will affect very different areas of his life in various ways. When setting the goals, it is legitimate to make the necessary preconditions for such a process of change the object of critical discussion. The patient's motivation, his personal orientation, his curiosity about psychology, and his ability to utilize object relationships are among the factors which play a decisive role in the current discussion of indications for classical psychoanalysis.

Kuiper (1968) professes a restrictive approach to the establishment of indications and points out, quite rightly, that young analysts' enthusiasm for the standard technique leads them to apply it uncritically. There can, for example, be highly unfavorable consequences if the analyst treats silence and stereotyped nonanswering of questions as indispensable components of the standard technique and employs them with patients for whom this technique is not suitable. Note that we designate the technique unsuitable, not the patient. We thus agree with Kuiper that the standard technique is very limited in its applicability, but accentuate the necessity of modification and adaptation to fit each individual patient. Kuiper even puts forward a motive for the tendency toward excessive application of the standard technique: Analysts have invested a lot of energy, time, and money in learning it, and now they want to try it out exclusively and intensively with as many patients as possible. The inevitable disappointments then lead, via reaction formation, to dismissal of other, "nonanalytic" aids (Kuiper 1968, p. 261). At the same time, idealization of the standard technique removes the analyst's own doubts about it; instead of thinking about modifying his technique, he blames the patient for turning out to be unsuitable after all.

All too often, it emerges that the characteristics described as necessary or adequate for the acceptance of the responsive or analyzable patient for classical psychoanalytic treatment simultaneously form goals of the treatment process:

> The patient must have a sufficient degree of intelligence, an ability to tolerate painful affects and be capable of sublimation. His object relationships will be relatively mature and his capacity for reality-testing will be more-or-less well established. His life will not be centred around his analysis so that he becomes unduly dependent on it, and his moral character and educational achievements will have assured him of a good position in life with adequate rewards. It would seem that we may be in the paradoxical position of finding that the patient who is ideally suited for analysis is in no need of it! (Tyson and Sandler 1971, p. 225)

Rather than drawing the conclusion that minor deviations from this ideal must be tolerated, we prefer to examine the interactional quality of those characteristics. "Healthy enough to stand it" refers after all to the psychoanalytic situation which patient and analyst must create and maintain. Kuiper believes that the question of who analyzes whom in what way and to what end cannot be taken seriously enough. Defining what the analyst must and can do in every individual case to make an analytic process possible should bring to an end the persistent debate concerning analyzability. In a review of the difficulties regarding analyzability, Bachrach (1983, pp. 199-200) reduced the problem to three groups of patients:

1. "Reflective persons of basically reliable ego who are able to adapt to the expected range of differences among analysts and make the most productive use of their analytic opportunities"
2. Ego-weak patients who display an infantile character and are "unable to participate in the work of analysis"
3. Patients described by Bachrach as "borderline" cases (not in the diagnostic sense), "for whom the fate of the analytic work often more heavily depends upon the person and special talents of the analyst"

Although it is plain what Bachrach is trying to express in the words "basically reliable egos," we consider it more advantageous and strategically more appropriate to examine the interactional configuration in every therapeutic situation. The basic reliability of which Bachrach speaks is as much a fiction as Hartmann's "average expectable environment," which led the theory of ego psychology up a blind alley (Fürstenau 1964). The importance of the psychoanalyst's ability to vary his approach in response to each individual patient's needs and conflicts has grown by the same extent to which the main symptoms have been shifted from circumscribed disturbances to more diffuse personality problems (Thomä and Kächele 1976). The existence of two complementary techniques, which Cremerius (1979) described for solely didactic reasons as opposing poles, is an expression of the fact that "the boundaries of analyzability are not the boundaries of the patient and his psychopathology, as claimed by Freud (1937c), but the boundaries of the analyst" (Cremerius 1979, p. 587). We believe that the concept of "analyzability" has lost every last scrap of specificity and could be beneficially replaced by "treatability." If "analyzable" comes to refer to what a psychoanalyst can do and endure, then indications can become the object of discussion and research only within the framework of the bipersonal foundation of the therapeutic process.

The conception of indication in the initial interview thus changes from *prognostic* (static) to *adaptive* (dynamic), expressly referring patient and analyst to one another (Baumann and von Wedel 1981). A successful example of this thinking is given by S.H. Shapiro (1984), who proposes a genuinely psychoanalytic approach to ascertaining the most suitable treatment method. Instead of a trial analysis — which we also consider no longer appropriate, for many reasons — Shapiro has an exploratory phase in the course of which he tells the patient about the method of free association. We agree with his assessment of the potential of a *diagnostic phase of therapy*, which is not a trial analysis in the conventional sense followed by the decision regarding suitability, but rather has the purpose of finding out what changes can be achieved under what therapeutic conditions. The wide scope of the current forms of psychoanalytic therapy allows room for many ideas, which do not even have to be restricted to the field of psychoanalysis in the stricter sense.

If we apply Balint's recommendations to general practitioners to the pschoanalytic initial interview, and develop the conception of a longer relationship to the patient extending beyond one single meeting, the many possibilities offered by patient-oriented indications open up various paths to change which the patient can follow immediately or at a later date (Hohage et al. 1981).

Analysis of the many aspects of the problem of indication must include both the recognition of the subjective elements in the decision (Leuzinger 1981, 1984; Dantlgraber 1982) and consideration of institutional factors affecting psychoanalytic activity. The interaction of the two is often very difficult to discern, as they are easily concealed by the strategies the analyst employs to justify his procedure.

The influence of theoretical assumptions on the decision is great, but still greater is the effect of practical circumstances, which influence the determination of indications now just as they did in Freud's time. Alteration of such circumstances — such as the inclusion of psychodynamically oriented and analytic psychotherapy in the services covered by health insurance — enlarges the circle of patients who can undergo treatment. Class-specific factors nevertheless continue to play a significant role in decisions on indications, as is shown by all empirical studies on this topic. The bias in selection is concealed behind criteria of suitability which thus in many places impose iatrogenic restrictions on the range of psychoanalysis.

Social changes and the covering of costs by health insurance have brought us nearer to the goal of attracting patients from a broad range of social and nosologic backgrounds by means of flexibility in the structuring of the initial interview. It is easy enough to start an analysis with a highly motivated individual, even if the treatment turns out to be difficult; the art of the initial interview lies in awakening a hesitant patient's interest in the therapy he urgently needs. The development of many different forms of psychoanalytic therapy which can be tailored to the individual patient means that Freud's metaphor of gold and copper has to be revised. Today therapy can be planned and structured to meet the individual patient's needs. This perhaps brings us to the central problem concerning the initial interview: We are in a situation where we must make decisions relating to the patient that are no longer defined by the old familiar dichotomy of psychoanalysis vs. analytic psychotherapy. We have to consider how the most favorable conditions for the patient's development can be created and which psychoanalyst is the best for this task. At the end of the first meeting, if not before, the analyst must face the questions: What happens now? Which external conditions have to be satisfied if treatment is to take place? How can a therapy be harmonized with the patient's personal and professional life?

The adaptive approach to indications — the one we regard as commensurate with our present state of knowledge — does not reduce the great responsibility which goes along with the acceptance of a patient for therapy, regardless of frequency and duration. It avoids, however, the particular strains which arise when far-reaching temporal and financial commitments have to be made simultaneously with the assessment of analyzability. We also believe that when discussing the arrangements for the analysis, stress should be laid right from the outset on defining the duration of therapy in terms of the desired and achievable goals, rather than in terms of years or number of sessions. This robs the information concerning the duration of analysis of its depressing effect, and the patient can hope for improvement or cure in less than 1, 2, or X years. Since deterioration, improvement, and cure — the analytic process in its entirety — also depend on the analyst's professional competence, the duration of treatment is also a dyadically determined quantity depending on many factors.

The analyst must always take into consideration the fact that the patient is at liberty to interrupt or terminate the treatment at any time. Attention must therefore be paid to suggestive undertones in remarks about frequency and duration. On the other hand, both participants know that the patient's ideal freedom of choice is in reality restricted — by external circumstances, by self-deceptions based on unconscious motivations, and by the relationship and transference conflicts of the analytic process. Thus there are many factors determining how long treatment should ideally continue and how long it actually lasts.

In the transition from initial interview to therapy, it is important to leave as much room for flexibility as possible and to create an atmosphere of freedom which arouses hope (Luborsky 1984). At the same time, a framework must be established which ensures good working conditions. There is no simple solution to this problem. However, our seemingly banal experience is that patients generally continue to attend as long as there is a positive balance between investment and return. There are good reasons for attaching central significance to the patient's personal assessment of investment and return and thus for according his decisions the consideration they deserve. In this way an ideal scope for development is at least envisaged, however many restrictions actually emerge in its realization. The matter never rests at purely subjective weighing up of pros and cons. Even a multimillionaire who retreats to a desert island like a modern Robinson Crusoe with his analyst Dr. Friday in order to undergo interminable analysis will have to reckon on his analyst assessing the relationship of investment to return differently than he does. There is no need to let this fictive situation spur us on to further fantasies, as nowhere in the world does the patient have sole control of investment and return, of frequency and duration of treatment. The analyst also has a say, and the latently present third parties express their opinions too, directly or indirectly — the effect being particularly incisive in the case of third-party payment.

Enormous differences are possible in the assessment of what we have for the sake of brevity referred to as investment and return. Too many combinations are conceivable for us to be able to discuss them individually here. Our choice of economic terminology is quite deliberate, although we realize it may well alienate the reader. We must not allow the enthusiasm over the frequently liberating effect of psychoanalysis to divert us from the involvement of the patient's family and the investment in terms of time and money. Klauber (1972b, p. 99) placed particular emphasis on the great influence of the cost in time and money and the involvement of the latently present third parties, the patient's family. In West Germany and West Berlin the great majority of analyses are paid for in full by the public health insurance companies. Even most so-called private patients (i.e., those not in public health insurance schemes) receive third-party support from private health insurance companies or the state. The only analysands who genuinely pay out of their own pockets are future analysts undergoing training analyses. Since over 90% of the population are compulsorily insured by public health insurance companies, most patients undergoing analytic psychotherapy suffer no financial privation as a result. Patients come to the initial interview with a certificate for treatment guaranteeing that the costs will be borne by their insurance company. We will return to this theme later (Sect. 6.6), but first we will discuss the patient's relatives, who are always latently present in the initial interview and are not infrequently really present. The analyst's attitude to the patient's family colors the way the dialogue is conducted, and is another factor which can have an often totally unnoticed influence on the direction of the analysis.

## 6.5 The Patient's Family

Freud (1940a, p. 145) described the earliest endeavors in psychoanalysis as the study of "the individual development of human beings." In the Enlightenment tradition, he strove to explore the connections between a patient's widely varying actions and his inner afflictions, and to achieve a cure through self-recognition. Freud sought to effect the expansion of an individual's consciousness by enabling him to gain insight into his unconscious psychic life, seeing in this an essential contribution of psychoanalysis to enlightenment.

The request for psychoanalytic treatment must come from the patient alone. Any agreement between therapist and patient has ethical and legal implications. Discretion and professional confidentiality contribute to a basis of trust between the two parties. In considering whether and when to consult members of the family, we must have the patient's well-being in mind. Only in emergencies may we contact them without the patient's permission, for instance if the patient is not in a position to supply reliable anamnestic information to enable the doctor to make a diagnosis and decide on the appropriate form of treatment. An example of such an emergency is a psychotic or suicidal patient, i.e., one who is not in control of himself. Otherwise the analyst must follow the rule of giving the family no information about the patient.

Generally the psychoanalytic method makes it unnecessary to involve the patient's family. The psychoanalyst relies on what he observes in the sessions with the patient. It is assumed that a patient in analysis has relationship conflicts with the analyst similar to those with his spouse and closest friends and relatives. The analyst needs no direct contact with the patient's family because with the development of the transference neurosis, if not before, he can experience for himself how the patient behaves toward those close to him and unconsciously provokes actions and attitudes for or against himself.

An analyst with an interactional understanding of transference and countertransference can on the one hand gain insight into the way the patient sees things, and on the other, understand the behavior of the relatives, whose reactions may bear similarities to his own countertransference. To these two dimensions can be added at least one more, i.e., the analyst's professional knowledge of human interaction.

The psychoanalytic method raises specific questions concerning the way the analyst deals with the patient's relatives. The method is dependent on the dyadic relationship. In comparison with a surgical operation, the situation is complicated by the real presence of a third person. The commitment to a two-person relationship entails differentiation between internal and external relationships. The psychoanalytic method is a dyad, but could more correctly be termed a "triad minus one," as a third party is always present in some sense, even when no member of the family actually takes part in the treatment. This real absence but latent presence of the third party has major consequences for all concerned.

Glover's survey of 29 British psychoanalysts (Glover 1955) included questions on how they saw and dealt with the problem of patients' relatives. He asked, for instance, whether they had contact with relatives, and if so, with or without their patients' knowledge: "All speak to members of the family, most unwillingly, and at the patient's request. With few exceptions (severe psychoses, children), interviews are arranged with the knowledge of the patient" (Glover 1955, p. 322).

The subsequent literature contains scant reference to the technical management of this problem, although it has broad clinical relevance; indeed, it plays an important role in every therapy. This includes training analyses, where in most cases the analysand's families have no direct contact with the training analyst or institution, although both inwardly and outwardly they are deeply involved. It is not uncommon for the partners to enter therapy themselves or form their own discussion groups.

Freud wrote that he was "utterly at a loss" in face of the problem of how to treat the patient's relatives. His advice runs as follows:

> I must give a most earnest warning against any attempt to gain the confidence or support of parents or relatives by giving them psycho-analytic books to read, whether of an introductory or an advanced kind. This well-meant step usually has the effect of bringing on prematurely the natural opposition of the relatives to the treatment — an opposition which is bound to appear sooner or later — so that the treatment is never even begun.
>
> Let me express a hope that the increasing experience of psycho-analysts will soon lead to agreement on questions of technique and on the most effective method of treating neurotic patients. As regards the treatment of their relatives I must confess myself utterly at a loss, and I have in general little faith in any individual treatment of them. (1912e, p. 120)

As we know, Freud later expected his analysands to have read his works, but did not wish to give their relatives access to the same information. He resigned himself to "the natural opposition of the relatives to the treatment." His optimism had hardly increased by 1917:

> Psycho-analytic treatment may be compared with a surgical operation and may similarly claim to be carried out under arrangements that will be the most favourable for its success. You know the precautionary measures adopted by a surgeon: a suitable room, good lighting, assistants, exclusion of the patient's relatives, and so on. Ask yourselves now how many of these operations would turn out successfully if they had to take place in the presence of all members of the patient's family, who would stick their noses into the field of the operation and exclaim aloud at every incision. In psycho-analytic treatments the intervention of relatives is a positive danger and a danger one does not know how to meet. (1916/17, p. 459)

These remarks have to be seen in part against the background of Freud's technique at that time, which was concentrated on the exploration of the unconscious and of infantile sexuality. The comparison of the psychoanalytic situation with a clean, aseptic operative field leads logically to descriptions of relatives as a source of danger. The ideal of the clean field is expressed explicitly in Eissler's (1953) description of parameters. For him, the intrusion of a family member into the dyadic situation represents a deviation from the basic model technique. This technique views relatives as a confusing and disturbing factor in an otherwise apparently ideal space between doctor and patient.

In an earlier discussion of the problem of the patient's relatives (Thomä and Thomä 1968), we took the view that there are two reasons for analysts' "unwillingness" to involve them, one general and one specific. We see the *general* reason in the wish to protect the "working alliance" (Greenson 1967) with the patient. The "working team" of doctor and patient (Heimann 1966, pp. 333-334) can only function if interference by relatives remains limited. In the effort to ensure discretion and gain the patient's trust, the analyst pushes the family too far out toward the periphery. Richter (1970) mentions further aspects of excessively rigid adherence to the two-person relationship:

> Psychotherapists know that treating an individual is generally less arduous than working with the clustered problems of the whole family group. It is easier to comprehend the difficulties of a single patient than the knot of interactional conflicts involving several members of a family. In addition, it is easier to bear, and work on, the transference of a single patient than the complex tangle of emotions of a whole group of people in the grip of neurotic tensions. (p. 122)

Patients feel the analyst's unwillingness to change the setting, and this leads to specific manifestations of transference/countertransference. The relatives then feel all the more excluded, and their mistrust grows. They tend to react by either idealizing or totally rejecting the analyst. This again depends on what the patient reports about the analysis and what he keeps to himself. Since the development of the transference neurosis depends to a high degree on the analytic technique, it is very likely that the patient will act out intensively outside the analytic relationship and that the persons affected will react with counteroffensives. The consequent professional attitude distances the analyst from the patient's relatives and can be viewed as the specific reason for his reluctance to deal with them.

### *6.5.1 The Burden on the Family*

Hans Thomae (1968, p. 89) stressed that for Freud and his followers, the way an individual acts and feels is determined above all by the conjunction of a need and a specific constellation of environmental factors within a more or less circumscribed critical phase. The connection between the patient's *individual fate* and its impact on the environment characterizes the tension between the patient and his family. Psychoanalytic treatment affects the relatives as well as the patient, and these consequences of the psychoanalytic process cannot be taken too seriously.

The family has a correspondingly strong interest in the patient's treatment. Nothing could be more natural than the desire to see the analyst and get to know him, or at least learn something about him. In the early phase of analysis some patients will bring a close relative (usually the spouse) with them, unannounced and with noticeable hesitation, in order to bring about at least a superficial acquaintance. Probably many more relatives than we suppose have seen the therapist or heard something about him.

The relatives' interest in the analyst and the treatment arises from their realization that not only the patient's life will be changed, but theirs too. Some try to escape these changes by claiming that the problem lies wholly with the patient, whom they "hand over for therapy." Mostly, however, they notice that an individual's development processes also affect the people around him, changing the relationships between them. Grunberger (1958) illustrated the links between the lines of development with the example of the restructuring of the patient's superego. The inevitable structural modifications of the superego in the course of the psychoanalytic process disturb the existing arrangements regulating life within the family.

Lidz et al. (1965; Lidz and Fleck 1985) provided a striking account of how closely the psychic conflicts of severely disturbed patients are interwoven with the psychic problems of their relatives. It is precisely when the patient's relatives are emotionally disturbed themselves, or at least contribute to maintaining the patient's neurosis, that unconscious motives can lead them to lend only partial support to the treatment. In such a case the analyst should consider whether the interpersonal conflict should be made a goal of therapy, although then the question arises of whether the members of the family should be included only during one certain phase of therapy, or whether treatment of a couple or of a whole family seems to be indicated and the two-person therapeutic setting should be abandoned.

Patients often base important decisions concerning their professional and private lives on what they have discovered about themselves in the course of analysis. When this happens, it is essential that the analyst give the patient's relatives the feeling that he is aware of the burden on them and recognizes that the psychoanalytic process has repercussions on them too. In our view, this means not just thinking about the intrapsychic conflicts but also considering the patient's relationships with other people, in order to achieve a balance between the external and the internal, between interpersonal relationships and intrapsychic object relationships. The positive change in the psychoanalyst's attitude to the patient's family and environmental situation has modified the management of this problem in the way we have described.

Few empirical studies have been published on how partners or other family members change during or after psychotherapeutic treatment. In a study on 39 hospital inpatients with severe psychic disturbances, Kohl (1962) wrote that all the partners also suffered some form or another of mental illness and endangered the success of the therapy. Bolk-Weischedel (1978) relativized this statement. In a semistructured follow-up study of the spouses (15 women and 35 men) of 50 patients treated on an outpatient basis, she found that 13 previously symptomatic individuals became symptom-free and experienced positive structural change during their partners' treatment. Eleven previously symptom-free spouses became symptomatic, six of them with subsequent positive structural development. Ten spouses suffered so much during the treatment that they sought advice or therapy for themselves. Ten patients decided on separation or divorce during the course of the treatment; this corresponds to the figures on the divorce rate during psychotherapeutic treatment given by Sager et al. (1968). The majority did not regret taking this step. Bolk-Weischedel interprets this appearance or alteration of symptoms as an indicator of a lability, induced by the treatment, which first makes progressive development possible.

### *6.5.2 Typical Situations*

Great sensitivity is needed in dealing with the patient's relatives. The keynote is always the creation of a therapeutic situation which gives the patient faith in the therapy and in the analyst. In other words, the principle we follow when making our decisions is that whatever we do, the vital point is to create for the patient "the best possible psychological conditions for the functions of the ego" (Freud 1937c, p. 250). In occasional cases the inclusion of one or more members of the patient's family can promote the psychoanalytic process by combating stagnation. It is not merely a matter of expanding the basis of observation to gain more information; the presence of the relatives enables added concentration on the interpersonal relationships between them and the patient. The observation of this interaction serves diagnostic purposes (for example, the degree of real dependence must be evaluated), but therapeutic influence can also be exerted.

There are basically three situations in which we have to decide whether or not to take up direct contact with a patient's family: (1) during the initial interview; (2) in an emergency (accident, suicide risk, committal to hospital); (3) in the course of the treatment.

It is well known that the *initial interview* can take many forms. One essential element in the assessment of the patient's condition is the behavior of the relatives — whether they do not appear at all, stay in the background (outside the house, in the waiting room, etc.), or arrange it so that they come into the office with the patient. Depending on the analyst's approach, various things can happen. Relatives who remain in the background and hesitate to approach the analyst are unconsciously reinforced in their reserve; those who appear unexpectedly are rebuffed with analytic neutrality and distance. The opportunity to recognize the interpersonal dynamic and analyze it with an expert eye can then be lost. For various reasons, it is difficult to behave in a natural way (Heimann 1978).

It is common knowledge that some patients decide on separation or divorce from their partners during the course of psychoanalytic treatment. Because prospective patients and their partners know their marriage might be endangered, they often seek a therapist whose own marriage is said to be stable by the friends who recommend him. Conversely, would-be patients with extramarital relationships tend to choose therapists with similar life styles, because they believe that such therapists will understand them particularly well. Patient and partner may raise urgent questions on this topic at the time of the initial interview.

In the initial interview we inquire about the patient's relationships, distinguishing between present and past ones. At the beginning of therapy it is useful to note how the persons close to the patient react. Reports by friends and relatives on their past treatment have a decisive influence on the patient's initial attitude to his own therapy. The analyst can answer many urgent questions by tendering information about psychoanalytic treatment.

*Emergency situations* form an exception to the normal rule that every contact with a relative must be discussed with the patient. Such situations may be uncovered in the initial interview or may first reveal themselves during the course of treatment; for instance, suicidal tendencies in a psychotic episode demand swift action which often necessitates the cooperation of the patient's family. It is very unusual to have to commit a patient to a psychiatric hospital against his will; usually we can obtain his consent, though often only with the help of his family.

The patient's partner can enter the *treatment situation* at the wish of the patient or the analyst, but also at his or her own request. The question of what (apart from emergencies) precipitates interaction with relatives leads to the definition of the ideal patient: someone able and willing to include the neurotic element of his relationship disturbances in his transference in such a way that his conflicts are renewed and can be resolved — in other words, someone who is suffering but who works through his conflicts in the analysis. The reaction of the patient's family obviously depends on how he reports his experiences in the analysis. The psychoanalytic method demands a high capacity for introspection on the part of the patient and his family. Often, however, not all the parties involved initially possess this. The progress of a treatment may even set something in motion in the patient's partner with which neither of them can come to terms; one or the other then requests the analyst's assistance in mastering this problem.

In all considerations of what help the psychoanalyst can offer, it must be remembered that the therapeutic situation revives infantile behavior patterns in both the patient and his relatives. This forces us to weigh up very carefully just what and how much we say to any family member who is brought in. If one talks to a relative alone, every word and every scrap of information will be passed on to the patient in a subjective manner. If for particular reasons a joint session with both patient and relative does not seem advisable, we recommend telling the patient what has been said to the relative. Menninger and Holzman (1958) favor telling the patient in advance what will be said to the relative, but this probably has no decisive effect on the patient's reaction. More important is the decision whether one can talk to the two of them together. One then reduces the risk of the information being distorted, but may succumb to the temptation of regarding the descriptions of the patient's relationships as objective. Greenacre made the following comment on this subject:

> While it is undoubtedly true that an analyst's vision of the total situation may at certain points be seriously impaired by his need to stick to the microscopy of his work or by an overidentification with the patient, still it seems that this is in the long run less distorting ... than if the analyst succumbs to the pressure of outside information, which is sometimes not in the least objective. (1954, p. 682)

Greenacre never gives or requests specific information concerning the patient without the latter's knowledge and consent, and only does so at all at the patient's request.

We will now discuss ways of looking at this issue. Dealing with relatives raises two types of complications for the psychoanalytic technique: those from inside to outside, and those from outside to inside.

If the patient's conflicts are not included in his transference, they manifest themselves outside the transference in all his activities and relationships. This compulsion toward repetition outside the therapeutic situation takes the place of the impulse to remember, and is acted out mainly within the family. The analyst must then try to ascertain whether the patient who behaves in this way is avoiding working through his conflicts in the doctor-patient relationship by using his relatives as substitutes, or whether his acting out is so egosyntonic that he cannot include his suffering in the transference relationship; whichever is the case, therapeutic influence is obstructed. It is often difficult to achieve clarity on this point. Even if we define acting out simply as those forms of behavior outside the treatment sessions which take the place of remembering and working through within the analysis — repetition in actions — the kind of relationship the patient has with his partner will in part determine, for example, how much he tells his relatives about the analysis. Provision of adequate information to the partner guarantees confidentiality of the patient's relationship to the analyst, but also reinforces his loyality to his partner. If patients talk too much about the analysis, their relatives may become anxious and be tempted to intervene. On the other hand, relatives who are told little about the therapy feel excluded, and any pre-existing skepticism concerning the analyst is reinforced. This acting out must be interpreted if a change in the patient's behavior is to be induced.

The patient's anxiety that he will change but that his partner will not is often so strong that no progress can be made. In this case, the analyst must accede to the patient's wish and arrange to have an explanatory talk with the partner. Such a talk can be very effective in a situation where the patient is placed under strain by the partner's feeling of being excluded.

Here too, it is important to distinguish whether a relative is brought in at the wish of the patient or is driven by his own anxieties to seek contact with the analyst. If a patient withdraws into the analysis and tells his family little about it, this behavior may strengthen their justifiable sense of exclusion, and they tend to counterreact. These complications are particularly delicate; on the one hand we have to preserve the patient's regression, but on the other, too great a retreat into an infantile dyad may indicate an exaggerated regressive tendency. The analyst must carefully elucidate the patient's degree of readiness to exclude external reality, and must sometimes head off exaggerated regressive tendencies by means of technical intervention (for example by confronting the patient with reality). If this fails and a relative intervenes from outside in the therapeutic process, a joint discussion may release the tension. In some cases, though, it may be important to preserve the two-person relationship, in which event the tension that arises must be endured.

Special attention must be paid to the wish or demand, from partner and/or patient, that the partner should also undergo therapy. Coming from the patient it may arise from guilt feelings, coming from the partner it may be an expression of jealousy, helplessness, or the desire for revenge. However, it is also possible for the patient's progress in the course of the treatment to awaken the partner's own previously suppressed wishes for therapeutic help, and such wishes must be taken very seriously. Occasionally, the analyst has to consider enlarging the therapy to include the partner. In such a case the interpersonal relationship will relegate the individual intrapsychic conflicts to the background. A large proportion of such therapies are indeed direct continuations of individual therapies (Bolk-Weischedel 1978). It may also seem appropriate to offer the partner separate treatment or even to refer him or her to another analyst. The latter is preferable if the couple is considering a separation.

Although the problem of relatives seems to have been neglected in the literature, we believe we can discern a trend toward *inclusion* of members of the patient's family in the therapy plan. This certainly results in part from the broadening of the spectrum of indications for psychoanalysis. A higher proportion of those seeking treatment are people with developmental problems or narcissistic personalities, borderline cases, or psychotics. Among these, some also have alcohol and drug problems, and many have marital difficulties, with all the consequences. Correspondingly, the 1976 survey by the American Psychoanalytic Association revealed an increasing number of psychoanalytically oriented psychotherapies which include partners and other family members.

The inclusion of relatives is necessary not only in treatment of children, psychotics, and patients with inadequate ego structures, but also with some compulsive neurotics. A friend or partner, for instance, can serve as "auxiliary ego" (see Freud 1909d, p. 175).

The attitude of analysts has also changed in recent years, becoming increasingly more patient- than method-oriented; they now pay more attention to family and environment. Pulver's (1978) overview contains hints of greater flexibility. The change in the clientele demands changes in the methods of treatment; thus more emphasis is being placed upon interpersonal relationships.

## 6.6 Third-Party Payment

### *6.6.1 Psychoanalysis and the German Health Insurance System*

Nearly all patients consulting a psychoanalyst in the Federal Republic of Germany (FRG) have medical insurance. Over 90% of the population are members of compulsory insurance programs. Persons earning more than about DM 50 000 (ca. $20 000) annually are no longer compelled by law to insure themselves against illness, but are free to do so voluntarily. At the time of the initial interview, most patients have no clear idea of whether, or to what extent, their insurance company will agree to cover the costs. Only the cautious few who plan long-term and have been considering the possibility of a psychoanalysis for some time have inquired in advance and have a realistic payment plan. Those who are members of the various public health insurance organizations have mostly been officially referred by their family doctors and assume this means they will not have to pay. They know that they have the basic right to treatment free of charge by the doctor of their choice, but the majority have extremely vague conceptions of psychotherapy and psychoanalysis.

Many patients do not know that psychodynamically oriented and analytic psychotherapy are recognized by the insurance companies and that the analyst is thus remunerated for his services according to a fixed scale. Their insecurity is correspondingly great, with a very broad spectrum of attendant reactions. Depressives tend to assume that analytic psychotherapy is not covered by their insurance and that they will not be able to afford the fees themselves. Others take it for granted that they will receive free treatment for their marital and other problems, even if these cannot be construed as illnesses. Patients referred to a psychoanalytic outpatient clinic ask the receptionist about payment by the insurance company. As all people with public health insurance know from previous visits to the doctor, the official referral guarantees treatment free of charge. The doctor is not entitled to charge these patients any additional fee on top of his remuneration from the insurance company.

When agreeing on the therapy, if not before, the patient should be informed of the regulations covering psychoanalysis, including payment in the context of public or private health insurance. Because the subject matter is so complex and is immediately complicated further by the subjective and unconscious meanings which the patient attaches to it, the analyst should not confine himself to giving only limited information. Above all, he must himself be acquainted with the way in which psychotherapeutic care fits into the German health insurance system. We regard it as essential to inform the reader about the current regulations, although they form only the external framework of therapy. In cases of third-party payment, it is extremely important that analyst *and* patient be fully informed about the part played by the third parties, in order to be able to grasp both the unconscious meaning of this arrangement and the interaction between inside and outside. Neglecting to provide information *and* to supply continual interpretations brings about confusion which endangers the analytic process.

We have to familiarize the reader with the banal facts of the mode of payment and with the regulations for the use of analytic psychotherapy within the German insurance system. The less patient and analyst know about the legal framework and its historical development, the more difficult it is to analyze the many and varied unconscious meanings attached to third-party payment.

Every third-party payment, whether by the health insurance company or by the patient's family, brings problems which have both external and internal — material and psychic — aspects. We are clearly talking primarily about the situation in West Germany, but we are not addressing ourselves exclusively to the German reader. The recognition of psychoanalysis as a valid form of treatment for mental illnesses has led in many countries to a situation in which health insurance companies cover the expenses. This is reflected in the international currency of English terms such as "third-party payment" and "peer report." The arrangements for payment via health insurance, involving an application by the treating analyst and peer review by a second analyst on behalf of the insurance company, vary greatly from country to country, but we believe that some typical problems are universal and thus that readers of all nationalities can pick up some ideas on treatment technique from this section. Our knowledge of the situation in many other countries has also convinced us that Germany — a country whose history has not often been characterized by successful compromises — has arrived at a system of third-party payment for analytic therapy through health insurance which is not only effective but leaves a great degree of flexibility for the individual case. Third-party payment and the peer report system, which have proved successful in West Germany over the past decade, are now attracting interest in many other countries, and for this reason our experience merits international attention.

Critics from other countries, such as Parin (1978), Parin and Parin-Matthèy (1983b), and Mannoni (1979), have not taken the trouble to examine the West German system in detail before condemning it. Lohmann (1980) — by no means a lover of institutionalized psychoanalysis — repudiated the assertion made by Mannoni (of the Lacan school) that there is a connection between socialization and payment, and described many of Mannoni's invectives as ignorant and grotesque. Ironically, Lohmann's arguments also apply to Parin's (1978) ideological prejudice against psychoanalysis as conducted in the context of the West German health insurance system. De Boor and Moersch (1978) have also advanced pertinent arguments to counter Parin's view. The discussions between representatives of the various European associations of psychoanalysis in recent years show how difficult it is to absorb information and dismantle prejudices. Groen-Prakken (1984) has summarized the debate. She stresses the undeniable advantage of patients in some countries now being able to obtain psychoanalytic treatment independent of their means, but overall this is outweighed by the fear of interference on the part of those providing the financing. "Interference," not "assistance," is the word most frequently used in these discussions. Since third-party payment can be provided by various agencies — insurance companies, the state, or a national health service — there are different contractual partners in different countries; in the western world, however, one can assume that democratic governments and insurance companies, which exist to serve the common good, are not interested in invading the private sphere and will respect the statutory and professional ethical provisions on confidentiality. The important thing is thus to find solutions which on the one hand guarantee the rights of the individual, and on the other are compatible with the statutory responsibilities of the insurance companies. The current international debate on third-party payment reminds us vividly of the controversies preceding the introduction of the present system in West Germany. Thanks to the efforts of certain doctors, including some analysts, it was possible to establish a set of agreements between the *Kassenärztliche Bundesvereinigung* (KBV; the national corporate organization of physicians regulating matters of public health and the payment of medical care) and the health insurance companies. These contain lucid guidelines that exclude manipulative interference and make analytic psychotherapy available to the insured to an extent which was previously unthinkable. Up to the 1960s, following the example set at the Berlin Psychoanalytic Institute (1920-1933), psychoanalysts had treated quite a few of their patients on a low-fee basis out of a sense of social responsibility (de Boor and Künzler 1963).

We will first discuss the external framework of the system of third-party payment by the public health insurance companies. The insured patient makes no direct payment; the analyst receives his fee via his branch of the KBV. However, the patient does have a substantial monetary interest in this transaction, since he pays a fair proportion of his earnings to his health insurance company as cover for general health care, including the eventuality of an illness whose costs would be too great for the average individual to pay alone. A typical person insured with one of these public companies pays about DM 5000 (approximately $2000) annually. There are no further charges at time of use. It should be emphasized that the patient's right of legal redress is directed not at the state but at the health insurance company, an arrangement dating back to insurance regulations implemented by Bismarck. The West German social insurance system is supervised by the state, but it is not a national health service in the sense of, for example, the system in the United Kingdom.

The patient knows how much is deducted from his salary or wages as his health insurance contribution, and he can calculate how much he has paid in over the years and how often he has availed himself of services. He has a free choice of doctor. Just as the public health insurance companies together form a corporate entity, nearly all doctors are members of the KBV.

The fees for doctors' services are negotiated between these two corporate organizations. Expressed simply, this means the following: The insurance companies have a duty of payment toward the regional physicians' organizations, which together comprise the KBV. The physicians, in return, have a duty to provide medical care for the members of the public insurance companies, i.e., for over 90% of the population. The regional sections of the KBV represent the interests of the doctors in the financial negotiations with the insurance companies. Obviously, the agreements on the fee rates for medical services involve compromises in which political factors play a part and the general economic situation must be considered. And indeed, in many respects, the specific regulations covering psychodynamically oriented and analytic psychotherapy, including the guidelines on payment, represent such a compromise.

Most analysts are reluctant to concern themselves with the topic of payment by insurance, and naturally, the less one goes into them the more complicated they seem. The latent presence of the third party financing the treatment is seen as a source of interference in the ideally purely dyadic psychoanalytic process. It is thus no wonder that nostalgia for the good old days, when settling the fees was a purely private matter, grows with third-party financing.

The advantages of the old system are, however, exaggerated. The true state of affairs can be seen by looking at the situation in countries where analytic psychotherapy is still not covered by health insurance. As far as psychoanalytic care is concerned, the good old days were only good for a very small proportion of the mentally ill. For the majority they were very bad old days. And in countries where the health insurance companies contribute nothing or not enough to the costs of psychoanalytic treatment, it is still true today that only the well-off can afford an analysis. The same conditions prevail which Freud bemoaned in his famous speech in Budapest at the end of the First World War: broad strata of the population suffer from severe neuroses without anything being done about it. At the same time, he predicted, "at some time or other the conscience of society will awake and remind it that the poor man should have just as much right to assistance for his mind as he now has to the life-saving help offered by surgery" (Freud 1919a, p. 167).

In some western countries Freud's prediction has been at least partially fulfilled, and third-party payment, as shown by the controversies of recent decades, has become a hotly debated aspect of treatment technique. Surprising, though, is that third-party payment has only now become a problem; the severely ill, married women, adolescents, and children without inherited wealth or a high income were always reliant on third parties. The biggest such group, and the most dependent on third parties for payment, are children and adolescents. In this section, as in this book in general, we restrict ourselves to the treatment of adults, but at this juncture we would like to stress the great importance of the fact that analytic psychotherapy of children and adolescents is included in the agreements between West German health insurance companies and doctors' organizations. Provision of the necessary funds ensures the treatment of financially dependent children. The early treatment of crises typical for particular phases of development and of neurotic manifestations was made possible by the inclusion of psychodynamically oriented and analytic psychotherapy in the medical treatment covered by health insurance. It is plain that the treatment of infantile neuroses at the time they arise is of tremendous psychosocial significance.

The complications which can arise from dependence on a spouse, other relatives, or wealthy acquaintances, even if they are required by law to provide financial support, are discussed in Sect. 6.6.2. Other problems of treatment technique can arise when financially independent patients pay out of their own pockets with money they have not earned themselves. Freud's Wolf Man is a good example. Originally very rich, he was impoverished by the Russian Revolution; nevertheless, Freud continued his treatment free of charge and even indirectly supported him. It is our belief that most patients, and thus also their analysts, were always dependent on direct or indirect financing by third parties.

For obvious reasons the self-payment by the minority was idealized. Those who genuinely finance their own therapy avoid many complications that inevitably accompany financial dependence on a third party. Therefore the ideal (interminable) analytic process was conceived of as one with a patient whose success in professional life demonstrated good — though neurotically limited — ego functions and who was in a position to remunerate the analyst adequately from his own resources. Even the financially independent patient nowadays usually claims, as a matter of course, the (partial) third-party payment to which he is entitled. The problems which occur in the psychoanalytic treatment of the rich and powerful are, as is made plain by Cremerius et al. (1979), much greater than the idealization of the self-payer would indicate. Even the very wealthy almost always have private health insurance, and expect — realistically — that their application for at least partial payment of the costs, accompanied by a report from the analyst, will be successful. The medical treatment of civil servants is subsidized to the extent of approximately 60%.

About 50 years after Freud's Budapest address (1919a), neuroses were at last recognized as diseases by West German public insurance companies. Far too little attention has been paid to the fact that the road leading to broad application of psychoanalysis was paved by the work in the 1920s at the outpatient clinic of the Berlin Psychoanalytic Institute, where poor patients were treated for very low fees, which did not even cover costs and were paid to the clinic, not to the therapist. The Institute, the first of its kind in the world, was thus kept going not only by the generosity of its benefactor, Max Eitingon, but also by the idealism of its members and trainees, who gave much of their time free of charge. The clinic was not very large, but the treatment of a relatively small number of patients sufficed to allay one anxiety which Freud had expressed in the Budapest address. Although he believed that the most important and effective elements of strict, disinterested psychoanalysis would be adopted in psychotherapy for the masses, he feared that "the pure gold of analysis" would have to be freely alloyed with "the copper of direct suggestion" (1919a, p. 168). Hypnosis and even an integration of psychic and material support would have a place in this future broad-based psychotherapy.

Freud's clear distinction between strict, disinterested psychoanalysis and the mass application of the method, expressed in his metaphor by the stark contrast between the pure gold of analysis and the copper of suggestion, has made a lasting impression right down to the present day. This makes it all the more important to repeat the finding of the report on 10 years work at the Berlin Psychoanalytic Institute (Radó et al. 1930): that the broad — though by no means mass — application of psychoanalysis did not lead to a relapse into simple suggestion. Freud's foreword for this report (1930b) underlined the threefold importance of the Institute as a center for teaching, research, and treatment. Simmel (1930, p. 11) stressed that the *outpatient* treatment of working-class and insured patients differed in no way from that of well-off, self-paying patients.

In 1946, amid the ruins of postwar Berlin, Kemper and Schultz-Hencke broke new ground by founding the Central Institute for Psychogenic Illnesses, which was financially sponsored by the local insurance society, the later General Communal Health Insurance (*Allgemeine Ortskrankenkasse*). Baumeyer (1971) and Dräger (1971) rightly emphasize the great social significance of this pioneering advance: "This was the first step in the recognition of neurosis as illness by a German public institution. For the first time one of the institutions in the social insurance system paid the costs of psychoanalysis and other psychotherapeutic treatment" (Dräger 1971, p. 267). For the first time, insured patients were able to receive psychodynamically oriented therapy at no direct cost, and this on a far greater scale than in the outpatient clinic at the old

Berlin Psychoanalytic Institute. Great credit is due to Dührssen (1962) for her pioneering analysis of the follow-up of 1004 patients who had received analytic psychotherapy at the Central Institute, in which she showed the effectiveness and efficiency of the treatment.

Baumeyer (1971) correctly stressed that the work of the Central Institute for Psychogenic Illnesses made a significant contribution to overcoming the resistance of the social insurance system to psychodynamic treatment: "The Central Institute for Psychogenic Illnesses provided the German Society for Psychotherapy and Depth Psychology with many of the arguments which after long and weary years of negotiations finally led to success" (i.e., to recognition of psychoanalysis by the health insurance companies) (p. 231).

The recognition of neuroses as illnesses was a precondition for the inclusion of the so-called standard psychotherapy in the program of the major health insurance companies in 1967, followed by the other public organizations in 1971 (Haarstrick 1976; Faber 1981). Some limitations were imposed by the obligations of the public and private health companies. The health insurance system exists to enable the necessary outpatient or inpatient medical treatment at the time of need for people from all strata of society, regardless of their financial situation. Apart from a few special circumstances, the patient pays no more than his regular insurance premium (approximately 14% of his income). The legal constraints thus do not permit the health insurance companies to demand from the patient any direct contribution toward the costs of analytic therapy. Whether this will change in view of the explosive growth in the cost of providing health care remains to be seen. In passing, we would like to state that a socially just regulation of the degree to which each patient should bear the costs directly would entail practical problems that could be exceedingly difficult to solve. For the time being, at least, the present legal framework will remain in force, and psychotherapy will continue to be available free of charge to members of public health insurance organizations whose illnesses fit the existing guidelines. It is to these guidelines that we now turn our attention.

In the latest version (March 1984) of the guidelines for the use of psychodynamically oriented and analytic psychotherapy, the methods of the two forms of therapy are defined and the indications for them laid down. The most important passages are as follows:

Psychodynamically oriented and analytic psychotherapy, as defined herein, are types of etiologically oriented psychotherapy in which the unconscious psychodynamics of neurotic disturbances with psychic and/or somatic manifestations is made the object of treatment. Techniques of psychotherapy which are not in accordance with the following descriptions of psychodynamically oriented and analytic psychotherapy will not be funded.

a) *Psychodynamically oriented psychotherapy* includes forms of therapy which treat currently active neurotic conflicts but strive for a concentration of the therapeutic process by means of restriction of the aims of treatment, use of a conflict-oriented procedure, and limitation of regressive tendencies.

b) *Analytic psychotherapy* includes the forms of therapy which treat not only the symptoms of the neurosis, but also the neurotic conflict material and the patient's underlying neurotic structure, in the course of which the therapeutic process is set in motion and continued with the help of the analysis of transference and resistance, involving the exploitation of regressive processes.

Psychodynamically oriented psychotherapy encompasses the short-term focal therapies and the dynamic psychotherapies which expose and work on conflicts. These short therapies, which originated from the psychodynamic derivatives from psychoanalysis, have proved their worth (Malan 1976; Luborsky 1984; Strupp and Binder 1984). Kernberg's (1984) expressive psychotherapy, based on the Menninger Foundation's follow-up study (Kernberg et al. 1972; Wallerstein 1986), is the equivalent of what is known in Germany as the psychodynamically oriented, conflict-revealing techniques of treatment.

The definition of the method of *analytic psychotherapy* fully incorporates the factors Freud regarded as the cornerstones of psychoanalysis, i.e., resistance, transference, and the therapeutic use of regression.

The application of the two forms of therapy in the framework of the health insurance system is restricted in principle to illnesses whose course can be influenced for the better. The therapist must satisfy the analyst acting as peer reviewer that the intended therapy has the potential to alleviate, improve, or cure the neurotic or psychosomatic disease in question. In the application form (from which we quote below), a conditional prognosis has to be stated and supported. The conditions which give the symptoms the status of an illness and the factors maintaining the symptoms must be set out. The decisive factor as regards prognosis is constituted by the *conditions for change* which the two parties, patient and analyst, must bring about. The analyst must in each individual case assess what he and the patient can achieve after he has aroused the patient's hopes by accepting him for therapy and taking on the responsibilities involved. In the situation we are concerned with here he must explain the prognostic criteria to a fellow analyst acting as peer reviewer, i.e., specify why he expects an improvement to occur.

In the above-mentioned guidelines the indications for the two forms of therapy are laid down as follows:

1. Psychoreactive psychic disturbances (e.g., anxiety neuroses, phobias, neurotic depression)
2. Conversion neuroses, organ neuroses
3. Autonomic functional disturbances with established psychic etiology
4. Psychic disturbances consequent on emotional deficiencies in early childhood; exceptionally, psychic disturbances related to physical injuries in early childhood or to malformations
5. Psychic disturbances resulting from severe chronic illness, as long as they offer a basis for the application of psychodynamically oriented or analytic psychotherapy (e.g., chronic rheumatic conditions, particular forms of psychosis)
6. Psychic disturbances due to extreme situations which evoke grave personality disturbances (e.g., a long prison sentence, severe psychic trauma)

The indications are further defined by a list of circumstances under which the health insurance organizations will *not* cover the costs of psychotherapy:

Psychodynamically oriented and analytic psychotherapy are not covered by public health insurance if they do not have the potential to bring about cure or amelioration of a disease or lead to medical rehabilitation. This applies especially to measures intended exclusively for professional or social adjustment, to child-rearing guidance, and other similar measures.

In the area of rehabilitation the following points have to be observed:

If indicated exclusively as a means to medical rehabilitation, psychodynamically oriented or analytic psychotherapy can only be applied under the condition that psychodynamic factors play an essential part in the psychic disturbance or in its effects and that with the help of psychodynamically oriented or analytic psychotherapy the patient can be integrated, if at all possible long term, into the working situation or into society.

The use of psychodynamically oriented and analytic psychotherapy is thus limited in a variety of ways. The range of application is defined in terms of method and nosologic orientation (indications), but at the same time is very adaptive. Each individual patient's motivation and adaptability must be assessed with regard to the possibility or probability of treatment being successful. Here we run up against the triad of necessity, effectiveness, and economy which governs a doctor's diagnostic and therapeutic action in Germany; he is obliged to review his chosen therapy and to justify it, in terms of the triad, to the insurance company.

The treating analyst argues the case for his therapy plan in an application in which the patient's personal data are encoded. This application is checked for form and content by an independent peer reviewer, also an analyst, who has to judge whether the above-mentioned preconditions (type of illness, indications) are fulfilled. The reviewer thus has no personal influence on the treatment process or the way treatment is conducted, but his very function means that he may have a significant effect on the patient's transference, especially at the time of applications for extension of therapy. The fact can then no longer be overlooked that the analytic dyad is in this sense a triad including a latent third party.

Complications inevitably ensue if analyst and analysand forget that they are in many respects only two sides of a triangle. The less the role of the peer reviewer in the therapy is clarified and interpreted, the better he serves as a projection screen. One cannot behave as if the reviewer were not there; whether therapy is extended or not depends on his assessment. In making his decision, he has to heed what the guidelines have to say on the subject of treatment duration: "Analytic psychotherapy should as a rule achieve a satisfactory result in 160 sessions, in special cases up to 240 sessions." Extension to 300 sessions is possible in exceptional circumstances, but must be supported by detailed arguments. Even 300 sessions is no absolute limit, and in the discussion of applications for extension we will present the conditions which have to be met in order for treatment to be continued within the guidelines. The compromise in the guidelines on psychodynamically oriented and analytic psychotherapy obviously has many different aspects. Our positive evaluation of this compromise will become still clearer in Sect. 6.6.2, in which we examine the consequences of the contractual agreements on the psychoanalytic process.

At this point, however, we would like to draw attention to an aspect of professional politics. The introduction of analytic psychotherapy as a form of treatment covered by the public health insurance system means that appropriately qualified doctors can be authorized to provide the specific psychotherapeutic services set out in the guidelines. It is thus unusual for doctors who offer psychoanalysis to be fully active in other areas (general practice or specialties). Their contract with the KBV — their authorization — is limited to psychoanalysis and psychodynamically oriented psychotherapy. Also involved in providing psychoanalytic care to the members of the public health insurance organizations are nonmedical psychoanalysts, who, after completion of a course of academic study (nowadays a degree in psychology is a prerequisite), spend several years in psychoanalytic training at an accredited institution. It is misleading to describe these nonmedical analysts as lay analysts. Sixty years ago, the prosecution of Reik, himself a psychologist trained as a psychoanalyst, on a charge of quackery led Freud to publish *The Question of Lay Analysis* (1926 e). The charge against Reik was dropped, but nonmedical psychoanalysts were not licensed to practice within the Austrian health insurance system (Leupold-Löwenthal 1984). The incorporation of nonmedical analysts into the network of services covered by health insurance in West Germany is exemplary in the history of psychoanalysis.

A consequence of the recognition of neuroses as diseases was that the psychoanalytic treatment goal had to be guided by the medical concept of illness. The health insurance companies are obliged to take over the costs only when the symptoms constitute an illness and the triad of necessity, effectiveness, and economy is also satisfied. Both in diagnosis and in treatment, the West German doctor must have these criteria in mind. He must also remember that neuroses are on a continuum with characterologically determined disturbances, which are not covered by health insurance, and that a smooth transition from one to other may occur.

### 6.6.2 *The Impact on the Psychoanalytic Process*

The psychoanalytic process is determined by a multitude of factors, which we will discuss in detail in Chaps. 8 and 9. At this juncture we will restrict ourselves to presenting a few typical consequences of third-party payment by insurance companies. We would like to begin by putting forward a thesis derived from our experience with the guidelines from the point of view of the patient, the treating analyst, and the peer reviewer. *Every* third-party payment affects the course of the therapy in a typical way, leading to problems which do not crop up when the analysand alone finances the treatment. These typical complications can, however, be solved by analytic means, i.e., by means of interpretation. Our experience confirms Eissler's (1974) expectation; the classical technique can also be applied when treatment is financed by health insurance.

Working through oral and anal themes is more complicated when payment is indirect, but not impossible. Ehebald (1978) and Cremerius (1981 a) have provided well-grounded refutations of the widespread view, most clearly expressed by Kemper (1950, p. 213), that direct payment is nothing less than the moving force of analysis.

Obviously the guidelines also involve restrictions, and it is vital that the social parameters be incorporated into the interpretive work. It can then be seen that the financing of treatment by health insurance, despite its limitations, creates most of all a great degree of freedom for patient and analyst, in that for a period they are relieved of all financial constraints. Their dependence on third-party payment grants them the *freedom* without which neither the necessary conditions for the psychoanalytic cure nor the material existence of the analyst would be assured. Without payment by the public health insurance organizations, the majority of those in need of analytic psychotherapy would have no access to it, and the psychoanalyst would depend on a small number of self-financing patients. We would like to stress once more that since 1967 every publicly insured person in West Germany who has neurotic symptoms constituting an illness has a *right* to etiologically oriented psychotherapy. The patient without means of his own is no longer dependent on the generosity of a well-off friend or relative. Analysis thus no longer depends on the economic factors which used inevitably to exert an unduly great influence on the decision-making process. Less than appropriate remuneration of the analyst for the time-consuming and highly skilled service he provides brings significant difficulties for both parties. These problems vary in degree, for a wide range of reasons. Freud reported unfavorable experience of gratis treatment, but on the other hand stated that "one does occasionally come across deserving people who are helpless from no fault of their own, in whom unpaid treatment does not meet with any of the obstacles that I have mentioned and in whom it leads to results" (1913c, p. 133).

Payment by the insurance company makes the patient independent of the benevolence of the analyst. Many countries still rely on self-sacrifice on the part of analysts. There, the social responsibility is borne by outpatient psychoanalytic institutions, where young analysts or trainees treat patients for fees so low they do not even cover their own costs. In many places, experienced analysts earning their living from private practice act as unpaid supervisors. In countries where no solution resembling the West German system has been found, the situation remains similar to that at the old Berlin Psychoanalytic Institute.

The contrast between the current situation in West Germany and the position in countries with no such provision for financing by insurance companies is striking. A West German analyst presently receives DM 70–80 per hour and thus has an income which, although secure, is limited, especially considering that the training is long and costly.

In general, the regulations on fees still undervalue the personal service that doctors provide; this is particularly true for the psychoanalyst, whose work is highly specialized and time-consuming. This reflects, among other things, a widespread idealization that goes hand in hand with a simultaneous devaluation. Psychotherapy is raised to a higher, nonmaterial level and glorified. It may not be defiled by worldly things, certainly not by anything so tainted as money, and should therefore not be practiced on a professional basis. On the other hand, both laymen and doctors dismiss psychotherapy in the same terms: "They don't do anything but talk; that can't do any good, so it shouldn't cost anything."

Idealization and devaluation take their toll on the patient. If he does not pay the analyst out of his own pocket, he loses the experience of an immediate symbolic reward. Thus it is essential to remember, and to interpret, the indirect compensation of the analyst by the patient's insurance company. The function of the third party has a great bearing on the interaction between patient and analyst, and must be elucidated continuously throughout the analysis in order for the analyst to be able to reverse any disappointments and projections of components of his own self. The association of idealization and devaluation and the role of payment form but one example among many we could give. Cremerius (1981 a) carried out a systematic investigation of many aspects of the influence that payment by health insurance companies exerts on the relationship between patient and analyst and on the development and configuration of the transference neurosis. Of course, the acceptance of psychoanalysis as a recognized treatment also increased the profession's social standing. Without a doubt, this had a favorable effect on the patient as well as the analyst, even though the trusting therapeutic relationship is actually established principally in other dimensions.

The financing of analytic therapy by health insurance companies has made the analyst independent of self-financing patients who pay punctually. He can now conduct initial interviews (up to six sessions as a basis for the application) in a purely patient-oriented manner, because his decision as to which form of psychotherapy to employ is no longer influenced by how much money the patient has (Ehebald 1978). The analyst practicing in West Germany today also no longer has to strike a balance between the number of patients he treats free of charge, or for reduced fees, and his desired standard of living. Freud had this to say on the subject: "It must be remembered ... that a gratuitous treatment means far more for the psychoanalyst than to any other medical man; it means the sacrifice of a considerable portion ... of the working time available to him for earning his living over a period of many months." A second free treatment has a detrimental effect on the analyst's earning power "comparable to the damage inflicted by a severe accident." Freud then asks "whether the advantage gained by the patient would not to some extent counterbalance the sacrifice made by the physician" (1913 c, p. 132).

We interpret this as meaning that it is important to find a solution which is acceptable to both parties. For this reason, we have stressed that the patient partly finances the treatment himself through his health insurance contributions, and that payment of the balance by the insurance reinforces his sense of being part of society. In contrast to the problems which arise in treatment conducted free of charge or for very low fees in outpatient clinics, and which are extremely difficult to solve analytically, the complications emerging from the fact that the patient need pay nothing directly out of his own pocket can be overcome interpretively. The analyst's countertransference is disturbed much less if his services are adequately recompensed, and in this respect the source of the payment is irrelevant.

The situation is different, however, for the trainees and young analysts carrying out treatment practically free of charge in the outpatient clinics of psychoanalytic institutions, who sometimes even have to pay their own supervision fees. The severe problems to which they are exposed often become apparent at the conclusion of their period of training, which is frequently followed swiftly by the termination of such analyses. Despite the serious difficulties in treatment technique which may occur, we share Cremerius' (1981 a) view that indirect payment represents no grave obstacle to the psychoanalytic process. The complications inherent in the psychotherapy guidelines lie in another area, as we will now demonstrate.

The difficulties arise in connection with the binding of psychotherapy to the medical *concept of illness* and with the fixing of *time limits* for the financing of the treatment, defined in terms of necessity, effectiveness, and economy. The guidelines reflect a compromise between the exigencies of psychoanalytic therapy and the statutory norms. Let us first examine the area of *agreement* between the guidelines and psychoanalytic practice. Sections 6 and 9 of the application form for the financing of therapy require the following:

6. Psychodynamics of neurotic condition. An account of the development of the neurosis and the intrapsychic conflicts, including the resulting neurotic compromises and symptoms. The time of onset of the symptoms, the precipitating factors, and the psychodynamic development are to be described.
9. Prognosis of psychotherapy. Assessment of the patient's motivation, and awareness of the problem, capacity for forming a therapeutic relationship, reliability, and partial coping with life. In particular, assessment of the capacity or tendency for regression, degree of fixation, flexibility, potential for development, and insight into the illness ....

The guidelines demand from the analyst nothing other than a rational justification of his therapy plan according to the principles of the etiologic theory of psychoanalysis. The peer reviewer refers to the general level of knowledge within psychoanalysis and to his own experiences in deciding on the *plausibility* of the psychodynamic connections described by the analyst. His principal task is to determine whether the symptoms constitute an illness. He can also form an idea of the persuasiveness of the connections between the neurotic compromise and symptoms and the analyst's treatment priorities. The peer reviewer cannot, of course, determine whether the descriptions correspond with reality or whether the treating analyst is orienting himself on his outline in conducting his treatment. Nonetheless, he does form a certain impression of the course of the therapy, because the analyst is obliged, in every application for extension of the financing for the further 80 sessions, to summarize the course so far and to describe the change in the symptoms in relation to transference and resistance. The revised prognosis with regard to regression and fixation is one of the most important items in the application for continuation of treatment.

It will have become apparent that fundamental principles of psychoanalytic theory are contained in the scheme of indications and course within which the treating and reviewing analysts interact. Without this common basis, no peer report system could function. Even Beland (1978), in an otherwise critical paper, conceded that the peer report system has proved its worth. The reviewer's clearly defined function does not permit him to intervene in his colleague's treatment. His position becomes more difficult if he cannot follow the processes described in the application. Every application is expected to display a certain persuasiveness and coherence, and an application for continuation must state how the transference neurosis is developing and what changes in the symptoms (improvement or deterioration) are resulting. The peer system has led to reviewers talking to their treating colleagues in cases of doubt, and thus to an intensification of the dialogue between analysts.

These observations concerning an important aspect of the guidelines may already suffice to support the following view: In the application for the initiation or continuation of psychodynamically oriented or analytic psychotherapy, like in every seminar on technique, it is important to demonstrate that the psychodynamic appraisal and the treatment steps undertaken are in accord. The patient's reaction to the therapy so far must also be described, as the correctness of the treatment as a whole is shown by his progress.

Thus it is advisable not just for legal reasons, but also on grounds of technique, to write every application in such a way that the patient can, if he wishes, read and understand it. It is probably not harmful for a mature patient to share in the analyst's reflections unless these deviate considerably from the insights conveyed in interpretations. If the discrepancy between the content of an application and the patient's experience of the therapy cannot be bridged in the dialogue about the application, the chances of gaining knowledge in the dyad are poor. According to psychoanalytic theory, the prospects for achieving a cure are then also very low.

The guidelines demand from the treating analyst a kind of self-supervision. Most analysts agree that it is essential occasionally to reflect intensively on the development of the therapy in the light of analytic criteria. In the case of the peer review procedure, a second analyst with a precise, narrowly defined function gives his opinion on the result of this relection — incidentally, with the right of veto on the part of the analyst making the application. If the self-supervision can be seen as the beginning of scientific work in practice, the review procedure can even be regarded as an extended form of self-supervision. In many respects, applications for continuation represent a store of knowledge which is far from exhausted. The descriptions they contain mirror the treating analyst's view of psychoanalytic practice in the framework of the psychoanalytic scheme formulated in the guidelines.

It is a truism that the psychoanalytic process takes time, but it is for just this reason that applications for continuation and the imposition of a limit on the number of sessions throw up such great problems of principle and of treatment technique. We would like to go into this topic at some length.

The components of the compromise are as follows:

1. On one hand, since the first, methodologically inadequate statistics were gathered at the old Berlin Psychoanalytic Institute, it has been demonstrated that satisfactory results can also be achieved with psychodynamically oriented and analytic psychotherapy of limited duration.
2. On the other hand, analyses have been growing in length since the early 1950s. The forerunners of the "supertherapy" (Balint 1954, p. 158) are the ever longer training analyses.
3. The goals of these analyses are moving ever further away from the treatment of symptoms amounting to illness as defined in medical terms, and from the proof of necessity, effectiveness, and economy.

An improvement in the symptoms on the basis of partial structural changes is as a rule accompanied by a change from neurotic distress to a state of general happiness, albeit not entirely free from unhappiness and tragedy (Freud 1895d, p. 305). When this state has been reached is a matter of judgment.

Despite the limitations applied, the guidelines impose no absolute upper limit. However, as one of us (H.T.) has been able to establish in his capacity as peer reviewer, it relatively rarely happens that applications for confirmation beyond the standard duration are supported in the way Freud recommended for particularly deep analysis (see Chap. 10). More often, the argumentation employed shows that it is not easy to achieve a balance between the time frame and the therapeutic utilization of regressive processes. We will go into this utilization of regressions in detail in Chap. 8, contenting ourselves here with saying that in analytic psychotherapy within the framework of the guidelines it is very important always to bear the social and economic realities in mind. These permit no regression for its own sake. The situation of the insurance companies and their members plays a role. This brings us to a further component of the compromise:

4. Financial considerations on the part of the health insurance organizations played a part in the limitation of the duration of treatment because the insurers foresaw numerous insoluble dilemmas, including financial problems, in the extent of deviation from the medical definition of illness and the extension of responsibility to cover financial assistance in the relief of social and domestic problems or the raising of the so-called quality of life in general.

Beland has this to say on the matter:

> Every patient, every analyst, and every reviewer can understand and accept such a restriction – it is honest and needs no justification based on neurosis theory. The dilemma facing this system of insurance, namely having to legitimize the limitation of the service provided by means of a theory of treatment, rather than by a lack of money, is a miserable state of affairs with harmful consequences for the reviewer, the therapist, and above all the patient. It is therefore desirable for reviewers to free themselves from the responsibility of having to justify the termination of the service after 240 or 300 hours. (Beland 1978, p.9)

It emerges from what we have said that the theory of treatment underlying the guidelines sets no absolute limit. This theory is established in a strictly psychoanalytic manner, and thus empirical proof is necessary, as laid down by Freud (see Chap. 10). As we have already stated, however, the limited means (among other factors) have played a role in the restriction of services. First, it has been shown that in many cases a lasting improvement in symptoms can be achieved within 300 sessions, which may well indicate an at least partial alteration in structure. We do not want at this juncture to go into the difficulty of proving this to be the case. Second, it has also been demonstrated that a good number of the analyses which are continued further lead to an enrichment of the quality of life going beyond the medical concepts of "healthy" and "ill." We would recommend that both the treating analyst and the peer reviewer give serious thought to Beland's criticisms and our reflections; it is essential that the social reality be considered in interpreting the transference neurosis, and the flexibility of the guidelines should not be forgotten.

There is little point in talking about the duration of the treatment in the initial sessions, whether with regard to the limitations embodied in the guidelines or in respect of the utopian vision of interminable analysis. It can even be antitherapeutic to do so. However, it is indispensable to include time and money — and thus the role of the peer reviewer — into the interpretation of transference in the context of applications for extension. If there is the risk of suicide at the expiry of the treatment period financed by the health insurance company, the analyst should reflect on how he has conducted the treatment before criticizing the restrictions imposed by the guidelines. Fortunately, our experience is that the majority of patients treated within the framework of the guidelines experience a favorable alteration in the symptoms and that the emphasis shifts away from the illness and toward difficulties in coping with life, which Freud did not count as neuroses. The guidelines even allow for long analyses for severely ill patients, provided the prognosis is reasonable.

In summary, most psychodynamically oriented and analytic psychotherapies can be terminated within the limits set out in the guidelines, i.e., after 50 (sometimes extended to 80) sessions or 240 (300) sessions respectively. It would of course be very useful to know the results of therapy, and with regard to third-party payment it would be interesting to learn the reasons why patients finance extension of the therapy themselves; however, in both cases we have to rely on estimates. The findings of research indicate the probability that about two-thirds of patients leave psychotherapy cured or with a considerable improvement in their symptoms, the remaining third showing no improvement.

It remains unsolved whether these latter patients could be improved or cured by further therapy under the same conditions (same analyst, third-party payment) or altered conditions (e.g., self-payment) without variation or modification of the method or a change of analyst. Nevertheless, we believe it is possible to specify fairly reliably the circumstances under which patients are prepared to continue the therapy at their own expense after third-party payment has been discontinued. It is necessary to go back to the beginning of the therapy and examine the general influence the psychoanalytic process has on thinking and experiencing. Initially, all patients hope and expect to become healthy and lead productive lives, and thus take an interest in the efficacy of analytic therapy. The growing insight into relationship conflicts and their association with fluctuations in the symptoms can, of course, lead to expectations which have little to do with the medical concept of health and illness or with the guidelines based on this concept.

The difficulties in coping and the expectations which analysands develop in the course of treatment often agree only marginally with the medical concept of illness and health. Faber (1981) points out, with all respect to the utopian element of the wish for self-discovery with the aid of analysis, that illusionary utopian elements in analytic goals must be grasped as transference and countertransference phenomena. He argues that one should work toward justified psychoanalytic utopias soberly and steadily: "It is a work of culture — not unlike the draining of the Zuider Zee" (Freud 1933a, p. 80).

We estimate that 10%–20% of the patients in the average psychoanalytic practice finance a continuation of the analysis out of their own pockets after discontinuation of third-party payment. This group is very heterogeneous, and the patients' goals are extremely varied. One category in this group is formed by those who have sought analysis because of the severity of their symptoms.

In the light of what we have said above, we believe that scientifically grounded applications could secure approval for continuation of treatment in many of these cases.

Another category of these secondary self-financers includes those who expect continuation of analysis to give their life a deeper meaning, independent of medical considerations. Some can only endure their work or their life with the help of their relationship to the analyst. How much this deeper meaning is worth to the analysand is related to his material means. On balance, a wealthy patient and his analyst can reach the decision to continue with the analysis much more easily than, for example, a middle-ranking civil servant who lives entirely off his salary.

Therefore the switch to self-financing often means having to reduce either the frequency of sessions or the analyst's fee. In case of the latter, the issue is not only how much the patient can afford, but also what level of payment is still acceptable to the analyst without the inevitable restrictions and sacrifices placing so much stress on the analytic relationship that the therapeutic work suffers. Any significant reduction in fees for a patient who has four sessions weekly, for example, involves a not inconsiderable decrease in the analyst's earnings. On the other hand, private financing of further therapy can affect the living standard of the patient and his family. Additional conflicts with the latently present third parties can be expected, and ultimately some sort of balance must be struck with them.

Thus many factors must be taken into account in order to reach a productive arrangement with the third parties — family, health insurance company, and reviewer — and achieve a reconciliation with oneself.

# 7 Rules

## 7.1 The Multiple Functions of Psychoanalytic Rules

Freud compared the rules of psychoanalytic treatment with the rules of chess: both give rise to an infinite variety of moves which are limited only in the opening and closing phases:

> Among them there are some which may seem to be petty details, as, indeed, they are. Their justification is that they are simply rules of the game which acquire their importance from their relation to the general plan of the game. I think I am well-advised, however, to call these rules "recommendations" and not to claim any unconditional acceptance for them .... The plasticity of all mental processes and the wealth of determining factors oppose any mechanization of the technique; and they bring it about that a course of action that is as a rule justified may at times prove ineffective, whilst one that is usually mistaken may once in a while lead to the desired end. These circumstances, however, do not prevent us from laying down a procedure for the physician which is effective on the average. (Freud 1913c, p. 123)

The comparison with chess is an obvious one when seeking to illustrate the diversity of the ways in which treatment can be conducted. The complex interactional sequences which, in a certain form, underlie defense or the end game in chess bear similarities to the strategies used in conducting treatment. Recommendations can be formulated which express strategic considerations in the form of rules. The actual rules of play in chess, e.g., those which lay down how the pieces may be moved and which have, as it were, the function of laws, have to be understood differently, since if they are not followed, there is no game at all.

In chess it is simple to differentiate between moves which are against the rules and those which are inexpedient, but in psychoanalysis such distinctions are more difficult. This is due on the one hand to the historical development of psychoanalytic theory and technique, on the other to the different functions that psychoanalytic rules have. As is well known, in analyses conducted by Freud the psychoanalytic situation had very much the character of an association experiment serving the purpose of exploring the genesis of the neurosis. Even in his later cases, Freud retained elements of this experimental situation (Cremerius 1981). His strictest and most unequivocal directions related to the parameters for this situation. The rules seemed to produce a "social null situation":

> For Freud, however, the psychoanalytic situation was not simply his own version of contemporary professional trends; it was essential to both his working technique and his theorizing.

It allowed him to confront both the patient and the scientific public — Freud's double audience — with the fact that the patient's productions could not be dismissed as artifacts of the particular situation, nor as having been induced by the therapeutist, but had, instead, to be explained on the basis of the patient's own psychic activities. (De Swaan 1980, p. 405)

It became clear long ago that this ideal is not appropriate for the social sciences. It has never been possible to produce the social null situation in a concrete form, although in its role as the leading utopian fantasy of psychoanalysis, it has had a detrimental influence on practice. The strict handling of the parameters can be attributed to the fact that analysts construe them predominantly as *rules*, not as means to a more favorable *treatment strategy*. Wittgenstein dealt aphoristically with the question of how reliably even such apparently clear rules lead to the desired goal.

A rule stands there like a sign-post. Does the sign-post leave no doubt open about the way I have to go? Does it shew which direction I am to take when I have passed it; whether along the road or the footpath or cross-country? But where is it said which way I am to follow it; whether in the direction of its finger or (e.g.) in the opposite one? And if there were, not a single sign-post, but a chain of adjacent ones or of chalk marks on the ground — is there only *one* way of interpreting them? So I can say, the sign-post does after all leave no room for doubt. Or rather: it sometimes leaves room for doubt and sometimes not. And now this is no longer a philosophical proposition, but an empirical one. (Wittgenstein 1953, pp. 39-40)

Referring to Wittgenstein's concept of rules, Habermas (1981) elaborated the connection between the introduction of rules and the resultant possibility of producing an identity of meaning and intersubjective validity for simple symbols:

Both aspects marking the use of simple symbols are united in the concept of rule: identity of meaning and intersubjective validity. The general quality which constitutes the meaning of a rule can be portrayed in any number of exemplary actions. (Habermas 1981, vol. 2, p. 31)

Rules create an identity of meaning, because they ensure that phenomena following the rules can be sought out as constants from among the multitude of events. They produce "the unity in the multiplicity of their exemplary manifestations, different forms they take in reality, or application" (Habermas 1981, vol. 2, p. 32). These considerations are of great importance for the understanding of the psychoanalytic situation and the rules which constitute it; they emphasize that the meaning of the behavior of analyst and patient is bound to the existence of common rules. The pettiness of some rules, spoken of by Freud in the quote above, is the result of the striving after identity of meaning, even beyond the boundaries of the given treatment situation. Precisely in the field of psychoanalysis, marked by so many uncertainties and contradictions, rules have acquired the function of keeping the group together and stable. In this context the fact that all psychoanalysts follow the same rules serves as a sign of professionality. This explains, for example, why the use of the couch and the frequency of the sessions have become important criteria of whether a treatment may be termed "analysis."

The meaning of rules derives from their interpersonal acceptance. In fact, one important function of rules is to enable an intersubjective exchange to take place. This is particularly true in psychoanalysis. A uniform framework ensures that findings are comparable, etc., thus enabling standardization of the psychoanalytic process (Bachrach 1983). Standardization is necessary in order for an analyst to be able to compare clinical data and generalize observations; he would otherwise merely observe and describe phenomena from a random standpoint. Patients react in many different ways, for example to the couch and to lying down, but the analyst has a certain breadth of experience with these reactions and can therefore draw diagnostic and therapeutic conclusions. However, the standardization of the external framework often provides only the appearance of uniformity, since the impact of the rules depends largely on additional factors. Standardization must not be carried so far that it obstructs the therapeutic process. To use Wittgenstein's term, we are dealing here with empirical propositions concerning comparisons between rule, way, and goal. And indeed we do modify the rules if they are counterproductive, for example, if lying on the couch inhibits the patient.

The diversity of the parameters is also the reason why psychoanalytic treatment rules do not form a closed, structured system, but are rather a collection of directives in various areas and of differing imperative content. Freud's most important treatment recommendations are spread among at least a dozen of his works. A study group at the Sigmund Freud Institute has listed 249 such recommendations and attempted to categorize them. The classification into 11 categories, ranging from rules for behavior to rules for determining indication, highlights their diversity in content and in degree of abstraction (Köhler-Weisker 1978; Argelander 1979).

It is difficult to ascertain how many of these numerous guidelines constitute the core of real rules of psychoanalytic chess. In contrast to chess, there are no rules whose only effect is that two people meet for a game. Psychoanalytic rules are always also rules of strategy which must be negotiated and continually confirmed in every individual relationship. This differentiates psychoanalysis from chess, in which game rules and rules of strategy are clearly separated.

Treatment rules are fundamentally goal oriented; as stated by Tafertshofer (1980), they can be conceived as individual steps in the psychoanalytic method and thus compared with other scientific methods. However, this goal orientation forbids just that canonization of rules which is self-evident in chess. Freud was aware of this problem, and gave priority to efficacy.

We have the impression that critical analysis of the efficacy of rules is still rather poorly developed in psychoanalysis. All too often, rules are justified not by their usefulness, but by the fact that they are anchored in psychoanalytic theory. This theoretical anchoring of rules is a tricky business. Westmeyer, in a critical review of behavior-therapy rules, raised considerations which are also valid for our understanding of the rules governing psychoanalysis. He demonstrates that the logical derivation of technological rules from the findings of basic science is a utopian illusion: "Technological rules are therefore also not true or false, like laws and statements of scientific theories, but rather more or less efficient or effective — in the degree to which the target states ensue after realization of the measures recommended" (Westmeyer 1978, p. 123). We will discuss this problem in more detail in Chap. 10.

As for psychoanalysis, one can see that while the theories are predominantly concerned with the determinants of genesis, the rules of technique are oriented toward achieving the necessary and sufficient conditions for change: psychoanalytic technique is not simply application of theory.

The relationship between rule function and strategic function in every individual treatment rule is in a constant state of flux. The analyst's need for security and problems of identity encourage him to absolutize the rules. Difficulties arising in the therapeutic process often compel one to scrutinize the appropriateness of the method and thus to question the treatment recommendations. Patients contribute to this fluctuation. It cannot escape the notice of an alert patient that the analyst proceeds according to certain rules, even when he does not say that he is doing so. The patient himself often queries the legitimacy of proceeding in this way. It is therefore only a matter of time until the parameters of the analysis are themselves questioned critically. They then temporarily lose the status of framework and are fiercely disputed until the unconscious determinants leading the patient to call them into question have been understood and resolved, or the parameters modified accordingly. Treatment rules have a natural tendency to become the scene of the conflict between patient and analyst; this is an experience which cannot be avoided, and which perhaps even should not be avoided.

Using the example of patients with superego disturbances, Cremerius (1977) demonstrated convincingly that patients conversely make their analysts' rules their own and begin to treat them as absolute. It is hardly necessary to point out that the effectiveness of the treatment is endangered just as greatly by absolutization of the rules as by unrestricted questioning of every agreement contributing to the structure. Therapeutically, it is indispensable that the analyst vary the rules according to the situation and the individual patient's disturbances. To paraphrase the proverb, in psychoanalysis exceptions are the rule. Whether and how the analyst explains the rules he has introduced is determined very largely by the character of the therapeutic relationship. We agree that the therapeutic purpose of rules should be painstakingly explained, without playing down the advantages for the analyst in his work or the disadvantages for the patient's current well-being. The analytic process develops in an interplay of questioning of treatment rules and their reestablishment in reinforced form. Optimally, in the course of this interplay analyst and patient develop an understanding of the rules which is the best for the analysis in question.

We have already mentioned that psychoanalytic treatment recommendations mirror the whole spectrum of basic theoretical assumptions, purposive ideas, and clinical experience. We do not want to attempt to provide an exhaustive description of all important treatment rules; rather, we want to discuss a few particularly crucial recommendations, among which the advice on the problem of abstinence has a special place, as it embodies a basic principle of treatment technique. We refer to this in various places: in the Introduction, and in the chapters on the initial interview, transference, countertransference, and the psychoanalytic process (Chaps. 2, 3, 6, 9). Abstinence is of course an important factor in the fundamental rule of psychoanalysis and in the analyst's evenly suspended attention, which we will look at more closely in Sect. 7.2.3. The problem of abstinence, however, will be dealt with here, because it demonstrates particularly clearly the multiple functions of psychoanalytic rules and the difficulties which arise from them.

There are two aspects to abstinence in psychoanalysis: as a rule it aims to impose specific limitations on the patient, as a recommendation of analytic neutrality it aims to place restrictions on the therapist. Laplanche and Pontalis (1973) define the principle of abstinence as the "rule according to which the analytic treatment should be organized so as to ensure that the patient finds as few substitutive satisfactions for his symptoms as possible" (p. 2). Neutrality is "one of the defining characteristics of the attitude of the analyst during the treatment" (p. 271). Substantively, the two aspects belong together; they are based on the one hand in the characteristics of all professional relationships, on the other in the peculiarities of the analytic situation. Cremerius (1984) has described the destiny of the concept and rule of abstinence in striking terms. He points out that Freud's first resort to this rule was necessitated specifically by the problems Freud encountered in treating women suffering from hysteria. Their wishes for concrete love-relationships threatened the professional relationship. First of all, then, the commandment of abstinence has the function of a "game rule" to ensure the continuation of the analysis: "The love-relationship in fact destroys the patient's susceptibility to influence from analytic treatment. A combination of the two would be an impossibility" (Freud 1915a, p. 166). Freud cites in this context the generally accepted morality, which he wanted to replace by methodological considerations. Strictly speaking, it is a matter not so much of general morality as of a quite specific norm which establishes the framework of the relationship between analyst and patient in the manner of a game rule.

However, the rule of abstinence receives its outstanding significance from Freud's attempt to replace normative argumentation with one oriented on his method. While medical ethics would urge strict rejection of the patients' feelings of love, Freud recommends that their development should not be disturbed, but rather that they should be used in order to reach and better analyze the suppressed wish impulses. Not only on grounds of medical ethics, but also on grounds of method, he stated that the erotic wishes should not be satisfied:

> The treatment must be carried out in abstinence. By this I do not mean physical abstinence alone, nor yet the deprivation of everything that the patient desires, for perhaps no sick person could tolerate this. Instead, I shall state it as a fundamental principle that the patient's need and longing should be allowed to persist in her, in order that they may serve as forces impelling her to do work and to make changes, and that we must beware of appeasing those by means of surrogates. (Freud 1915a, p. 165)

The purpose of this recommendation is to maintain a favorable tension potential, which is assumed to keep the therapeutic process in motion. It should be stressed that Freud bases his argument on plausibility: the appropriateness of maintaining tension can be investigated and proved in the individual case. The warning to therapists not to appear to comply with the patient's wishes, whether out of kindness or from therapeutic motives, is also based on plausible arguments which can be supported by clinical observation.

Matters did not rest here, however. These technical arguments became allied with the assumptions from instinct theory which underpin abstinence and the corresponding attitude of strict neutrality on the part of the analyst. Freud himself played an essential part in this development. Four years after his first exposition of the rule of abstinence, he wrote:

> *Analytic treatment should be carried through, as far as possible, under privation — in a state of abstinence ....* You will remember that it was *frustration* that made the patient ill, and that his symptoms serve him as substitutive satisfactions. It is possible to observe during the treatment that every improvement in his condition reduces the rate at which he recovers and diminishes the instinctual force impelling him towards recovery. But this instinctual force is indispensable; reduction of it endangers our aim — the patient's restoration to health .... Cruel though it may sound, we must see to it that the patient's suffering, to a degree that is in some way or other effective, does not come to an end prematurely. (Freud 1919a, pp. 162-163)

In this context, he recommends that the analyst should "re-instate it [the patient's suffering] elsewhere in the form of some appreciable privation," detect "substitutive satisfactions," and "require him [the patient] to abandon them," in order that "the energy necessary to carrying on the treatment" cannot escape. This is especially necessary in the case of secret transference gratifications. In contrast to 1915, when he recommended only a favorable tension potential, Freud now opts for the maximum possible tension, thus greatly strengthening the rule of abstinence. This rule is justified both by the theory of symptom genesis and by economic considerations.

We have already explained that derivation of rules from theory is utopian and often harmful, because the question of the suitability of the rules is relegated to the background. The rule of abstinence is a particularly good example, having had clearly unfavorable effects on the development of psychoanalytic technique. Cremerius (1984) points out that the specific features of the treatment of hysteria were, without justification, incorporated into the treatment of other forms of neurosis. Wishes that are quite characteristic of resistance in women suffering from hysteria can have completely different meanings in obsessives, phobics, and anxiety neurotics. The analyst's concern that a patient might find secret substitutive gratification in the transference leads to a defensive approach. The function of the rule of abstinence is no longer to produce a favorable tension potential and thus actuate development, but rather to prevent developments which are viewed with apprehension. The conception that necessary frustration constitutes the motive force for change has become more than questionable and has above all distracted attention from the unfavorable consequences which exaggerated neutrality on the part of the analyst has on the therapeutic process.

Arguments derived from instinct theory are not necessary to justify the demand for neutrality on the part of the analyst, as it can also be substantiated methodologically. The call for neutrality refers to various areas: with regard to work on the material offered by the patient, the analyst should not pursue his own advantage; with regard to therapeutic ambition, the analyst should renounce suggestive techniques; with regard to the problem of goals, the analyst should not pursue his own values; and finally, with regard to the problem of countertransference, the analyst should reject any secret satisfaction of his own instinctual wishes.

As a fundamental principle of the psychoanalytic method, the neutrality rule had from the outset immense significance in ensuring objectivity and establishing a psychoanalytic identity. The scientific ideal played a decisive role. For these reasons, hardly any other analytic rule is in so much danger of being absolutized, although meanwhile a widely based countermovement has formed. In 1981, none of the participants in the panel of the American Psychoanalytic Association favored unconditional affirmation of strict analytic neutrality (Leider 1984). The experience that sometimes more and sometimes less gratification had to be allowed moved Freud to take a flexible attitude toward the rule of abstinence. We also have nothing against pragmatic compromises, as long as they are compatible with medical ethics and can be vindicated methodologically. We would like to go a step further, and believe that nowadays psychoanalysts can, for fundamental reasons, face the rule of abstinence with greater assurance. As we have already pointed out, the professional concern about possibly allowing the patient too much gratification is considerably reinforced by the principles of instinct theory. Under their influence the ideal of complete abstinence was established, with the aim of raising endopsychic pressure by way of denying oedipal gratification and redirecting the psychic energies (whose discharge is thus blocked) into the revitalization of memories. Despite the continuing use of the jargon, most analysts have taken leave of the theory of cathexis (that is, of the principle of economy) in their clinical work. This process began decades ago when Balint (1935), referring to Freud's neglect of the alternative theory of tenderness, credited tenderness with an importance of its own. As long as approval and gratification are not misunderstood as sexual stimuli, the analyst's anxiety that the slightest concession could lead down the wrong path is unfounded. The liberation from the chains of the rule of abstinence can be seen most clearly in Kohut's technique of narcissistic gratification. In view of our strong doubt about the existence of an independent narcissism, we would assume that narcissistic gratification might have an oedipal connotation, so that it will definitely have a bearing on libidinal transference. Nevertheless, Kohut is right when he says that the rule of abstinence must today be understood differently. In view of the multiple functions of rules, which we have discussed, changes in one single area are sufficient to set in motion a correction of the whole.

## 7.2 Free Association: The Fundamental Rule of Therapy

### *7.2.1 Features and Development*

It is not only in the hierarchy of the rules that free association takes first place. In a letter to Stefan Zweig on February 7, 1931, Freud (1960a, pp. 402-403) mentioned — and clearly agreed — that the technique of free association was regarded by many as the most important contribution made by psychoanalysis. Jones (1954, p. 265) counts the devising of the method of free association as "one of the two great deeds of Freud's scientific life, the other being his self-analysis through which he learned to explore the child's early sexual life, including the famous Oedipus complex." Jones bases this view on the fact that in the interpretation of dreams, free association helps to find the way to the latent dream thoughts. Dream formation can be reconstructed because "when *conscious* purposive ideas are abandoned, *concealed* purposive ideas assume control of the current of ideas" (Freud 1900a, p. 531). The associations are seen as indicators of those purposive ideas and fantasies which the patient cannot reach without the analyst's interpretative assistance because they are located in the psychodynamic unconscious.

Free association was only later expressly accorded the status of fundamental rule. In a third-person account of his own technique, Freud described its development as follows:

> The writer therefore endeavoured to insist on his *unhypnotized* patients giving him their associations, so that from the material thus provided he might find the path leading to what had been forgotten or fended off. He noticed later that the insistence was unnecessary and that copious ideas almost always arose in the patient's mind, but that they were held back from being communicated and even from becoming conscious by certain objections put by the patient in his own way. It was to be expected — though this was still unproved and not until later confirmed by wide experience — that everything that occurred to a patient setting out from a particular starting-point must also stand in an internal connection with that starting-point; hence arose the technique of educating the patient to give up the whole of his critical attitude and of making use of the material which was thus brought to light for the purpose of uncovering the connections that were being sought. (Freud 1923a, p. 238)

Strictly speaking, there are significant differences in meaning between the two German words *Einfall* and *Assoziation*, which are both customarily rendered as "association" in English and are indeed often used synonymously in German. A good *Einfall* (spontaneously occurring idea) has a creative quality about it, whereas the word *Assoziation* stresses a connection. At least for subjective experience, an *Einfall* is the spontaneous expression of thought processes which lead to a new configuration. The patient's *Assoziationen*, however, are assembled by the analyst into a meaningful whole. An *Einfall* has an integrating function that comes close to insight, as Niederland (see Seidenberg 1971) pointed out.

Strachey discussed the difficulty of rendering *Einfall* in English in a footnote to his translation of the chapters on parapraxes in the *Introductory Lectures on Psycho-analysis*:

> If a person is thinking of something and we say that he has an *Einfall*, all that this implies is that something else has occurred to his mind. But if we say that he has an "association," it seems to imply that the something else that has occurred to him is in some way connected with what he was thinking before. Much of the discussion in these pages turns on whether the second thought is in fact connected (or is necessarily connected) with the original one — whether the "*Einfall*" is an "association." So that to translate "*Einfall*" by "association" is bound to prejudge the issue. Nevertheless it is not always easy to avoid this, more especially as Freud himself sometimes uses the German "*Assoziation*" as a synonym for "*Einfall*," especially in the term "*freie Assoziation*," which must inevitably be translated "free association." Every endeavour will be made in the present discussion to avoid ambiguity, even at the cost of some unwieldy phraseology; later on, the need to avoid the word "association" will become less pressing. (Freud 1923a, p. 48)

The contexts of discovery and of origin regarding free association are — how could it be otherwise — inextricably interwoven into the history of ideas. We will limit ourselves to a few remarks on the contemporary historical context. It was a part of the tradition of the Helmholtz school, in which Freud (through his teacher Brücke) stood, for psychic phenomena to be included under the postulate of continuous psychic determinism, to which Freud then also ascribed free associations. Equally strong was the influence Herbart and Fechner had on psychology in the last century; Freud was familiar with it through his teacher Meynert and the latter's association theory. Herbart even formulated concepts such as "inner apperception" and "freely rising ideas" as dynamic entities, i.e., from the point of view of their mutual inhibition. In order to at least hint that the history of free association is not limited to scientific thought, we would like to mention a completely different source: Bakan (1958) conjectures that the origin of free association could lie in the meditation techniques of Jewish mysticism.

This is not the place to define the originality of free association vis-à-vis various forerunners. What is certain is that Freud's technique developed gradually out of hypnosis and Breuer's cathartic methods. In his self-analysis, Freud was greatly helped by free association. It is no exaggeration to say from today's viewpoint that in the experiment on himself Freud discovered by means of association the importance of fantasizing in the recognition of unconscious psychic processes (Freud 1926c).

Association psychology played godfather during the introduction of the method of free association. It emerged that the patient's associations, which can be fitted together into series with linkages and junctions, are steered by "unconscious complexes." One could in brief say that the "complex" conceived by Jung (1906), which steered the reactions in the experimental association studies, found its earliest counterpart in Freud's thought in the conviction that all psychic phenomena are determined by unconscious wishes. In an early comment on this topic (1906c, p. 112), Freud said: "The aim of psycho-analysis is absolutely uniform in every case: complexes have to be uncovered which have been repressed because of feelings of unpleasure and which produce signs of resistance if an attempt is made to bring them into consciousness." Freud attempted to get to these complexes by means of hypnocatharsis, the pressure procedure, and finally free association. He commented that Jung's association studies made it possible "to arrive at rapid experimental confirmation of psycho-analytic observations and to demonstrate directly to students certain connections which an analyst would only have been able to tell them about" (Freud 1914d, p. 28).

The method of free association — the fundamental rule of psychoanalysis — is in Freud's opinion in the tradition of Wundt's experimental psychology, which was continued in Jung's association experiments. Critical historical appraisal of the theory of associationism has had considerable consequences for our understanding of the fundamental rule (Rapaport 1974; Bellak 1961; Colby 1960; Wyss 1958). We learn from Zilboorg's study (1952, p. 492) not only that Freud was familiar with the English school of associationist psychology — it is well known that he translated a work by John Stuart Mill — but also that he may have known about a first self-experiment by no less a scientist than Galton.

Since therapy consists in integrating the parts into a whole, connecting the elements like the pieces in a jigsaw puzzle, the gestalt psychological principles set forth by Bernfeld (1934) were implicated from the very beginning. Because of the importance of this relatively unknown and, as far as we know, not previously translated piece of work, we would like to quote from it at length:

> Dream interpretation, the therapeutic process of psychoanalysis, every individual session of analysis, and extensive areas of applied research work by psychoanalysts are all based on series of thoughts, images, actions and affects which are in essence present in words and sentences presented to the therapist or researcher. His task, or preliminary task, is to get to know the law these sequences follow. On the basis of this law he can then explain, interpret, and influence. In the impoverished terminology of earlier psychology, "idea" [*Vorstellung*] was the word used to describe the research material of psychoanalysis — an imprecise term even then, but one which served an initial purpose. The sequences whose law the analyst has to discover can thus be roughly termed associations of ideas. In the early days of psychoanalysis it was all the more justified to speak of associations, in that the sequences were generally not object-related, but rather determined by "inner" forces and goals. But by no means does this make psychoanalysis an "associationist psychology." (Bernfeld 1934, p. 43)

The transition from theme-centered to free association took place in the light of experiences Freud had in the treatment of his patients, experiences which led him to recognize "resistance" and "transference" as constituent features of the patients' unconscious dispositions. Material which in hypnosis was completely hidden (and thus unavailable for therapeutic elaboration) could, with the introduction of the new method, be understood as essential. We are referring here to the close intermeshing and interrelationship between the substance and the method of psychoanalysis and to the fruitful consequences which free association was to have on Freud's further theoretical deliberations. A notable factor is the help Freud got from his patients in the development of free association. Emmy von N., for example, responded to the insistence with which he sought the origin of a symptom by saying that he shouldn't always ask where this and that came from, but let her say what she had to say (Freud 1895 d, p. 63). The conversation, then conducted increasingly in the manner of free association, was not "so aimless as would appear. On the contrary, it contains a fairly complete reproduction of the memories and new impressions which have affected her since our last talk, and it often leads on, in a quite unexpected way, to pathogenic reminiscences of which she unburdens herself without being asked to" (Freud 1895 d, p. 56). This "unburdening" seems to be next door to abreaction. From then on, Emmy von N. spontaneously contributed her thoughts to the conversation as a "supplement to her hypnosis," as Freud noted (1895 d, p. 56). With the discovery of free association, the "talking cure" was born as an expression of personal spontaneity and freedom of opinion. In addition came the turnabout from the patient's previous passivity — answering questions or abreacting under hypnocatharsis — to his active participation in the structuring of the dialogue. This extension of treatment technique facilitated free association. Freud stressed (1900 a, pp. 102-103) that some patients find it difficult to impart the thoughts which come to them. At the same time, however, he reported: "Nevertheless, ... the adoption of an attitude of uncritical self-observation is by no means difficult. Most of my patients achieve it after their first instructions" (p. 103). Free association, in contrast to earlier hypnotic techniques, developed toward "a conversation between two people equally awake" (Freud 1904a, p. 250).

### *7.2.2* ***Instructing the Patient About the Fundamental Rule***

The context in which the patient is instructed about the fundamental rule demands *special* attention. Often, the formalities of the treatment, i.e., the restrictive arrangements regarding payment, appointments, and holidays, none of which arouse particularly pleasurable feelings in most people, are discussed in the same session and almost in the same breath as the fundamental rule. And in fact the various aspects of the agreement become so closely associated that the fundamental rule is very often seen mistakenly as almost equivalent to a contract, like the arrangements concerning fees and the procedure to be followed in the event of interruptions and missed sessions. The patient's already existing anxieties are strengthened by the unaccustomed prospect of having to disclose his best-kept secrets to a stranger. While being informed about the fundamental rule, many patients think of something which they decide to keep to themselves, which if we are lucky we hear about later. Initially, at any rate, not much remains of the pleasure in telling stories. Freud attempted to make it clear by means of an anecdote why the patient cannot be allowed to make an exception and keep a secret: if an extraterritorial refuge in St. Stephan's Church had been created for the tramps of Vienna, that is exactly where they would have stayed (Freud 1916/17, p. 288).

The fundamental rule leads to a conflict with the patient's preexisting ideals and behavior norms, which are functions of the superego. The patient classifies the demand for free association in the same category as a whole series of old precepts (on whose acceptance powerful counterforces had gone underground). Is it really inevitable that there will be a struggle over adherence to the fundamental rule, as A. Freud (1937) expressed it? What is decisive is how the patient experiences the fundamental rule, and this experiencing is obviously not a preexisting quantity, but situative and processual: the more sacrosanct the fundamental rule, the more powerful the counterforces! Words have their own weight, which creates realities. Talking in terms of a struggle brings a struggle into being. Should one struggle at all, when just mentioning the word wakes counterforces because the patient would like to win for once at last? There are many methods of self-assertion. Analytic experience teaches that a great deal can be symbolically linked with the *reservatio mentalis*: many patients keep some secret for a long time or for ever. According to analytic theory, derivatives of this secret and its unconscious roots have to enter treatment *indirectly*. In this case we would perhaps even expect symptoms pointing to a psychodynamically effective, i.e., pathogenic, focus. Freud permitted no exceptions to the fundamental rule and made his patients commit themselves to absolute honesty; in his opinion experience showed that it does not pay to make exceptions. In one case where he did allow an exception, the patient, a senior official bound to secrecy by his oath of office, was satisfied with the outcome of the treatment; however, Freud himself was not, and attributed his dissatisfaction to the fact that he had made the exception (1916/17, pp. 288-289). But what sense is there in obliging a patient to be honest if at the same time one knows that complete honesty is prevented by inner resistances? The demand for absolute honesty augments the patient's bad conscience and his unconscious feelings of guilt, leading to reactions which have a negative effect on the therapy. We have repeatedly found that it can pay not to fight over the fundamental rule, but rather to permit exceptions, in the hope and belief that the establishment of a relationship of trust will finally give the patient enough security to tell us even his well-guarded secrets. Freud seems to have had similar experiences: "How small is the effect of such agreements as one makes with the patient in laying down the fundamental rule is regularly demonstrated" (1913c, p. 135).

Our criticism of authoritarian formulations of the fundamental rule should not be taken as a plea for its abolition. We hope, though, that our arguments contribute to an application of the rule which increases the patient's freedom and capacity for associating. Gill (1984, personal communication) has drawn our attention to the fact that it is no sign of tolerance to use the patient's associations for purposes of interpretation without having familiarized him with the point of the fundamental rule, but rather a sign of concealed authoritarianism. The patient must know that he can contribute to the progress of the treatment and make the analyst's task easier — or harder. The *conscious* bracketing out of certain themes and the suppression of associations is a complication which is often *iatrogenically* reinforced: the patient struggles against the caricature that the analyst has drawn.

The call for free association seems to lead to a dilemma. As far as his conscious endeavor and his freedom of decision go, the patient is in the position to say anything. The rule should encourage him to forsake conscious selection in favor of a spontaneous free play of thought. If the feelings and thoughts now described by the patient are considered from the point of view of their determination, they seem *unfree* in the sense that they are motivated. The patient cannot control the latent context of motivation because the unfolding of the unconscious and preconscious thoughts and wishes is interrupted by the so-called censorship. Interpretive assistance in the overcoming of censorship helps the patient to experience his dependence on unconscious wishes and imperative needs, as well as the enrichment which results when he regains access to them. Free association thus does not lead to a genuine or even insoluble logical paradox, although it does of course manifest contradictions inherent in the tension between dependence and autonomy. The rule could even be viewed as a symbol of contradiction: we become freer when we reconcile ourselves to our dependence on our bodies and their demands and on the fellow men we all rely on.

In communicating the fundamental rule to the patient, one technique which suggests itself is to use *metaphors* which can lead from the strict obligation of "you *must* say everything" to the inner freedom of "you *may* say everything."

Whether this function is fulfilled by the metaphors reported in the literature — some of which we would now like to discuss — is dependent on many factors, not least on their semantic import.

We begin with Freud's famous travel metaphor:

> What the material is with which one starts the treatment is on the whole a matter of indifference — whether it is the patient's life-history or the history of his illness or his recollections of childhood. But in any case the patient must be left to do the talking and must be free to choose at what point he shall begin. We therefore say to him: 'Before I can say anything to you I must know a great deal about you; please tell me what you know about yourself.'
>
> The only exception to this is in regard to the fundamental rule of psycho-analytic technique which the patient has to observe. This must be imparted to him at the very beginning: 'One more thing before you start. What you tell me must differ in one respect from an ordinary conversation. Ordinarily you rightly try to keep a connecting thread running through your remarks and you exclude any intrusive ideas that may occur to you and any side-issues, so as not to wander too far from the point. But in this case you must proceed differently. You will notice that as you relate things various thoughts will occur to you which you would like to put aside on the ground of certain criticism and objections. You will be tempted to say to yourself that this or that is irrelevant here, or is quite unimportant, or nonsensical, so that there is no need to say it. You must never give in to these criticisms, but must say it in spite of them — indeed, you must say it precisely *because* you feel an aversion to doing so. Later on you will find out and learn to understand the reason for this injunction, which is really the only one you have to follow. So say whatever goes through your mind. Act as though, for instance, you were a traveller sitting next to the window of a railway carriage and describing to someone inside the carriage the changing views which you see outside. Finally, never forget that you have promised to be absolutely honest, and never leave anything out because, for some reason or other, it is unpleasant to tell it.' (1913c, pp. 134-135)

This metaphor shows what is meant by "free," namely not excluding anything consciously and deliberately. While Freud uses a metaphor of travelling great distances, Stern (1966, p. 642) prefers the analogy of a dangerous journey in a confined space. He tells the patient that the analyst's office is like the control room of a submarine, and asks him to look through the periscope and describe everything he sees outside. No analyst will have any trouble in supplying associations here, reaching perhaps from Lewin's (1946) "blank dream screen" (the wide open sea) to projective identification (an enemy warship), to say nothing of Ferenczi's "thalassal regressive trend." But how will the patient feel in a cramped control room? He might first enjoy the metaphor, because he has seen a cartoon in the *New Yorker* representing Kohut's unconscious "twinship transference" in terms of two submarine commanders watching each other's progress through their periscopes in order to steer identical courses. However, it is more likely that no stress-relieving joke like this will occur to him, quite apart from the fact that the cartoon is our own invention.

Let us assume that the patient has never been in the control room of a submarine and has equally little personal experience of the analytic situation, and further that he is not too inhibited and has a modicum of gumption. What would the analyst answer if the patient's first free association were to ask the commander of the submarine to show him how the periscope works because he has no experience with it and cannot see anything? The analyst can now make it easy for himself and wait for further associations, using the opportunity to familiarize the patient with another rule, the one stating that questions are generally not answered, but clarified through further associations, i.e., by the patient himself. We leave it to the reader to decide whether the patient's trust in the commander will have grown or shrunk by the end of this imaginary dialogue. Obviously, our reaction to this metaphor of the fundamental rule is ironic.

Apparently most analysts do not find it easy to translate the "sacred rule" (Freud 1916/17, p. 288) into a productive, secular form. One can see this from the fact that the various preferred formulations of the rule have been discussed in minute detail. We will give a few examples. Altmann (1976) tells the patient: "You are entitled to say anything here." Glover (1955) voiced criticism:

> The form of the association rule most frequently communicated to patients seems to be: 'Say what is in your mind'. And this is taken by the patient to mean: 'Say what you are thinking'. Whereas if the instruction were: 'Tell me also all about your *feelings* as you observe them rising into your conscious mind', in a great number of cases the ideational content would follow of necessity. (p. 300)

Schafer's (1976) statement of the fundamental rule conveys the sense of: "I shall expect you to talk to me each time you come. As you talk, you will notice that you refrain from saying certain things" (p. 147). Schafer goes on to say: "Similarly, rather than 'What comes to mind?,' the kind of question that is conceptually and technically exact according to the action model is, 'What do you think of in this connection?' or 'What do you now connect with that?' or 'If you think of this, what do you think of next?'" (p. 148). He spurns formulations like "'Say everything that comes to mind' and its variants, 'What does that bring to mind?' 'What comes to mind?', and 'What occurs to you?'," saying that their content increases passivity and encourages regression. He sees such formulations as remnants of hypnosis which go along with the patient's disavowal of responsibility for his own mental rehearsal of actions. By addressing himself to the acting, thinking patient, Schafer extends the patient's responsibility from the outset to include his unconscious motives. The patient is thus no longer the passive recipient of his associations, but their active creator. Schafer's action language therefore extends the individual's sphere of responsibility to include unconscious wishes.

Spence (1982b) criticized Schafer's formulations because they intensify the already strong superego aspect of the fundamental rule. Just because our character is revealed by our associations does not mean that they can be counted as motivated actions for which we are responsible as for our deeds. This responsibility exists only in the wider sense, as Moore (1980) explains. One does not reach the level of responsibility for unconsciously motivated speech acts until the associations are *appropriated* as part of one's own ego. The therapeutic problem is thus how the analyst can facilitate this process of appropriation, i.e., how he conducts the struggle over adherence to the fundamental rule. It is decisive that the analyst succeed, step by step but as quickly as possible, in familiarizing the patient with the fundamental rule to the point where he follows it willingly, because with the analyst's help his associations lead him to make enriching discoveries about himself. Morgenthaler (1978) has supplied some striking examples and contrasted them with the deformation that results when the fundamental rule is communicated to the patient in a manner that reinforces the superego.

One patient even completely misunderstood the widespread question: "What are you thinking of?" Instead of seeing it as an encouragement, she took it as a rebuke: "What *are* you thinking of?" This unusual misunderstanding draws our attention to the unconscious overtones this question can have for many patients. It is to be hoped that Morgenthaler's arguments will change attitudes to the fundamental rule and put an end to the controversies which have continued over the decades, although Little (1951) put forward a similar argument over 30 years ago: "We no longer 'require' our patients to tell us everything that is in their minds. On the contrary, we give them permission to do so" (p.39). E. Kris (1956a, p.451) attributed far-reaching consequences for the structure of the analytic situation to this change in emphasis: the situation is made more personal when the analyst no longer requires free association but permits it, like a parent who does not object to bad behavior.

We do not consider it sufficient to impart the fundamental rule only once, but we also put little stock in a kind of trial analysis with an introduction to free association, as suggested by Greenson (1967). Greenson's aim is to assess the patient's capability for free association, which varies enormously and is unquestionably dependent on the patient's illness. Therefore, typical restrictions and resistances to association have been described in the literature. Consistent with our general approach, the aspect which particularly interests us in the discussion of the fundamental rule is what the analyst does to make it easier — or even possible — for the rule to be followed.

Despite the provocative title of his article — "Psychoanalysis Without the Fundamental Rule" — Schlieffen (1983) does not recommend doing away with free association; without it the analyst would be lost. Rather, with reference to Morgenthaler (1978) he shows that strict enforcement of the fundamental rule can have an effect on the patient's capacity for association which is nothing short of deforming. We would like to elucidate this point of view by asking whether, from the association theory point of view, Stern's metaphorical introduction (described above) of the fundamental rule is more likely to facilitate or to hinder free association and the development of therapeutic regression. Since the analyst's office generally bears little resemblance to the control room of a submarine, transference-neurotic associations relating to the analyst's professional surroundings will be hindered. The metaphor puts the patient in a completely foreign situation, making him even more helpless than he is in any case. Of course, regarding treatment technique, the question is not only how the analyst introduces the fundamental rule, but also what he later does to make free association easier or more difficult.

Freud's statements concerning the fundamental rule, which — strangely, considering his skepticism about abiding to agreements — never wavered in strictness from his technical writings right up to his description of the conclusion of a "pact" (1940a), must today be analyzed as to their effects ["never forget that you have promised to be absolutely honest" (1913c, p. 135)]. It is not sufficient for the analyst to do what Epstein (1976) suggests and talk of a "basic condition" rather than a "basic rule." Epstein holds that in contrast to "condition," the word "rule" relates clearly and expressly to superego functions. However, it is certainly not just a matter of toning down the superego aspect of the fundamental rule by changing terminology: one can, like Altmann (1976), doubt whether the patient can ever be made to feel so at home in the therapeutic situation that the initial anxiety disappears. Hardly any patient will think of the pleasurable aspect of association when the fundamental rule is revealed to him.

How what the analyst says comes across to the patient depends on both timing and choice of words. The more superego, the less free association — it is on this formula that we base our advice that the analyst familiarize the patient with the rules step by step, paying particularly close attention to timing, choice of words, and above all the patient's reactions. All the analyst's statements on rules are important for the transference relationship, and the way in which he reacts to questions from the patient, particularly those concerning the fundamental rule, has repercussions on both transference and the working alliance.

For the evaluation of the specific context, one can, as we have already described, draw profitably on association theory. How is a patient supposed to learn to take pleasure in telling stories when he simultaneously hears about the restrictive obligations concerning payment and attendance which he will have to observe for an indefinite length of time. Discussing holidays and the duration of the treatment — again, there are many ways of doing this — changes the cluster of meanings which form around the various formulations of the fundamental rule.

In a panel discussion (Seidenberg 1971, p. 107), Greenson said that he gives quite detailed information, stressing the advantages of the couch-chair position and the avoidance of eye contact. Greenson also answers the patient's questions generously. Clearly this willingness to oblige moved an unnamed analyst in the auditorium to pose the probably sarcastic question of what Greenson does when a patient asks him to demonstrate free association. Greenson answered that he would do so only after he had tried to find out what had motivated the patient to make the request.[1]

One of our patients understood the statement that he could follow his fantasies more freely lying on the couch than sitting in a chair as meaning that he was not permitted to direct his critical gaze at the analyst. This drastic misunderstanding, to which the analyst contributed, was not cleared up until late in the analysis. Correction of the repercussions on the patient's unconscious defense mechanisms was laborious and time-consuming.

For the reasons described, care must be taken to avoid unfavorable concatenations. The formulation we recommend therefore runs roughly as follows: "Please try to say everything you think and feel. You will find that this is not easy, but it is worth the effort." We place particular importance on recommending that the patient *try* to say everything; the rest seems to us to be of secondary significance. The advantage of a certain standardization is that the analyst

[1] We deal with the answering of questions in Sect. 7.4, where we explain why we find Greenson's hypothetical answer wrong. Knowledge of motivation would yield no elucidation which can be achieved clearly, given the division of tasks. The patient must know that, and why, free association is his task, not the analyst's.

can refer back to a fixed point of departure if the patient begins to discuss the changing "misunderstandings" or the way he has understood the rule. On the other hand, precise stipulations contain the danger of ritualization, of no longer considering how the manner of imparting the fundamental rule should perhaps be varied for a particular patient. So-called lower class patients are particularly likely to be deterred by stereotyped formulas (Menne and Schröter 1980).

We hope that we have shown how important it is for the analyst to consider from the very beginning what he can do to make free association easier for the patient. The establishment of the therapeutic relationship and the interpretations together enable continuous correction of unfavorable courses taken at the beginning of the therapy.

### *7.2.3 Free Association in the Analytic Process*

According to one very widespread view, the patient develops the ability to associate freely only late in the course of treatment. Often it is said that when a patient is genuinely in the position to associate freely, his case is closed (Merloo 1952, p.21).

The structure of the first sessions and the manner in which free association is explained cannot neutralize even the conscious resistance of the patient, much less his unconscious resistance. Nevertheless, one should realize the possible unforeseen side effects that strict rules can have if they are sucked into the wake of compulsive confession and the desire for punishment. At issue in the struggle over adherence to the fundamental rule (A. Freud 1937) are both free, spontaneous, and nonselective communication by the patient and his resistance to it. The theory of resistance concerns the relationship between association and the conscious or unconscious opposition to association. The later typology of the forms of resistance and the differing explanations for them (which we have dealt with in Chap. 4) all go back to the observation of association resistance.

Freud writes:

> Thus a psychical force, aversion on the part of the ego, had originally driven the pathogenic idea out of association and was now opposing its return to memory. The hysterical patient's 'not knowing' was in fact a 'not wanting to know' — a not wanting which might be to a greater or less extent conscious. The task of the therapist, therefore, lies in overcoming by his psychical work this resistance to association. (1895 d, pp.269-270)

We would be moving too far away from treatment technique if we were now also to discuss the theories which Freud used in his attempt to explain the association resistance he observed. He soon realized (1904a) that inner resistance, in the role of censor, has a deforming influence on all mental processes.

An important measure of the freedom a patient has won is indeed his ability to give himself up to his associations in the protected environment of the analytic situation. Considering that observations of this are an everyday occurrence for the analyst, it is amazing that there are so few painstaking studies of association. We base this statement on the comprehensive account by Mahony (1979), to whom we are also indebted for other important suggestions. Mahony complained that the relevant psychoanalytic literature consists largely of free association on the subject of free association. The examples given by A. Kris (1982) are probably representative; most analysts view everything the patient communicates, verbally and otherwise, as free association. Like Kanzer (1961), Kris includes everything in the process of free association: the agreement of appointments and fees, the entering and leaving of the consulting room, the position the patient takes on the couch, etc. Everything can be seen as an expression of free association.

A. Kris thus has a comprehensive understanding of the method and process of free association: it is a shared process, the patient trying to verbalize all his thoughts and feelings, the analyst — guided by his own associations — helping him to fulfill this task (A. Kris 1982, pp. 3, 22). The ability to associate freely (or more freely) can be viewed as an expression of inner freedom and thus as a desirable treatment goal. So far, so good. However, it is not the analyst's accompanying associations or evenly suspended attention as such which eases the patient's progress. How helpful interpretations originate in the analyst and what effect they have on the patient are of essential importance. Directly after every kind of intervention, which, true to the word's etymological provenance, interrupts the patient's flow of speech, the theme of the intervention is continued for the time being: it is precisely when the patient ignores the proposed interpretation that he will set the analyst thinking. Now it is the analyst's evenly suspended attention which concentrates on the theme. The more polymorphic the patient's associations are and the more he changes the subject, the more difficult it gets to find any meaning in what he says. Is the method then being taken *ad absurdum*? No, because it only now becomes properly clear that the patient cannot ignore the presence of the other person, the analyst. So he simply communicates nonsense to him.

Of course, the analyst quite rightly finds a meaning even in genuine or feigned madness. In fact, jumbled association often serves to restore the balance of forces, as no good gestalt can be constructed out of miniscule fragments of information. The analyst is at his wits' end, checkmated. This fact itself is not changed by our seeing a deeper meaning in the situation. This has to be recognized in order to make the patient grasp what power he has and how very dependent on him the analyst is. However great the inequalities in the division of power and dependence may be, they are reduced to bearable proportions when patients realize, in these and other situations, how much the analyst depends on them. Not infrequently, such experiences mark a therapeutic turning point. It is therefore advisable, on the one hand, to consider what the patient says from the point of view of continuity — Which theme from the last session is being continued today? — and on the other hand to regard the present session as a unit — Which problem is the patient trying to solve today?

We will now discuss a study of case reports where one would strongly expect to find descriptions of free association. The reports we are talking about are those with which young German analysts demonstrate their qualification for the profession. In a representative sample, Schlieffen (1983) found not a single description of the way in which the fundamental rule is introduced or of the consequences of the various formulations of the rule. How about the more important question: How does the association process unfold in the course of an analysis, and how is it described? In ten reports chosen at random, we found no descriptions of association sequences, nodal points reached by the patient in the sense of association resistance, or their interpretation. There is also no evidence to indicate that patients become more spontaneous in the later stages of the analysis as shown by the increasing freeness with which they make associations. Whereas there is an almost constant lack of revealing chains of association leading analyst and patient to latent meanings, we find many *indications* that the patient had individual spontaneous ideas. One could say that Freud preferred to speak of spontaneous ideas. His own self-analysis and Farrow's years of self-experiment (1942) could be considered as examples which have still not found a fitting place in the history of medicine (Schott 1983).

Only occasionally in the psychoanalytic literature is any attempt made at systematic investigation of connections between individual spontaneous ideas (Thomä 1961; Hohage and Thomä 1982). In our opinion this is linked to problems of method which are very hard to solve: Where is the line to be drawn between free association and the not-so-free statements made during treatment? If spontaneous ideas lead to a deeper meaning, this indicates that they may constitute free association. Spontaneous ideas about dreams are still those most frequently gathered. However, many analysts these days are plainly rather cautious concerning the individual dream elements, i.e., cautious about gathering spontaneous ideas in a theme-centered way in the sense of Freud's classic technique.

The analyst's reserve makes it easier for the patient to say everything that occurs to him. But where do his communications lead? And should we consider everything which could be a pointer toward latent meanings as a free association? Or do we wait until the patient himself recognizes his unconscious wishes? If this were the case, self-knowledge could be achieved by conducting a sufficiently long monologue under the conditions of free association. The analyst does not expect the patient to supply ever more meaningless associations and finally come so close, in self-hypnosis, to a primary process mode of thinking that his ego becomes his id and his id becomes his ego. No, he listens until something occurs to him which, after careful deliberation, he believes he can communicate. In *An Outline of Psycho-Analysis* we read:

> We reflect carefully over when we shall impart the knowledge of one of our constructions to him [the patient] and we wait for what seems to us the suitable moment — which is not always easy to decide. As a rule we put off telling him of a construction or explanation till he himself has so nearly arrived at it that only a single step remains to be taken, though that step is in fact the decisive synthesis. (Freud 1940a, p. 178)

Whether one calls the patient's communications free association or not, in every case the analyst's interpretations add a new element, even when he tries (like Rogers' extremely nondirective, client-centered therapist) to add nothing and only stress one or another part of a sentence in an encouraging way. Even a parrot-like repetition adds something. The more a patient sinks into an apparent monologue and moves away from verbalizing and toward a hypnogogic state, the more important becomes the analyst's manner of sustaining the relationship. In all such regressive states, however, the appearance of a monologue is deceptive. These retreats into certain forms of monologue in the presence of the analyst have several aspects. M. M. Gill (1982) has pointed to the aspect of resistance in them. Even in regression, the patient remains within the transference relationship. He may perhaps be seeking a transitional object that the analyst can put a name to, even when it belongs to the prelinguistic period of development.

Freud's travel metaphor also raises the question of the transformation of images into words. Spence (1982a) particularly draws attention to this aspect of free association and to the loss of information involved in description (p. 82). He emphasizes that the patient is not merely a passive viewer of images, but actively constructs them. In addition, sentences that have been begun follow the rules of grammar, even when the psychoanalytic dialogue proceeds in a relaxed fashion. According to Spence, the fundamental rule contains two contradictory instructions. As partner in the dialogue, the patient cannot simultaneously be introspective, and when he gives himself over to his most secret thoughts he cannot participate in a conversation. Spence believes that this paradox in therapy is solved, in successful treatments, by each of the two participants contributing to the development of a language differing from their everyday language (1982a, p. 85). Our experience also shows that meaningful metaphors develop in many analyses, and that they are unique to the respective dyads.

We hardly need to point out that free association — like everything else — can be used as resistance. It is no coincidence that Freud described this problem in compulsive neurotics. The translation of thoughts into words always involves a selection, and only a patient who pours everything out quickly and without thinking would appear to adhere fully to the fundamental rule. The thoughtful patient has the occasional association, and will, when he speaks, reject or defer the occasional word or partial thought. The deferred material is not lost to free association, but the highly ambivalent compulsive neurotic shows that rules can be taken *ad absurdum*. Indeed, two different thoughts cannot be expressed simultaneously.

We do not want to get involved here, however, with what patients make out of the fundamental rule on the basis of their individual pathology. Rather, we want to consider what the analyst contributes to their particular understanding of the rule. Many patients understand free association as a demand for disconnected, unordered, or nonlogical thinking or for them to conduct a monologue in the presence of a silent analyst. In any case, the imparting of the fundamental rule is the occasion for many misunderstandings which need both elucidation and interpretation. If a patient reacts to the analyst's stimulus by conducting a monologue, one must ask what the analyst has contributed to this state of affairs. In this connection anecdotes are revealing. Loewenstein reports a patient who said: "I was going to free-associate, but I'd better tell you what is really on my mind" (Seidenberg 1971, p. 100).

The patient's ability to free-associate might increase as the treatment goes on. Eissler, though, points out that "it is questionable whether anyone has ever lived up to [this requirement] completely" (1963b, p. 198). Certainly, every patient has at some time during the therapy planned to hold something back. Particularly portentous are preconscious processes of selection which restrict the patient's flow of associations because he has discovered that his analyst has sensitive spots which seem to be genuine sources of irritation (see Chaps. 2, 3). Finally, we can add one further approach to the study of the motivational contexts of decision-making processes, i.e., of their determined nature, looking at them from the point of view of ego autonomy. Let us assume that a patient has resolved to keep something back and sticks to his decision. Has the analyst then lost the struggle over adherence to the fundamental rule? We believe the answer is no, because we assume that the patient's behavior can be seen as displaying a certain reserve, a *reservatio mentalis*, as a documentation of inner freedom. Kanzer (1961, 1972) has long stressed that with many patients it is inappropriate, even a mistake, to insist on the fundamental rule. The need to differentiate the self from others is in his view one part of healthy individuation, and even a necessary developmental step for patients with disturbances of separation. Giovacchini (1972) shares this view when he concedes the patient the right to keep a secret from him. The patient understands that the analyst does not envy his autonomy and concedes him the right to withdrawal and demarcation. The right to hold something back means that the patient does not have to be constantly and rigidly on guard against an all-devouring imago projected on the analyst.

Eissler's statement above can only be interpreted to the effect that the *reservatio mentalis* (the partial refusal to tell everything) is an expression of self-determination. We may conjecture that the reason that no one can fulfill the demands of free association completely is that this would be the equivalent of total self-relinquishment. But why does the patient balk at one particular revelation? Why does he anchor his autonomy to precisely one part of his experience and memories? Analysis of the motivation for this resistance must be pursued ever further. On the other hand, the patient understandably seeks to establish a foothold in the one area where he can assert his independence from the analyst: in bracketing out one theme or another entirely.

Dewald, however, in his book *The Psychoanalytic Process* (1972, p. 613), took the view that free association leads to the primary process: "In essence, the form and content ... of free association tends ... in the direction of the primary-process mode of thinking, and hence further to foster the process of regression in the service of the ego." Both Holt's investigations into the primary process (1967b) and clinical experience argue against the view that free association becomes less structured as the analytic process goes on. We even hesitate to express the expectation that all patients will have more creative and spontaneous associations at the end of the treatment than at the beginning. Greater inner freedom can express itself in a multitude of ways — in silence, in speech, and in action.

## 7.3 Evenly Suspended Attention

Freud (1912e, p. 115) described the close links between the analyst's evenly suspended attention and the patient's free association. The complementary nature of the two processes is underlined by some writers' preference for the term "free floating attention," although this is an incorrect rendering of the original German *gleichschwebende Aufmerksamkeit.*

The analyst who follows this rule remains open for all the patient's associations and leaves him complete freedom to unfold his ideas and fantasies. Most important of all, he does not permit himself to be influenced by his abstract theoretical knowledge, but sees every patient as unique and incomparable and is eager to hear and experience something new. He deliberately avoids drawing comparisons in order not to hinder his access to the unknown. If he follows Freud's recommendation (1912e, p. 114), he swings over "according to need from the one mental attitude to the other" and postpones the "synthetic process of thought" to the end of the treatment. As long as the treatment continues, new material can constantly emerge which can correct the previous image, i.e., the provisional reconstruction. The technique of evenly suspended attention should remind the analyst that every case could turn out differently than one would be led to expect by the general (and always provisional) theory and by one's limited personal experience.

While listening passively, the analyst tries to let everything impress him to the same degree and — his attention evenly suspended — not to select. In the process he discovers his own limitations, which exist on two levels. His evenly suspended attention is disturbed by his countertransference (in the traditional sense), such as results from his personal presuppositions regarding particular human problems. This disturbance occasions self-reflection and self-analysis. In the newer understanding of countertransference, such disturbances of evenly suspended attention can be made therapeutically productive (see Chap. 3). In addition, the analyst notices that his evenly suspended attention is steered involuntarily in certain directions: not everything can be kept suspended evenly. When an interpretation comes to mind, he has chosen one of many possibilities, for both the patient's free associations and the analyst's interpretations are motivated.

On the basis of these considerations, we see the rule of evenly suspended attention as containing the demands — far from easy to fulfill — for self-critical examination of one's own attitude to this patient at this moment and for constant grappling with the general and specific problems of psychoanalytic theory and treatment technique. We also share Freud's opinion (1915c, p. 117) that we always listen actively, inasmuch as our understanding of what we observe is affected by preexisting ideas. Therefore it is in principle impossible to devote the same attention to everything, and we do not do so in practice. However, it is both possible and necessary to account for our ideas, and for what lies behind them, to ourselves and to the scientific community, and to correct presuppositions in light of observations. The exchange with the patient contains numerous possible occasions for this, especially when assumptions that the analyst has expressed as interpretations are revealed to be erroneous.

You may say, "Surely it should be plain to analysts, of all people, that they should not approach the patient with fixed prejudgments. There's no need for a rule! And analysts do not need to be reminded that they have many and varied ideas on the phenomena, because that is where the controversies between the various schools began. In this way the psychoanalytic routine reflects one aspect of the philosophical notion that all observations are theory-laden."

We could content ourselves with these remarks on evenly suspended attention and count on agreement from all sides when we say that the analyst should strive for openness and that his attention should not be determined by presuppositions or even prejudgments. However, the story does not end there; the consequences of an alternative tradition of thought, developed by Freud with a metaphorical explanation of evenly suspended attention, reach right down to the present day. Freud attributed to the analyst's unconscious the special ability to act as a receiving organ for the transmissions of the patient's unconscious:

Just as the receiver converts back into sound waves the electric oscillations in the telephone line which were set up by sound waves, so the doctor's unconscious is able, from the derivatives of the unconscious which are communicated to him, to reconstruct that unconscious, which has determined the patient's free associations. (Freud 1912e, p. 116)

This statement provided a foundation for the rule of evenly suspended attention as well as for the requirement that the analyst be purified of countertransference (see Chap. 3). Freud conceptualized this capacity to receive the unconscious according to the then usual model of sensory perception. It was assumed that external reality was perceived directly and correctly. This model was therefore later also called the "mirror theory" or the "doctrine of immaculate perception" (see Westerlundh and Smith 1983).

It was thus in keeping with the zeitgeist to explain perception of the unconscious with the mirror or telephone metaphor. Only recently has the direction of research into the early mother-child relationship been determined by the fact that even a baby does not assimilate its world passively, but constructs it (Stern 1977). Freud's metaphor thus seemed at first to solve a whole series of practical and theoretical problems so well that it founded a tradition of psychoanalytic thought and practice which is still influential today. Evenly suspended attention was popularized through Reik's "third ear," which contains important elements of the specific empathy around which Kohut (1959) later established a school. Isakower technicized evenly suspended attention as an "analyzing instrument" (Balter et al. 1980). A special location within the analyst's psychic apparatus was now postulated as accounting for his ability to hear his patient's unconscious. At the same time, Spence (1984) called his critical essay "Perils and Pitfalls of Free Floating Attention"; the title speaks for itself. After a psychoanalytic investigation of the process of understanding and empathy which incorporates concepts from the philosophical hermeneutics of Gadamer and Habermas, he comes to the conclusion that evenly suspended attention as *passive* listening *without* preconception does not exist.

By replacing the hermeneutic term "preconception" with "idea," we can easily draw a parallel with Freud's above-mentioned description. If the analyst listens *actively*, he can by all means keep his ideas, his fantasies, his feelings, his preconceptions evenly suspended and remain open for new experiences. Spence even provides convincing psychoanalytic arguments to show that it is precisely self-deception which opens the way for immaculate perception of the unwitting, unconscious — and therefore not easily accessible to reason — projection of one's own ideas.

The myth of evenly suspended attention — that is how Spence regarded ostensibly theory-free passive listening — has many functions, like all the myths which could be construed as prototheories in the history of science. Evenly suspended attention is indeed a hybrid which we have now separated into its two original components. It owes its survival to just this mixture of well-grounded rational elements — radical openness instead of reserve — and mystical expectations of fusion and unity, connecting one's own unconscious with the other's, as in Freud's telephone metaphor. Looked at soberly, the rule of evenly suspended attention contributes to the patient's feeling that he is understood and therefore helps to create a *rational* basis for the treatment. However, in order to come closer to the process of exchange between patient and analyst, we must forfeit a degree of fascination, as we will show when we discuss Kohut's concept of empathy in Chap. 8 and in the discussion which now follows on listening with Reik's "third ear."

We begin by introducing the third ear and its functions in Reik's own words:

Psychoanalysis is in this sense not so much a heart-to-heart talk as a drive-to-drive talk, an inaudible but highly expressive dialogue. The psychoanalyst has to learn how one mind speaks to another beyond words and in silence. He must learn to listen "with the third ear." it is not true that you have to shout to make yourself understood. When you wish to be heard, you whisper. (1949, p. 144)

and

One of the peculiarities of this third ear is that it works two ways. It can catch what other people do not say, but only feel and think; and it can also be turned inward. It can hear voices from within the self that are otherwise not audible because they are drowned out by the noise of our conscious thought-process. (1949, pp. 146-147)

The third ear is, according to Reik, closely related to evenly suspended attention:

Do you picture the psychoanalyst as a man leaning forward in his chair, watching with all five senses for minute psychological signs, anxious lest one should escape him? I've talked about tiny signals, the faint stimuli that flit and waver, slip past, and attain such suggestive significance for the conjecture of unconscious processes. In the face of such differentiated data, so hard to take hold of, you would think that the keenest attention is called for. Do you imagine the analyst not just attentive but tense?

The picture is false, and the analyst's attention is of a different kind. Freud defines this particular kind of attention as *"gleichschwebend."* The word is difficult to translate; simultaneously with its connotation of equal distribution, it also has the meaning of revolving or circling. The closest I can come to the German is "freely floating." Another possibility, which emphasizes the psychological balance rather than the motion, would be "poised attention." Two factors induced Freud to recommend such free-floating attention.

It saves tension, which, after all, it is not possible to maintain for hours, and it avoids the dangers that threaten in the case of deliberate attention directed toward a particular aim. If we strain our attention to a certain point, if we begin to select from among the data offered and seize upon one fragment especially, then, Freud warns us, we follow our own expectations or inclinations. The danger naturally arises that we may never find anything but what we are prepared to find. If we follow our inclinations, we are sure to falsify the possible perception. The rule that we must note everything equally is the necessary counterpart to the demand we make upon the patient to tell everything that occurs to him without criticism or selection. (1949, pp. 157-158)

Reik goes on to say

And now, how can free-floating attention and taking note be brought into consonance? If from the wealth of a mass of passing data we want to take note of something, we must direct a keen gaze upon special points, turn our attention to them in particular, must we not? How can I take a note of anything, if I do not direct my whole attention to it, if I treat insignificant detail in exactly the same way as that which is important? Perhaps it will be said that the notion of "poised" attention aims precisely at taking note of everything and remembering everything. But is not that notion self-contradictory? Attention is always directed only to particular objects. Attention, we have always been taught, implies selection. How can we avoid the danger of selection, if we want to be attentive? (1948, pp. 158,159)

As is well known, Reik suggested solutions for these contradictions in that he described different kinds of "attention":

The quality of the attention in psychoanalysis may be well illustrated by the comparison with a searchlight. Voluntary attention, which is restricted to a narrow sector of our field of experience, may be compared in its effect to the turning of the searchlight upon a particular piece of ground. If we know beforehand that the enemy is coming from that direction, or that something is going to happen upon that field, then we have anticipated the event, as it were. It is advantageous to illuminate that particular sector brightly. Let us assume a different case, that something, for instance a noise, has turned our attention to a particular zone. Only then do we turn the searchlight upon it. Our attention did not rush on in advance of the perception, but followed it. This is the case of involuntary attention. If we drive at night along a road near New York, we may notice that a searchlight in the middle of the road is scouring the surrounding country uninterruptedly. It illuminates the road, is then directed to the fields, turns toward the town, and swings in a wide curve back to the road, and so repeats its circuit. This kind of activity, which is not confined to one point but is constantly scouring a wide radius, provides the best comparison with the function of free-floating attention. (1949, p. 163)

In this metaphor the third ear corresponds to a third eye which sees and assimilates everything around it without the slightest preexpectation. The third ear and the third eye are a tabula rasa, ideally completely blank and absolutely free of preexpectations.

Reik's solutions themselves lead to contradictions, because the exploratory, selective character of evenly suspended attention must, sometime and somewhere, halt the motion of the searchlight. Evenly suspended attention stays suspended only until it alights. From the point of view of perceptual psychology, the psychology of thinking, and the theory of knowledge, Reik's suggestion is naively positivistic, and he overlooks the fact that behind the beam of the searchlight is the observer's whole personal perceptual and thinking apparatus, including his theoretical expectations: his perception is "theory-laden."

Our rather casual statement that the suspension of attention only continues until the analyst offers an interpretation — whether accepted by the patient or not — passes over the preconscious (intuitive) or conscious processes of selection which precede it. One can see the psychoanalyst's receptive function as part of a fourfold process of passive and active listening, experiencing, perceiving, and interpreting (Thomson 1980). We make our perceptions, observations, and resulting interpretations in light of conscious and unconscious theories. This principle also applies to prescientific experience, however naive its expectations may be. Thus we find that patients' perceptions fit the theory that is a fixed scheme in their unconscious, and that their expectations are thus fulfilled.

We go along with the explanations the patient gives for his fears and inhibitions, and enter his world without reservation. How else could we understand him? We listen for undertones, we notice interruptions. Yet in situations where the patient is bewildered, where he cannot comprehend compulsive symptoms or phobias, we would also get no further if we were equipped with no more than ordinary common sense. But the receiver and the third ear would also not get any more sense out of the patient's association without the many programs stored there which provide the analyst with comparative explanatory models. The third ear and the receiver would in any case not be able to hear anything of the unconscious if they were not the organs of an analyst who has absorbed as much knowledge and gathered as much experience as possible. Flexibility in listening is not guaranteed by a third ear with extrasensory faculties. On the contrary, every mystification which leads to the unconscious fixation of presuppositions must be an obstacle to the scientific legitimation of psychoanalysis.

The notion that the third ear hears best when the analyst otherwise behaves as if he were deaf has retained a certain mysterious fascination. Thus for Bion (the "psychoanalytic mystic" according to Grotstein 1982), the passive, receptive analyst's self-emptying takes on mystical qualities. In order to attain the state of mind he believes essential for the practice of psychoanalysis, Bion avoids all memorization, resisting any temptation to remember the events of a particular session or to go strolling in his memory. He chokes every impulse to remember anything that has happened previously or any interpretations he has made on earlier occasions (Bion 1970, p. 56). At the same time, he demands that the patient must be shown the evidence behind an interpretation, even if it relates to a period of several years of acting out (p. 14). In one way, the idea of a final conquest of all countertransference in both the specific and the general sense also underlies this notion, since Bion refuses to let any wishes or yearnings enters to his thought.

Since a balanced relationship between the two attitudes — feeling and thinking — is not easy to achieve, this problem continues to be discussed by every successive generation of psychotherapists and analysts. Fenichel's (1934) criticism of Reik's one-sidedness remains as valid as ever and is now, in the context of the current discussion of empathy, once again topical. Fenichel quoted Ferenczi, who had said:

> Analytic therapy, therefore, makes claims on the doctor that seem directly self-contradictory. On the one hand, it requires of him the free play of association and phantasy, the full indulgence of *his own unconscious* .... On the other hand, the doctor must subject the material sub-

mitted by himself and the patient to a logical scrutiny, and in his dealings and communications may only let himself be guided exclusively by the result of this mental effort. (Ferenczi 1950 [1919a], p. 189)

Finally, we hardly need to point out that we have drifted further and further away from the concept of evenly suspended attention as a rule of treatment and toward the analyst's complex process of cognition. Indeed, a direct line can be drawn from Freud's evenly suspended attention via Reik's third ear to Kohut's (1959) introspective empathic kind of psychoanalytic observation (Cohler 1980, p. 81). Another line leads to those aspects of feeling and thinking that are described today as processes of inference within the analyst (Ramzy 1974; Meyer 1981a; Kächele 1985). All these themes will be pursued further in the following chapters.

## 7.4 The Psychoanalytic Dialogue and the Counterquestion Rule: To Answer or Not to Answer, That Is the Question

Is it unduly dramatic of us to use a paraphrase of Hamlet's "To be or not to be, that is the question" in the title of this section on the problems posed by patients' questions and the appropriate responses from the analyst? Is it permissible to attribute the significance of "to be or not to be" to the questions that crop up in the course of analysis? Indeed it is: we would not have chosen this wording if we had not believed that an element of drama is inherent in the psychoanalytic dialogue. The patient comes to the analyst seeking answers to questions he cannot solve by himself. In none of his many discussions — with friends and colleagues, with clergymen, doctors, and quacks — has he been given satisfactory answers, i.e., answers which cure his symptoms. The last resort is then psychoanalysis, in which it can literally be a matter of to be or not to be, life or suicide. We have already spoken of the profound, agonizing questions which the patient cannot formulate but which his unconscious conflicts confront him with. It no longer needs to be emphasized that ultimately the *clarification* of these unanswered questions constitutes the beneficial effect of the analysis. However, what about the questions the patient can and does ask? How should they be dealt with? Let us first give some examples: Will the treatment cure or at least improve my symptoms? How does it work? How long will it last? Have you treated similar illnesses before? Do I have the same illness as my father? Soon the patient takes an interest in the analyst's private life and family, wants to know his holiday address or — for emergencies — his home telephone number.

If the reader puts himself in the place of the analyst, he will sense something of the tension these questions create. They force the analyst's hand: the patient has urged him to give an answer, and will understand everything he now does as a response. Even silence is in this sense an answer.

Through the patient's questioning, the initiative passes to the analyst, whether he likes it or not. The compulsion arises from the fact that analyst and patient have entered into a dialogue and are therefore subject to rules of discourse, on which they must be in at least partial (tacit) agreement if they want to be in any position to conduct the dialogue in a meaningful way. It is in the nature of a question that the person asking it wants an answer and views every reaction as such. The patient who is not yet familiar with the analytic situation will expect the conversation with the analyst to follow the rules of everyday communication. If questions are left unanswered, he may take this as a sign that the analyst cannot answer, is not willing to answer, or both.

The question is thus a means by which one person can induce another to enter into a verbal exchange, a dialogue. Since psychoanalysis lives from conversation, from the "interchange of words" (Freud 1916/17, p. 17), it is extremely important what and how the analyst replies — and not just to questions. Questions serve here as an excellent example of a broad spectrum of direct and open attempts by the patient to involve the analyst ad hoc in an exchange; requests and criticisms are further examples. Questions can also contain hidden attempts of this nature, as our examples above will probably already have shown; also, something which initially seems to be purely a question to obtain information can later turn out to be, for example, an accusation. Questions are difficult to deal with because they invite interaction in such a multiplicity of ways. What mother has not occasionally been exasperated by her child's insistent inquisitiveness! The analyst's situation is no different when questions put him under pressure.

One rule of treatment which has ossified into a frequently encountered stereotype seems to cut through all difficulties like Alexander's sword through the Gordian knot. This stereotype is to respond to a question from the patient with a counterquestion: "What leads you to ask that question?" For example, if a treatment report mentions that a given question came up and was "analyzed," one can be fairly sure that the patient asked a question which was then thrown back at him with a request for the thoughts behind it. Such information is also often invited indirectly by silence. This answering of questions with questions is, for the general public, one of the characteristic features of analysis. Indeed, the text on the jacket of the German edition of J. Malcolm's book *Psychoanalysis: The Impossible Profession* (1980; *Fragen an einen Psychoanalytiker*, 1983) contains the following: "The author asks the questions which every patient always wanted to ask, but to which he knew the analyst would only respond 'What occurs to you when you ask yourself why you wanted to ask me that question?'" We, too, followed this stereotype for many years, until the unfavorable consequences taught us better. We discovered how deeply entrenched in the professional superego this rule can be from the guilty conscience we suffered when we disregarded it, and we assume that many other analysts may have had the same experience. As can be seen from the following anecdote, the stereotype is obviously passed on from one generation to the next through training and control analyses, on the assumption that answering questions with questions plays a not insignificant part in ensuring a particularly profound and rigorous analysis. Be that as it may, this anecdote, which in essence is not fictive, shows that candidates follow this rule especially strictly. Shortly before the end of the preliminary session, a candidate says to his first analysand: "If you have any more questions, please ask them now. From the next session onward, I'll be bound by the principle of abstinence and will no longer be able to answer your questions."

The following overview of the literature (Sect. 7.4.1) will show that this stereotype derived from the discharge model of mental functioning. It is assumed that the withholding of an answer will result in the patient more quickly expressing thoughts which will lead to the latent meaning of the question. Thus the rule is justified by the hoped-for gain in therapeutic insight. An unintended result, however, is that the patient often interprets the failure to answer his question as a rejection. What influence does this rejection have on the transference relationship and on the desired process of restructuring the patient's self- and object-representation? We believe that we have to assume that only a few patients have an ego so intact that they experience the rejection represented by the stereotyped nonanswering of questions without feeling offended and without all the implications this has for unconscious defense mechanisms.

At least in the introductory phase, a patient will not be able to see any sense in the counterquestion — as we will refer to it from now on for the sake of brevity — and the rejection and offense he experiences can arouse unconscious defense mechanisms which lead to imperceptible transformations of the thoughts he contributes. Thus the analyst's withholding of answers, intended to stimulate the patient's flow of associations, achieves the opposite.

From studying the literature and from personal experience we have come to the conclusion that the counterquestion rule, far from ensuring the depth of self-recognition, in fact disturbs, and can even occasionally destroy, the very basis of self-recognition, namely the dialogue. This conclusion is supported by another result of the following investigation — by the exception to the rule. With which patients may the analyst waive the counterquestion rule? With those who do not have an intact ego with a high threshold of tolerance, i.e., with a large proportion of the patients who consult an analyst! What happens, then, when the analyst no longer follows the rule? Are the patient's questions simply answered? By no means. We merely abandon rigid adherence to a rule which can no more be reconciled with the bipersonal theory of psychoanalytic process than it can with experience in practice. Just as ego- or self-development is tied to the principle of dialogue, therapeutic self-discovery and further development of the ego are tied to the response of the new object. In this respect the exceptions to the rule predominate. However, it is not only with those patients who display insecure object relationships that we have become skeptical of previous practice. Since in analysis all objects are constituted principally through the verbal agency of a responding subject, we can explain why the variation of a time-honored rule is called for to make the psychoanalytic dialogue more fruitful. It is not a matter of simply answering the questions; rather, the counterquestion rule must be replaced by a reasonable attitude, as described by Curtis (1979, p. 174): "It is of course a matter of analytic judgment whether an answer, explanation, or acknowledgement of a patient's question about the analyst is in the best interest of the analytic process." Since the counterquestion rule provides an apparently easy way of dealing with a complicated problem, it is not surprising that it has survived for decades. Let us now examine the foundation of the stereotype and its history.

### *7.4.1 The Foundation and History of the Stereotype*

One justification for the stereotype of not answering the patient's questions seems to derive from the rule of abstinence: the answering of a question is said to represent an unacceptable gratification of the patient's instincts, hindering the progress of the analytic process. It is assumed that if the analyst has given an answer once, there might be a danger that the patient will ask more and more questions, with his questioning eventually developing into a resistance which the analyst himself has induced.

Another problem is posed by the personal questions the patient asks in order to find out something about the analyst. It is assumed that answering such questions destroys the analyst's therapeutic incognito or reveals his countertransference, disturbing the development of transference.

Because of these fears, the nonanswering of questions has become a stereotype of therapeutic technique. This did not originate with Freud, who was flexible in this respect. In his report on the introductory phase of the analysis of the Rat Man (Freud 1909 d), we find that he answered his patient's many questions concerning the mechanisms of the psychoanalytic treatment and the prognosis directly, without making the patient's questioning an object of interpretation.

Blanton (1971) relates that during his own analysis he often asked Freud about his scientific views. According to Blanton, Freud answered his questions directly, without making any interpretations. Neither in his specifically analytic writings nor anywhere else in his oeuvre did Freud explicitly address the technical problem of how to deal with patients' questions, apparently because for him it was not a problem.

To our surprise, our survey of the literature revealed that it was Ferenczi who, in 1918, formulated the rule of never answering patients' questions:

> I made it a rule, whenever a patient asks me a question or requests some information, to reply with a *counter interrogation* of how he came to hit on that question. If I simply answered him, then the impulse from which the question sprang would be satisfied by the reply; by the method indicated, however, the patient's interest is directed to the sources of his curiosity, and when his questions are treated analytically he almost always forgets to repeat the original enquiries, thus showing that as a matter of fact they were unimportant and only significant as a means of expression for the unconscious. (1950 [1919 a], p. 183, emphasis added)

Ferenczi believed that counterquestioning enabled him to arrive quickly at the unconscious determinants, the latent meaning, contained in the question. We are not of the opinion that this assertion can claim universal validity. To start with, there is no small likelihood that a rigid application of this rule will discourage the patient from asking questions altogether, leading him to withhold not only the questions but also the related thought processes, without this necessarily being clear to the analyst. Moreover, conventional answering by the analyst of questions from the patient on the level of everyday communication does not automatically entangle them in a question-and-answer game whose unconscious determinants are inaccessible to further analysis. Our experience was the opposite, namely that well-considered answers according to the rules of everyday discourse help a patient for the first time to talk about the feelings of rejection he has experienced as a result of an all too inflexible application of the counterquestion rule. Our subsequent interpretation of his avoidance of questions then enabled the patient for the first time to ask further, profounder questions, which could then be comprehended as deriving from hitherto unconscious tendencies and interpreted.

Many analysts have had similar experiences and varied their technique accordingly, and for this reason Ferenczi's rule has not won universal acceptance. This is shown by Glover's survey (1955, pp. 261ff.), which was carried out in the 1930s but whose results Glover regarded as still representative in the 1950s. Among other things, he asked his colleagues whether they would admit their moods, anxieties, or illnesses to their patients. The majority were prepared if necessary to confirm the patient's observations to this effect. Some made their decision according to the conjectured effect on the patient, i.e., were flexible in this respect. Only a small minority had made it a rule to neither confirm nor deny patients' speculations or questions. As for nonpersonal questions, a large majority in this survey were prepared to give information on sexual and nonsexual matters, although for only a quarter of the analysts questioned was this unproblematic. There was widespread agreement that questions should be analyzed, but it was felt that it would be a mistake to make a question the point of departure for an analysis of motivation if giving an answer were realistically justified. The stereotyped analysis of questions was thought to increase the patient's indifference or resistance and also to be a sign of inappropriate anxiety on the part of the analyst.

The results of this survey show that psychoanalysts are flexible in how they respond to questions from the patient. However, only rarely does one find in the literature a statement opposing the stereotype of ignoring questions which is as clear as that by Kohut (1971, p. 89):

> To remain silent when one is asked a question, for example, is not neutral but rude. It goes without saying that — given specific clinical circumstances, and after appropriate explanations — there are moments in analysis when the analyst will not pretend to respond to the patient's pseudorealistic requests but will instead insist on the investigation of their transference meaning.

A high regard for interpretations, which we fully share, has led a good many analysts to overlook the fact that a positive therapeutic climate is created when the patient's questions are taken seriously on the manifest level. In our view analysts resort to the counterquestion technique because they fear that patients could otherwise remain at a superficial level. We find an example of this in Dewald's study (1972) of the course of an analysis, which, by virtue of verbatim protocols, has the particular merit of permitting exact inspection. At the end of her first session the patient asked what she should do if she were pregnant. Dewald replied that it was necessary to understand what lay behind the question in order to be able to recognize meanings other than those contained in the question itself. The meaning of the question on the manifest level remained obscure, and the analyst made no attempt to find out anything on that level.

As Lipton remarks in his critique (1982), by using this technique Dewald influences the patient in such a way that her utterances take on a disconnected and illogical character; this is what Dewald strives for, because he hopes in this way to gain the material for his purely historical genetic interpretations. He achieves this by signaling to the patient with his response to her first question that the manifest meaning of the question is of no interest to him and by repeatedly interrupting her in the course of the session, almost always only to ask for thoughts or details. We agree with Lipton that the analyst can comprehend hidden, latent meanings only when he has understood what the patient is saying to him on a manifest level. Through his form of counterquestioning and his insistence on additional associations before even the manifest meaning of the patient's question was clear, Dewald deprived himself of the possibility of understanding and interpreting the transference aspects of the question. To do this, it would have been necessary to understand what the patient's question meant on a manifest level and to know which situational precipitating stimuli had induced her to ask it. In this case, however, the counterquestion rule was directly to blame for the fact that material which would have been highly significant for the patient's current transference remained inaccessible to analysis. It emerged much later that the patient was already 2 months pregnant when she asked Dewald her question.

Our misgivings about the counterquestion rule do not, however, rest only on the fact that it is by no means always conducive to deeper understanding. Rigid application of the technique can also lead to serious complications in the development of transference.

Greenson (1967, p. 279) describes a patient whose previous analysis had been unsuccessful, probably because the analyst had employed a very rigid technique whose features included not answering questions and never explaining this course of action to the patient. Greenson was able to structure the analysis more productively by telling the patient why he could not answer his questions. Greenson's recognition that patients have a right to an explanation of the strange — in comparison to the everyday situation — rules of discourse in analysis enabled this patient to talk about the profound feelings of humiliation and of being ignored that he had had with his previous analyst. In this way, the patient's negative transference, which had led to deadlock in the previous analysis, became accessible to elaboration and interpretation.

The reader will probably be astounded to learn that Ferenczi, the very analyst who was the first to believe that deficiency states and defects of early origin could be corrected, pleaded the case for rigidity in such a sensitive area of communication. At the time (1950 [1919b]), he formulated the counterquestion rule, he was of course firmly oriented on the discharge model of therapy and advised forced fantasies or heightened tension as part of the nascent active technique. Is it futile to speculate on a connection between rigidity on the one hand and mothering of regressed patients on the other? No, because our present knowledge indicates that it is very probable that the refusal to answer questions can, in patients so disposed, precipitate severe, psychotic-like regressions. Of course, we are not claiming that Ferenczi's counterquestion rule was solely responsible for the severe regressions suffered by the patients he treated in the 1920s. Assuming that he followed the rule strictly when treating severely ill patients — as indeed he did — on the basis of our present knowledge we can say almost with certainty that iatrogenic regressions were inevitable.

Particularly instructive in this respect are the findings discussed by a panel on "severe regressive states during analysis" (Weinshel 1966). Numerous case reports by leading analysts in the course of this discussion led Frosch (see Weinshel 1966, pp. 564, 567) to refer to silence on the part of the analyst as the most important of the factors which can precipitate a severe regression and to recommend that analysts should "speak more often" and "answer questions more readily" when working with patients at risk. This conclusion became obvious after it had been recognized that rigid application of the counterquestion rule and the use of silence, either as a general technical expedient or by ignoring an individual question or request, were partially responsible for iatrogenic damage. For various reasons, however, the appropriate flexibility is not easy to realize. If you simply treat according to rules, you delegate your responsibility to them. If you accept rules without further ado, you overlook the tendency toward manipulation which is always inherent in them. Only when you forsake strict adherence to the rule and decide for yourself whether, how, and why you answer a patient's question do you become conscious of your responsibility. Seen from the point of view of the exponents of the rule system, however, the flexible analyst manipulates even if he justifies his decisions pragmatically and scientifically. Even that which is advisable or has been proven beneficial for the patient becomes manipulation. Accordingly, Frosch described his recommendation that the analyst demonstrate flexibility in the treatment technique of patients at risk, by saying that this involves "manipulation" (e.g., staying seated during treatment sessions, giving one's private telephone number, prescribing psychotropic medication, or changing the frequency of sessions). However, the rule system does not have the last word:

> If the climate, the attitude, and the thinking are analytic from the outset, I believe that the smooth, imperceptible shift to the classical psychoanalytic technique will be absolutely natural and that the beginning of the treatment will merge continuously and organically into the subsequent therapy. (Weinshel 1966, p. 567)

Since the counterquestion rule in the context of a rigid rule system, as advocated for example by Menninger and Holzman (1958), can have unfavorable side effects in every phase of therapy — and not just in patients at risk — the cultivation of the kind of analytic climate described by Frosch is always crucial. In each individual case the prescribed mixture of therapeutic agents must be adjusted in order to be able to realize the aim of psychoanalytic treatment, namely to achieve structural changes through the interpretation of transference and resistance. There will then be some psychoanalyses in which the analyst leaves many questions unanswered, and others which are more strongly supportive. The classification of therapies into supportive, expressive, and strictly analytic becomes questionable. Let us consider the following short exchange reported by G. and R. Blanck (1974, p. 330):

*Mr. Forrester*: I feel as though I hate everyone today, especially all women. (Pause.) You never seem to mind when I say that. (Pause.) You're a cool cookie. I feel sad. Why don't you say something? *Therapist*: I will. I don't mind when you say what you feel.

Important here is not the content of the intervention, but the Blancks' statement that in the treatment of a borderline patient it is permissible, *contrary to the psychoanalytic technique*, to accede to the request for a comment. Our experience with the counterquestion technique up to the present day speaks against viewing it as a sound technical rule.

### *7.4.2* ***Rules Governing Cooperation and Discourse***

Asking questions and giving answers are verbal behavior aimed at creating a dyadic structure, in contrast to the more monologue-like patterns of verbalization when the patient free-associates. The counterquestion rule has the purpose of transforming an interactive pattern of verbal action initiated by the patient back into a monologue. In order to be able to grasp the implications of a digression from everyday rules of conversation, it is appropriate to take a look at some of the rules governing cooperation and discourse which form the bounds of experience and expectation for each person. We will limit ourselves to those patterns of verbal action which belong to the theme of question and answer.

Austin (1962), in his theory of speech acts, proceeds from the observation that things get done with words. In the patterns of verbal action, there are specific paths of action available for interventions to alter reality (Ehlich and Rehbein 1979). However, speech, if it is to become effective as a means of action, is dependent on the existence of interpersonal obligations which can be formulated as rules of discourse. These rules of discourse depend partly on the social context of a verbal action (those in a court of law differ from those in a conversation between two friends), and conversely, a given social situation is partly determined by the particular rules of discourse. Expanding this observation psychoanalytically, one can say that the implicit and explicit rules of discourse help to determine not only the manifest social situation, but also the latent reference field, i.e., transference and countertransference.

If any kind of meaningful dialogue is to take place, each partner must be prepared (and must assume that the other is prepared) to recognize the rules of discourse valid for the given social situation and must strive to formulate his contributions accordingly (the general principle of cooperation enunciated by Grice 1975). If the discourse has been disturbed by misunderstandings or breaches of the rules, metacommunication about the preceding discourse must be possible which is capable of removing the disturbance. For example, one of the participants can insist on adherence to the rule (e.g., "I meant that as a question, but you haven't given me an answer!"). In such metacommunication, the previously implicit rules which have been broken can be made explicit, and sometimes the occasion can be used to define them anew, in which case the social content and, we can add, the field of transference and countertransference can also change. In Greenson's above-mentioned case (1967, p. 279), we see the analyst's intervention as an example of this type of communication about the discourse: the counterquestion rule is explicitly introduced and explained, and in this way the analyst frees the patient of the anxiety that the analyst is dealing with him in an arbitrary way, i.e., not adhering to the general principle of cooperation. The transference relationship is then relieved of a source of aggressive tension.

In every speech act, the general principle of cooperation is supplemented by further specific rules according to the intention of the speech act; this allows the addressee to identify it (e.g., to distinguish questions from requests or from accusations) and to determine the appropriate reaction. Thus, for example, the appropriate reaction to a question is either an answer or the reason for not giving an answer. We would now like to consider silence and counterquestioning against the background of some rules of discourse.

When the analyst responds to a patient's question with silence, the silence is accorded a meaning. Since silence can be interpreted in any number of ways, the patient has a multiplicity of possibilities, and his choice depends on the situational context and on the current form of the transference relationship. In view of the rules of discourse, the patient must assume either that the analyst does not wish to observe the general principle of cooperation, or that the analyst wants to tell him silently that one of the prerequisites which would make his utterance a question is not fulfilled. If the patient assumes the former, this can lead to treatment being broken off. This does not happen if the patient is ready, because of transference, to accept the definition of the relationship by which the analyst may behave arbitrarily. In this case the analyst has, through his silence, contributed to the formation of this transference pattern of submission to an arbitrary regime, or at least reinforced it. Yet also if the patient assumes that the second possibility is in fact the case, he will quite likely find the silent way in which the information is "communicated" particularly rude, which will also inevitably have repercussions on the transference relationship.

A relatively favorable situation can still develop if the patient interprets the analyst's silence as meaning that the latter is not in possession of the information requested. In this case the repercussion on transference could take the form of the patient reducing his overidealization of the analyst.

Ferenczi's counterquestion technique — especially if used without explanation — may be understood by the patient as meaning that the analyst does not want to impart the information requested although he has it. There are indeed social contexts in which the relationship between speaker and addressee is asymmetrical (often corresponding to an imbalance of power), and this is expressed in the absence of willingness to convey information. For example, in a court case the defendant is not permitted to ask the judge for information (except perhaps to ensure verbal understanding), but the converse is certainly permissible. Ferenczi's rule (even in Greenson's modification) boils down to explaining the analytic situation as a field of interaction in which no genuine questions of information from the patient are permissible. The patient incorporates this into his transference phenomena, the exact manner depending on his disposition. One possibility would be that he fantasizes the analytic situation as a court scene. If he has the appropriate transference disposition, he can also assume that the general cooperation principle is not being adhered to. We have already dealt with this above in the discussion of silence on the part of the analyst. This danger is especially great in the introductory phase, when the patient still cannot grasp the sense of the rules of psychoanalysis.

A somewhat different situation emerges if the analyst follows Greenson's suggestion and explains to the patient the purpose of the counterquestion technique. Such explanations do not have a long-lasting effect, but do strengthen the working relationship, especially if the information about rules is enriched interpretatively.

We would like to summarize our reflections prompted by speech act theory as follows: The patient enters the analysis with a largely preconscious knowledge of rules of discourse, mainly from his everyday experience. Irritations and corresponding influences on the transference pattern set up by the patient can result whenever the analyst diverges from everyday rules of discourse or implicitly or explicitly introduces new rules of discourse. By doing this, the analyst guides the patient in the direction of a transference pattern which fits the new rules of discourse. Which transference pattern then emerges depends on the patient's transference dispositions.

### *7.4.3 Object Finding and Dialogue*

Our reference to speech act theory, specifically to the verbal pattern of question, answer, and response, has shown that the rules of discourse form a very differentiated system of interrelated reactions on the part of the dialogue partners. Similarly, interrelated and coordinated patterns are known at the level of nonverbal interaction between mother and child. René Spitz (1965) called this mother-child behavior a dialogue and worked out the significance of this dialogue as a precondition for the child being able to gain internal object constancy. The natural next step is to apply Spitz' considerations to the verbal dialogue in analysis, which is after all supposed to lead to the restructuring of self-representations and object representations.

According to Spitz, not only the patterns of action interconnect in the dialogue between mother and child, but also their previous and current affects. It is not the case that the mother could or even should maximally fulfill the child's every wish, but the dialogue must proceed gratifyingly for the child often enough to enable the development of the image of a good object relationship (*nihil est in intellectu quod non prius fuit in sensibus*).

On the other hand, the child's patterns (his image of the object relationship) also become differentiated, in that the mother avoids fulfilling all the child's wishes and the child thus learns to gain control of his impulses and to cope with the (initially only temporary) absence of the real person without affective overflow.

The analogy of the preverbal dialogue, as Spitz described it, with the verbal pattern of question-answer-response is clear. Stretched between direct answer and response is the arc between gratification and frustration. Like the mother, the analyst must find the right mixture of the two if he wants to promote his patient's development. Here it becomes plain that rigid application of the counterquestion rule represents too simple a solution to the problem. Some questions must be answered at the level thematized by the patient if we want to facilitate the development of a sound working relationship. There are bound to be some frustrations, for a variety of reasons, for example because the analyst does not know the answer or because he wants to protect his private sphere (just as the mother must protect herself against excessive claims made on her by her child), and also because wholly natural frustrations promote a differentiation of the patient's relationship patterns which is appropriate to reality. In this way the analyst remains entirely within the framework of the everyday rules of discourse.

We do not want to suggest that the analyst should follow the everyday rules of discourse when answering patients' questions, or indeed at all in the therapeutic setting. However, we do want to emphasize that the explicit and implicit rules introduced by the analyst by means of his technique are essential determinants of the form taken by the patient's transference. Flader and Grodzicki (1978) conjecture that the fundamental rule and the rule of abstinence induce transferences which repeat the child's relationships to the people it was dependent on. Of course, there is probably no mother who evades or leaves unanswered all her child's questions, and thus the iatrogenic component must be borne in mind in the repetition (see Chap. 2). Moreover, the repetition takes place under more favorable conditions. The stereotype discussed above does not create a fruitful climate for the patient to find better answers today than he has found in the past. The analyst must carefully assess how much a patient can bear in the way of digressions from the everyday rules of discourse according to the foreseeable consequences on the transference relationship.

The unique possibilities of the analytic dialogue derive from the fact that its rules of discourse are in certain respects wider in scope than those of everyday discourse. The purpose of this widening of scope, with interpretation as the single most important component, is to enable the unconscious to be brought into the sphere of the conscious. This is also the purpose of the counterquestion rule, which is, however, not achieved when the rule is applied rigidly. Thus the analyst has not done his job properly if he simply answers the patient's questions conventionally; he must understand what is unconsciously behind the question. Flader and Grodzicki (1978) state that he must ultimately answer questions that the patient cannot yet even ask consciously. An example will make this clear: The child, afraid of being alone, asks the departing mother, "When will you be back?" The mother will answer the question and perhaps add a few words of consolation. The patient who asks his analyst the same question at the beginning of the summer holidays will possibly get the following interpretation in reply: "You are asking that now to make sure that I will come back and that your anger about me going away doesn't endanger our relationship."

In this way the analyst partially avoids answering the question (although in this example it is answered insofar as the analyst implicitly says that he will come back). This evasion contains frustration. Thus the analyst instead begins a special kind of metacommunication with the patient with the intention of throwing light on the unconscious components of the patient's relationship to him in an interpretation of transference, thereby providing an answer to the question which the patient cannot pose: "Why am I so aggressive, and why can't I express my aggression?"

To the extent that he feels the analyst has understood him in this interpretation and that he thus learns to understand himself better, the patient gets something which certainly contains a measure of gratification, but which beyond that helps him to overcome his conflicts. In this way he is more than compensated for the frustration caused by the analyst's refusal to answer his question directly. However, in order for this stage to be reached, i.e., in order for the analyst to be able to make a helpful interpretation, a therapeutic relationship with conscious, unconscious, and transference components must first develop. The analyst contributes to this development with everything he does or leaves undone. In patients at risk, rigid adherence to the counterquestion rule increases the danger of malignant regression or limits the accessibility of the patient for interpretations. On the other hand, the therapeutic objective will also not be achieved through simple adherence to the everyday rules of discourse. It is essential that the analyst strive for clarity concerning what his interventions have precipitated and that he take the patient's reactions into account in further interventions.

# 8 Means, Ways, and Goals

## 8.1 Time and Place

The structure of numerous social events is based on the categories of time and place. The regular club evenings, the Wednesday meetings in Freud's apartment, church on Sunday, and summer vacations at the same place every year are just a few examples of the biologically and socially based rhythm of life. Regularity can reinforce identity. We now want to examine the issue of the frequency of treatment from this perspective about the organization of experience.

Even though Freud introduced his "principle of leasing a definite hour" for pragmatic reasons, the daily session was nonetheless important to prevent treatment from "losing contact with the present," by which he meant a patient's life outside analysis (1913c, pp. 126-127). Yet we also must take into consideration the fact that the treatment itself can become a patient's present, i.e., the decisive factor in his life. More recently it has become possible to observe a tendency away from daily sessions, as Freud practiced them, and toward analyses of varying intensity. This tendency is motivated by strategic considerations, that is by the attempt to be flexible in finding solutions:

> The specialized yardstick for the temporal intensity of treatment is one which registers which combination of structuring, confrontation, and assimilation is optimal for the dynamic of treatment, given the observation and participation of the analyst and taking into consideration relevant events and the patient's experiences outside the analytic situation, his assimilation of them between sessions, and the goals of treatment. (Fürstenau 1977, p. 877)

Alexander and French (1946, p. 31) suggested controlling the intensity of transference by varying the frequency of sessions — which met vehement resistance. What is it, then, that moves us to retain the frequency originally chosen and to alter this arrangement only after long and careful reflection? This raises an interesting point: on the one hand, the frequency of sessions is viewed as a variable dependent on the optimal combination of structuring, confrontation, and assimilation, but on the other hand, once settled it takes on the character of an independent variable, that is it becomes part of the setting and an object on which conflicts in the relationship can crystallize. The time agreed upon becomes the scene of struggle involving very different motives — on both sides. It can be just as much an occasion for conflict as the analyst's silence. Since adherence to the schedule of sessions in the analyst's office is an important general condition, it is an especially attractive target for the patient unconsciously to attack. This is a sensitive area because the patient can threaten the analyst's autonomy by attacking his use of time as a basis for organization. The more uncompromising the analyst is in defending the established frequency, the more intense the struggle can become.

The arrangement of frequency is an issue which can be derived from the theory of technique only to a limited extent. Deciding on six, five, four, three, two or even only one hour per week does not in itself enable us to make predictions about the consequent scope for the maneuvers that can make therapy possible under extremely variable conditions, such as were described by Rangell (1981) in his retrospective on twenty-five years of professional experience. Frequency does, of course, influence the amount of space available for unconscious processes to unfold. This leads us to the stage metaphor, which we, like Sharpe (1950, p. 27) and Loewald (1975) before us, take seriously. While the size of the stage, i.e., the space available for enactment, provides a general frame, more is demanded of the director than simply putting actors on the stage. Loewald (1975, pp. 278-279) speaks of transference neurosis as a drama that the patient creates and enacts together with the analyst. In addition, we are especially interested in the question of the length of time that the individual patient requires to enact his unconscious conflicts in the analytic relationship. Today it seems obvious that standardized policies, e.g., that four hours is a minimum to enable transference neurosis to develop, are the remnants of an orthodox understanding of psychoanalysis. It can be shown that whenever a reduction in the weekly number of hours has been necessary for real economic reasons — such as in France, where as a rule analyses are conducted in three sessions a week — the substance of the analytic activity does not necessarily depend on this external factor. In occasional cases it may be possible to establish and maintain a therapeutic process only if treatment is very frequent (five or six sessions a week). In such circumstances this frequency is justified. We believe, however, that a myth of uniformity currently obscures psychoanalytic thought, preventing any objective discussion of the individual case — such as the number of sessions per week a patient requires.

We regard the argument that it would be possible to determine the differences between patient's reactions to the standardized situation more satisfactorily if all patients had the same frequency of sessions to be the expression of a false and restrictive understanding of the rules. In his comparison of psychoanalytic procedure with the preparation of a specimen for microscopic study, which requires that the correct procedure be followed in order to ensure the comparability of the results, Bachrach (1983) committed the fundamental error of assuming that identical data could also be accumulated in a social situation by employing a prescribed set of external procedures. Bracketing out the specific meaning of such external procedures creates an illusion, as we have made clear in discussing the issue of analyzability.

The significance of the frequency and the desired intensity of treatment can only be adequately understood, however, if the question of how an analysand comes to terms outside analysis with his experiences in analysis is included in the theoretical and clinical discussion. Patients who require a long time to create a connection between individual sessions — who retreat into a kind of defensive capsule and who obstruct the development of the self-analytic process — obviously require a greater frequency of treatment than patients who develop this ability early and are able to use it. The "analytic space" (Viderman 1979) thus also refers to the intrapsychic world of experience opened by the analytic process and not just to the concrete treatment periods themselves. Freud wrote in this regard that "for slight cases or the continuation of a treatment which is already well advanced, three days a week will be enough" (1913c, p. 127).

Candidates in training are exposed to special burdens; they are, for example, required to adhere to a prescribed frequency of four sessions a week. If a patient desires to reduce the frequency to three or even two sessions, after thorough consideration of the situation it is often impossible to evade his questions of whether fewer sessions would not be sufficient and what the reasons are that a reduction cannot even be attempted. In most cases and situations there are no convincing arguments; the candidate in training, in contrast, must stick to four sessions in order to obtain formal recognition as a psychoanalyst. He is faced with a difficult decision. If he were to accept the reduction, the analytic process would proceed under altered conditions and might often even be more productive, because the patient has increased autonomy. Yet the candidate might then have to bear a considerable burden: analysis with only three sessions per week will not be recognized and consequently the length of his training would be increased considerably, possibly by three years or even more. Worst of all is when the struggle over frequency leads to termination. However, if the patient submits to the regulation without being convinced of its correctness, the analytic process is subject to a severe strain, at least temporarily, and therapeutic effectiveness is endangered.

The duration of an individual session is almost always 45–50 minutes. "Occasionally, too, one comes across patients to whom one must give more than the average time of one hour a day, because the best part of an hour is gone before they begin to open up and to become communicative at all" (Freud 1913c, pp. 127-128). It seems to be unusual for us to meet such patients today, or do we not want to meet them? The complaint that a 45–50 minute session is too short is not uncommon.

How the time is experienced subjectively is determined by what has or has not been achieved in therapeutic work in the time available; it is determined by the interaction. Even though, obviously, the analyst cannot simply comply with nagging wishes but must analyze them, there is still Freud's reference to "the average time of one hour a day." The word "average" implies there is variation around a mean. Deviation from the hourly session in modern practice is probably minimal, however, although time is money. Greenson, in particular, has criticized the analyst's material interest in maintaining an exact schedule of sessions; he pointed especially to the practice of not taking a suitable break between sessions.

I believe that the decline of the 50-minute hour is symptomatic of a materialist trend in psychoanalytic practice, at the expense of a humanistic and scientific point of view. It is obvious that taking patient after patient on an assembly-line schedule is an act of hostility, subtle and unconscious though it might be. (Greenson 1974, pp. 789-790)

Greenson's criticism expresses the necessity for the analyst to create sufficient distance from the subjective world of one analytic process to enable him to pay undivided attention to a new patient. In view of the great diversity in style of work, we believe that each analyst should decide individually on the duration of the break that he requires.

The manner of experiencing time that stems from the anaclitic-diatrophic phase of development is viewed as an essential factor in the success of the patient's fundamental experience in the psychoanalytic situation (Stone 1961). Kafka (1977, p. 152) points out that the psychoanalyst's special interest in time feeling may arise from the fact that he is continuously observing how past experiences are structured in the present. However, special sensitivity to the temporal aspects of psychoanalytic activity is necessary. It is difficult to answer theoretically the question of how old, schematically stored knowledge with an inherent, condensed temporal structure is transformed into the current flow of time (Bonaparte 1940; Ornstein 1969; Schachtel 1947; Loewald 1980). The "psychopathology of time" represents another important area for the analyst (Hartocollis 1985). The work of Schilder (1935a), who attempted to apply the phenomenological studies of Straus (1935), von Gebsattel, and Minkowski (1933) to psychoanalysis, has unfortunately been forgotten. Loewald has rekindled this theoretical discussion, whose relevance for actual treatment is greater than often assumed (Loewald 1980, pp. 138-139).

Kafka (1977, p. 152) makes a special reference to the following points: "The patient's analytic hour" is an "extended 'time out' (from work, from usual activity, from usual style of behavior, and from usual style of communication)." One factor which determines the nature of this time out, i.e., the degree to which the patient can step out of his everyday activity and time feeling, is the analyst's manner of using the hour, including the true function of the analyst's silence:

The world outside the room is put into the background. The quiet acts like a lampshade modifying a too bright light. The pressing nearness of material reality becomes remote. It is as if the silence of the analyst already marks the beginning of a quieter, less immediate way of looking at others and at oneself. (Reik 1949, p. 123)

The analyst's silence, if well dosed, can support the patient's time out and help him to turn to his inner, subjectively experienced time feeling. The regularity of sessions, which provides the structure for frequency-specific rhythms, makes it possible for patients to develop their own analytic time feeling, i.e., a personal understanding of time outs. For the analyst the session is an "extended and relatively usual 'time in'" (Kafka 1977, p. 152). How the analyst uses it is determined both by his personal equation and by the rhythm which develops in the relationship. In other words, the analyst's use of the analytic hour is determined by his personal conceptions of time, of the time available, and of the sensual quality of unconscious timelessness. "The analyst, more than the patient, assumes that contiguity of communication (and of experience) has *possible* 'meaning' implications transcending contiguity as such" (Kafka 1977,

p. 152). The analyst has his own theory-dependent hypotheses about the temporal structure which is contained in the patient's material in a linear temporal way. He can view utterances made at very different times as "meaningful connections." This constructive activity is at first relatively new to the patient, who must first be convinced of the truth of this view of the matter. Kafka thus refers to the analyst as a "'condenser' and 'dilator' of time."

The patient is supposed to internalize this bold, constructivistic form of gaining access to the dimension of time, in the sense of the assimilation of life history as described by Habermas.

I think that the process of connecting events and feelings differently — in a sense, bringing new information to bear on episodes reexperienced during psychoanalysis — permits a reorganization and reinterpretation of time feeling. The reorganization may enhance the sense of continuity and facilitate the widening of temporal perspective and its extension into the future. (Kafka 1977, p. 154)

The individual time outs of analytic sessions combine to form a period of time, the duration of which is difficult to predict, especially at the beginning of treatment. "An unwelcome question which the patient asks the doctor at the outset is: 'How long will the treatment take? How much time will you need to relieve me of my trouble?'" (Freud 1913c, p. 128). Freud's ingenious advice was to refer to Aesop's fable:

Our answer is like the answer given by the Philosopher to the Wayfarer in Aesop's fable. When the Wayfarer asked how long a journey lay ahead, the Philosopher merely answered 'Walk!' and afterwards explained his apparently unhelpful reply on the ground that he must know the length of the Wayfarer's stride before he could tell how long his journey would take. This expedient helps one over the first difficulties; but the comparison is not a good one, for the neurotic can easily alter his pace and may at times make only very slow progress. In point of fact, the question as to the probable duration of a treatment is almost unanswerable. (1913c, p. 128)

If we look at current practice, we find laconic comments about the so-called standard procedure, for example that "it takes place in four or five sessions per week, usually lasts four to five years, rarely lasts less than three years, and can even last longer than six years in certain cases" (Nedelmann 1980, p. 57). Even though the majority of the forms of psychoanalytic therapy are conducted in a much shorter period of time, the question of why the neoclassical technique has led to such an increase in length of treatment that the effort and result are in such a precarious balance is nonetheless timely. When Freud mentioned "long periods of time," he meant "half a year or whole years — of longer periods than the patient expects" (1913c, p. 129)

In Sect. 8.9 we will discuss in greater detail the factors which have contributed to an increase in the length of psychoanalytic treatment. We would like to point out at this juncture, however, that discussion of the period of time required for psychoanalytic treatments tends to contain the danger of confusing the subjectively experienced time (Minkowski 1933) with the objectively transpired period of time. Precisely for these reasons, we have subjected the policies which we take to be expressions of a reified understanding of the psychoanalytic process (according to Gabel 1975) to critical examination.

> Time is a dialectical dimension not only because, contrary to space, it is impossible to conceive of it in a state of rest, but also because its progression effects a dialectical synthesis constantly being reborn from its three dimensions: present, past, future. It is a totality which can be dissociated by reification of the past or the future .... (Gabel 1975, p. 107)

The study of the psychoanalytic space, in contrast, must start from the concrete space and describe its extension in meaning metaphorically. The patient molds the analytic space on the basis of his subjective experience, i.e., his individual scheme of apperception, and expects to meet the analyst in this space. Viderman (1979, p. 282) phrased it in the following way:

> The transference neurosis does not develop in a space devoid of affects .... The analytic process is possible only in a specific environment created by the technical rules in which the affects and counteraffects of the two organizers of the analytic space interact.

The analyst's office forms the external framework in which the therapeutic process unfolds. Secluded and safe behind a sign saying "Do not disturb," a space is created for the dyadic activity which is temporally limited and whose physical features can have a positive or a negative influence.

Although there is very little in the literature about the room in which treatment takes place, the photograph of the room Freud used is familiar to all psychoanalysts. It has been described in detail by Engelman (1976); for H. Doolittle (1956) it was the sanctum. Freud stimulated the development of transferences by means of his person and his treatment room, and did not understand the mirror metaphor in the sense of a blank screen. In contrast, anecdotes are told about analysts who attempt to standardize all external influences by using a very monotonous room, having a tailor make them the same suit over and over, and trying in other ways to become a perfect mirror. This attitude attracted Fenichel's criticism (1941, p. 74).

If we apply the maxim that the analyst must feel comfortable in the analytic space so that the patient can also sense it, then the actual arrangement of the space may vary considerably. The specific arrangement can then be studied to determine the extent to which it expresses a congruence between the analyst's attitude and behavior. The prime feature of the analytic space is the analyst himself, who sits still or moves around and who personally furnishes his office. Goffmann's (1961) studies on role theory are relevant for understanding the analytic space as the setting for treatment. A multitude of minor details regarding the analyst's use of the therapeutic relationship have repeatedly been made the object of extensive discussions; this is a clear indication that the reality of the relationship is part of the system of roles in a model describing how specialized services are provided (Goffmann 1961). The analyst decides where analysis is to take place, i.e., where a psychoanalytic relationship can develop, and makes himself an object of discussion as a result of how he has arranged the setting. The treatment room should have the quality of a "facilitating environment." We attribute the analyst the capacity for "concern" (Winnicott 1965), and the ability to sense the room temperature and whether the patient needs a blanket. Difficulties resulting from understanding the space as an extension of the real analyst are less frequent with neurotic patients, whose curiosity about objects in the room or the furnishings can be answered and handled in accordance with our recommendations for dealing with questions (Sect. 7.4). Difficulties arise where severely disturbed patients experience the treatment room as a transitional object. Greenson illustrated this with the experience of one patient who, by stroking the wallpaper, was able to find comfort that Greenson was unable to provide with his voice: "Even the analyst's office may take on extraordinary power in serving the patient as a haven against the dangers in the external and internal world" (Greenson 1978, p. 208).

The explicit use of the analyst's office as a facilitating environment implies, furthermore, the importance of the analyst being continuously aware of the separation process. If the patient treats the room and the objects in it as if they belonged to him, and if the analyst does not act quickly enough to clear up the patient's confusion of "mine" and "yours," the result is repudiation of the fact that the patient's share in the room is temporally limited and in principle incomplete. Misunderstandings then result which impede the therapeutic process. In this way ego boundaries, an abstract theme in Federn's (1952) theory, become technically relevant. They are, of course, of supreme importance in all borderline cases. The problems involved in making meaningful demarcations are often difficult for the practicing analyst to answer in his office because the demarcations have to be made individually. In institutions, in contrast, there are sometimes difficulties in making a room available which the analyst has personally arranged.

The patient's perceptions in the analyst's office are an important precondition for him to be able to enrich his limited identifications with human features and personal experiences by forming transitional objects. The patient also detects thresholds and boundaries, and thus the analyst's autonomy and personal space, everywhere. If the analyst's office is in his home, the personal rooms are not accessible for the patient, while in institutions patient and analyst might meet in the toilet. A tension results between the patient's inquisitive desire to share in the analyst's private life and his respect for the analyst's personal space. By setting spatial and temporal limits, the analyst provides an example for individuation and autonomy. In order to be able to reach this goal, the patient voluntarily sacrifices part of his independence for a while in order to attain an autonomy which is greater and freer of anxiety.

## 8.2 Psychoanalytic Heuristics

"Eureka — I've found it!" This is what the Greek mathematician Archimedes is said to have cried on discovering the law of displacement. Heuristics is defined as an art of discovery and as a methodological guide to the discovery of something new. Taken together, a patient's small triumphs amount to discoveries of great therapeutic significance, even if they affect only the situation of one person and his close relatives, and do not go down in history like Archimedes' exclamation. If the patient has worked his way to a new insight, the analyst is pleased that an idea which he conceived on the basis of his professionally trained empathy fell on fruitful ground.

Despite his pleasure that the joint search has been successful, the analyst remains reserved, for several reasons. He does not want to relativize the patient's pride and satisfaction in the creative accomplishment of having found an unusual and surprising solution. And perhaps he will wait a little too long to signalize his agreement with the patient, because he views even limited confirmation as an improper additional suggestive influence. In such a moment he might even think of the saying that one swallow doesn't make a summer. And finally, heuristics is plagued by the complex question as to the foundation of the conviction that something important has been identified or even discovered. In any case, the issue is to determine the plausibility of the presumed connection by considering it critically from completely different perspectives. In Freud's words,

> we give the patient the conscious anticipatory idea and he then finds the repressed unconscious idea in himself on the basis of its similarity to the anticipatory one. This is the intellectual help which makes it easier for him to overcome the resistances between conscious and unconscious. (1910d, p. 142)

We agree with Boden (1977, p. 347) that "a heuristic is a method that directs thinking along the paths most likely to lead to the goal, less promising avenues being left unexplored." Algorithmic strategies can be described, in contrast, as systems of rules which can be prescribed or defined in a step-by-step manner; nothing can go wrong if the algorithm is followed in the prescribed way. If situations exceed a certain degree of complexity, the steps prescribed by algorithmic strategies become increasingly intricate; in this case the use of heuristic rules is advantageous.

Freud's chess metaphor makes it clear that he was aware of the complexity and indeterminacy of the psychoanalytic situation. Although he did not distinguish between the algorithmic and heuristic methods, his technical recommendations nonetheless largely correspond to our understanding of heuristic strategies. An algorithmic quality foreign to the essence of the psychoanalytic technique is present to a degree proportional to the loss of flexibility in the application of these recommendations. Understanding the fundamental rule as a heuristic strategy emphasizes our conception that the psychoanalytic situation is a complex situation with several meanings, which can be understood only if the analyst obtains more information than is initially available.

The primary purpose of heuristic strategies is to collect and organize the relevant information. Good heuristic strategies reduce insecurity, complexity, and ambiguity, and increase the probability of understanding what is important at any particular moment. These procedures start from the assumption that the information they collect can add to the knowledge we have already gathered, and that criteria for including or excluding material emerge from the search process itself. The algorithmic procedure reduces complexity and identifications in a manner which is artifical and much too rapid. It attributes meaning to material on the basis of prior knowledge, and thus terminates the search process in an artificial and unacceptable way.

It is possible to extract from Freud's works a large number of technical rules, i.e., recommendations for treatment which are intended to direct immediate activity, as demonstrated by a study group in Frankfurt (Argelander 1979, pp. 101-137). If technique is understood as the means and ways of applying the method (see for example Rapaport 1960), it is possible to classify rules into types according to their function in the analytic process.

Strategies which promote the process of participant observation, i.e., concern the attitude toward psychoanalytic perception, recommend that the analyst stay very close to the patient's emotional experiencing and at times identify with the patient in order to participate in his subjective experience. The analyst's general rule of maintaining evenly suspended attention and passing everything that the patient tells him to *his own unconscious mental activity* defines precisely the kind of participant observation which promotes the perception of unconscious motivations. The significance of the analyst's "free association," which has to occur within his evenly suspended attention, emphasizes the necessity for him to enrich the patient's fragmentary descriptions with his own experience (Peterfreund 1983, p. 167).

There are strategies for speaking, in addition to those for listening, which the analyst can employ to help the patient emphasize the significance of his statements. The analyst supplements these general strategies, aimed at promoting the subjective aspect in the patient's comments, by directing his and the patient's attention particularly to unusual, rare, or unique phenomena which are not part of the everyday flow of experience. In this regard, Argelander (1979) refers to the Dora case, where only "certain details of the way in which she expressed herself" provided a guide (Freud 1905e, p. 47). Manifestations termed "interference phenomena" occur when statements organized according to primary and to secondary processes coincide. These strategies lead to an interruption in the evenly suspended attention, then to a condition of readiness, and finally to a focussing of attention (Chap. 9): the readiness for analytic perception becomes the readiness for analytic action. Following the heuristic search, inner mental processes review the new information from different points of view. The analyst calls upon the case-specific, individual, and generalized working models at his disposal, and prepares an intervention.

We will now consider the form the underlying processes take in theory. Starting from a discussion of the concept of empathy, Heimann (1969) expanded her ideas about the analyst's cognitive process to include three functional states; she referred to suggestions made by Greenson (1960), who had spoken of a working model which the analyst devises for himself. It is noteworthy that Heimann was stimulated to these ideas by a review article in which Holt (1964) discussed the state of cognitive psychology. We consider this to be one of the interfaces where it is possible to recognize the influence of cognitive psychology on the revision of psychoanalytic metapsychology. The development of cognitive psychology and of research on artificial intelligence (Lindsay and Norman 1977) led to substantial differentiation of the concepts that Greenson used in his working model, which we now want to describe following Peterfreund (1975, 1983).

Many analytic concepts are based on ideas about the organization of memory. In cognitive psychology this dynamically structured system is referred to using the terms "maps," "models," "representations," "knowledge structures," "schemata," or "scripts." Peterfreund employs the term "working model." The information constituting the different working models is based on the data the organism has selected and organized in the course of its life. Learning can be grasped as the establishment of working models. Although innate genetic programs form the basis of these models, they continue to develop throughout life. The systems constituting working models can be described using terms such as "information," "data processing," and "stored programs." When a working model is activated, most processes occur at a preconscious level.

A large number of different working models are plausible, extending from "general knowledge about the world" to "knowledge about one's own life history." It is also useful to differentiate "cognitive models for the ideas of developmental psychology" from a "cognitive model about the therapeutic process."

These working models are not contained one within the other, like a set of Russian dolls, but must be understood as parts of a networklike structure with numerous temporal and spatial cross-references. The analyst usually works with these models at a preconscious level; they presumably function like schemata in cognitive psychology (Neisser 1976). They are immersed in the flow of experience, and at the same time determine what the subject accepts:

> A schema is that portion of the entire perceptual cycle which is internal to the perceiver, modifiable by experience, and somehow specific to what is being perceived. The schema accepts information as it becomes available at sensory surfaces and is changed by that information; it directs movements and exploratory activities that make more information available, by which it is further modified. (Neisser 1976, p. 54)

The establishment and dismantling of the structures of experience take place at different rates and under different conditions in the different working models. The abstract concepts of metapsychology are stable because they can never be seriously threatened by experience. In contrast, working models closer to experience are influenced by clinical verification. The development of the theory of hysteria shows vividly how Freud was only able to realize the full potential of his conceptual approach by replacing real trauma with the fantasized trauma of seduction (Krohn 1978).

## 8.3 Specific and Nonspecific Means

### *8.3.1 General Points of View*

Since its beginnings psychoanalysis has distinguished between different means of therapy. In fact, the psychoanalytic method was constituted by its differentiation from *suggestion* and by its emphasis on *insight* and *remembering* on the part of the patient, supported by the analyst's interpretations. Despite the doubts arising from the meaning assigned to the concepts "specific" and "nonspecific" (Thomä 1980; Cheshire and Thomä 1987), therapeutic means are better classified within this frame of reference than in the contrast between object relationship and interpretation.

Half a century ago psychoanalysis became polarized, the effects of which can still be felt, moving Cremerius (1979) to ask whether there are two psychoanalytic techniques. He referred on the one hand to classical *insight therapy* with its emphasis on interpretation, and on the other to *therapy based on emotional experience*, which credits experiencing in the object relationship with the essential therapeutic function. This polarization goes back to the contrast drawn by Ferenczi and Rank (1924) between the therapeutic effect of experiencing and that achieved by a certain interpretation fanaticism; they even described the psychoanalytic form of experiencing as therapeutically superior to reconstruction by remembering. There are many indications that, in reaction, advocates of the classical technique tended to counter the overemphasis on experiencing right up to Freud's late study on *Constructions in Analysis* (1937d).

At the beginning of the 1950s experiencing was again discredited, this time as a result of the manipulative use of corrective emotional experience in the technique propounded by Alexander, who in 1937 had been one of Ferenczi and Rank's strongest critics (Thomä 1983a). The extremes moved even further apart when Eissler (1953) introduced the basic model technique with its guiding concept of the "parameter." In Sect. 8.3.3 we will provide a more detailed description of insight therapy centered on pure interpretation, but first we must point out that even more problems are associated with this rigid contrast between the two techniques. One element in the controversy was the claim that the therapy of emotional experience was especially effective in correcting preoedipal defects, i.e., those which originate in the preverbal phases of development. Thus Balint refers to a contrast between interpretation, insight, and object relationship (see Sect. 8.3.4). Even Kohut's self psychology retains the scheme of disturbances of oedipal or preoedipal origin, or for short, two- or three-person psychopathology. Although Kohut's understanding of the empathic compensation for self defects differs greatly from Ferenczi's therapy of deficiency, they have many practical aspects in common. These similarities are located where previously insufficient mothering should be balanced in some way. Since in the purely interpretative technique the therapeutic effectiveness of confirmation and gratification is underestimated and these actions appear to violate the norm of abstinence, "empathy" became, in reaction, a collective term describing deep, averbal, and confirmatory understanding beyond, prior to, or independent of the interpretation.

In the development of the technique there were instances of negligence and underestimations on both sides, with corresponding consequences on practice. In one version the therapeutic function of confirmation and gratification is given as a nonspecific factor, which is contrasted to specific interpretations (Heigl and Triebel 1977). In the other version the wordless look of narcissistic admiration becomes the remedy for a damaged self image. Simple processes of finding new values and meaning by means of interpersonal agreement during critical discussions of realistic perceptions in the here-and-now take on a mystical quality.

Obviously, classification according to specific and nonspecific factors may lead to a dead end if they are not viewed as interactive. Depending on the situation, a factor which is generally nonspecific and forms part of the silent background may move to the forefront in a certain moment of the interaction and become a specific means. It seems obvious that this change should be conceptualized as a figure-ground inversion, as it is termed in gestalt psychology.

Bibring (1937) attributed the silent background a stabilizing effect independent of the interpretive technique.

Even if these anxieties are later resolved analytically, I would still like to believe that the experience of the certainty of not losing the analyst's support *immediately* consolidates the feeling of security which was not acquired, or only too weakly, in childhood, perhaps as a result of not having such an experience of certainty. However, such immediate consolidation has lasting value only in the context of the analytic process, even though it is actually not part of the analytic therapy. (Bibring 1937, pp. 30-31)

As already indicated (Thomä 1981, p. 73), the analysts's contribution to the patient's security and consolidation is an essential part of the psychoanalytic situation; it stands in a complementary relationship to specific means. Strupp (1973, p. 35) also emphasized that the specific and nonspecific factors are not given, opposing quantities, but that they are interdependent.

### *8.3.2 Remembering and Reconstruction*

We would like to begin with the therapeutic effect of remembering:

Strictly considered — and why should this question not be considered with all possible strictness? — analytic work deserves to be recognized as genuine psycho-analysis only when it has succeeded in removing the amnesia which conceals from the adult his knowledge of his childhood from its beginning (that is, from about the second to the fifth year). This cannot be said among analysts too emphatically or repeated too often. The motives for disregarding this reminder are, indeed, intelligible. It would be desirable to obtain practical results in a shorter period and with less trouble. *But at the present time theoretical knowledge is still far more important* to all of us than therapeutic success, and anyone who neglects childhood analysis is bound to fall into the most disastrous errors. The emphasis which is laid here upon the importance of the earliest experiences does not imply any underestimation of the influence of later ones. But the later impressions of life speak loudly enough through the mouth of the patient, while it is the physician who has to raise his voice on behalf of the claims of childhood. (Freud 1919 e, pp. 183-184, emphasis added)

There is still controversy as to which partial processes of the complex event should be considered necessary conditions and which sufficient conditions. Some remembering is accompanied by few affects and does not lead to a change either in or outside therapy. There is also emotional abreaction of no lasting import. Apparently something essential must be added to remembering and abreacting in order to achieve a therapeutic effect. Is it the security of being able to deal differently and better with pathogenic experiences than in the traumatic situation? How does the patient become more self-secure in order to overcome his helplessness, like the dreamer who finally masters his repeated nightmares? Is it the presence of an understanding psychoanalyst, with whom the patient identifies, which provides him with additional strength by letting him use the psychoanalyst as an auxiliary ego? Is understanding, wordless communication sufficient? Do identification with the psychoanalyst and establishment of a working alliance provide the patient so much security that emotional remembering becomes possible without this itself having much additional therapeutic significance? Are abreaction and remembering secondary manifestations of a favorable course of therapy instead of its precondition? We confront these questions when evaluating the therapeutic value of insight in the therapeutic process. Does insight fall like fruit from the tree of knowledge, and does the change follow in consequence? As the necessity of working through demonstrates, this is plainly not the case.

It is essential in attempting to achieve integration and synthesis that the patient's regression does not exceed what his ego can endure; only then are the conditions for integration and synthesis favorable. In our opinion, Freud's view that the synthesis occurs on its own after analysis cannot be maintained. We believe that the psychoanalyst must never lose sight of the goal of creating the best possible preconditions to facilitate the patient's integration and synthesis.

Kris (1956b) emphasized, in his study on the recovery of childhood memories, that reconstruction can at the very best achieve an approximation of the actual facts. The fact that, according to Kris, the primary goal of interpretations is not to elicit memories has very important consequences for technique. For Kris, their task is to create favorable conditions to enable the patient to remember. The patient's task is eased if a certain degree of similarity between a current and the earlier situation can be created by means of interpretation. Kris distinguishes between dynamic interpretations, which relate to the current conflicts, and genetic interpretations, which relate to archaic impulses or early unconscious fantasies. One goal of analysis is to establish a continuum connecting the dynamic and genetic interpretations (Fine et al. 1971, p. 13). This theme is implicit in the interpretation of transference and in the controversy about the here-and-now and the then-and-there (Sect. 8.4).

The meaning of the relevant component parts of the act of remembering is probably dependent on the particular state of the ego's synthetic function. Because the transformation and development of the ego depend on the unfolding of both affective and cognitive processes, and because both, despite their reference to the past, occur in the present and point to the future, it is obvious that more weight has been attached to the here-and-now of emotional experience since Ferenczi and Rank's (1924) important study. Nonetheless, its importance is still neglected compared to that of reconstruction. There are more substantial reasons for the controversies, and it is impossible to trace them back to Alexander's manipulative creation of a corrective emotional experience. The strong reaction to Alexander's interventions in the course of transference neurosis could hardly be comprehended if a problem central to the theory and technique of psychoanalysis were not involved. We will now turn to this problem.

The diversity of ways that the psychoanalytic process can reflect both childhood development and the analyst's theory of childhood development was demonstrated recently at the International Psychoanalytical Congress in Helsinki in 1981. All four main speakers — Segal (1982), Solnit (1982), Etchegoyen

(1982), and Schafer (1982) — mentioned this interdependence. Schafer in particular drew consequences which we would like to utilize to support our line of argument. The reconstruction of memories does not become truer because the psychoanalyst adheres to the idea that they are independent of his theory, are not influenced by his behavior and interventions, and manifest themselves in pure form in transference. On the contrary, his theories and actions are instrumental in determining the psychoanalytic process, whose features are the reconstruction of the pathogenesis on the basis of the patient's verbal and nonverbal communication in transference, and the uncovering of the patient's memories. Because the general theories of neurosis are referred to in ideographic reconstructions, i.e., in case descriptions, the plausibility of each reconstruction depends in part on the degree of validity that the general theories can claim.

For Freud and his followers, the archaeological model was decisive for the analytic process. Although the psychoanalyst has more difficult methodological problems to solve than the archaeologist, Freud believed that the task of psychoanalysis is easier because we are able to communicate in the present with the person suffering from injuries which occurred in the past. Freud made comparisons to archaeology and the study of classical antiquity in numerous places. His discussion in *Civilization and Its Discontents* (1930a, p. 69) is a representative example. The assumption that "in mental life nothing which has once been formed can perish — that everything is somehow preserved and that in suitable circumstances (when, for instance, regression goes back far enough) it can once more be brought to light" is his starting point for a comparison with the development of the Eternal City. His vivid description of Rome's development and his attempt to present the "historical sequence in spatial terms" makes it possible for him to reach the particular features of mental life:

> The fact remains that only in the mind is such a preservation of all the earlier stages alongside of the final form possible, and that we are not in a position to represent this phenomenon in pictorial terms.
>
> Perhaps we are going too far in this. Perhaps we ought to content ourselves with asserting that what is past in mental life *may* be preserved and is not *necessarily* destroyed. It is always possible that even in the mind some of what is old is effaced or absorbed — whether in the normal course of things or as an exception — to such an extent that it cannot be restored or revivified by any means; or that preservation in general is dependent on certain favourable conditions. It is possible, but we know nothing about it. (1930a, pp. 71-72)

If the issue is to find new ways and seek new solutions, everything which occurs to the patient in the present moves to the center of attention and the reconstruction of the past becomes a means to a goal.

Freud always retained his belief in the great resemblance, even identity, between the reconstructive work of the archaeologist and the psychoanalyst, "except that the analyst works under better conditions and has more material at his command to assist him, since what he is dealing with is not something destroyed but something that is still alive" (1937d, p. 259). The analyst also "works under more favourable conditions than the archaeologist" because he can rely on "repetitions of reactions dating from infancy" in transference (1937d, p. 259).

It has been shown with regard to the reliability of reconstructions that precisely the fact that the analyst deals with something which is still alive, initially assumed to be an advantage, creates considerable complications. It is beyond doubt that the idea of how something might have been related or might have fit together originates in the archaeologist's mind on the basis of extant knowledge, and that the resulting construction provides convincing proof for his idea's validity. Unidentified pieces have no active role, but are adapted to the construction and fill the gaps. In contrast, for the psychoanalyst the patient has the last word and the reconstruction is not an end in itself. "The analyst finishes a piece of construction and communicates it to the subject of the analysis so that it may work upon him" (Freud 1937d, p. 260).

Thus the ideas of the two processes must be adjusted to each other, but the successful re-creation of an interrupted process of mental development does not uncover a figure that had been buried. First, a meaningful connection is discovered. But have the parts that the psychoanalyst collects and fits together from associations ever formed a whole? Has the idea of this whole been retained in the patient's unconscious, or do we use memories in order to be able to make changes through a comparison with the present? The archaeologic model of psychoanalysis unites reconstruction of the past with a cure.

Freud's analogy with sculpture, as a model for therapy, contains a different principle, that of creative change (1905a, p. 260). It always remains important to know the regularities according to which mental formations petrify. Yet if the point is to seek other solutions and find new ways, everything which occurs to the patient in the present moves to the center of attention. Freud introduced the sculpture model to distinguish psychoanalysis from the technique of suggestion. He compared the work of the painter and that of the sculptor in order to describe the therapeutic model of psychoanalysis:

> Painting, says Leonardo, works *per via di porre*, for it applies a substance — particles of colour — where there was nothing before, on the colourless canvas; sculpture, however, proceeds *per via di levare*, since it takes away from the block of stone all that hides the surface of the statue contained in it. In a similar way, the technique of suggestion aims at proceeding *per via di porre*; it is not concerned with the origin, strength amd meaning of the morbid symptoms, but instead, it superimposes something — a suggestion — in the expectation that it will be strong enough to restrain the pathogenic idea from coming to expression. Analytic therapy, on the other hand, does not seek to add or to introduce anything new, but to take away something, to bring out something; and to this end concerns itself with the genesis of the morbid symptoms and the psychical context of the pathogenic idea which it seeks to remove. (1905a, pp. 260-261)

We would now like to turn to Loewald's (1960, p. 18) interpretation of this comparison, which can be summarized as follows: In analysis we bring the true form to the surface by removing the neurotic distortions. Like the sculptor, we need to have an image, if only a rudimentary one, of the goal. The analyst does not only reflect on transference distortions. His interpretations contain aspects of the reality that the patient begins to grasp hand in hand with the transference interpretations. This reality is communicated to the patient by chiseling away the transference distortions, or as Freud described it, by using Leonardo da Vinci's elegant expression, *per via di levare* as in sculpture, and not *per via di porre* as in painting. A sculpture is created by removing material, a picture by putting something on a canvas.

The attentive reader will have noticed that Loewald employs Freud's analogy in the context of working through transference. The real questions relate to the quality and source of what is new. In sculpture nothing is found in the stone which was already there in a certain shape or which could have let us imagine the final shape. Everything was in the sculptor's mind. The situation is different for a psychoanalyst, who discovers something in the unconscious, intervenes, and thus changes the appearance and nature (externally and internally) of the original substance. His ideas, his images, and his way of communicating them lead to transformations.

The two models share a basis in unconscious preforms. The difference between them is that the psychoanalyst as sculptor exerts a much greater influence on the formation than the archaeologist could possibly do with his material. Since no comparison is perfect, we can, in summary, say that the psychoanalyst contributes to the changed and new forms in a genuine way. The work of both the sculptor and the archaeologist is based on the ideas with which they form the material. Yet the ideas have very different scopes for influence: The marble block is unformed, the fragments of a vase are given. The psychoanalyst is an artist sui generis: the material he encounters is present in a flexible and not yet petrified form.

It is fascinating to discover that all stages, and not just the final form, are retained in psychic processes. The natural regression in sleep promotes the tendency of the dreamer to remember images from long-forgotten periods which are stored in the long-term memory. The apparently ahistorical elements are those containing fixations which are visited in regression. The early fixations stimulate motivations for the formation of symptoms and stereotypical behavior. Repetition compulsion and the rigidity of typical character structures represent descriptions which lead to genetic explanations if the relationship between the preliminary stages and the final form can be clarified.

Psychoanalysis has concerned itself especially with the reconstruction of the preconditions of illnesses, and has in the process moved further and further back in life, as far as early childhood. Problems resulting from the clarification of the relationship between the early stages and the final form are discussed in Chap. 10.

### *8.3.3 Intervention, Reaction, and Insight*

The reestablishment of "severed connections" (A. Freud 1937, p. 15) is the primary goal of analysis, and the analyst's interpretations facilitate the synthesis. The classical psychoanalytic technique is thus characterized by the fact that interpretation is its most important instrument or means. Whether the analyst does something or not, whether he explains the patient a rule or stays silent, whether he utters a significant or meaningless "hm" or makes an interpretation, his mere presence has an effect, even if he acts in a completely inobtrusive way. It is helpful to understand interventions as referring to everything that the psychoanalyst contributes to the course of analysis, especially that which helps the patient to gain insight. Among the different kinds of interventions, interpretations occupy a qualitatively prominent position and are characteristic of the psychoanalytic technique. We share the enthusiasm of a patient who once said, "If such connections are established, then I expect I will be able to say, 'Okay, goodbye, I'm healthy.'"

What constitutes an interpretation? Why does an analyst intervene at a particular moment? How do we evaluate the effect of our interventions? If we agree that an intervention has been effective, how was it effective? These questions make it obvious that we cannot get very far in examining interpretations and other interventions without taking the patient's reaction into consideration. This leads us to the subject "insight." How can we distinguish between insight and other reactions? Can we classify the kinds of reactions? What is insight, and what role does it play in the therapeutic process (Fine and Waldhorn 1975, p. 24)? Such questions cannot be avoided when interpretations are examined (Thomä and Houben 1967; Thomä 1967b). For the sake of better orientation, we first refer in general to technical variations such as interpretations of transference and resistance, and deep interpretations (Loch 1965b). Freud distinguished between the interpretation of isolated parts of a patient's material, e.g., a parapraxis or a dream, and the reconstruction of important events in a patient's past, suggesting the term "construction" for the latter (Freud 1937d).

In passing, we would like to mention the division of the interpretation process into preparation (Loewenstein 1951), confrontation (Devereux 1951), and clarification, in the sense of the word used by Bibring (1954). The more complete the protocol of a session, the easier it is to recognize which kinds of interpretation an analyst favors in a particular case or in general. Transcriptions of tape recorded sessions allow detailed studies by independent researchers.

Since transference interpretation is credited, correctly, with the greatest therapeutic effectiveness, and yet since it also raises special problems, it is discussed in detail in Sect. 8.4.

It is possible to distinguish different aspects of an analyst's interpretations. They provide a preconscious or unconscious context for the patient's associations. It is useful to distinguish several types of problems: How does an interpretation originate? How does it work? How can its accuracy be recognized? Combined consideration of association and interpretation makes it possible to draw consequences about the *accuracy* of an interpretation, i.e., about the connection between the analyst's idea, the formulation of the interpretation, the goal of the interpretation, and the effect of the interpretation. This takes us to a level accessible to everyone, from which it is also possible to draw conclusions about inaccuracies. Thus, *indirectly* something is discovered about the origin of the interpretation, and it can be assumed that in this indirect way something can be learned, especially about highly conflictual processes within the analyst (e.g., caused by intensive countertransference). Yet regardless of how a single interpretation originated — whether primarily through unconscious or preconscious intuition or through theoretical deduction, from below or from above — knowledge of its origin does not provide any indication of its accuracy.

Since interpretations constitute the analyst's most important means of intervention, the response they evoke from the patient is decisive. Isaacs (1939, pp. 153-154) summarized the patient's reactions to interpretations as a criterion of their accuracy and effectiveness; her catalogue provides a basis for orientation:

1. The patient may give verbal assent ....
2. There may now be conscious elaboration of images and the meaning of images, with conscious co-operation and appropriate effect.
3. There may be further associations which from their specific nature confirm our view ....
4. There may be a change of associations and of attitude .... E.g. there may be a conscious repudiation, in such terms as to provide a confirmation, if it expresses guilt and terror such as would be felt and only felt if our previous interpretation had been correct.
5. The patient may on the following day bring a dream which carries on and elaborates and make much plainer the unconscious phantasy or intention which had been interpreted. Not only so, but he may recount a dream immediately upon our interpretation, one which he had not told us up to that point ....
6. Memories of past real experience may be recovered as a result of interpreting present unconscious trends, memories which link these trends to real experiences and make both intelligible.
7. Inferences as to external situations which had previously been rejected by the patient may be admitted, or voluntarily brought up by the patient ....
8. One of the most important tests of the correctness of our specific interpretations is the resulting diminution in specific anxieties. This may be shewn in a number of different ways. E.g. there may be bodily signs of relief from anxiety, such as relaxing of rigid muscles, stilling of restless or stereotyped movements, change in tone of voice ....
9. The resolution of anxiety is seen also in the patient's associations, which may shew that the whole unconscious phantasy situation has been changed, with new material emerging as a result of the right interpretation ....
10. These changes in amount and direction of anxiety have their greatest significance in the transference situation. It is what happens in the transference situation, indeed, which provides us with an acid test of the correctness of our perceptions. A valid interpretation may change the phantasy picture of the analyst from a dangerous to a helpful figure....If interpretation has been both true and adequate, phantasies will unfold more richly, and memories stir more freely ....

Although these features are indications for the accuracy of interpretations, they cannot be taken as proof (Thomä and Houben 1967). In addition to them, according to Isaacs (1939, p. 155) the following general rules also apply to interpretations referring to earlier feelings and actions in the attempt to reconstruct the patient's life history:

*Confirmation* of these inferences then comes in various ways: E.g. (a) New memories, either not yet told to us or long forgotten by the patient, emerge as a result of our interpretations; (b) such memories may directly corroborate what has been inferred, may be new instances of the same kind, or whilst different, may yet be linked with our inferences, historically or psychologically; (c) further associative material may arise which makes intelligible the *forgetting* of this and other experiences, as well as present attitudes; (d) corroboration may be gained from outside sources such as friends and relations. Such corroboration from outside is not necessary for the analytic work itself, but it is useful from the scientific point of view, as an additional and independent proof.

Our introductory comments on nonspecific and specific means explain our reasons for attributing interpretation a special position in the psychoanalytic technique. On the other hand we view interpretation in interaction with the nonspecific background, which can move to the foreground at certain moments of therapy and then has a special effectiveness. This is the reason that we maintain a critical distance to Eissler's interpretive purism. Eissler (1953) introduced the basic model technique in his attempt to detect *the* decisive and truly psychoanalytic variables from among the numerous variables which characterize or determine the analytic process and the cure. For the time being we will adopt this position, because we agree with the analysts who believe that "interpretation is the most powerful and consequential intervention at our disposal" (Eissler 1958, p. 222).

Eissler goes even further. In his opinion, the classical technique of psychoanalysis is a therapy "in which interpretation remains the *exclusive* or leading or prevailing tool" (Eissler 1958, p. 223, emphasis added). This technique does not exist anywhere in pure form; in Eissler's own words, "no patient has ever been analyzed with a technique in which interpretations alone have been used" (1958, p. 223). Eissler introduced the concept of the parameter from mathematics, where the term is used to describe values in equations which either remain unknown or are kept constant and which appear *in addition to the true variables.* Eissler borrowed the term to describe everything beyond interpretation, the true psychoanalytic variable.

The conditions of the basic model technique are still fulfilled, according to Eissler (1953, pp. 110-113), if a parameter satisfies four criteria:

> (1) A parameter must be introduced only when it is proved that the basic model technique does not suffice; (2) the parameter must never transgress the unavoidable minimum; (3) a parameter is to be used only when it finally leads to its self-elimination; that is to say, the final phase of the treatment must always proceed with a parameter of zero .... [(4)] The effect of the parameter on the transference relationship must never be such that it cannot be abolished by interpretation. (1953, pp. 111, 113)

In the same study Eissler refers to two other parameters that might be essential in the therapy of schizophrenics or seriously ill neurotics; they are *goal construction* and *reduction of the symptoms.* These two parameters do not satisfy the four conditions, and in employing them the analyst abandons the basic model technique and cannot return to it. Yet interpretations in fact also contain a final aspect, i.e., a goal, and the purist technique thus becomes adulterated. Eissler demonstrates the features of what he calls parameters by referring to the deviations from the basic model technique that Freud resorted to in response to one patient's (the Wolf Man) personality structure and symptoms. He illustrates the first of the above-mentioned criteria for parameters with reference to Freud's active interventions in the therapy of phobic patients.

The fact that the basic model technique has caused more problems that it has solved in the history of psychoanalysis is associated with the fact that attention was not paid to the context. The restrictive perspective based on this technique determined from then on the view of practice as it *should* be. Yet, as Eissler also had to admit, since a systematic description of psychoanalytic hermeneutics had not yet been written (1958, p. 226), the analyst is provided with a set of tools which must get filthy when used and whose hermeneutic technology cannot be systematically worked out until the therapeutic function becomes the center of attention. Interpretive purism can prevent a therapeutically favorable atmosphere from developing. Insight then lacks affective depth.

The concept of "insight" is, on the one hand, central to psychoanalytic theory, which claims to be able, in contrast to other forms of therapy, to achieve changes by means of insight. Interpretation, the most important instrument of therapy, is directed at the patient's ability to achieve a change in his disturbances by means of insight. On the other hand, in recent years insight has increasingly been contrasted with the curative effect of the therapeutic relationship. The reservations regarding the leading role of insight come from two different camps. Kohut's school is rather skeptical about the concept of insight because it is allegedly irresolvably linked to the therapy of psychic conflict, and the curative factors in the self-psychological theory of cure are decisively dependent on the internalization of the psychoanalyst's empathic understanding. The second reservation stems from the fact that the concept of insight is attributed to one-person psychology; in the critical evaluation of the latter, the accentuation of the curative effect of the therapeutic relationship displaces even insight (Appelbaum 1975, 1976; Eagle 1984). This happens by virtue of the fact that the curative effect of the discovery of a new object is made dependent on the internalization of the analyst's functions or on learning in the framework of a new relationship (Loewald 1960; Thomä 1981).

Among the large number of authors who continue to believe in the significance of the concept of insight, there are major controversies about substantive questions, which have so far made it impossible to arrive at a uniform definition. The definition given in the Glossary of Psychoanalytic Terms seems to be unsatisfactory to many; according to it, insight refers to "the subjective experience or knowledge acquired during psychoanalysis of previously unconscious, pathogenic content and conflict" (quoted in Blacker 1981, p. 659).

Looking at the different implicit and explicit definitions of insight in the considerable literature on the subject, it can be noted that they are influenced by the interaction of at least three different points of view.

1. For Freud, insight is linked with the discovery of unconscious reality (Bush 1978). Here insight proves to be the capacity to explain present behavior on the basis of earlier events, as Fisher and Greenberg (1977, p. 350) demonstrate. Insight refers to unconscious pathogenic childhood conflicts and their subsequent derivatives and consequences (Blum 1979, p. 44). Wherever, in therapy or research, insight is defined in this way, separate proof must be supplied that the cognition of unconscious processes is actually linked with a curative effect.
2. In the examples given by many authors, becoming aware of something that had been unconscious is understood in a different sense. Becoming conscious often means that psychic contents are given a new meaning. Blum (1979) quotes in this connection the definition of insight given in *Webster's Dictionary*: penetrating into or apprehending the inner nature of things. Noy (1978) emphasizes the connection between insight and creativity.
3. The fact that therapeutic insight and the desired therapeutic change are frequently far apart — a circumstance that Freud had also complained of — has led to attempts to limit the concept of insight by linking it with therapeutic

change. Yet each change has to prove itself in concrete behavior or in acts. In this approach the concept of insight is linked very closely with behavior and action.

The intensive study of the phenomenon of pseudoinsights has strengthened the tendency for analysts not to view those moments in which a patient's aha experience solves major problems as being prototypical for insight. Instrumental in this regard was a study by Kris (1956a), who described insight in a framework of a "good hour" and grasped it as a process. He thus corrected a false conception which had its origin in Freud's *Remembering, Repeating and Working Through* (1914g). Freud had thought that insight is the decisive cognitive act and that working through is subsequent to it, while in fact insight and working through are intimately connected and are part of the therapeutic process from the very beginning.

Kris' study also emphasizes the trend toward not attaching the concept of insight only to contents but also to the patient's accessibility to his thoughts. While Strachey (1934) stated firmly how the patient must see the analyst if an interpretation is to have a mutative character, authors like Reid and Finesinger (1952), Richfield (1954), Kris (1956a), and Hatcher (1973) describe in minute detail the access that patients have to their thoughts in phases of insight. It is important to be alert to the fact that the dichotomy of content and patient's access refers to different, though related phenomena. The word "insight" suggests that some mental content is seen and understood in a different way. The moment of internal change in a patient *cannot* be directly observed by the analyst; it can only be indirectly deduced. When reference is made to an altered access, it would be better to speak of "seeing in" than of insight. This distinction might possibly end the old controversy about whether insight is the cause or effect of the psychotherapeutic process. "Change," if viewed as a fictive instantaneous event, refers to a result, while "seeing in" and "changing" characterize a process.

The discussion about pseudoinsights led very quickly to a correction of the idea that change is achieved exclusively by means of cognition. Fenichel (1941) continued to rely on the polarity of feeling and thinking. Almost all authors commenting on the concept of insight express the opinion that "true" insight or seeing in lies between the poles constituted by emotions and intellect. There are differences in how these poles are described. Reid and Finesinger (1952) refer to them as emotions and cognitions. Richfield (1954), in contrast, describes two forms of knowledge. Valenstein (1962) uses the German word *Erlebnis* to refer to the emotional pole. Finally, Hatcher (1973) distinguishes "experiencing" self-observation from a more reflective form.

The insight process is described as connected with an act of integration, which contains the potential for new solutions and thus for change as well as for creativity. Differences result from the ways that this integration is conceptualized. For Kris (1956a) and Reid and Finesinger (1952) certain psychic *contents* are integrated. Kris describes this process as the ego's integrative function and discusses the relationship between this function and Nunberg's (1931) concept of the synthetic function of the ego. Myerson (1965) also considers the reintegration in the context of the synthetic function of the ego. For authors like Pressman (1969) and Valenstein (1962) it is more an issue of a specific, i.e., integrated, *access* to thought contents. Although the difference appears insignificant at first sight, it marks two different ways of conceptualizing integration: either as the union of psychic entities or as an activity recombining a certain psychic content, which had been split into separate aspects, under a more general point of view. Scharfman (see Blacker 1981) emphasizes the integrative function. In the psychoanalytic process, insight fulfills the function of "bridging different levels of mind."

Understanding insight as an integrating psychic activity makes it possible to grasp the points where the psychoanalytic concept of insight and the various experimental results on gaining insight intersect. We find integrating activities, e.g., the combination of different psychic entities under general points of view, in very greatly varying fields of mental activity. The special features of the integrating activity in the psychoanalytic process of insight are the result of the fact that the different psychic levels, in Scharfman's sense, are in opposition. The integration of opposing mental levels is a special psychic accomplishment requiring the mastery of a state of tension. Integration of the experiencing and intellectual forms of access to one's own internal processes, which is a prominent topic in the psychoanalytic literature on insight, differs from cognitive insight experiments principally in that experiencing and intellectual forms are in opposition and are liable to produce conflicts.

### *8.3.4 New Beginning and Regression*

Balint related his theory of the genesis of psychic and psychosomatic illnesses to the technical concept of the new beginning in his book *The Basic Fault: Therapeutic Aspects of Regression* (1968). New beginning and basic fault are the two sides of one coin: the new beginning is a therapeutic concept, the basic fault an explanatory one. For Balint, the basic fault is a necessary condition for every serious psychic or psychosomatic illness. New beginning referred ultimately for him to all of those processes which can be observed in the therapeutic elimination or inactivation of the conditions causing the illness, i.e., in the resolution of the basic fault. Basic fault and new beginning comprise a theory of the genesis and treatment of psychic illnesses (Thomä 1984).

The basic fault belongs to the area of the early mother-child relationship. Intrapsychic conflicts which are tied to the oedipal three-person relationship do not arise in the small child. Balint describes the basic fault as a defect in the psychic structure, specifically in the sense of a deficiency (Balint 1968, pp. 21-22). Starting from the theory of a basic fault, neuroses and character difficulties, and perhaps even psychoses and psychosomatic illnesses, are explained as symptoms of one and the same etiology. Since everyone experiences this earliest and fundamental deficiency, it could thus be viewed as a necessary condition of any and every illness.

The deficiency hypothesis can be found in many psychosomatic theories, whose common denominator is that they locate the genesis of the deficiency in an early, preoedipal phase of development. If the psychoanalytic treatment technique is restricted to the interpretation of intrapsychic conflicts, it is inapplicable where these conflicts cannot yet be present. It now becomes clear why preverbal empathic understanding and wordless experiencing receive special attention in the elimination of deficiency states. In contrast, the therapeutic means of remembering and insight via interpretation move to the background. The balance between insight and emotional experience — the two prime components of the therapeutic process — is altered in favor of experience.

The new beginning is achieved, according to Balint, by means of *regression* in the psychoanalytic situation. Regression, too, is not a process that occurs in the patient naturally or on its own (Loch 1963). Balint reminded us that

> regression is not only an intrapsychic phenomenon, but also an interpersonal one; for its therapeutic usefulness, its interpersonal aspects are decisive. In order to understand the full meaning of regression and to deal with it in the analytic situation, it is important to bear in mind that the form in which the regression is expressed depends only partly on the patient, his personality, and his illness, but partly also on the object; in consequence it must be considered as *one* symptom of the interaction between the patient and his analyst. This interaction has at least three aspects: the way (a) in which regression is recognized by the object, (b) in which it is accepted by the object, and (c) in which it is responded to by the object. (1968, pp. 147-148)

We will now discuss the relationship of the new beginning to those regressive states which lead behind the traumatization and which Balint described within the framework of object relationship psychology. These states are inaccessible to associations and interpretations. In Balint's opinion the most important of the additional therapeutic means

> is to help the patient to develop a primitive relationship in the analytic situation corresponding to his compulsive pattern and maintain it in undisturbed peace till he can discover the possibility of new forms of object relationship, experience them, and experiment with them. Since the basic fault, as long as it is active, determines the forms of object relationship available to any individual, a necessary task of the treatment is to inactivate the basic fault by creating conditions in which it can heal off. To achieve this, the patient must be allowed to regress either to the setting, that is, to the particular form of object relationship which caused the original deficiency state, or even to some stage before it. (1968, p. 166)

This deficiency state "cannot be 'analysed' out of existence," but remains as a scar (1968, p. 180). It is obvious that the description of the attitude which is desirable for the analyst, which can lead to a compensation of the deficiency state, depends on the theoretical understanding of the crises which precede or accompany the basic fault.

Balint's impressive images of permeation, entwinement, and fetal harmony make it possible for him to postulate the unconscious longing to regain this unity. With regard to the accuracy of his theory, Balint adds:

> If my theory is correct, then we must expect to come across all these three types of object relationships — *the most primitive harmonious interpenetrating mix-up, the ocnophilic clinging to objects, and the philobatic preference for objectless expanses* — in every analytic treatment that is allowed to regress beyond a certain point. (1968, pp. 71-72)

The phenomena as such are not controversial. There are certainly very few people to whom the feeling of being part of the world, the pleasure in holding on to objects, and the joy in the depth of space are foreign. Balint himself mentioned many striking everyday examples of ocnophilic and philobatic ways of experiencing in *Thrills and Regressions* (1959). Philobatism and ocnophilia are suited to serve as poles of a typology in which mixed forms predominate.

Here, just as with the new beginning, we are dealing with problems that result from Balint's attempts not only to describe certain phenomena but also to explain them by means of his psychoanalytic object relationship theory. The comprehensive concept of regression links object relationship psychology both with dream theory and with lying on the couch, which at least invites regression and, together with free association, could even be termed a regressive act. According to the theory devised by Balint, who himself was not unaware of its contradictions (1968, p. 129), a new beginning can take place if a primitive, preverbal object relationship develops between the analyst and the deeply regressed patient (1968, pp. 165-167).

Balint distinguishes chronologically and phenomenologically between three forms of primitive object relationships:

> (a) the most primitive, which I called *primary love*, or primary relationship, a sort of harmonious interpenetrating mix-up between the developing individual and his primary substances or his primary object; (b) and (c) *ocnophilia* and *philobatism* which form a kind of counterpart with one another; they already presuppose the discovery of fairly stable part and/or whole objects. For the predominantly ocnophilic individual, life is safe only in close proximity to objects, while the intervening periods or spaces between objects are felt as horrid and dangerous....In contrast, the predominantly philobatic individual experiences the objects as unreliable and hazardous, is inclined to dispense with them, and seeks out the friendly expanses separating the treacherous objects in time and space. (1968, p. 165)

Although the new beginning in the here-and-now takes place in a favorable object relationship and in principle cannot be derived from the then-and-there, it is still understood as regression to an early pretraumatic phase of development. The unsolved problem of the relationship between reconstruction and therapeutic change immediately becomes apparent if we focus on one significant point from among Balint's criteria for the new beginning: a new beginning always takes place in transference, i.e., within the object relationship, and leads to a transformation in the patient's relationship with his objects of love and hate and, consequently, to a considerable reduction in anxiety. Transference is not understood here in a narrow sense, as repetition, but rather as a comprehensive type of relationship with substantially new elements.

Innovative experiences in the new beginning are beyond repetition compulsion, and they also cannot be explained by means of theoretical recourse to the pretraumatic harmony which existed before the basic fault developed. By attributing the earliest "object relationship" a special therapeutic role in the new beginning of regressed patients suffering from a basic fault, Balint neglected the situational and creative elements in the therapeutic situation. The concept of the new beginning receives its comprehensive meaning in the theory of therapy when it is understood as an event in the here-and-now which is made possible by the analyst (Khan 1969).

For this purpose, both of the technical means (interpretation and object relationship) are essential, presumably in different dosages and in connection with further curative factors. The division of all of psychopathology into two classes, with the basic fault a condition of every serious illness, is not satisfactory. Of course it is possible for us to project all our creative potential and every new beginning back to the earliest moment in our development and ultimately to find our true selves there in a retrospective utopia. Having shifted the original creative phase to the beginning of life, Balint succumbed to his own theoretical prejudices and localized the new beginning there. We, in contrast, conceive the new beginning as a creative process which is linked to many psychic acts, trial actions, and their realization, which must be tried repeatedly (Rothenberg 1984).

Using this conception, we attempt to link two views of regression, that of ego psychology and that of object relationship theory. The danger that regressions will degenerate in a malignant way is very large inasfar as they are *not* in the service of the ego (Kris 1936). Alexander (1956) pointed this out emphatically. In general, neither works of art nor cures result from regression alone; otherwise there would be many more artists and far fewer emotionally disturbed individuals.

## 8.4 Transference Interpretations and Reality

Since Strachey's studies (1934, 1937) transference interpretations have been considered the mutative instrument par excellence. Since the mutative effect of the transference interpretation, i.e., the change, is tied to the exchange between patient and analyst, Strachey's innovation became the prime example for therapeutically effective exchange processes and for object relationships and their impact on intrapsychic structures.

According to Strachey, in mutative interpretation there is an exchange of superego contents; the attitudes which the analyst communicates by means of his interpretations are internalized by the patient as new and mild parts of the superego. The result of this exchange is thus that the patient partially identifies with the psychoanalyst. Since identification plays such a significant role in therapy, we will discuss it later in detail. Strachey described a type of transference interpretation which alters the patient's experiencing and behavior. The patient arrives at his new identifications because the analyst assumes the functions of an auxiliary superego.

The concept of mutative interpretation directed attention to exchange processes and thus became the pattern for an interactional understanding of therapy. This evaluation of Strachey's paradigmatic work is the result of independent studies presented by Klauber (1972a) and Rosenfeld (1972). Both of these authors emphasize that Strachey's innovation has had a lasting influence on psychoanalytic treatment technique. The contents of mutative transference interpretations have since been substantially extended. Strachey had assumed that especially parts of the superego are projected onto the analyst. Yet the important issue in the theory of projective and introjective identification is no longer the superego, but good and evil parts of the self. Rosenfeld (1972) therefore supplemented the contents of Strachey's mutative interpretation according to the interpretive contents of the Kleinian school.

At the level of the relationship the psychoanalyst functions as more than merely an auxiliary superego, whose stepwise introjection by means of mutative interpretations is, for Strachey, the condition for a cure. Using the terminology of the structural theory of psychoanalysis it is possible to call the psychoanalyst an auxiliary ego. In this function, he helps the patient to gain new insights and thus to interrupt the neurotic repetition compulsion. Although the analyst contributes to an immediate dissipation of anxiety, it would be wrong to equate his function as auxiliary ego with direct support of patients who have weak egos. Strachey limited himself to describing the psychoanalyst's introjection into the patient's superego, but we are today moving toward a two- and three-person psychology as a consequence of the development of psychoanalytic object relationship psychologies, which assign the patient's identification with the analyst a central position. While it was once possible to assume, in working with a patient displaying superego pathology, that a reliable relationship would develop on its own because the healthy parts of the patient's personality would form a link with the task of analysis despite resistance and repression, in many of today's patients this is no longer possible. It speaks for itself that Kohut (1977) attributes the analyst a function of a selfobject. Here we are dealing with exchange processes in the sense of a primary identification, which creates something shared as the basis for reciprocity and mutuality.

The discovery of the patient's readiness to enter into a therapeutic relationship with the psychoanalyst, to work together to some extent, and to identify with him was paradigmatic. Strachey expressed his surprise

> at the relatively small proportion of psycho-analytical literature which has been concerned with the mechanisms by which its therapeutic effects are achieved. A very considerable quantity of data have been accumulated in the course of the last thirty or forty years which throw light upon the nature and workings of the human mind; perceptible progress has been made in the task of classifying and subsuming such data into a body of generalized hypotheses or scientific laws. But there has been a remarkable hesitation in applying these *findings* in any great detail to the *therapeutic process itself.* (Strachey 1934, p. 127, emphasis added)

This observation can be explained by the fact that no specifically psychoanalytic vocabulary was available to describe the curative factors, i.e., those processes that lead *out* of transference neurosis. The description was thus necessarily vague. Some use was made of the terminology of preanalytic, hypnotic psychotherapy, which was not free of the disrepute attached to suggestive influence. In the model of mutative interpretation, Strachey established a new foundation for the analyst's influence even if it was limited to the exchange of superego contents. Thus it was no longer necessary to borrow elements from preanalytic theories or from general concepts to explain therapeutic change in certain respects.

How much is still unclear and controversial can be seen from the contradictions in the theories of the therapeutic process and from the difficulties that have been encountered in trying to transform them into practical steps. What does the psychoanalyst contribute toward the creation of a common basis? How does he make it easier for the patient to identify with the joint task and with the analyst, who sheds new light on his problems in coping with life and on his symptoms? An answer to these questions cannot be found by relying on the working relationship in general, but requires that this relationship be translated into individual technical steps. The same is also true for the application of the theory of identification to therapeutic exchange processes. Mutative interpretations are today recognized as belonging to a larger category of interventions. To ease comparison, we would like to refer to two representative passages from a study by Strachey:

> It is not difficult to conjecture that these piecemeal introjections of the analyst occur at the moments of the carrying through of transference-interpretations. For at those moments, which are unique in the patient's experience, the object of his unconscious impulses simultaneously reveals himself as being clearly aware of their nature and as feeling on their account neither anxiety nor anger. Thus the object which he introjects at those moments will have a unique quality, which will effectually prevent its undifferentiated absorption into his original super-ego and will on the contrary imply a step towards a permanent modification in his mental structure. (1937, pp. 144-145)

Strachey then compares the therapeutic effects of the analyst with those of a therapist who employs suggestion:

> It is true that the analyst, too, offers himself to his patient as an object and hopes to be introjected by him as a super-ego. But his one endeavour from the very beginning is to differentiate himself from the patient's archaic objects and to contrive, as far as he possibly can, that the patient shall introject him not as one more archaic imago added to the rest of the primitive super-ego, but as the nucleus of a separate and new super-ego. ... He hopes, in short, that he himself will be introjected by the patient as a super-ego — introjected, however, not at a *single gulp* and as an archaic object, whether bad or good, but little by little and as a *real person*. (1937, p. 144, emphasis added)

It is improbable that Strachey actually hoped to be consumed as a real person. On the contrary, he probably hoped for a *symbolic internalization*, which coincidentally is said to be characteristic of many cannibalistic rituals (Thomä 1967a, p. 171). In the course of such internalizations both the relation to reality and the self-feeling undergo a change. It is thus possible to say that reality changes as a result of the symbolic interaction.

The current phase of psychoanalytic technique is characterized, according to Klauber (1972a, pp. 386-387), by the attempt to distinguish transference from nontransference elements and to describe more precisely the *reality* of the analytic situation. We hope that the discussion in this section will contribute toward this goal.

Klauber gives the following description of the phases since Strachey's unusually influential work. In the *first* phase, attention was directed by what may be the most creative of all the subsequent studies — A. and M. Balint's paper "Transference and Countertransference" (1939) — to the fact that every analyst has an emotional need to do his work in a way which conforms to his personality, and that he thus creates a totally individual and characteristic atmosphere. The question was thus raised whether it were at all possible for the analyst to have a mirrorlike attitude, as recommended by Freud. The *second* phase began after World War II. The therapeutic significance of the analyst's reaction was especially emphasized by Winnicott's study "Hate in the Countertransference" (1949) and by Heimann's paper "On Countertransference" (1950). Central for the *third* phase were the descriptions by Searles (1965) and Racker (1968) of the complex interaction between patient and analyst.

Both mutative interpretations and Strachey's thesis that the analyst in his benign role is introjected into the patient's superego put special emphasis on the problem of reality in the therapeutic situation and on the question of how the analyst's "real person" has an effect. These issues are as old as psychoanalysis itself. Now, in the midst of the *fourth* phase, it appears to be becoming possible to resolve them technically. We regard the present development as a major step toward integration of the here-and-now and the then-and-there.

We begin by referring to those solutions mentioned by Strachey and emphasized by Klauber, who exhorts us not to overestimate the content and specificity of interpretations, because they have to be seen in the context of a relationship. The analyst's attitude signalizes, "I will stay friendly anyway and will not act like the old object; I behave differently than the obsolete anxiety conditions would lead you to expect." The analyst does not adhere to the principle of an eye for an eye and a tooth for a tooth, thus making it possible to interrupt the *circulus vitiosus* that Strachey so forcefully described. After all, in the theory of ego development the concept of the superego stands for ways of experiencing and acting that belong to the category of commandments, prohibitions, and ideals. The reevaluation of these norms is the goal of mutative interpretations according to Strachey. Klauber's argument that this process means the internalization of parts of the psychoanalyst's value system is convincing. A cautious formulation of this view can even be found in some of Strachey's comments.

The real person of the psychoanalyst manifests itself as a "new object" in the second phase of Strachey's mutative interpretation. In this phase the patient's sense of reality plays a decisive role, and the analyst becomes an archaic transference object during the development of anxiety. The result of the second phase of interpretation depends on the patient's

> ability, at the critical moment of the emergence into consciousness of the released quantity of id-energy, to distinguish between his phantasy object and the real analyst. The problem here is closely related to one that I have already discussed, namely that of the extreme lability of the analyst's position as auxiliary super-ego. The analytic situation is all the time threatening to degenerate into a 'real' situation. But this actually means the opposite of what it appears to. It means that the patient is all the time on the brink of turning the real external object (the analyst) into the archaic one; that is to say, he is on the brink of projecting his primitive introjected imagos on to him. In so far as the patient actually does this, the analyst becomes like anyone else that he meets in real life — a phantasy object. The analyst then ceases to possess the peculiar advantages derived from the analytic situation; he will be introjected like all other phantasy objects into the patient's super-ego, and will no longer be able to function in the peculiar ways which are essential to the effecting of a mutative interpretation. In this difficulty the patient's sense of reality is an essential but a very feeble ally; indeed, an improvement in it is one of the things that we hope the analysis will bring about. It is important, therefore, not to submit it to any unnecessary strain; and that is the fundamental reason why the analyst must avoid any real behaviour that is likely to confirm the patient's view of him as a 'bad' or a 'good' phantasy object. (Strachey 1934, p. 146)

This hesitation to react, whether in the sense of a good or a bad object, should make it possible for the patient "to make a comparison between the fantasy external object and the real one" (Strachey 1934, p. 147). The patient's sense of reality is strengthened as a result of this comparison between the different imagos projected onto the analyst and a more realistic perception. Thus, according to Strachey, there is adjustment to external reality and recognition that the current objects are not good or bad in the archaic sense. Strachey apparently means that differentiated insight relativizes the infantile perceptions, and concludes his argument with the following comment:

> It is a paradoxical fact that the best way of ensuring that his ego shall be able to distinguish between phantasy and reality is to withhold reality from him as much as possible. But it is true. His ego is so weak — so much at the mercy of his id and super-ego — *that he can only cope with reality if it is administered in minimal doses.* And these doses are in fact what the analyst gives him, in the form of interpretations. (Strachey 1934, p. 147, emphasis added)

The technical problems of Strachey's theses may well be rooted in the contradictions attached to the definition of reality in the analytic situation. Indeed, it is not only in Strachey studies and the discussion of them that this problem is unsolved. The general difficulties result from the fact that

> Freud assigns an important part to the notion of *reality-testing*, though without ever developing a consistent theoretical explanation of this process and without giving any clear account of its relationship to the reality principle. The way he uses this notion reveals even more clearly that it covers two very different lines of thought: on the one hand, a genetic theory of the learning of reality — of the way in which the instinct is put to the test of reality by means of a sort of 'trial-and-error' procedure — and, on the other hand, a quasi-transcendental theory dealing with the constitution of the object in terms of a whole range of antitheses: internal-external, pleasurable-unpleasurable, introjection-projection. (Laplanche and Pontalis 1973, p. 381)

Strachey had apparently thought in terms of antithetical regulatory principles, i.e., in the framework of the pleasure and reality principles. Since, according to theory, the pleasure principle is merely modified by the reality principle, the search for gratification on a real (material) object remains the determining factor. On the other hand, *psychic* reality is molded by unconscious wishes and fantasies. Freud believed it necessary to assume a contradiction between these realities, because the incest taboo and other inevitable frustrations limit material gratification while at the same time constituting the actually desired reality:

> It was only the non-occurrence of the expected satisfaction, the disappointment experienced, that led to the abandonment of this attempt at satisfaction by means of hallucination. Instead of it, the psychical apparatus had to decide to form a conception of the *real circumstances* in the external world and to endeavour to make a *real alteration* in them. *A new principle of mental functioning was thus introduced*; what was presented in the mind was no longer what was agreeable but what was real, even if it happened to be disagreeable. (Freud 1911 b, p. 219, emphasis added)

Assuming that the object relationships are regulated by the pleasure and reality principles, then the experienced reality is determined by the dominance of the one or other principle. It is characteristic of psychoanalytic theory to view the pleasure principle as the primary and archaic fact, which is inexhaustible and derives from the unconscious, the id. It certainly makes a big difference whether I only imagine something or whether I can actually grasp an object or in some way immediately perceive it (Hurvich 1970; Kafka 1977). Yet this is not a contradiction between different realities, which would have to be taken into consideration and would inevitably lead to the irresolvable problem of "why the child should ever have to seek a real object if it can attain satisfaction on demand, as it were, by means of hallucination" (Laplanche and Pontalis 1973, p. 381). Since transference interpretations also involve the analyst as an individual, we have to add a few more comments on psychic reality. Referring to the *real* person of the analyst precipitates concerns, as if psychic levels were supposed to be sacrificed and replaced by materialization, i.e., wish fulfillment.

Reflection on the theory of psychic reality is necessary. Like McLaughlin (1981), we believe that we can come closer to a solution to these problems by viewing the analytic meeting from the perspective of *psychic reality*, i.e., as a *scheme* which is both comprehensive and contains different meanings. Patient and analyst naturally experience the situation very concretely, with their subjective wishes, affects, expectations, hopes, and ways of thinking. As soon as we reflect on our different psychic states, a plan develops for ordering our experiences and events with regard to space and time. To a great extent a person follows his subjective schemata for thinking and acting, which thus govern his behavior, without reflecting on them. He experiences the fact that psychic reality is constituted situationally in interpersonal relations. Psychic reality in McLaughlin's sense refers both to concrete subjective experiences and to their unconscious roots. The analyst constructs a patient's psychic reality within the framework of the psychoanalytic theory he uses. Such constructions are aids to orientation. McLaughlin also includes the analyst's countertransference in his comprehensive understanding. The many levels of meaning of the concrete psychic realities, including the underlying theories held by both the patient and analyst, are interrelated and understood interactionally. The security which the analyst could have drawn from the mirror analogy is thus lost. McLaughlin shows that reflection on psychic reality is very productive, even though the analyst may initially have to put up with insecurity since, according to McLaughlin, he can no longer proceed from an understanding of himself as a real person who enters into a realistic relationship with the patient. Everything is relativized by the patient's perspective. Reality develops in this two-person relationship by means of an interactive process in which the participants' subjective perspectives are continually tested and a certain consensus is reached. Patient and analyst learn to make themselves understood. The result of a successful analysis is a gradual and mutual confirmation of the psychic realities and their authentication, a term McLaughlin uses to describe a process of change. In this way both participants acquire *relative* security with regard to their perspectives.

The analyst is affected by the critical discussion that takes place in the psychoanalytic dialogue. He is the expert, not only employing common sense but also expressing opinions that he has acquired during his training. His professionalism has molded his thinking. His view of a patient's psychic reality (as well as his experience of his own) is not independent of the theories that he uses. In testing authentication we have to go further than McLaughlin and raise the question of whether the indirect source of some of the problems we face should not be sought in Freud's theories on psychic reality.

We are dealing with a region of high tension between poles marked by the antithetical concepts of psychic reality vs material reality, reality principle vs pleasure principle, pleasure-ego vs reality-ego. Ultimately we arrive at reality testing as the act that distinguishes between internal and external, or between what is merely imagined and what is actually perceived. Freud opposed psychic reality to material reality after he was forced to give up his theories of seduction and of the pathogenic role of real infantile traumata. Fantasies not derived from real events possess the same pathogenic value for the subject which Freud originally attributed to unconscious memories of actual events. The contrast between the two realities is thus linked to contents characterizing the realities. Psychic reality is the world of the subjective, conscious, and unconscious wishes and fantasies, and material reality is characterized by the actual gratification or nongratification of instinctual needs on objects.

According to Laplanche and Pontalis (1973, p. 363) psychic reality designates the "unconscious desire and its associated fantasies." Is it necessary to attribute reality to unconscious desires? Freud asks this question in the context of dream analysis, answering:

> If we look at unconscious wishes reduced to their most fundamental and truest shape, we shall have to conclude, no doubt, that *psychical* reality is a particular form of existence not to be confused with *material* reality. (1900 a, p. 620)

Thus there is both psychic reality and material reality. The decisive sentence with regard to the psychoanalytic view of the genesis and nature of neuroses reads: "The phantasies possess *psychical* as contrasted with *material* reality, and we gradually learn to understand that *in the world of the neuroses it is psychical reality which is the decisive kind*" (Freud 1916/17, p. 368).

In Freud's theory, psychic reality is regulated by the pleasure principle, which itself is molded in human development by life's necessities by means of the reality principle. Reality testing is subordinate to the reality principle. The growing child learns to postpone immediate gratification in order to find a more realistic gratification of its needs, i.e., one based on mutuality and congruence with the needs of fellow man. The tension between psychic and material realities is thus based on the assumption that there is a surplus of desires continually seeking gratification but not finding it because of life's necessities in general and the incest taboo in particular. To create more favorable conditions a certain amount of gratification in the therapeutic situation is necessary; otherwise the old frustrations would simply be repeated. The problem of frustration and gratification in the analytic situation becomes easier to solve if the theory of psychic reality is deepened and not linked with *frustration* in a one-sided fashion. In fact, it is necessary and essential therapeutically that the patient be enabled to reach many joyful congruences with the object, i.e., the analyst, and to discuss differences of opinion. This facilitates the path to the frustrated unconscious childhood desires seeking gratification in the present.

The purpose of these comments is to indicate the consequences of a comprehensive conception of psychic reality. The patient seeks and hopes for an improvement or cure of his symptoms and difficulties, that is, he hopes to achieve a positive change with the help of an expert. His attempt to relate all of his feelings and thoughts reveals a multifaceted image of the world in which he lives. He describes different views of his world depending on his mood and on the predominance of different desires, expectations, hopes, and anxieties. Although the patient also distinguishes between his perceptions of people and things and his ideas about them, he does not divide reality into a psychic sphere and a material one. This is true despite his awareness that his desires and ideas may conflict and that he is dependent on external objects in his search for pleasure and gratification. Very diverse processes take place in the analyst when he listens and lets his emotions and thoughts reach a conclusion. If the analyst intervenes at any point with a comment, the patient is confronted with information. Yet, as Watzlawick et al. (1967) say, it is impossible not to communicate, since negative information, e.g., the analyst's silence, also constitutes a communication, particularly when the patient expects some kind of response. The psychoanalyst's comments introduce points of view that the patient must confront in some manner — he can ignore them, accept them, reject them, etc. Sooner or later there will be joint reflection on various issues. Present during this reflection, either consciously or unconsciously, are many third parties: family members, other relatives, and people the patient knows, works with, and lives with. The analyst's own experiences, desires, longings, old anxieties, and current struggles are constantly touched on. Since he himself is not the one who is suffering, he can for the good of the patient find a distance from which he can presume the existence of a wish when the patient momentarily reacts with anxiety. The emotional and intellectual burdens of this activity on the analyst would of course be too great to bear if he did not have a wealth of explanatory sketches at his disposal which reflect typical conflict patterns. They facilitate his orientation during therapy.

Relating these points to Strachey's understanding of reality, we find the following. In his statement that "the analytic situation is all the time threatening to degenerate into a 'real' situation," Strachey refers to the pleasure principle in a wide sense of the term (Strachey 1934, p. 146). He starts from introjected imagos that are then projected onto the analyst without taking situational precipitating factors into consideration. Noteworthy is that Strachey assumes fixed quantities both here and when speaking of the real, external object, i.e., the psychoanalyst. It is clear from the passage quoted above that Strachey believed it possible to use *withdrawal of reality* to reinforce the patient's capacity for differentiation when *testing reality* at the time of the mutative transference interpretation.

By following the mirror analogy, the analyst may get involved in a role conflict which keeps him from confirming the patient's rather realistic perceptions in transference interpretations and thus prevents him from working against new denials and repressions. Heimann (1956) did not notice, despite her early innovative contribution on countertransference (1950), that it is impossible to be, on the one hand, a mirror having no self and no independent existence, but only reflecting the patient, and on the other, a person who is part of the analytic situation and of the patient's problems both at a realistic level and at a fantasy one. It suffices if the analyst demonstrates some restraint, enabling the patient to reenact in transference the relationship patterns which have remained active unconsciously.

In the context of the extension of the theory of transference (in the sense of a comprehensive concept of transference) our considerations have to lead to the view that the analyst's so-called reality is constituted during the patient's constant unconscious and conscious testing. In the instant he makes a mutative interpretation, the analyst also reveals something of himself, as Strachey emphasizes. This certainly does not refer to just any personal confession. What is directly or indirectly expressed in helpful interpretations is enriched by the analyst's professionalism and by the fact that his experience is independent of an overly narrow subjectivity. The analyst's professional knowledge facilitates a cognitive process which opens up new avenues for the patient to find solutions. These are by no means personal confessions, but communications — whether nonverbal or in the form of interpretations — about how the analyst views a patient's problem, how he himself feels and thinks in this regard, and what and how he is in regard to the patient. In this sense we agree with Rosenfeld (1972, p. 458) that the psychoanalyst's interpretations may reflect very clearly what he is.

Especially important in this regard is the *spontaneity* of the analyst, as Klauber emphasizes:

> Various technical consequences follow from this emphasis on spontaneity. Spontaneous exchanges humanize the analytical relationship by the continual interchange of partial identifications. It is this human quality of the relationship which is the antidote to the traumatic quality of transference as much or more than the acceptance of impulses by an analyst who reinforces the benign qualities of the superego. (1981, p. 116)

The precondition for this cognitive process which includes the other ego, the analyst, is of course that the analyst does not withdraw by proffering purely reductive transference interpretations. Gill's (1982) systematic analysis of the factors precipitating transference and, especially, resistance to transference (see Chaps. 2 and 8) following very plausible preconscious perceptions makes it possible to provide an answer to the question of what the analyst is as a real person in the therapeutic situation. The here-and-now must be considered in its interrelationship with the then-and-there, and in the process new and innovative perspectives are opened. Freud (1933 a, p. 74) contrasted the immutability of the repressed, the so-called timelessness of the unconscious, to analytic work, which overcomes the power of the past. The here-and-now is linked with the then-and-there in the process in which something becomes conscious, and precisely this is the mutative effect of transference interpretations.

The analyst must be patient, because it takes some time before unconscious processes manifest themselves in transference in such a way that therapeutically effective interpretations are possible. This is what is meant by Freud's statement that from "the physician's point of view I can only declare that in a case of this kind he must behave as 'timelessly' as the unconscious itself, if he wishes to learn anything or to achieve anything" (1918b, p. 10). Note that "timelessly" is in quotation marks; from the context it is clear that transferences also develop in severe cases if the analyst waits patiently. *Once* the timelessness of the unconscious has been overcome, it even becomes possible to significantly reduce the length of treatment for such severe illnesses, according to Freud, because it enables the analyst with increasing experience to make helpful transference interpretations, i.e., those linking the past with the present. The repetitions create the impression that time is standing still. The dreaming ego also has time feeling and is aware of objections (Freud 1900a, p. 326; Hartocollis 1980). It is therefore misleading to speak of the timelessness of the unconscious when referring to the time feeling at different levels of consciousness.

Our line of argument is important for understanding the mutative effect of transference interpretations because they link past and present. In Freud's view, past, unconsciously preserved wishes lose their effect when they reach consciousness. This leads to the conclusion that transference interpretations which assume that the patient's perceptions and experiences in the here-and-now are ahistorical repetitions miss the point just as much as interpretations of the here-and-now which ignore the unconscious dimension of the individual's life.

The emphasis on the ahistorical quality of unconscious processes and their interpretation in the here-and-now often goes together with a very strict application of the mirroring function. Ezriel's (1963) studies start from the assumption that the ahistorical reenactment in transference is more complete the more passive and abstinent the well-analyzed analyst is. Such an analyst directs his interpretations at the object relationships which are unconsciously sought or avoided. Ezriel recommends a type of transference interpretation oriented on the object relationship which is sought but anxiously avoided. For this reason his interpretations always contain an explanatory "because," as in the sentence, "You are now avoiding this wish to relate that fantasy *because* you fear rejection."

Close examination of Ezriel's work leads to the realization that his description of the psychoanalytic method as ahistorical is not justified. It is true that the therapeutic effectiveness of the psychoanalytic method is related to the here-and-now and to the knowledge that can be acquired in the analytic situation. Yet Ezriel's conception is based on the assumption that the unconscious is ahistorical. Thus the patient's present realistic perceptions also do not play an independent role even though only here-and-now interpretations are given; such interpretations refer exclusively to seemingly ahistorical, momentarily effective, unconscious forces and constellations. Mutative qualities could not be in the here-and-now if the unconscious constellations were timeless, excluded from the individual's past, and ahistorical. We have highlighted Ezriel's work here because he assigned the here-and-now a special methodological significance; however, his studies failed because, among other factors, he neglected to give the analyst's situational influence the same importance in practice as he did in theory.

The inclusion of personal influence and realistic perceptions in transference interpretations is the central issue distinguishing Freud's reconstructive genetic transference interpretations from the innovations which followed upon Strachey's publications. If the corrective object relationship in the analytic situation is referred to, as Segal (1973, p. 123) does, then the analyst is bound to include the influencing subject (the analyst) and the patient's realistic perceptions of the analyst in the formulation of transference interpretations. The importance of psychic reality and unconscious fantasies is by no means diminished by the discovery that realistic observations, for example the analyst's countertransference, play a role in their genesis.

The patient participates in the psychoanalyst's value system whenever it is of consequence for new solutions to neurotic conflicts. This identificatory participation, which Strachey described in his reevaluation of the superego, commandments, and proscriptions, is not only inevitable, it is therapeutically necessary. Trying to avoid it leads to a strained atmosphere which may be characterized by anxious avoidance of therapeutically necessary participation.

The findings of research in the social sciences make it essential that great importance be attached to the psychoanalyst's influence on the situational origin of perceptions and fantasies. The theories about the handling of real relationships also affect the structuring of the therapeutic situation. Since in Freud's theory the reality principle is secondary to the pleasure principle and real gratification is always sought — even though gratification may be delayed for varying periods of time — tension develops in the therapy as a result of frustration and renunciation. Creating an atmosphere of this kind can provide relief to a group of inhibited patients because alone empathy and tolerance toward the aggressions produced by frustration can lead to some alleviation of the superego. The transformation of an excessively strict superego into a mild one does not create the kind of therapeutic problems that have to be solved in the repair of defective ego functions or the construction of previously underdeveloped ones. The patient's identification with the psychoanalyst plays a decisive role in this. It seems as if this category of patients is increasing in number, and it is therefore important to determine the conditions under which identifications are formed.

The relationship of transference interpretations to the other aspects of the therapeutic relationship received too little attention in the one-sided reception of Strachey's position. Klauber's (1972a) work is the most outstanding of the few exceptions. Strachey had ascribed these other components, such as suggestion, lessening anxiety, and abreacting, an important role in treatment. The problem, however, of how the analyst presents his real self to the patient in small doses has not been solved.

As in the discussion between Greenson, Heimann, and Wexler (1970), controversies continue as to how the analyst should handle realistic perceptions in the here-and-now. Some analysts fear that this could ultimately lead to the gratification of needs and mean that treatment would no longer be conducted in a state of *frustration* and *abstinence*. These problems of technique can be solved constructively and to the advantage of therapeutic change if we understand their origin in the psychoanalytic theory of reality. In discussing this point we will start from the following observation by Adorno:

> On the one hand, "libido" is for it [psychoanalysis] the actual psychic reality: gratification is positive, frustration negative because it leads to illness. On the other hand, psychoanalysis accepts the civilization which demands the frustration, if not completely uncritically, then at least in resignation. In the name of the reality principle it justifies the individual psychic sacrifice without subjecting the reality principle itself to rational scrutiny. (Adorno 1952, p.17)

Although the reality principle that the analyst represents is relatively mild, it should cause enough frustration "to bring this conflict to a head, to develop it to its highest pitch, in order to increase the instinctual force available for its solution" (Freud 1937c, p.231). This statement from one of Freud's later texts shows that technical problems result from the psychoanalytic theory of reality.

Subjecting the reality principle to rational scrutiny can only mean, with regard to technique, that the patient's perceptions must be taken seriously. In the moment that this takes place, an intentional act finds its object, thus creating reality. We will return to this topic later when discussing the relationship between historical truth and perception in the here-and-now. Since the individual's conception of reality is determined in a sociocultural context, neither the one nor the other can be taken as absolute. The reality of the psychoanalytic situation is thus constituted in the exchange, assimilation, and rejection of opinions.

Neither the analyst nor the patient starts from a completely valid standpoint when testing reality. In the one case we would end up adjusting to the existing conditions, in the other in solipsism. At the one extreme the individual declares that his family or society is insane and the cause of his illness, at the other the individual is dependent on and made ill by external factors. Carrying this polarization to its limits, society as a whole could be declared insane and the emotionally disturbed could be considered to be the healthy individual revolting against sick society. Successful therapy would then adjust this person to the sick society without noticing it. Adorno goes this far when he writes, "By becoming similar to the insane totality, the individual becomes truly sick (1972, p.57).

A mutative interpretation seems to have a special effect if it is devised to strengthen the working relationship, i.e., the patient's *identification* with the psychoanalyst in his role as *auxiliary ego*. As a result of the great influence exerted by Strachey's work a new form of "interpretation fanaticism" developed. This had been previously criticized by Ferenczi and Rank (1924), on the grounds that it referred to genetic reconstructions which neglect experience in the here-and-now and are thus therapeutically ineffective. Strachey (1934, p.158) also examined this unsuccessful interpretation fanaticism and pointed to the emotional immediacy inherent in his mutative interpretation (as transference interpretation) at the decisive moment of urgency. At the same time he emphasized that the majority of interpretations do not refer to transference.

Nevertheless, a new form of interpretation fanaticism developed, this time with reference to "transference" in the sense of pure repetition. This limited the therapeutic effectiveness of psychoanalysis for a different reason than excessive intellectual reconstruction did. The consequence of understanding everything that occurs in the analytic situation or is mentioned by the patient primarily as a manifestation of transference is, as Balint (1968, p. 169) emphasized, that "the principal frame of reference used for formulating practically every interpretation is a relationship between a highly important, omnipresent object, the analyst, and an unequal subject who at present apparently cannot feel, think, or experience anything unrelated to his analyst."

The inequality which develops can lead to malignant regressions if the external circumstances of a patient's life are neglected in favor of ahistorical transference interpretations. Such interpretations refer to those interpretations which exclude the present in all its forms — the analytic situation, the analyst's influence, and external circumstances. If the present is viewed solely as repetition of the past or of unconscious schemata derived from the past, which Freud described as templates or clichés, transference interpretations do not refer to a genuine situation which has a basis in the present reality. Strictly speaking, the here-and-now is then nothing more than a new imprint of an old pattern or template.

In contrast to the ahistorical conception of transference and the interpretations associated with this view, authentic interpretations of the here-and-now provide new experiences because they take the present seriously. The psychoanalyst fulfills here a genuine task that cannot be reduced to that of father or mother. Heimann (1978) used the expression "supplementary ego" to describe this function, traced it back to the mother, and also called it the "maternal function." Because of the danger of a reductionist misunderstanding, we do not want to call the therapeutic supplementary or auxiliary ego maternal, but only to adopt the designation of the *function*, which is the essential aspect.

> The mother [in the person of the analyst], as supplementary ego, offers the child [the patient] concepts that it does not have itself. The mother teaches the child new concepts of thinking and thus sets it on the path of progress. (Heimann 1978, p. 228)

Freud's technical demand that "the patient should be educated to liberate and fulfill his own nature, not to resemble ourselves" seems to contradict the great therapeutic significance of the patient's identification with the analyst (Freud 1919a, p. 165). Another passage (Freud 1940a, p. 181) reads, "We serve the patient in various functions, as an authority and a substitute for his parents, as a teacher and educator." On the other hand, Freud warns:

> However much the analyst may be tempted to become a teacher, model and ideal for other people and to create men in his own image, he should not forget that that is not his task in the analytic relationship, and indeed that he will be disloyal to his task if he allows himself to be led on by his inclinations. (Freud 1940a, p. 175).

At a symposium on the termination of treatment, Hoffer (1950) described the patient's capacity to identify with the psychoanalyst's functions as the most important component of the therapeutic process and its success. This topic thus has fundamental significance for understanding the therapeutic process, if for no other reason than it closely associates the psychoanalyst's *functions* with the patient's *identifications.*

Consideration must be given to a whole series of theoretical and practical problems which we would now like to outline by formulating a few questions. What does the patient identify with? What are the consequences of the psychoanalytic theory of identification for the optimization of practice, with the goal of making it easier for the patient to assimilate the functions mediated by the analyst? What does the psychoanalyst mediate, and how does he do it? With regard to the patient's experience, is it possible to distinguish the functions from the person who has them? How does the psychoanalyst indicate that he is fundamentally different from the expectations which characterize transference neuroses and the consequences they have on the processes of perception? Does it suffice for the patient to recognize that the way the psychoanalyst thinks and acts does not conform to the established patterns of expectations? Does it suffice for the analyst to define himself negatively, i.e., by not conforming to the patient's unconscious expectations? In our opinion, such a lack of conformity does not suffice to interrupt neurotic repetition compulsion and the therapeutic function is rooted in the fact that the psychoanalyst works in an innovative manner, introducing new points of view and enabling the patient to find previously unattainable solutions to problems.

The innovative elements occupy such a natural role in therapy that they have, almost unnoticed, become part of the point of view that a *synthesis* takes place apparently on its own. Yet the psychoanalyst's interventions in fact contain at least latent goals which help to determine how the released elements are reassembled. The fundamental therapeutic function of the psychoanalyst is that he is effective as a "substitute." Regardless of whether he is viewed as an auxiliary superego or an auxiliary ego, and however the current school-determined language of theory and practice deviates from Strachey's, it is a generally accepted psychoanalytic experience that support initiates the exchange processes which lead to new identifications. The result is a lack of independence on the part of the patient, leading among other things to the necessity that he speak his therapist's language, as Balint (1968, p. 93) described the situation, showing great understanding for this connection between language, thinking, and acting.

Learning from a model — or in psychoanalytic terminology, identification — has a significance in every therapeutic process which can hardly be exaggerated. Since the very different psychoanalytic object relationship theories of the various schools became a focus of attention, all concepts referring to the relationship of internal to external and of subject to subject (or object) are of special technical interest (Kernberg 1979; Meissner 1979; Ticho, according to Richards 1980). In his introduction to a conference on object relationship theory, Kanzer (1979, p. 315) calls special attention to the fact that the emphasis given to object relationships has made it possible to develop a dyadic understanding of the traditional treatment of adults. He also refers to numerous authors who have furthered this development (Balint 1950; Spitz 1956; Loewald 1960; Stone 1961; Gitelson 1962).

Common to internalization, identification, introjection, and incorporation is that they all refer to a movement from without to within, involving assimilation, appropriation, and adaptation (Schafer 1968; Meissner 1979; McDevitt

1979). Regardless of the meaning attached to these words — e.g., incorporation taken literally and too concretely, identification as symbolic equating — their common feature is that they refer to an object relationship. Balint (1968, pp. 61-62) therefore pointed out that it is not possible to talk about identifications in a narrow sense of the word unless there is a certain distance between within and without or between subject and object. Freud's fundamental anthropological observation deserves to be mentioned in this connection; he noted that relinquished object relationships are expressed in identifications (1923b, p. 29). It hardly needs to be emphasized how significant this aspect of identification is in separation, bereavement, and the termination of analyses.

We believe that it is now possible to solve the old problem concerning reality in the psychoanalytic situation, and that fifty years after Strachey's important article psychoanalytic technique can and will considerably expand its therapeutic potential. Transference interpretations play a special role in this development. In our argument we have so far distinguished the following aspects:

1. Here-and-now interpretations can be taken to include every kind of reference to the analytic situation, but not to the patient's current circumstances outside of analysis or to those prior to analysis. The extension of the concept of transference, which we discuss in Chap. 2, creates two classes of intervention: one relates to everything that is outside the analytic situation, the other includes all interpretations concerning the here-and-now in the comprehensive understanding of transference. In the traditional form of transference interpretation, the analyst assumes there is a *repetition* and thus focusses his attention on the *genesis*. These statements are based on the assumption that there is a conditional relationship between current experiencing and behavior and earlier experiences. In other words, such transference interpretations read something like, "You are anxious because you are afraid that I will punish you just like your father did."
2. It is possible for transference interpretations to be directed more toward the genesis and toward the *reconstruction* of memories. In contrast, it is also possible for the here-and-now to move to the center of the interpretation if *unconscious processes* are assumed to be *ahistorical*. Of course, the subject matter of this kind of transference interpretation is the analyst as an *old* object. Furthermore, the momentary dynamic is nearly identical to the conserved (ahistorical) genesis. In the here-and-now interpretations, the differences between the material which has been transformed from the past into the present and the analyst's contribution to transference are levelled out. There is no investigation of the affective and cognitive processes creating the momentary psychic reality. The purpose of the analyst's mirrorlike attitude is to manifest the ahistorical unconscious fantasies and the unconscious defense processes directed against them in the purest form.
3. We come finally to the type of transference interpretations in the here-and-now which realize both the potential for dyadic knowledge provided by the psychoanalytic method *and* its therapeutic effectiveness. We are thinking of all those transference interpretations which consider in a comprehensive manner the impact of the patient's more or less realistic perceptions on the unconscious processes. In this context we can refer to Klauber's conception

that one task of psychoanalysis in the current phase is to distinguish the transference from the nontransference elements in the psychoanalytic situation. In the meantime, however, transference theory has expanded so much that speaking of nontransference elements creates misunderstandings. Of course, it is essential to distinguish between the imaginative decorations and the wishful image of the world facilitated in the analytic situation, on the one hand, and the realistic elements of the analyst's behavior, on the other. This process of differentiating the kinds of dyadic knowledge constitutes the mutative effect of transference interpretations.

We can now mention Arlow's (1979) view that transference develops by means of metaphoric thinking. On the basis of unconscious schemata (Freud's templates), psychic reality is formed from the points of view of contrast and similarity. The patient compares the psychoanalytic situation and the psychoanalyst with current and previous experiences. If transference is viewed as a manifestation of metaphoric thinking and experience, as Arlow does, it is necessary to assume that the *similarity* makes it possible to establish a connection, to carry something from one shore to the other, i.e., from a previous to the current situation. Precisely from the therapeutic points of view, therefore, Carveth's (1984b, p. 506) criticism must be taken seriously. He points out that the analyst's *confirmation* of the similarity is *the* precondition for changing the transference templates, which according to psychoanalytic theory have been formed by the necessity to deny realistic perceptions and to repress affective and cognitive processes. Freud's unconscious templates are very similar to the linguistic category of "dead metaphors" (Weinrich 1968; Carveth 1984b). These can come to life, i.e., manifest themselves out of the dynamic unconscious, if similarities (in the sense meant by Gill) are admitted and acknowledged in transference interpretations. Otherwise there is a repetition of acts of denial, and the old templates maintain their influence. The moment that similarities are identified also marks the discovery of the here-and-now and the then-and-there. This differentiation of kinds of dyadic knowledge makes it possible for the mutative interpretation to exert a corrective emotional experience.

Finally, we would like to point out that our view draws its therapeutic application from Freud's fundamental assertion that "a fragment of *historical truth*" is contained in all emotional disturbances (1937d, p. 269). Freud emphasizes that if this historical truth were acknowledged, then:

> The vain effort would be abandoned of convincing the patient of the error of his delusion and of its contradiction of reality; and, on the contrary, the recognition of its kernel of truth would afford common ground upon which the therapeutic work could develop. That work would consist in liberating the fragment of historical truth from its distortions and its attachments to the actual present day and in leading it back to the point in the past to which it belongs. The transposing of material from a forgotten past on to the present or on to an expectation of the future is indeed a habitual occurrence in neurotics no less than in psychotics. (1937d, pp. 267-268)

It should be clear how we would like to make this conception therapeutically useful. The common ground can be found in the *recognition of the kernel of truth* in transference interpretations. In doing this, it is as a rule sufficient to acknowledge the general human disposition, as we suggest in Chap. 3. Constructions of historical truths are, in contrast, dubious; they lack the power of conviction emanating from current experience. We believe that the patient, in comparing the here-and-now and the then-and-there, ultimately establishes a distance to each, freeing himself for the future. We would therefore like to paraphrase a statement of Freud's (1937c, pp. 231-232) to the effect that the analytic work proceeds best when the patient establishes distance between himself and both past experiences and current truths, which then become history.

## 8.5 Silence

Speech and silence are the two sides of every conversation; the participants must either speak or remain silent. Specifically, either one participant speaks, or both are silent, or both speak at the same time. The moment one person speaks, the other can only remain silent or interrupt him, and if both are silent, a space is created which is claimed by each and which only one of them can seize in order to speak for an indefinite period of time. The analyst's silence provides the patient with an opportunity to speak. (Incidentally, the doctor's office is called in German a *Sprechzimmer*, or room for talking.)

There are good reasons to encourage the patient to initiate the dialogue. A one-sided distribution of speech and silence, however, contradicts the rules of everyday communication. Deviations from the expected course of dialogue thus lead to surprises, irritations, and finally helplessness. For example, if the analyst behaves very passively in the initial sessions, he exerts an unusually strong influence on the patient, whose expectations have been formed by previous visits to physicians. The patient expects questions about his complaints and their history, usually phrased directly so that he can provide concise answers. The more the discussion deviates from his expectations and from the patterns of speech and silence characteristic of everyday communication, the greater the surprises.

These few comments should suffice to demonstrate clearly that the effects of employing silence as a tool vary greatly. It is impossible to make a general recommendation in this regard, since whether the silence is experienced as rejection or benevolent encouragement depends on many situational circumstances. It is thus all the more surprising that the view that psychoanalysts sit silently behind the couch is not limited to caricatures. On the contrary, analysts often make a virtue out of silence, as if the profession followed the motto "speech is silver, silence is golden."

There are in fact good reasons, from analytic points of view, to be reserved in the dialogue and not to ask importunate questions which hinder the patient from getting to the topics that are important to him. The patient can be invited in this way to take the first steps toward free association. By showing restraint, the analyst can motivate the patient into attempting to say everything that he feels a need to say and is currently able to express. In the long term, the analyst's silence also promotes the patient's regression, which is not self-serving but a part of the therapeutic process. For this reason alone, the dosage of silence and speech is of preeminent significance.

In view of the practical necessity to be just as prudent in using silence as the spoken word, the fact that a stereotype is made of silence is a real cause of concern. It is not unusual for this stereotype to lead the analyst to behave in an extremely restrained fashion even in the initial interviews, i.e., to use them as a kind of miniature trial analysis in order to determine whether the patient is suited for the planned therapy.

Pauses are an essential part of therapy for both diagnostic and therapeutic reasons, and provide the patient with opportunities to introduce a new important topic. This can also be used as a means of gaining a first impression of the extent to which the patient tolerates the analyst's silence.

Since we oppose using this method to determine the suitability of a patient for analysis, and urge instead that it be adapted to the patient, it is important to examine the question of how it was possible for the analyst's silence to become a stereotype. Factors which contributed to this situation include, in our opinion, the high regard for free association and regression as self-curative processes, and the overemphasis on self-cognition as a means of therapy. Freud, for example, recommended that the analyst avoid making an interpretation until the patient himself has almost arrived at the same insight into a previously inaccessible constellation:

> We reflect carefully over when we shall impart the knowledge of one of our constructions to him and we wait for what seems to us the suitable moment — which is not always easy to decide. As a rule we put off telling him of a construction or explanation till he himself has so nearly arrived at it that only a single step remains to be taken, though that step is in fact the decisive synthesis. (Freud 1940a, p. 178)

This recommendation unites two points of view into one ideal: first, the principle that the patient be disturbed as little as possible, and second, the experience that the patient's own insight has a greater therapeutic effect than information provided by the analyst. Freud clearly indicates that there is an ideal moment or a particularly favorable junction between internal and external factors, and that it is important for the analyst to find this favorable moment for breaking his silence. The dichotomy of silence and speech is thus transformed into the polarization between silence and interpretation. This occurs, if at all possible, without the intermediate stages which naturally occur in every psychoanalytic dialogue even though they do not really fit into the ideal picture of psychoanalysis.

We now arrive at a surprising result: hand in hand with the highly stylized view that interpretation should be the analyst's only form of verbal communication, a high, even mystical, value has been attached to silence. Silence has become the inconspicuous, sheltering, and supportive origin of interpretation. We reject mystification, although it is beyond doubt that some momentary agreements between patient and analyst are based on deep, unconscious communication, as if interpretations were previously agreed upon, i.e., as if patient and analyst had exactly the same thoughts. We agree with Cremerius (1969) that silence based simply on custom, with no critical foundation, must be rejected. Silence is one of the tools, one of several technical operations, which have to be applied according to the situation to promote the analytic process.

The fundamental rule and its counterpart, evenly suspended attention, are rules of treatment constituting a special type of dialogue, which in the actual course of treatments is rarely as asymmetric as the theoretical discussion would seem to suggest. Verbatim protocols of analytic dialogues reveal that the analyst usually participates actively, even though according to the literature the quantitative ratio of verbal activity varies between 5:1 and 4:1 in favor of the patient. In this evaluation, pauses are generally considered part of the patient's time, a consequence of the fundamental rule and the fact that the issue of the analyst's interventions has not been formally regulated. We do not accept this approach and believe it more appropriate to consider longer pauses as joint discursive activity. The fundamental rule is effective for only a limited period of time if the dialogue has been exhausted. At some point the analyst is then faced with the question of whether he should end the silence. During longer periods of silence the intrapsychic processes of the partners in the dialogue do not stand still. Patients have numerous motives for remaining silent, covering the entire spectrum of the theory of neurosis; similarly there are many reasons for the analyst not to speak. A resistent silent patient may bring about a countersilence in the analyst. If both partners are silent, the processes of nonverbal communication become more prominent and are also perceived.

Cremerius (1969, p. 98) reported one patient who oriented himself on the number of matches the analyst lit during the breaks in speech: few matches were a sign of harmony, many matches indicated a disturbance of the communication.

A psychology of silence, the beginnings of which are now available, would contribute to establishing a technical basis for distinguishing the level of subject-object fusion from the level of refusal to communicate. In both cases, the capacity to follow the fundamental rule reaches its limits. Nacht (1964) views silence as a kind of integrative, mystical experience shared by patient and analyst, and believes that this exchange without words may represent a reexperience (or new experience) of the state of fusion and total amalgation from early development. He thus ties silence to the idea of reparative change, i.e., of a cure by means of pregenital love as propounded by Ferenczi, in whose tradition he must be seen.

The ego psychological standpoint also suggests that interpretation not be used as a means of achieving change. Calogeras (1967) has demonstrated this in the treatment of a chronically silent patient. However, we view the detailed justification for the introduction of the parameter "renunciation of the fundamental rule" to be an example of what we discussed with regard to the basic model technique (Chap. 1). In the same sense, Loewenstein (see Waldhorn 1959), Zeligs (1960), and Moser (1962) argue in favor of allowing the silent patient the time he needs. Freud's guideline is also applicable here: all technical steps should be directed at creating the most favorable conditions for the ego.

In addition to the general aspects of the function and consequences of the analyst's silence, we would like to deal with the special topic of *power* and *impotence* in the psychoanalytic relationship. We believe that the analyst's silence, if used in a stereotype manner and brought to an end by interpretations which may be very far from what has occupied the patient's attention in the long period since either he or the analyst last spoke, may contribute in a highly unfavorable manner to a polarization of impotence and power between patient and analyst. Here is an example (composed of notes and a statement by the analyst):

A longer analysis. The patient is often silent for long periods of time. So far no satisfactory explanation of this behavior. One day she relates that her mother was often silent for long periods and that this silence always announced trouble and made her afraid. After the patient was then silent for quite a while, the interpretation was made:
A: You are announcing trouble and want to make me afraid, just as your mother did to you when she was silent.
The patient agrees with the interpretation, but is then silent for a long time. Later she says that she was very hurt by the interpretation because she had to acknowledge that in a certain respect she is similar to her mother, whom she hates intensely. (Flader and Grodzicki 1982, pp. 164-165)

Since we want to use this example to support the thesis that precisely the constellation of obstinate silence on the part of the analyst followed by a sudden transference interpretation leads to a polarization of omnipotence and impotence, we must emphasize that Flader and Grodzicki believe this to be a good example of a transference interpretation for which it is possible to describe the discursive mechanisms of psychoanalytic interpretations. "In the above example of a transference interpretation the patient first accepted the interpretation and then relapsed into silence, probably for the purpose of assimilation" (Flader and Grodzicki 1982, p. 173).

We do not share this positive interpretation of the patient's reaction. Independent of the fact that the transference interpretation and the subsequent silence by the patient are linked to the defense mechanism of identifying with the aggressor — she acts like her own mother and treats the analyst like the child she herself used to be — the fact that the patient immediately accepts the interpretation implies that she subordinated herself rapidly to the analyst's unmediated intervention. Interpreting the subsequent long period of silence as an act of assimilation hardly meets Isaac's criteria for positive reactions to interpretations. It may well have been the silence of assimilation, but what the patient had to assimilate was probably her bewilderment at discovering that she resembles her hated mother. In this sense, the analyst's notes contain the comment that the interpretation hurt her very much, not that it moved her. This difference is important, especially in the context of a passage presented by a team consisting of a linguist and a psychoanalyst. One of the reasons that we chose this example is that it reminds us of our own unfavorable experiences with this technique.

The analyst's silence and subsequent sudden awareness of the answer to the question that the patient had not even raised — in the above example, "What am I really doing, and what do I really want?" — can lead in this way to a polarization of impotence and omnipotence which is both bipersonal and intrapsychic. The analyst becomes omnipotent and the patient impotent; the patient's unconscious fantasies of omnipotence are strengthened to the extent that he experiences humiliation in the psychoanalytic situation. Whenever somebody is made to feel impotent and helpless — whether by denying him a vital gratification or in some other way slighting his self feeling — there are attempts at compensation, which may begin simultaneously or at some later time.

Experiences of impotence may be compensated by fantasies of omnipotence. Pathological omnipotent behavior, in contrast to the fleeting omnipotence fantasies familiar to everyone, is generally a desperate attempt to defend oneself against overwhelming dominance and arbitrariness. The polarization following upon stereotypical silence and sudden interpretations is not immediately comparable with the situation of children, although in the course of normal development they too experience impotence and the unequal distribution of power between adults and children and have compensatory fantasies of grandeur. Indeed, we must go further and raise the question of whether additional severe mortifications might be created precisely by this analogy. Specifically, if the analyst views these compensatory fantasies as *distorted perception* derived from transference, he rejects the patient's criticism of his own extreme silence. In addition, the next step is that the compensatory fantasies of grandeur or omnipotence are interpreted as the consequence of a preserved infantile narcissism.

We thus have every reason to structure the psychoanalytic situation in such a way that the impotence-omnipotence polarization does not shift further in favor of reactive fantasies in the course of therapeutic regression.

How can a patient understand that his behavior, e.g., his silence, constitutes a question and that the analyst's interpretation is an adequate response? Flader and Grodzicki (1982) were able to show that the analyst can only detect the wish or motive contained in the patient's silence by breaking the rules of everyday communication. In a similar vein, Schröter (1979, pp. 181-182) described interpretations as negations of everyday forms of interaction.

> Interpretations are the analyst's comments on the patient's utterances and actions. In them, he attempts to bring out the unconscious meaning of the utterances and actions, or specifically, the unconscious fantasies, desires, and anxieties which are implied in them. Thus the patient is implicitly defined as not completely knowing what he says, at least with regard to the interpreted meaning of his utterance.

Since, as Schröter himself notes, the patient experiences this to be extremely foreign, anomalous, or even threatening, the maxim must be that deviations from everyday communication should be dosed according to the consequences on the analytic process. This recommendation is based on our experience that all patients — and not only those with narcissistic personality disorders — react with great sensitivity to violations of the normal form of everyday dialogue and that this is especially true if they are in a situation in which they require help. Schröter (1979, p. 181) notes that interpretations are very commonly experienced as criticism, slights, or humiliation, and we extend this mutatis mutandis to include silence. Therefore, a manner of conducting the dialogue must be found which is optimal with regard to treatment technique and which keeps unfavorable consequences to a minimum.

## 8.6 Acting Out

The general issue of action in psychoanalysis and the generally negative appraisal of acting out are good indications that it is easier for us to deal with the word than with the actual deed. Despite the efforts of some psychoanalysts to provide an adequate treatment of acting out from, for example, the points of view of developmental psychology and psychodynamics, the term is still used to refer to forms of behavior which are undesirable and may even endanger the analysis. Specific phenomena in the psychoanalytic situation have made this concept necessary and given it its negative image.

We have to analyze why acting out takes place and why it is considered a disturbance. In other words, which forms of behavior does the analyst evaluate negatively, i.e., in the sense of acting out? We choose this formulation to draw attention to the fact that the psychoanalyst (including the factors he takes as given, e.g., framework, policies, fundamental rule) exerts a significant influence, although apparently only the analysand can question or reject the rules that have been agreed upon and deviate from the desired structure of the dialogue and the relationship, specifically with *words* and by *remembering*.

Freud discovered the phenomenon he termed acting out in the context of Dora's transference, and described it in his *Fragment of an Analysis of a Case of Hysteria* (1905 e). Acting out did not take a meaningful place in psychoanalytic technique until after the publication of *Remembering, Repeating and Working Through* (1914 g), in which Freud derived it from the psychoanalytic situation and transference. Freud compares the psychoanalytic technique with hypnosis, mentions several complications, and then continues:

> If we confine ourselves to this second type in order to bring out the difference, we may say that the patient does not *remember* anything of what he has forgotten and repressed, but *acts* it out. He reproduces it not as a memory but as action; he *repeats* it, without, of course, knowing that he is repeating it. (1914 g, p. 150)

Kanzer (1966, p. 538) therefore refers to "the motor sphere of transference."

The expression "acting out" has two meanings, as Laplanche and Pontalis (1973, p. 4) point out: Freud "fails to distinguish the element of *actualisation* in the transference from the resort to *motor action.*" The combination of these meanings is related, on the one hand, to the discovery of the concept in the Dora case, and on the other, to the model of cognitive affective processes as related to movement. The structure of the mental apparatus generally lets the psychic process run from the perceptual end to the motor end (Freud 1900 a, p. 537).

With regard to unconscious wishful impulses Freud comments that "the fact of transference, as well as the psychoses, show us that they [unconscious wishful impulses] endeavor to force their way by way of the preconscious system into consciousness and to obtain control of the power of movement" (1900a, p. 567). The description of both affective and nonverbal utterances in the psychoanalytic situation as acting out has resulted in confusion, as many authors have pointed out (Greenacre 1950; Ekstein and Friedman 1959; Rangell 1968; Scheunert 1973). In the words of Laplanche and Pontalis (1973, p. 5):

But inasmuch as Freud, as we have seen, describes even transference on to the analyst as a modality of acting out, he fails either to differentiate clearly or to show the interconnections between repetition phenomena in the transference on the one hand and manifestations of acting out on the other.

In his later studies, Freud still emphasizes primarily the connection between remembering and acting out: "The patient ... acts it out before us, as it were, instead of reporting it to us" (1940a, p. 176). Of course, acting out also takes place outside of transference as such:

We must be prepared to find, therefore, that the patient yields to the compulsion to repeat, which now replaces the impulsion to remember, not only in his personal attitude to his doctor but also in every other activity and relationship which may occupy his life at the time – if, for instance, he falls in love or undertakes a task or starts an enterprise during the treatment. (Freud 1914g, p.151)

Acting out is not only related to remembering and repeating, but also has meanings and functions which make a purely technical classification and differentiation appear insufficient. Laplanche and Pontalis (1973, p. 6) have therefore recommended that the psychoanalytic theories of action and communication be subjected to a reconsideration that would have to include the following topics: affective and impulsive abreactions and controls; blind acting out and goal-directed action; motor discharge and highly organized acts such as play and scenic representation, structuring of relationships, creative achievement, and other ways of resolving tensions and conflicts by means of differentiated and complex courses of movement and action; acting out as the result and resolution of defense and adaptation potentials in the repertoire of an individual in relationship to his environment.

There are a large number of unconscious conditions which may increase the tendency to acting out. They include early traumas with a deficient capacity for the formation of symbols, since memory and remembering are connected with the acquisition of word symbols, which themselves lead to a state in which the memory apparatus has a useful structure (Blos 1963). Disturbances of the sense of reality, visual sensibilization, fixations at the level of the "magic of action" are different kinds of conditions which may put emphasis on action language in contrast to verbal language. At the same time, fantasies and action are possible preverbal means of problem solving and communication.

Actions can cause a stronger and more immediate feeling of self-modification that words, and there is also a greater potential for influencing external reality and the world of objects. Acting out can have the function of mastering tension and creating (or recreating) the feeling for reality. Finally, acting out also is a way of exploiting the external world for ruthless maximization of pleasure (Blos 1963).

Acting out can help to ward off passive desires and the associated anxieties, and also to undo the effects of experiences of impotence and traumatic helplessness.

Blos (1963) described acting out as a common and appropriate solution for the problems of separation in adolescence. The ego impoverishment resulting from the withdrawal of libido from the important (parental) objects is compensated by overcathexis of the external world or of the possibilities for interacting with it (which is naturally a source of important new experiences). In our opinion, this experience also throws light on the role that acting out plays during separation from loved ones as well as in the stages of development and the consequent separation from the past.

It would be possible to continue the list of meanings and functions of acting out indefinitely. The list demonstrates the ambiguity of the concept and the difficulty of defining it in terms of treatment technique. Boesky (1982, p. 52) has recommended speaking of acting out only in connection with repeating and working through. We have referred to several meanings because a differentiated understanding of acting out makes it possible to recognize it both within and outside the analytic situation, to integrate it, and to make it accessible to analytic work. It also limits the negative meaning to forms of behavior having primarily destructive consequences, serving denial and confusion, or seriously threatening the therapeutic cooperation. The fact that this is a process burdening the capacity and tolerance of the analyst should in itself not lead to a negative evaluation. Whether such behavior and reactions in the individual case are habitual or accidental is secondary.

Expressed in technical terms, interpretations — not evaluations and rules — should be the primary means of restricting acting out in the transference, so that a fruitful treatment process remains possible.

For practical and prescriptive reasons, Freud continued to assert that "nothing takes place in a psycho-analytic treatment but an interchange of words between the patient and the analyst" (1916/17, p. 17). The *word* is *the* feature of psychoanalytic treatment. For Freud, the purpose of lying on the couch was to block the expressive-motoric field of experiencing and behavior, for precisely defined theoretical reasons: by limiting movement, he wanted to interrupt the external discharge and strengthen the pressure within, in order to facilitate *remembering*. Abstinence and frustration were intended to increase the internal pressure in order to revive memories.

Since regression promotes fantasizing, the result is a certain tendency toward acting out, toward repetition through acting out, which runs counter to the demand that the patient verbalize and mentally rehearse actions. Infantile feelings, conflicts, and fantasies are repeated in transference, but the analysand's ego is supposed to function under the mature conditions of verbalization and introspection — conditions which determine the course and vitality of the analysis. Increased tension (increased pressure resulting from a reduction in the sphere of action, from abstinence, and from frustration) also opens up additional ways for manifesting regression (discharge, adjustment, defense). Since gestures are more difficult in the lying position and there is no visual contact, speech remains the primary means of communication. It is not an effective substitute, however, for repressed or inhibited tendencies toward action. Blum (1976) particularly mentions preverbal experiences, which, just like certain affects, sensations, and moods, cannot be adequately expressed in words.

The conclusion is that analysis is not possible without some acting out. It is impossible for all aspects of experience (and of neurosis) to be expressed in words. Boesky (1982) refers to acting out as the potential for actualization inherent in the transference neurosis.

The skepticism toward acting out that is nonetheless present might also be connected with its discovery and description in the Dora case, to be specific, with the patient's discontinuation of treatment. We would now like to quote the following description in order to comment on current points of view. Dora's analysis, in the year 1900, lasted only eleven weeks.

> At the beginning it was clear that I was replacing her father in her imagination, which was not unlikely, in view of the difference between our ages. She was even constantly comparing me with him consciously, and kept anxiously trying to make sure whether I was being quite straightforward with her, for her father 'always preferred secrecy and roundabout ways'. But when the first dream came, in which she gave herself the warning that she had better leave my treatment just as she had formerly left Herr K.'s house, I ought to have listened to the warning myself. 'Now,' I ought to have said to her, 'it is from Herr K. that you have made a transference on to me. Have you noticed anything that leads you to suspect me of evil intentions similar (whether openly or in some sublimated form) to Herr K.'s? Or have you been struck by anything about me or got to know anything about me which has caught your fancy, as happened previously with Herr K.?' Her attention would then have been turned to some detail in our relations, or in my person or circumstances, behind which there lay concealed something analogous but immeasurably more important concerning Herr K. And when this transference had been cleared up, the analysis would have obtained access to new memories, dealing, probably, with actual events. But I was deaf to this first note of warning, thinking I had ample time before me, since no further stages of transference developed and the material for the analysis had not yet run dry. In this way the transference took me unawares, and, because of the unknown quantity in me which reminded Dora of Herr K., she took her revenge on me as she wanted to take her revenge on him, and deserted me as she believed herself to have been deceived and deserted by him. Thus she *acted out* an essential part of her recollections and phantasies instead of reproducing it in the treatment. What this unknown quantity was I naturally cannot tell. I suspect that it had to do with money, or with jealousy of another patient who had kept up relations with my family after her recovery. When it is possible to work transferences into the analysis at an early stage, the course of the analysis is retarded and obscured, but its existence is better guaranteed against sudden and overwhelming resistances. (Freud 1905e, pp. 118-119)

If we consider Freud's description of Dora's acting out on the basis of our current state of knowledge, we have to admit that Freud was prompted to wait patiently by his overestimation of the importance of unconscious traces of memories compared to the significance of the situational factor precipitating transference, which in this case had negative consequences. He realized this himself after the termination of the analysis: did she notice something about *him* that made her mistrustful, as with Herr K., or did she notice something about *him* that created an attraction, as previously with Herr K?

Based on the retrospective analysis of this case history by Deutsch (1957), Erikson (1964), and Kanzer (1966), it is probable that Dora's acting out was motivated by situational factors. Freud subsequently emphasized this, although he had not drawn the conclusions from this fact in 1905.

Freud was searching for the sexual fantasies of this hysterical girl, who had become ill after Herr K. had twice attempted to seduce her. He attempted to ascertain the unconscious "truth" of her (ultimately incestuous) fantasies. Dora's memories seemed to support such assumptions with regard to her agitation and her many and varied sensations after she had vehemently rejected the attempted seduction.

Dora, however, was concerned with another truth: she wanted to prove that her father and the other people around her were guilty of insincerity. Her father had an affair — secret, but known to Dora — with Herr K.'s wife, and when registering his daughter in Freud's office had emphasized that she was just imagining her scene with Herr K. Lidz and Fleck (1985, p. 444) have interpreted Dora's case history in terms of family dynamics. They show in detail that Freud, contrary to his own goals, did not pay sufficient attention to the purely human, social, and family relationships. They raise a number of questions, all of which indicate that Freud underestimated the consequences of Dora's complicated family relationships on her experiencing and illness. Freud did not consider, for example, the fact that Dora's father repeatedly violated the generation boundary, first using his daughter as a substitute for his wife and then as a means to distract Herr K., the husband of his lover. Lidz and Fleck raise other questions in connection with the concept of generation boundary, and reach the conclusion that Dora's parents, together with Herr and Frau K., repeatedly violated that boundary.

Erikson provided the following summary of the problem which resulted from the fact that Dora and Freud were searching for different truths:

> But if in the patient's inability to live up to his kind of truth Freud primarily saw repressed instinctual strivings at work, he certainly also noted that Dora, too, was in search of some kind of truth. He was puzzled by the fact that the patient was "almost beside herself at the idea of its being supposed that she had merely fancied" the conditions which had made her sick; and that she kept "anxiously trying to make sure whether I was being quite straightforward with her." Let us remember here that Dora's father had asked Freud "to bring her to reason." Freud was to make his daughter let go of the subject of her seduction by Mr. K. The father had good reason for this wish, for Mr. K.'s wife was his own mistress, and he seemed willing to ignore Mr. K.'s indiscretions if he only remained unchallenged in his own. It was, therefore, highly inconvenient that Dora should insist on becoming morbid over her role as an object of erotic barter.
>
> I wonder how many of us can follow today without protest Freud's assertion that a healthy girl of fourteen would, under such circumstances, have considered Mr. K.'s advances "neither tactless nor offensive." The nature and severity of Dora's pathological reaction make her the classical hysteric of her case history; but her motivation for falling ill, and her lack of motivation for getting well, today seem to call for developmental considerations. Let me pursue some of these.
>
> Freud's report indicates that Dora was concerned with the historical truth as known to others, while her doctor insisted on the genetic truth behind her own symptoms. At the same time she wanted her doctor to be "truthful" in the therapeutic relation, that is, to keep faith with her on her terms rather than on those of her father or seducer. That her doctor did keep faith with her in terms of his investigative ethos she probably appreciated up to a point; after all, she did come back. But why then confront him with the fact that she had confronted her parents with the historical truth? (Erikson 1962, pp. 455-456)

Important for Dora were her own opinion of herself and its realization. Blos (1963) wrote, on the basis of his experience with adolescents, that acting out has an important function in cases in which reality has been concealed from the child by its environment in some traumatic way. Acting out then serves to reestablish the sense of reality. After a treatment has been discontinued, it becomes impossible to work through the function of acting out. The events Freud subsequently described show, however, that serious consideration of Dora's concerns would have reduced the risk of acting out or of breaking off treatment. Her acting out was determined by a mistake in Freud's attitude, i.e., in his focussing. In the specific treatment situation that Freud refers to self-critically, his mistake was insufficient interpretive activity.

What is the consequence that *Freud* drew from the instant of therapy that preceded Dora's acting out, i.e., her unannounced absence? Dora had listened, without making any of her usual objections, as Freud had attempted to interpret at a deeper level the attempted seduction by Herr K. and her anger that her story was considered a product of her imagination: "I know now — and this is what you do not want to be reminded of — that you *did* fancy that Herr K.'s proposals were serious, and that he would not leave off until you had married him." Dora "seemed to be moved; she said good-bye to me very warmly, with the heartiest wishes for the New Year, and — came no more" (Freud 1905e, pp. 108, 109). Freud thus traced Dora's anger back to the fact that she felt her secret wish had been detected whenever he referred to her imagination.

In 1900 Dora was an 18-year-old girl in the phase of adolescent detachment. She was in a period of development in which, as we now realize, acting out (including interrupting treatment) is nothing unusual and even fulfills an important function in development (one similar to that of a trial action). Discontinuation of treatment must be judged in a different light, however, than those forms of acting out which do not threaten the therapeutic work or serve denial.

In this context the question remains unanswered whether even the discontinuation of treatment may in some circumstances constitute a kind of acting out that is the realistic form of action for a *patient* to follow (and is not only the result of the actualization of an unconscious conflict). Dora paid one further visit to Freud a year later because of "facial neuralgia," but she did not alter her decision to end treatment. She did, however, officially terminate her treatment — she "came to see me again: to finish her story" (1905e, p. 120) — and told Freud enough to enable him and us to reach certain conclusions. Dora's decision not to continue the treatment but to clarify what she considered to be the real issue seems to have been important to her.

An act becomes *undesired* acting out especially as a result of its *consequences*, whether they are (unconsciously) intended or not. The consequences are also the reason for the recommendation, which used to be common, that tha analysand not make any vital decisions for the duration of the analysis (Freud 1914g). This recommendation that important decisions be postponed may in fact have been sensible in short (several months) analyses, especially if the recommendation did not amount to more than a request that the patient reconsider his situation.

Today such an intervention is suspect. At any rate, it is indispensable that the consequences of such direct or indirect suggestions be followed carefully. Rules established to counteract acting out could have just the opposite effect and lead to unconsciously controlled substitute manifestations either within or outside the analytic situation which may be difficult to follow. In this way the analytic activity is inevitably further separated from the presumed transferred conflict, and the independent precipitants resulting from the current phase of the psychoanalytic relationship (e.g., Dora's disappointment with Freud) gain in significance.

As a result of his theoretical point of view, Freud had to assume that acting out is so intimately related to repetition that he consequently neglected his self-critical observation on the actual genesis of her disappointment and acting out in their relationship.

Today we are more aware for such developments because we know that the theoretical point of view (that emotionality and motor action precede remembering) runs counter to the model of treatment technique (remembering has priority). In addition, the increase in the duration of analysis can promote the regressions associated with the predominance of pre- and nonverbal modes of communication and action. In the history of the psychoanalytic technique, this tension has found its expression in the discussion of the therapeutic functions of experiencing and remembering ever since the book by Ferenczi and Rank (1924), as reflected in Balint's new beginning (1952 [1934]) and contemporary work (see Thomä 1983 a, 1984).

The emphasis put on repetition in transference and on its resolution by interpretation led to a neglect of the innovative, creative side of acting out (especially within the psychoanalytic situation). Balint describes these important components in the context of the new beginning. Viewed historically, this sanctioned the individual case of acting out (although under a different name).

A possible consequence of neglecting the innovative side is that patients are unintentionally forced into a blind form of acting out outside of analysis. Without a doubt, Freud's description is accurate:

> We think it most undesirable if the patient *acts* outside the transference instead of remembering. The ideal conduct for our purposes would be that he should behave as normally as possible outside the treatment and express his abnormal reactions only in the transference. (1940 a, p. 177)

But if the acting out in the psychoanalytic situation, and in transference in particular, precedes remembering and belongs to genetically older strata, then remembering can only take place as a second step. If it is taken as the first step in analysis, the result is an absence of affective depth. As a consequence, there is primarily rational reconstruction within the analysis and an acting out of emotions outside it.

Zeligs (1957) understands "acting in," i.e., acting out *in* the psychoanalytic situation, to refer to all nonverbal commmunications. If limited, for example by means of understanding, interpretation, and a suitable technique and attitude, acting in can be included much more easily in the interpretation than can acting out outside the analysis, and can then lead to insight and change. In this sense, acting out is close to the change Balint described as a new beginning. Just as the negative evaluation of acting out was related to the theoretical understanding of repetition, which was supposed to be overcome by means of remembering and insight, it is now clear that acting out is inevitable, even desirable, in therapy in the form of acting in. Much more takes place in treatment than simply an exchange of words: nonverbal communication does not stop despite the limitations on the sphere of action imposed by the rules. Thus the analyst has no choice but "to accept acting out as a means of communication," even for patients not suffering from regression (Balint 1968, p. 178). The unique advantages of the interpretive method of psychoanalysis are not endangered if the conditions for the dialogue are structured in a manner which allows the analyst to express understanding for acting out. How much room there is for variation is demonstrated by the fact that Eissler (1950) thought it essential that any modification serving the goal of structural change be adopted.

Each manner of structuring the analytic situation and the verbal dialogue, whether rigid or flexible, must be examined with regard to its consequences. Deprivation achieves a special intensity in the pure, neoclassical mirror technique, and according to theory, especially fruitful memories should be brought to light. Yet just the opposite is often the case; antitherapeutic acting out often reaches a disturbing degree. The exclusion of psychomotoric and sensual communication and the concentration on verbal exchange with a partner who is unseen and hides his identity contradict human nature. Self-presentations rely on feedback which is positive or negative and emotionally modulated, and they usually employ all the senses and subliminal perceptions. It cannot be denied that the overevaluation of remembering and the associated neglect of sensations linked with the body ego, which can manifest themselves even on the couch as rudiments of, for instance, a desire to move, promote *malignant* acting out. In such acting out, whether within or outside the analytic situation, the patient seeks with all his resources acknowledgement of the bodily self-feelings which have not been recognized or named. These self-feelings, by the way, take the form of participation by the somatic symptoms (Freud 1895d) and are closely linked to remembering. The classification into remembering and acting out has theoretically severed the original connection. Since acting out refers to bodily experiences, it is logical to use this term to describe nonverbal or unreflected behavior.

The negative connotations associated with acting out are too large, however, to be overcome by adding a corrective adjective, e.g., *benign* acting out. Nonmalignant acting out must even be therapeutically desirable. Yet it is very improbable that the majority of analysts would answer yes to the question of whether they desire acting out to take place. This fact indicates that the fixed opinions about this concept cannot be altered by adding some prefix. We have mentioned and discussed several theoretical and technical reasons for this negative attitude, indeed anxiety, of many analysts toward acting out. We believe that one of the most important reasons for this attitude is the fact that acting out – with its impulsive, complex, bodily, and regressive features which often result from unconscious motives which are difficult to follow – places considerable demands on the analyst as a person and in his role as analyst.

It is thus essential for analysts to realistically evaluate their competence and to retain a feeling of security in the treatment situation. One aspect of this is that the analyst needs to maintain an overview of what is happening in the analysis by limiting the number of variables and possibilities for expression. This is a precondition for the treatment that a patient is entitled to.

Whether the analyst allows acting out, how he works with it in the analytic situation, and how he makes new solutions possible probably depend to a large degree on the capacity and flexibility that the analyst demonstrates in confronting and reviewing the present analytic situation, and not only the psychogenesis. In other words, they depend on his ability to be receptive for phenomena in the current encounter — forms of behavior, ideas, and sensations — which are usually more difficult to thematize in the here-and-now than as repetitions from the past. By following this principle of paying attention to current dynamic and intensive affects and ideas, it may be possible to recognize the past better and thus to make the present "more present," i.e., freer of the past.

## 8.7 Working Through

Working through played an important role in Freud's clinical work as early as his *Studies on Hysteria.* Therapeutic working through is grounded in the overdetermination of symptoms and the narrowness of consciousness:

> Only a single memory at a time can enter ego-consciousness. A patient who is occupied in working through such a memory sees nothing of what is pushing after it and forgets what has already pushed its way through.(Freud 1895d, p. 291)

Thus even at that time the therapeutic procedure was conceived causally: if the pathogenic memories and the affects related to them reach consciousness and are worked through, then the symptoms dependent on them must disappear completely. The explanation given for the variation in the intensity of symptoms during therapy and for their final resolution was that the pathogenic memories were being worked through and that association resistance was encountered. The matter is not taken care of if a single item is remembered and a "jammed affect" is abreacted, or in today's terms, if a patient achieves insight into an unconscious connection:

> Thanks to the abundant causal connections, *every pathogenic idea* which has not yet been got rid of operates as a motive for *the whole of the products of the neurosis,* and it is only with the last word of the analysis that the whole clinical picture vanishes .... (Freud 1895d, p. 299, emphasis added)

Pathogenic ideas repeatedly cause new resistance to association; working through the resistance in moving from one stratum to the next toward the pathogenic core removes the basis for the symptoms and finally leads to the abreaction. This was Freud's initial description of the therapeutic process. Working through was then mentioned prominently in the title *Remembering, Repeating, and Working-Through* (1914g), although Freud discussed this problem of technique on only one page. This problem has not yet been conclusively solved (Sedler 1983).

The present controversies and the recommendations for resolving them revolve around questions that become more accessible if we look at the more important passages from Freud's pioneering study. It was shown to be a mistake to believe that "giving the resistance a name" would "result in its immediate cessation." Freud continued:

One must allow the patient time to become more conversant with this resistance with which he has now become acquainted, to *work through* it, to overcome it, by continuing, in defiance of it, the analytic work according to the fundamental rule of analysis. Only when the resistance is at its height can the analyst, working in common with his patient, discover the repressed instinctual impulses which are feeding the resistance; and it is this kind of experience which convinces the patient of the existence and power of such impulses. (1914g, p. 155)

The joint labors thus lead to resistance "at its height," where working through "is a part of the work which effects the greatest changes in the patient and which distinguishes analytic treatment from any other kind of treatment by suggestion" (1914g, pp. 155-156).

After the discovery that "giving the resistance a name" does not suffice, and that arduous working through is necessary to achieve permanent change, much of what Freud and subsequent analysts discussed remained obscure. There is a clear assertion about causality: once the resistance has been properly worked through, the symptoms must disappear like ripe fruit falling from the tree of knowledge. No new symptoms should take their place. However, we should know more exactly what the modifying change resulting from working through consists of. If the causally grounded therapeutic prognosis is accurate, then the following theoretical questions must be clarified and tested in therapy: What is the state of the joint labors? Did the analyst contribute too little or too much toward resolving the resistance? Is working through exclusively a matter for the patient? What is the relationship of working through to experiencing, to abreaction, and to insight? Where does working through take place — only in the therapeutic situation, or also outside it? Within and outside — does this antithesis indicate that working through refers apparently to the transformation of insight and self-knowledge into practical action and a change in behavior? This incomplete list of questions makes it obvious that we are in the middle of psychoanalytic practice and its theory of therapy; this also means trying to explain failures in order to improve practice.

The history of working through demonstrates that advances in theory and practice do not always go hand in hand. This is connected with Freud's attempts to explain the *failure* of working through, i.e., therapeutic failure. We are taking this indirect route because it makes the solutions being suggested today more plausible. Although therapeutically effective working through initially referred to the repetition of fixations from the patient's life history and their recurrence in transference (Freud 1914g), Freud attributed the failure 10 years later to resistance of the unconscious (1926d, pp. 159-160). We have already discussed this form of resistance and Freud's speculative explanation of repetition compulsion in Sect. 4.4. We have also explained why Freud's philosophical speculations on repetition compulsion are such a burden precisely for the depth-psychological understanding of working through, as Cremerius (1978) convincingly demonstrated.

The conservative nature of the instincts, the adhesiveness (1916/17), the inertia (1918b), or the sluggishness of the libido (1940a), and the tendency to return to an earlier state — the death instinct — appeared to impede therapy or even to prevent working through, in its role as an important act of change. These are, in fact, speculations about constitutional factors which may be present in one form or another without being accessible to examination by the psychoanalytic method. The limits to the therapeutic range of working through must be marked on the original field of the method. It must therefore be emphasized that because of the theory of the death instinct (which, incidentally, is not accepted by any reputable biologist — see Angst 1980) Freud neglected to clarify to the logical conclusion the psychological conditions for repetition and its working through both within and outside the analytic situation. What does this mean? It is important for us to investigate the approaches to explaining repetition compulsion which are contained in Freud's work and then to examine the analytic situation to determine whether its standardized form as an ideal type optimally mobilizes the potential for change in the average patient.

Therapeutically fruitful alternative explanations for repetition compulsion are available, for example, for the recurrence of traumatic events in dreams. Freud viewed this, just like the traumatic neurosis, as an attempt by the ego to reestablish the psychic balance. Originally Freud had assumed the existence of an "instinct for mastery" (1905d, p.193), which Hendrick (1942, 1943a,b) later attempted to revive. Examples of such an instinct are the acquisition of new skills, the intense curiosity of children, and the desire to move. Freud put repetition at the focus of his interpretation of childhood play but disregarded the pleasurable testing of new actions and perceptions which also take place; this neglect led to some one-sided views in the psychoanalytic understanding of theory and practice. Knowledge of the conditions leading to fixation and regression and to the repetitions associated with them is only one side of the coin. Freud's favorite object of scientific study was how and why people come to unconsciously seek and establish perceptual identities, i.e., to stick to their habits and pathological tendencies despite knowing better and wanting to change. On the other hand, there is the question of change. Pleasure seeks not only to become eternal and to repeat itself. We are anxious to learn and understand something new, and the greater the security that has formed or forms on the basis of interpersonally confirmed identities, the further we venture into the unknown.[1]

Since steps in an unfamiliar region may be accompanied by discontent and anxiety, it is essential that conditions favorable to change (the context of change) be created in the therapeutic situation (in contrast to the conditions of

[1] We disregard the pain and pleasure of lonely discoverers and inventors. It is perhaps possible to say that such individuals are successful largely independently of interpersonal confirmation. They find ascetic pleasure the moment they demonstrate that their expectation, contained in their fantasy, construction, or scientific understanding, coincides with a previously unknown reality, whether in external nature or human nature. It is not unusual for this aspect of reality to be named after the discoverer or inventor, who is then identified with what he discovered.

genesis — the context of discovery). Some developments in theory have influenced the psychoanalytic technique in a one-sided manner and limited its range. Working through was, for example, often neglected despite Freud's initial demands and although it had an integrating function: "The treatment is made up of two parts — what the physician infers and tells the patient, and the patient's *working-over* of what he has heard" (Freud 1910d, p.141, emphasis added). Hearing and telling are not enough; acting is what is important. Working through takes place at the junction between the internal and external and has an integrating function. Each point of view which is disregarded can make it more difficult for the patient to integrate the "severed connections" (A. Freud 1937).

Where Freud saw himself compelled to explain a failure by id resistance, we can today take full practical advantage of the continued theoretical development of his alternative idea regarding the meaning of repetition in playing, in the sense of mastery, as described by Loevinger (1966), White (1959, 1963), and Klein (1976, pp.259-260). Freud described this alternative idea in the following way:

> The ego, which experienced the trauma passively, now repeats it actively in a weakened version, in the hope of being able itself to direct its course. It is certain that children behave in this fashion towards every distressing impression they receive, by reproducing it in their play. In thus changing from passivity to activity they attempt to master their experiences psychically. (1926d, p.167)

According to Klein's comments on this alternative idea, the individual still has an unconscious intention to transform actively an event which was suffered passively and which has remained foreign to the experiencing self. Such events are traumatic, cause anxiety, and lead to repression. Attempts at self-cures fail because of the repression, since the consequences of unconscious intentions cannot be perceived in feedback loops. We must add that the analyst's interpretive assistance in working through lie in helping the patient to learn to perceive and control the unconscious intentions of his actions and behavior. For Klein, following Erikson, this mastery is no special, independent need striving for gratification, but a self experience — the self experiences itself as the initiator of an act. The self scheme is thus differentiated according to the processes of assimilation and accommodation and the other processes described by Piaget.

In 1964 a panel of the American Psychoanalytic Association on working through (see Schmale 1966) also referred to points of view from learning theory, which we will discuss in Sect. 8.8.

It is precisely a comprehensive understanding of theory and practice which raises questions about the nature of the relationship between resistance analysis and insight. Fenichel (1941) and Greenacre (1956) described working through as intensive and concentrated resistance analysis. Greenson (1965, p.282) put insight and change at the center of his definition of working through, as the following passage shows:

> We do not regard the analytic work as working through before the patient has insight, only after. It is the goal of working through to make insight effective, i.e., to make significant and lasting changes in the patient. By making insight the pivotal issue we can distinguish between

those resistances which prevent insight and those resistances which prevent insight from leading to change. The analytic work on the first set of resistances is the analytic work proper; it has no special designation. The analysis of those resistances which keep insight from leading to change is the work of working through. The analyst and the patient each contributes to this work.

This conception of working through resolves some of the technical difficulties. Its explanatory value lies in the fact that it makes it possible to comprehend the *effectiveness*, or lack of it, of the circular processes (insight — therapeutic benefits — ego change — new insight) described by Kris (1956a, b). However, there is not always progress around this circle. Insights are not regularly translated into changes. In Freud's words, "as you can imagine, there are likely to be difficulties if an instinctual process which has been going along a particular path for whole decades is suddenly expected to take a new path that has just been made open for it" (1926e, p. 224). Leaving old paths and finding new ones, i.e., separation and saying farewell — this aspect of working through suggests a comparison with the process of mourning.

Fenichel (1941), Lewin (1950), and Kris (1951, 1956a, b) have pointed out the similarities and differences between mourning and working through. We believe that the differences are even greater than Stewart (1963) assumed. He draws our attention to the fact that the task of mourning is to reconcile oneself with the loss of a loved object, while the purpose of working through is to change the form and goals of preceding gratifications and to find new ones. With a real loss, time also contributes to the healing process, and the dialogue with the dead changes with the conscious and unconscious process of mourning.

Neurotic processes are different. They are often not interrupted by insight alone because new confirmations of unconsciously anchored dispositions can be sought and found in the outer world over and over as a result of internal psychic conditions. Thus despite the patient's insight during the interviews, the symptoms can repeatedly stabilize outside analysis according to the old templates. We would like to emphasize our agreement with Ross (1973, p. 334) that working through does not take place exclusively in the analytic situation.

The division, indeed cleavage, into insight and action (into internal and external) can take place all the more easily if the analyst limits himself to transference interpretations or views working through primarily as a part of the terminal phase. Waelder (1960, pp. 224ff.) emphasizes that mourning and working through generally last 1–2 years. Yet if every inconspicuous step is viewed against the backdrop of separation and loss, the patient will also postpone working through until the final year of the analysis, when mourning and separation are prominent, instead of viewing it as a continuous task. The example of working through in the terminal phase that Waelder (1960, p. 213) gives is a patient's autosuggestive comment, "I should stop behaving this way and make peace with myself." The prospects for successful working through are not positive if at the end the proverbial good intention is the only thing left.

The purpose of working through is for insight to become effective. We are especially interested, therefore, in those cases in which insight leads no further than to good intentions, i.e., where the patient does not succeed in making peace with himself. Why does the insight gained through the analysis of resistance not lead to the changes that the patient desires and strives for? There are many answers to this question, most of which assert that the insight was simply not deep enough or that it lacked conviction because it did not result from interpretations within an intensive transference relationship.

Balint (1968, pp. 8, 13), for example, assumes that working through is linked to interpretations of resistance and is only possible in those patients who are accessible to words. Yet not everyone is willing to accept the gulf between verbal exchange and nonverbal relationship as a given fact. Indeed, Balint himself called for us to bridge the gulf. It is thus important to scrutinize resistance interpretations for implicit negative consequences. The latter seem to consist in an unresolved tension between the analyst formulating an image of the patient's unconscious wishes and potential and endeavoring to maintain neutrality and respect for the patient's liberty to make decisions by giving his interpretations in an open manner. This form of analytic behavior contributes to unsettling the patient and thus, in an indirect way, to a reaction which stabilizes habits.

On the other hand, the inequality between patient and analyst shifts even further in favor of the latter if primarily genetic interpretations are made. The patient then experiences the analyst, as Balint has shown, as omniscient with regard to the past and the origin of resistances. The analyst believes that all he has to do — in fact, that he may do nothing else — is to interpret resistances in the context of unconscious instinctual impulses and memories. In doing so he follows Freud's assumption that the synthesis, i.e., the creation of a new constellation of psychic elements, occurs on its own in analysis (Freud 1919a, p. 161).

It is true that interpretations can indirectly contribute to this synthesis because the new configurations which become possible are codetermined by the purposive ideas that the analyst has — and it is impossible not to have any. Yet an atmosphere is created which does not make it easier for the patient to overcome the *horror vacui* that may be linked with the new beginning and to translate his insight into real experience. The inevitable question is thus how many good insights and trial actions are necessary to attain a modification of symptoms and behavior in real life. Patient and analyst may feel so comfortable in the regression that they postpone the real test. There are always more or less plausible reasons for doing this, for example, because the patient does not believe that he is already able to change the forms of behavior tormenting him and those around him, and the analyst keeps looking in the past for deeper reasons for this inability.

Ultimately, working through is the process concerned more than any other with the patient bringing psychic acts to their conclusion and having positive experiences in doing so. Such positive experiences in analysis are all too comprehensible, and thus are discussed less than negative ones. This imbalance may increase just at those moments in working through when a good starting point for a trial action, i.e., confirmation and acknowledgement, is being sought. The fragile self-confidence which has just resulted from insight and experience is then lost again. Instead of working through leading to an increase in self-confidence, which could facilitate the patient's ability to cope with subsequent problems in "regression in the service of the ego" (Kris 1936, p. 290), it could lack any therapeutic effect and even result in a malignant regression. The structure of the psychoanalytic situation may constitute such a substantial factor contributing to this consequence that Cremerius (1978, p. 210) has recommended changing the setting in such cases. Still to be clarified is the analyst's contribution to the genesis of a malignant regression. Usually it is not too late to start over again by changing the technique or the setting. The criticism that the analyst manipulates the patient is inappropriate if he is frank to the patient and if changes are founded and handled interpretatively.

Working through has qualitative and quantitative aspects which can also be observed in learning processes, especially in relearning. Many patients ask themselves, as well as their analysts, how often they will have to endure a certain situation before they will be able to cope with it in a different and better way. For example, how many times must a patient have a positive experience when dealing with someone with authority in order to overcome his social anxiety and the more fundamental castration anxiety? Working through thus takes place both *within* and *outside* the analytic situation. We will discuss the points of view of learning theory in Sect. 8.8.

We believe that the problems posed by working through were relatively neglected in psychoanalysis in the last few decades because it also takes place outside the analytic situation and because learning theory must be taken into consideration to explain relearning. Our experience leads us to believe that Greenson's definition of working through — the analysis of the resistances preventing the transformation of insight into changes — is too narrow and one-sided. Even in working through the resistances which are manifest in the analyses of those patients who are *not* successful, the central issue is how to be successful within and outside the analytic situation.

What can the analyst do to ensure that the patient's hesitant attempts, his trial actions, will be successful and that, following the encouragement in analysis, he will continue his efforts outside? Patients have a greater desire and need for reassurance and the other interpersonal experiences which strengthen the ego than healthy individuals do. In the standard technique the patient receives little support, which is completely eliminated if at all possible. It seems that the patient can only accept those aspects of the analyst's interpretations that he unconsciously seeks or that relate to the internal forces keeping him from reaching his goal.

Many interpretations provide indirect encouragement. Yet if the analyst believes that he may not provide any support, he puts the patient in a predicament or trap. The analyst unknowingly creates, according to Bateson et al. (1963), a double bind by providing contradictory information. On the one hand, the interpretation of unconscious desires opens up new opportunities, and the patient agrees with his therapist. If, on the other hand, the analyst limits his approval because he fears influencing the patient, the security which has been gained can be lost again. The ambiguity of half-hearted interpretations perplexes the patient and impedes working through the transference relationship. Working through is no exception: views about it, just like those about transference neurosis, vary from school to school; and the analyst's contribution to it, just as to the specific transference situation, is not small even in very typical illnesses. Kohut (1971, pp. 86ff., 168ff.) deserves special credit for having pointed out the significant role confirmation plays in establishing and working through transference. As Wallerstein (1983) and Treurniet (1983) have shown, Kohut's technical suggestions are not tied to his views on narcissism and his self psychology. All patients have narcissistic personalities inasmuch as their self-feeling is dependent on confirmation, but this is true for every individual. The uncertainties which are inevitable in any working through to attain restructuring are easier for a patient to bear if his curiosity about his unconscious desires and goals is reinforced by a supporting relationship.

## 8.8 Learning and Restructuring

The limited explanatory value of Pavlov's model of learning became clear soon after the first attempts were made in the 1930s, when this was the most prominent model, to use the results of experimental research into learning psychology in order to improve our understanding of complex human learning. The later cognitive models of learning, which take, for instance, conceptual modifications and internal cognitive restructuring into consideration, are more helpful and stimulating for a comprehensive understanding of what happens in psychotherapy. The use of appropriate learning models seems advantageous especially where psychoanalytic thought is contradictory or incomplete, as in the case of working through. In this regard we would like to refer to French, who as early as 1936 expressed the hope that

> by always keeping the learning process underlying analytic therapy in mind we may be able to somewhat improve our perspective and sense of proportion about the significance and relative importance of the great multitude of unconscious impulses and memories that press toward the surface in psychoanalytic treatment. (French 1936, p. 149)

In this section we would like to focus attention on a few of the factors which support symptoms and on some of those which lead to therapeutic changes. The former play a special role in psychoanalytic treatment when we are concerned with their resolution, with therapeutic change, and with relearning, which is very close to working through. In this context we will disregard those processes and factors leading to the genesis of symptoms and neuroses; in doing so we are completely aware that we are introducing a somewhat artificial distinction between the genesis and the maintenance of symptoms. In the following, we refer to learning processes, or learning, for short, if there is a change in the likelihood that a certain behavior (act, thought, idea, affect) will manifest itself under comparable circumstances.

> If somebody repeatedly does something, or does not do it, in a certain situation although he previously would not have acted in this way under similar circumstances, or if his actions are more rapid and more secure than earlier, then we speak of a learning process. This is not the case if we have good reason to assume that the changed behavior is caused by other factors (e.g., intoxication, brain injury, or simply normal processes of maturation). (Foppa 1968, p. 13)

As is well known, there are three different paradigms for learning:

1. Classical conditioning (signal learning, stimulus-response learning), which is associated especially with Pavlov and (in psychotherapy) Eysenck and Wolpe
2. Operant or instrumental conditioning (learning by success), which is associated with the work of Thorndike and Skinner
3. Social learning (learning with models or by identification), as described by Bandura

In laboratory experiments it is possible to distinguish between these learning paradigms, and thus to study them separately, by varying the conditions. However, in real life, characterized as it is by a much greater multiplicity and complexity of internal and external conditions, learning processes seem as a rule to be determined according to the processes described by all three paradigms to different and changing degrees.

The most convincing paradigm of learning with regard to describing the course of psychoanalytic treatment seems at first to be learning with models, specifically, the analyst's model. This refers to how the patient accepts the analyst's ego functions — the manner in which the analyst identifies connections, common aspects, and differences in interpretations, which strategies he adopts to achieve affective and cognitive solutions to conflicts, how he phrases questions, and how he handles affects and the therapeutic relationship. The theory of social learning formulates a series of conditions which may influence the effects of social learning. Examples are the similarity between the model person (psychoanalyst) and the observer (patient) with regard to personal features such as social status, age, sex, and psychological personality structure; and the nature of the relationship between model person and observer, for instance, whether the observer desires the affection of the model person, fears its loss, or tries to avoid punishment by the model person.

Such conditions of interaction can determine to a large extent how the transference neurosis unfolds. This is by no means a reference to simple imitations of the psychoanalyst's manner of behavior or way of thinking, although they of course may also occur. More importantly, according to the findings of the theory of social learning we must expect sustained and internalized learning effects (changes), i.e., those which become integrated into the observer's entire repertoire of behavior and experiencing. This is especially true if the analyst's functions are mediated in a cognitive manner using symbols. This explanation shows that learning with a model goes far beyond the imitation of external forms of behavior, and emphasizes the similarities between this paradigm of learning and the processes of identification, as conceptualized in psychoanalysis. Empirical studies also reveal that the rapidity and permanence of model learning can be decisively improved by the mediation of verbal symbols.

The other two paradigms for learning exhibit a much less direct relationship to the events in psychoanalytic therapy. In the early 1930s several psychoanalysts (e.g., French 1933; Kubie 1935) applied the classical conditioning paradigm to the psychoanalytic treatment technique and attempted to use the former to justify the latter. These efforts were sharply rejected by Schilder

(1935b); in his opinion Pavlov's theory of learning could not be applied to more complex human learning processes and was thus unsuited to explain psychoanalytic thinking and action. Schilder instead attempted to describe a psychoanalytic understanding of conditioned reflexes, an approach which seems just as unproductive (see the fundamental study by Straus 1935).

Heigl and Triebel (1977) have reviewed several of the learning principles mentioned here with regard to their relationship to psychoanalytic therapy. They extended their usual psychoanalytic treatment technology to include those variants of "confirmation of even the smallest learning advances within the transference relationship" which are founded in learning theory, paying special attention to corrective emotional experience. Yet we have our doubts whether such global conceptions and the restricted therapeutic instructions derived from them are suited to significantly expand or deepen our understanding of the process of psychoanalytic therapy and of the analyst's influence on its course. Wachtel (1977) has provided a fundamental and comprehensive discussion of this issue.

We would like to direct our attention to a specific pair of concepts from learning theory that play a central role in all three paradigms for learning and also seem to be helpful for understanding learning processes in psychoanalytic therapy. These concepts are *generalization* and *discrimination*.

In accordance with the accepted learning theories, we understand generalization to refer, for short, to the tendency to react in a similar manner in comparable circumstances, and discrimination to the tendency in similar circumstances to notice the differences and to react accordingly, i.e., discriminatingly. Within the framework of the above-mentioned basic paradigms for learning theory we now want to attempt to use this pair of concepts to provide an exemplary description of transference phenomena.

In a strongly simplified form, *transference* in psychoanalytic therapy is characterized by the fact that the manner in which the patient forms and perceives his relationship, at least with regard to certain, conflict-specific aspects, to his analyst (not to mention to many others outside the therapeutic situation) is especially oriented on the patterns of the relationships to his mother and father, siblings, and other significant persons which he formed in early childhood (see Chap. 2). The external features of the analytic situation and the analyst's behavior should promote the development of transference; obviously, the analysis of transference, an essential component of psychoanalytic therapy, cannot begin until the transference has become sufficiently intense and differentiated. The features that are the same or similar in the transference relationship and in specific relationships outside of therapy are further clarified and given special emphasis by the analyst in the course of transference analysis. When the transference is full bloom, the differences between the therapeutic relationship, its genetic predecessors, and the relationships outside therapy become increasingly clear. By means of various activities the analyst offers the patient — at least indirectly, and surprisingly often unknowingly and unintendedly, yet always inevitably — an incentive and opportunity to develop and test alternative and, in particular, flexible patterns of relationships in the therapeutic situation. Ultimately the patient cannot avoid applying outside therapy the ability to form relationships in a different and flexible way which he has acquired and even tested in therapy and to adapt it to changing circumstances.

This brief description reveals similarities with the course of some learning experiments. The new learning experience is introduced by generalization processes; similarities are sought in different configurations of stimuli. If a stable pattern of responses has been formed in this manner, the experimenter can then promote discriminatory processes by changing the experimental conditions, especially the reinforcement scheme; the organism learns to respond differently to different configurations of stimuli. Yet before response patterns acquired in this way can be generalized to apply to the conditions outside the immediate experimental situation, it may be necessary for the patient to go through further learning experiences under nonexperimental conditions. Thus the psychoanalytic process and some learning experiments display a whole series of common features. French (1936, p. 191) even speaks of the "experimental character of the transference" and emphasizes

> the importance of reality testing in the transference. Striking as are the manifestations of the repetition compulsion, the transference is nevertheless not only a compulsive repetition of earlier events. It is also an experimental attempt to correct the infantile patterns.

Within the *basic* learning paradigms it is not possible to attain any substantial increase in knowledge from such analogies beyond such global statements. This concept of access via basic learning theory proves to be too cumbersome and not vivid enough to comprehend complex affective and cognitive learning processes. While it is possible to understand such very complex learning processes within the framework of the generalization-discrimination theory of learning, as emphasized by Mowrer (1960) in particular, a series of new ideas (e.g., the concept of secondary reinforcer and viewing the response as a discriminatory stimulus) would then have to be introduced. Although the learning theory model would then be complex, it would also be cumbersome and lack clarity. Thus we want to end our discussion of the basic learning model here and to select a level of verbal description which is high enough to allow examination of cognitive learning models and the restructuring processes that they should reflect.

When talking of learning, people also think of childhood learning and the sometimes vain efforts of teachers. Traditional teaching can be termed "superego education," as Balint (1952) emphasizes; children should be raised to be moral, decent individuals. Balint contrasts this to "ego education" in psychoanalysis, linking it with general considerations of the educational aspects of psychoanalysis. As can be demonstrated, the educational element in psychoanalysis was never completely rejected and achieved special importance in child analysis (A. Freud 1927).

Looking at the history of science, it is possible to draw a line linking the attempts to apply educational ideas in psychoanalysis and Piaget's "genetic epistemology." In experimental clinical investigations Piaget studied different stages of learning and development in childhood. His findings have recently been taken up by Tenzer (1983, 1984), who related them to some details of working through. Yet the precondition for this connection — that the process of working through unfolds in a manner analogous to the development and learning stages in childhood described by Piaget — is dubious. Of even greater significance for our understanding of working through seems to us to be Piaget's conception of the "cognitive scheme" made up of the developmental processes of accommodation and assimilation. We would now like to turn to these three concepts.

The cognitive scheme should be understood in the sense of a screen that structures perceptual and intellectual experiences and whose own structure and complexity is organized according to the developmental stages described by Piaget. The term "assimilation" is used when a new experience is incorporated into the existing cognitive scheme and increases the entire wealth of experience structured by the scheme. If a new experience cannot be incorporated into the existing cognitive scheme, the consequence may be a modification of the scheme (or, in contrast, the neglect or warding off of this alien new experience). The process of modification is called accomodation. It is not difficult to recognize how these concepts could be applied beneficially to our understanding of change in psychoanalytic therapy. Wachtel (1980) has demonstrated convincingly that this assimilation-accommodation approach can be productive for the theoretical and clinical understanding of transference phenomena.

We now want to undertake a similar attempt and try to clarify this theoretical approach with regard to *working through*. In this context we will also refer to the extension and expansion of Piaget's approach by McReynolds (1976) and, with reference to the psychoanalytic technique, by G. Klein (1976, pp. 244ff.).

The phase of *working through* begins after the patient has gained insight into the connections and processes marking the dynamics of previously unconscious conflicts. The goal is to use cognitive and affective insight to change behavior. While some patients achieve such behavioral changes without the analyst's assistance, this generally cannot be expected. We know from learning psychology that the different areas of cognition, autonomous processes, and psychomotoric ability can develop largely independently of each other (see Birbaumer 1973). Special processes of generalization are required to integrate endopsychic processes by means of feedback.

In psychoanalytic therapy this occurs in the process of working through. Deeper analysis of the unconscious past determinants of the genesis of the incapacity is postponed in favor of the integration or reintegration of psychodynamic details. Alexander's (1935) description of the integrative function of interpretation, based on the integrating or synthetic function of the ego (Nunberg 1931), deserves special mention in this context. Achieving this integration is the patient's task; he can rely on the analyst's support, although this could even turn into an obstacle.

It can regularly be clinically observed that the uncovering of unconscious material relevant to a patient's conflicts can create a substantial degree of destabilization, unrest, and anxiety. Such a lack of orientation can also be understood in terms of the conceptual framework of the processes of generalization and discrimination described above, and has been convincingly described and interpreted by McReynolds (1976) from the perspective of cognitive psychology. McReynolds formulated his theory of assimilation with reference to Piaget, distinguishing between congruent and incongruent ideas and perceptions. Cognitive congruence refers to the conflict-free assimilation (integration) of new perceptions into the existing structure, while incongruence refers to the transitory or persistent inability to assimilate new perceptions into the existing structure. It is possible for previously congruent, assimilated ideas or perceptions to be deassimilated as a result of changes in the cognitive structure. The relationship of unassimilated to assimilated ideas and perceptions is designated assimilation backlog; this backlog is viewed as a prime determinant of anxiety. Rules have been formulated for three elementary operations for the functioning of the cognitive-affective system:

1. The attempt is made to resolve cognitive incongruences.
2. The backlog in cognitive assimilation should be kept to a minimum.
3. Cognitive innovations (e.g., curiosity, suggestions, search for stimulation) should be kept at an optimal level.

These operational rules are described with regard to their utility for biological adaptation. Accordingly, there is an especially sudden and drastic increase in the assimilation backlog, and thus in anxiety, when cognitive changes at a higher level result in a deassimilation of previously congruent, integrated ideas, and consequently of the numerous points at which these ideas have contact with others.

With regard to working through in psychoanalytic therapy, assimilation theory provides an explanation for the fact that "striking" interpretations can create abrupt deassimilations accompanied by unrest and anxiety. In such a case the interpretation tears apart hierarchically superior, previously congruent ideas and thus contributes to the disintegration of subordinate ideas that were also congruent. This last effect can, however, also be achieved by integrating interpretations, for instance when distant and previously unconnected ideas are linked, possibly leading to the abrupt deassimilation of subordinate ideas. The analyst can help save the patient unnecessary unrest if his interpretations are well prepared and carefully dosed, for example by restricting them temporarily to hierarchically lower ideas. In an attempt to keep the assimilation backlog to a minimum, the patient may at times refuse to recognize or accept interventions which would have a deassimilating effect; this refusal is manifested clinically as resistance. The analyst's encouragement, acknowledgement, and reassurance that he will provide support in the work of assimilating integration may help the patient undertake the risky endeavor despite the anticipated disturbances.

It is necessary that such endopsychic cognitive restructuring be tested and tried out with regard to its viability for coping with the reality of life and for structuring relationships outside of therapy in a satisfactory way. We consider this to be an essential aspect of working through. The various transference configurations offer the patient a relatively risk-free chance to test different relationship patterns. With the analyst's support the patient will then transfer these reinforced activities to relationships outside therapy (generalization); he will then naturally become aware of the differences between the transference and working relationship in therapy and the more varied kinds of relationships outside of therapy (discrimination). The patient may have positive experiences, which strengthen and thus stabilize the modified cognitive scheme and the new pattern of behavior.

The patient's changed social behavior can, however, also lead to unexpected experiences for partners, friends, acquaintances, and colleagues as well as to negative experiences for the patient himself. The continued existence of the recently acquired and still insecure cognitive scheme is then endangered, and the patient is threatened by a relapse. In this case, the patient will look to the analyst for more confirmation and support in order to continue his uncertain endeavor of testing novel trial actions. The failure of the analyst to react appropriately can also have negative consequences for the patient and his efforts to try out new patterns of behavior. Here again, the patient's newly gained and fragile self-confidence can be lost. Such inappropriate abstinence by the analyst may frustrate the patient's need for security, even leading to malignant aggression, regression, or depression.

Alterations in the cognitive scheme, i.e., cognitive restructuring, cannot be directly observed, but must be inferred from lasting changes in observable behavior (see Strupp 1978). For this reason, the psychoanalyst's presumptions about the structural changes that have been achieved by a patient must in principle be empirically verifiable with regard to specific forms of observable behavior, including of course verbal behavior. Furthermore, such empirical verification must actually be performed. This means that it must be possible to derive verifiable predictions about the patient's future behavior, including how he will react in specific conflicts (e.g., strategies for conflict resolution, coping and defense mechanisms, symptom development, and structuring of relationships), from the presumptions about structural changes. Otherwise all discussion of structural change is meaningless (Sargent et al. 1983).

Thus it is often possible to close gaps in the psychoanalytic understanding of clinical phenomena by referring to concepts developed by other disciplines. Moreover, the psychoanalyst needs a good knowledge of neighboring disciplines to be able to use their concepts and consequently to attain a comprehensive understanding of his own theoretical concepts and clinical action.

## 8.9 Termination

### *8.9.1 General Considerations*

However long and arduous an analysis may have been, the terminal phase creates its own problems for both participants. Not infrequently there is an incongruence between the patient's and the analyst's conceptions of the goals of the treatment (E. Ticho 1971). Whether the analyst is successful in convincing the patient that the analytic work must be limited to goals accessible to treatment and that the terminable analysis be distinguished from the interminable has great practical significance. At the end of a psychoanalytic treatment the patient should have developed the capacity for self-analysis. This means simply that the patient learns and employs the special form of reflection that characterizes the psychoanalytic dialogue. Tied to this ability is the expectation that the capacity for self-analysis will work against the inclination toward regression which may still arise after analysis when new problems are encountered, and thus that the renewed development of symptoms will be hindered. This view is opposed quite often by "the myth of perfectibility," i.e., of the complete analysis, which molds the attitudes of some analysts toward the terminal phase as a result of the pressure exerted by their own exaggerated ideals (Gaskill 1980). It is not difficult to grasp that wealthy patients accept any offer such analysts make in order to continue the analysis.

It is possible to imagine which unconscious fantasies are associated with termination if we consider the metaphors used in the literature to describe the final phase. Weigert's (1952) comparison of the terminal phase with a complicated disembarkation maneuver in which all the libidinal and aggressive forces are in action clearly indicates that dramatic scenes can be expected. The danger of disillusionment does in fact exist if the entire course of treatment has been characterized by the striving for narcissistic perfection, the complete resolution of transference, and similar myths. This mythology of completeness has negative consequences if the analyst — measuring himself and the patient against ideal types — is disappointed about his work with the patient at the end of treatment while the patient, in contrast, expresses his gratitude. This demand for perfection denies the finite and limited nature of human actions and prevents the analyst from being proud and satisfied with his work. Moreover, the patient cannot separate himself because he consciously or unconsciously senses the analyst's disappointment. He will then make protracted efforts to convince the analyst of the success of the treatment or will identify with the analyst's disappointment. The literature sometimes contains reports describing just the opposite of this mutual dissatisfaction. More commonly, however, the inevitable imperfections of psychoanalytic practice, familiar to every one of us, are disguised in reports describing the termination of treatment in a way conforming to theory.

Referring to the final reports of 48 candidates in training, Gilman (1982) used a catalogue of questions to examine how they handled the terminal phase. All of these analysts reported a resolution of the symptoms and a complete working through of the neurotic conflict, although there was otherwise a large amount of variation. Furthermore, the termination was allegedly never initiated by external events such as changes in the patient's life or financial difficulties, but always by mutual agreement. These final reports serve a special function — to show that the analysts are worthy of admission to one of the professional associations — which in our opinion makes the conformist description of the terminal phase very comprehensible. In Earle's (1979) study of candidates in training, the criterion of mutual agreement on termination was satisfied in only 25% of the cases, a result which differs only slightly from the percentage reported for qualified analysts.

We would now like to end the discussion of perfection vs premature termination and to look for perspectives which can do justice to the multiplicity of reasons that psychoanalytic treatment may ultimately be terminated. Analyses should be terminated when the joint analytic work no longer produces significantly new insights. This makes it clear that the termination is a dyadic process, which in principle is incomplete if we assume that two persons will always have something else to say to each other. Disregarding external circumstances, we can assume that patients stop when the therapeutic exchange loses its importance and the burdens associated with the treatment are no longer balanced by an increase in knowledge. At this point even the interminable analysis will be terminated.

We must also overcome the idea that the right indications are a guarantee for a satisfactory terminal phase and a good conclusion, as Glover (1955) still assumed. The analytic process is determined by too many imponderables for the end to be predictable on the basis of the diagnosis (indication and prognosis) of an individual (see Chap. 6). The attitude linked with such a conception of predictability is closely associated with the basic model technique, whose erroneous fundamental assumptions have been the source of numerous faulty discussions of detailed issues. Successful and satisfactory termination always occurs, in both frequent and infrequent treatments, if a good working relationship has developed, creating the preconditions for regressive processes to be structured in productive fashion (Hoffmann 1983).

### *8.9.2 Duration and Limitation*

At no time has it been possible for the psychoanalytic procedure to promise the illusion of a rapid, miraculous cure. As early as 1895, Breuer and Freud reported that the procedure was arduous and time-consuming for the doctor. Yet since the psychoanalytic method was initially tried out "only on very severe cases" — on patients who had gone to Freud "after many years of illness, completely incapacitated for life" — Freud hoped that "in cases of less severe illness the duration of the treatment might well be much shorter, and very great advantage in the direction of future prevention might be achieved" (1904a, p. 254). Yet Freud also expressed mild skepticism toward setting an appropiate limit on therapy. Although such efforts required no special justification, Freud nevertheless wrote that "experience has taught us that psycho-analytic therapy — the freeing of someone from his neurotic symptoms, inhibitions and abnormalities of character — is a time-consuming business" (1937c, p. 216).

The use of the limitation of treatment as a technical measure was introduced by Freud in the case of the Wolf Man in reaction to a standstill in treatment: "I determined — but not until trustworthy signs had led me to judge that the right moment had come — that the treatment must be brought to an end at a particular fixed date, no matter how far it had advanced" (1918b, p. 11). Ferenczi and Rank (1924) took up this idea. Both of them considered termination, the "period of weaning," to be one of the most important phases of the entire treatment. Yet as early as 1925 Ferenczi revised this view; in the article "Psychoanalysis of Sexual Habits" (1950 [1925], pp. 293ff.) he greatly restricted the efficacy of using a fixed date as a means to expedite the termination of treatment and as "an effective means of hastening separation from the analyst." And in his paper "The Problem of Termination of the Analysis" (1955 [1928a], p.85) he argued that "neither the physician nor the patient puts an end to it, but ... it dies of exhaustion, so to speak." Ferenczi then continued:

> To put it another way, one might say that the patient finally becomes convinced that he is continuing analysis only because he is treating it as a new but still a fantasy source of gratification, which in terms of reality yields him nothing. When he has slowly overcome his mourning over this discovery he inevitably looks round for other, more real sources of gratification.

This point of view agrees with the two conditions Freud established for termination:

> First, that the patient shall no longer be suffering from his symptoms and shall have overcome his anxieties and his inhibitions; and secondly, that the analyst shall judge that so much repressed material has been made conscious, so much that was unintelligible has been explained, and so much internal resistance conquered, that there is no need to fear a repetition of the pathological processes concerned. (1937c, p.219)

According to Freud, the factors determining the possible result of psychoanalytic treatment are traumas, the constitutional strength of the instincts, and the alteration of the ego. Furthermore, the traumatic etiology of neuroses is the reason that the chances for a cure are especially high. "Only when a case is a predominantly traumatic one will analysis succeed in doing what it is so superlatively able to" (1937c, p.220). Successful integration of the instincts into the ego depends on their strength (whether constitutional or momentary). Yet Freud is skeptical whether analysis is successful in permanently and harmoniously integrating the instincts in the ego in certain circumstances since the instinctual strength can increase accidentally or as a result of new traumas and involuntary frustrations.

We know today that Freud, looking back at his analysis of Ferenczi, reached the conclusion that it is not possible in analysis to influence a dormant instinctual conflict, and he considered the manipulative activation of conflicts to be immoral.

> But even if he [the analyst] had failed to observe some very faint signs of it [negative transference] — which was not altogether ruled out, considering the limited horizon of analysis in those early days — it was still doubtful, he thought, whether he would have had the power to activate a topic (or, as we say, a "complex") by merely pointing it out, so long as it was not currently active in the patient himself at the time. (1937c, pp.221-222)

Thus although the strength of the instincts and its modification depend on unforeseeable imponderables, Freud put special emphasis on analysis of changes in the ego, by which he meant changes in the ego resulting from defense and from the distance to a fictive normal ego. Analysis is supposed to create the conditions most favorable for the ego functions. Freud thus took up ideas that A. Freud had included a year earlier in her book *Ego and the Mechanisms of Defense* (1937). Reich had pointed out as early as 1933 that resistance rooted in the individual's character, which Reich considered as acquired ego armor, often stands in the way of progress in analysis. The changes which occurred in psychoanalytic theory after the introduction of structural theory and the theory of defense mechanisms, together with the increased significance of analysis of resistance and character, due to Reich's influence, led to the increase in the duration of analyses.

Yet this lengthening of analysis actually has many causes. The opinion voiced by Glover, for many years responsible for research at the London Psychoanalytic Institute, is alarming:

> When coming to a decision on this question of length it would be well to remember that the earlier analysts were accustomed to conduct analysis of six to twelve months' duration which as far as I can find out did not differ greatly in ultimate result from the result claimed at the present day by analysts who spin their analyses to four or five years. (Glover 1955, pp. 382-383)

Balint's (1948, 1954) studies of the consequences of analytic training and the training analysis on the duration of therapeutic analyses deserve special mention because of their great frankness. Subsequent developments have confirmed Balint's findings. The increase in the duration of therapeutic analyses apparently depends the world over on the duration of training analyses. Balint showed that supertherapy goes back to a demand Ferenczi raised in 1927:

> I have often stated on previous occasions that in principle I can admit no difference between a therapeutic and a training analysis, and I now wish to supplement this by suggesting that, while every case undertaken for therapeutic purposes need not be carried to the depth we mean when we talk of complete ending of the analysis, the analyst himself, on whom the fate of so many other people depends, must know and be in control of even the most recondite weaknesses of his own character; and this is impossible without a fully completed analysis. (Ferenczi 1955 [1927], p. 84)

Balint referred to this fully completed analysis as "supertherapy" and used Freud's words to describe its goal:

> What we are asking is whether the analyst has had such a far-reaching influence on the patient that no further change could be expected to take place in him if his analysis were continued. It is as though it were possible by means of analysis to attain to a level of absolute psychical normality — a level, moreover, which we could feel confident would be able to remain stable .... (1937 c, pp. 219-220)

What is alarming is that, according to Balint, the formation of schools within the psychoanalytic movement and the burdens of the profession were the causes of the increased length of training analyses. The continuation of such analyses even after the official end of training coincided with the fact that this voluntary analysis (as a completely private matter) was held in high esteem. Balint reported that only the first shy protests had been heard about the correctness of supertherapy. According to them, the issue in supertherapy was then no longer therapy or even the immediate goal of training analyses, but rather pure self-knowledge.

According to Balint the first period in the history of training analysis was concerned with teaching, the second with demonstration, and the third with analysis as such; he also referred to a fourth period, concerned with research. In our opinion, the transformation into supertherapy for its own sake lacks everything commonly understood as research. Precisely what goes on in the prolonged training analysis has not been made the object of scientific study. The fact that the entire psychoanalytic movement was taken by the idea of the supertherapy, in fact thrives on it, is especially instructive. Training and supervisory analyses were the means by which schools constituted themselves around the various forms of supertherapy. The result is now exactly the opposite of what Ferenczi had hoped from the perfection of training analysis, which he called the second fundamental rule of psychoanalysis:

> Since the establishment of that rule the importance of the personal element introduced by the analyst has more and more been dwindling away. Anyone who has been thoroughly analysed and has gained complete knowledge and control of the inevitable weaknesses and peculiarities of his own character will inevitably come to the same objective conclusions in the observation and treatment of the same psychological raw material, and will consequently adopt the same tactical and technical methods in dealing with it. I have the definite impression that since the introduction of the second fundamental rule differences in analytic technique are tending to disappear. (Ferenczi 1955 [1928], p. 89)

Balint's comment on this was:

> It is a pathetic and sobering experience to realize that although this idealized, utopian description gives a fairly true picture of any of the present cliques of the psycho-analytic movement, it is utterly untrue if applied to the whole. Ferenczi foresaw correctly the results of *one* "supertherapy," but he had not even thought of the possibility that the real development would lead to the co-existence of several "supertherapies" competing with one another and leading to a repetition of the Confusion of Tongues. (1954, p. 161)

This competition would have to be decided on the basis of qualitative criteria. Since these, however, cannot be made the object of research in the case of private supertherapy, people resort to numbers: the longer analyses last, the better they are. The competition is decided by the duration of the supertherapy.

The identifications which develop in the course of training and supervisory analyses lead analysts to compare therapeutic analyses (and their duration) with their own experience. The result is that the duration of analyses of patients increases with that of training analyses. The latter is naturally not the only reason, but we have dealt with it here since this aspect of this unusually complex subject is not commonly discussed.

The discovery of preoedipally rooted pathological conditions is given as the primary reason for the increased length of therapeutic analyses. The use of object relationship theories in long analyses showed promise that narcissistic disturbances and borderline personalities could be treated successfully. This led indirectly to the lengthening of the treatment for neurotic patients, in whom narcissistic personality traits were now also being increasingly diagnosed. However much the theories about disturbances of early origin differ, they are all concerned with deep layers, which allegedly can only be reached with difficulty and after protracted work. A contradiction first pointed out by Rangell (1966) becomes immediately apparent here; he considered it impossible for early preverbal experiences to be revived in analysis. Therefore the analysis of deeper layers of psychic life cannot lead where object relationship theorists in the tradition of Ferenczi or Klein and where the self theorists in the tradition of Kohut believed it did. "Where are we then?" is the question that can be asked of every school with regard to the constantly increasing length of analytic treatment.

Freud clearly described a quantitative and qualitative relationship between the length of therapy and the chronic nature and severity of the illness:

> It is true that the treatment of a fairly severe neurosis may easily extend over several years; but consider, in case of success, how long the illness would have lasted. A decade, probably, for every year of treatment: the illness, that is to say (as we see so often in untreated cases), would not have ended at all. (1933a, p. 156)

Freud summarized the result in his terse statement, "An analysis is ended when the analyst and the patient cease to meet each other for the analytic session" because the patient is no longer suffering from his symptoms and "there is no need to fear a repetition of the pathological processes concerned" (1937c, p. 219).

If we take these justifications seriously, the length of an analysis is then tied to decisions which place high demands on the analyst's responsibility. Together with many other analysts, we urge greater frankness with regard to decisions about duration and frequency. Our recommendation is to let the severity of the symptoms and the aims of therapy be the guide. Of course, the severity of the illness and the frequency of treatment cannot simply be related quantitatively according to the equation that therapy must be more intense (and thus more frequent) the more severe the illness. The decisive factors are obviously the quality of what the analyst mediates and what the patient can accept and work through. Especially the severely ill, who seek much support, have great difficulties regulating their needs for closeness and distance. Critical questions of dosage then make it necessary to consider the situation qualitatively.

It is therefore particularly disturbing that quantitative aspects (length and frequency) play such an important role in analyses which take place within the framework of psychoanalytic training. Psychoanalytic societies set a minimum number of hours for such supervised treatment. The candidate's own interest in attaining his professional goal thus almost inevitably interferes with his decision as to the length and frequency of treatment that are in the patient's best interest. For example, the German Psychoanalytic Association set 300 hours as the minimum length for training cases at the time of the final examinatin; this is linked with the expectation that the analysis will continue thereafter. This requirement creates additonal complications because, under the limits imposed by the German health insurance system on the extent of psychotherapy and psychoanalysis, the financing of psychoanalytic therapy beyond 300 hours of treatment is subject to very special criteria (see Sect. 6.6). Under these circumstances it is difficult for any analyst, and not just candidates in training, to find satisfactory answers based on qualitative evaluation.

### *8.9.3 Criteria for Termination*

Analysts are always in danger of setting their criteria for termination and their goals according to personal and/or currently fashionable ideas and theories. Some limit the formulation of their goals to the level of metapsychology, where they are least open to criticism, while others orient themselves at the level of clinical practice.

The kinds of questions that analysts ask about goals determine the kinds of answers that they reach. Weiss and Fleming (1980) ask what state the patient's personality should be in when he leaves treatment. In their opinion, well-conducted analyses are characterized by the fact that the patient is freer from conflict and more independent than previously, and also has more confidence in his own capabilities. There is an increase in secondary process thinking and in the ability to test reality critically and to sublimate. There is an improvement in object relationships. The patient has developed a better understanding of the distinction between the analyst as a professional and as an object of transference.

A different kind of question concerns whether the patient has sufficient means and instruments to continue the analytic process independently. We would like to return to the topic of self-analysis because of its great significance. As we described with regard to the processes by which the patient identifies with the analyst (Sect. 8.4), we view identification with the analyst and his analytic technique as the most decisive step for the future progress of an analysis. We agree with Hoffer (1950), G. Ticho (1967, 1971), and E. Ticho (1971) that the acquisition of the capacity for self-analysis is a prime goal of psychoanalytic treatment. However, this goal stands in contrast to the fact that so far very little has been described in concrete terms about what actually goes on in the patient when he tries self-analysis after the termination of treatment. After interviewing colleagues, G. Ticho (1971) devised a scheme which is of assistance for further research. For Ticho, self-analysis is a process composed of different steps of work which have to be learned in sequence.

1. The ability is formed to pick up signals of an unconscious conflict; for example, an irrational or exaggerated response is perceived without having to overcompensate for it immediately with defense mechanisms such as displacement and projection.
2. Managing, without too much anxiety, to let thoughts run their own course, to associate freely, and to create a relatively free access to the id.
3. Being able to wait for a longer period of time to understand the significance of an unconscious conflict without becoming disappointed and giving up. The development of this ability is an indicator of how far the patient was able to identify with that part of the analyst which confidently waited during the analysis for the analysand to be ready to solve the conflict.
4. Following the insight that has been gained and attaining a change in himself [and/or in his environment]. This ability is formed as soon as the ego is sufficiently strong, and if the analysand was able in analysis to actually experience that insight can really lead to modifications of the ego. (G. Ticho 1971, p. 32)

We assume that the analysand acquires the capacity to self-analysis in a continuous, almost incidental learning process in which he identifies with the analytic functions (see Sect. 8.4). It is possible for the analyst to plan the end of treatment when he feels able to expect that the analysand has acquired the capacity for self-analysis. Once this goal has been achieved, other criteria for termination can be relativized. Firestein (1982) compiled a list of such criteria, including improvement of symptoms, structural change, reliable object constancy in relationships, and a fair balance between the realms of the id, the superego, and defense structures. *Relativization of these criteria* does not mean their rejection, but only *careful evaluation of them compared to the other goals that might be achieved given a lengthening of the analytic work.* Setting one's goals in terms of personality traits instead of abilities such as self-analysis fails to satisfy Freud's admonishing words in his essay "Analysis Terminable and Interminable" (see 1937 c, p. 250).

The ability to change is often more limited than we want to believe. Gaining knowledge of his own limits may often be more important to the patient than chasing after a utopia. This opinion may come as a surprise since we have referred throughout to the change as proof of the precious link between treatment and research (see Chap. 10). Yet "structural change" is a goal of treatment which seems to be one of the most difficult constructions of the psychoanalytic psychology of the personality to grasp, both theoretically and empirically; we therefore content ourselves with putting the patient in a position to structure his life in a way that it is more congruent with his desires and limitations than before treatment. Freud's (1933 a, p. 80) words "Where id was, there ego shall be" describe realistic goals of analytic treatment when the ego has reacquired insight and the ability to act.

### *8.9.4 The Postanalytic Phase*

The analyst's handling of his relationship to the patient after the termination of psychoanalytic treatment has received little attention. Comments on this topic are rather rare, even in verbal communication among psychoanalysts, in great contrast to the otherwise intense exchange of experiences. Our view of how Freud dealt with these questions is distorted by the fact that the reports on treatment conducted by him that have become known to the analytic world all come from patients in exceptional positions, e.g., Blanton, an analyst, or Doolittle, an author Freud held in high esteem. They thus do not permit us to draw conclusions about Freud's behavior in general. Today there is general agreement that the postanalytic phase has great significance for the further course and development of the processes of maturation initiated in the treatment. Yet in Menninger and Holzman's textbook (1958, p. 179), all we find is the matter-of-fact statement: "The parties part company. The contract has been fulfilled."

The subject of what occurs after the real separation of analyst and patient is an area in which "analysts, by falling so short of the scientific approach, have deprived themselves of the data and the contradictions so vital to the growth of psychoanalysis as a science" (Schlessinger and Robbins 1983, p. 6). Systematic follow-up studies were not common for a long time. The few thorough studies, that we will discuss, show more than clearly that our ideas about the postanalytic phase and the further reaching assimilation of the experience of psychoanalytic therapy belong to the gold mines that we have overlooked for too long. We must be very cautious in transferring the experience of self-analysis, as described by Kramer (1959), G. Ticho (1971), and Calder (1980), to patients. After training, analysts belong to a professional group, have constant contact to other analysts, and must always rely on self-analysis in their daily work. The conception of a postanalytic phase, as introduced by Rangell (1966), fits our understanding of events in the therapeutic process. The form that such postanalytic contacts should take is a matter of controversy and is determined by the inappropriate conception of the resolution of transference (see Chap. 2) and the corresponding anxiety regarding a revival of transference.

Is the analyst supposed to work toward a state in which the patient no longer seeks contact, with the goal that the analysis is so integrated into the patient's life that it succumbs to amnesia, like infantile memories? Or should the analyst stay open for renewed contacts? E. Ticho (according to Robbins 1975) supports the view that the analyst should not provide the patient the assurance that he is available for further consultation, because this would undermine the patient's confidence in himself. In contrast, Hoffer (1950) provides support to patients in this phase inasmuch as they require it. For Buxbaum (1950, p. 189), it is a sign of a successful analysis if the patient can say that he can take or leave the analyst. In her opinion, this is easier if the analyst permits the patient to renew contact if he wants to and thinks it necessary, even in the absence of symptoms. It is her experience that patients occasionally take up this offer but never abuse it. A strict "never more" would rather have a traumatic effect on the patient because it puts him in a passive position. Dewald (1982) suggests handling the question of postanalytic contact with intuition. While the refusal of further contact is a source of torment for some patients, such contact may be an unhealthy encouragement to be ill for others. Greenson (see Robbins 1975) experimented in one treatment by seeing one patient every four weeks for several months after the analysis. In this way the role of the analyst changed from psychoanalyst to listener to the former patient's self-analysis.

It seems obvious that the analyst should adopt a flexible attitude. If postanalytic contacts are clearly necessitated by the survival of some attitudes from transference neurosis, therapy in the form described by Bräutigam (1983, p. 130) seems appropriate. It is generally sensible to inform the patient that if his own self-analysis is insufficient to help him cope with current burdens, he can seek renewed contact to his previous or another analyst (see Zetzel 1965).

How the analyst handles real posttreatment contacts, whether coincidental or professional, is another matter. It is no longer appropriate and can only be inhibiting and harmful to maintain an attitude characterized by analytic distance. Yet the other extreme is characterized by the attempt to avoid neutrality by stimulating the patient into a premature and intensive familiarity; he often then reacts as if this were a dangerous temptation. The consequences of both attitudes are unfavorable, the first leading to inhibition and regressive dependence while the other precipitates confusion, anxiety, or hypomanic acting out. The best way to organize social and professional contacts after the termination of treatment lies somewhere between these extremes (Rangell 1966).

With regard to the further development of the analytic relationship following the termination of treatment, we would like to suggest that radical separation be generally replaced by the model of the unconscious structure characterizing an individual's relationship to his family doctor. As Balint demonstrated, the decisive aspect of the relationship to the family doctor is the feeling that he is available when needed. In our opinion, the analyst should lead the patient in working through the problems of separation on the basis of this feeling. To compare separation with death is an inappropriate exaggeration of the analytic relationship. This would only lead to artificial dramatization, so strengthening the unconscious fantasies of omnipotence and their projections that separation becomes even more difficult. It should remain possible to actualize the patient's latent readiness to enter a relationship, if it becomes necessary, because anyone can be so affected by changes in his life that he would like to turn to an analyst again. Whether this is the same analyst or, for external reasons, another one is secondary. Important is the basic feeling of having had a good experience, which gives people the confidence to again seek the help of an analyst.

Long-term observation following completed analyses is one of the neglected fields of study into which Waelder (1956) encouraged research. It is sensible to distinguish between unsystematic clinical investigations and systematic, empirical follow-up studies. Each has its own significance. The practicing analyst can make important long-term observations. The usually exaggerated concern about over an unnecessary revival of transference has excessively restricted analysts' curiosity and readiness for contact.

Pfeffer (1959) introduced a procedure of follow-up investigation which conforms to the self-understanding of psychoanalysis. This procedure took the form of psychoanalytic interviews, and its utility was confirmed by later studies (Pfeffer 1961, 1963). In each of the examined cases, the consequences of persisting unconscious conflicts — related to the originally diagnosed conflicts — were demonstrated clearly. The benefit gained from psychoanalytic treatment consisted primarily in the patient's ability to handle these conflicts in a suitable way.

Analysts seem to be gradually accepting the view that such follow-up studies not only provide external legitimation of psychoanalysis, but also represent a fruitful method of studying postanalytic change (Norman et al. 1976; Schlessinger and Robbins 1983). Previous case studies have demonstrated the stability of recurring patterns of conflict; such patterns are acquired in childhood and as such are relatively immutable. They form the individual product of the processes of maturation and development, structure childhood experiencing, and constitute the kernel of neurosis. Psychoanalytic treatment does not lead to the dissolution of these patterns of conflict, but to an increased capacity for tolerance and coping with frustration, anxiety, and depression based on the development of the ability for self-analysis. This capacity is established as a preconscious strategy to cope with conflicts by means of an identification with the analyst's endeavor to observe, understand, and integrate psychological processes. This is how Schlessinger and Robbins (1983) summarize the results of their follow-up studies. We believe that these findings remove a burden from us as analysts. They are also a source of satisfaction in that the analytic work can be portrayed more realistically and equitably by such follow-up studies than by any other method.

Systematic follow-up studies pursue other goals, especially those which have become possible at psychoanalytic outpatient clinics since Fenichel's (1930) first study of the results at the Berlin Psychoanalytic Institute (see Jones 1936; Alexander 1937; Knight 1941). Such studies attempt to evaluate the influence of different factors on the therapeutic process and its result, and are only possible with large samples of data (see, e.g., Kernberg et al. 1972; Kordy et al. 1983; Luborsky et al. 1980; Sashin et al. 1975; Weber et al. 1985; Wallerstein 1986). A survey of the state of research on the results of psychotherapy is given by Bergin and Lambert (1978).

Very few analysts have recognized the importance of such global evaluations of results despite their great value for social policy. In Germany, follow-up studies of this kind have contributed decisively to the inclusion of psychoanalysis in the treatment covered by health insurance (Dührssen 1953, 1962). Precisely because the current state of research on therapeutic outcomes goes far beyond simplifying procedures (Kächele and Schors 1981), systematic follow-up studies on the legitimacy of the inclusion of long-term psychoanalysis in the treatment covered by the public health insurance system is urgently required, especially in view of the impressive results achieved by psychodynamic short therapies (Luborsky 1984; Strupp and Binder 1984).

# 9 The Psychoanalytic Process

Although we have discussed various aspects of psychoanalytic treatment in the foregoing chapters, we have not focussed our attention on the role these aspects play in the therapeutic process as a whole. We have concentrated on segments of greatly varying duration within the course of treatment and alternated between macro- and microperspectives of the analytic process (see Baumann 1984). We have on the one hand used a magnifying glass to concentrate on small facets of treatment, such as the patient's questions, and on the other hand investigated the analyst's general treatment strategies — while maintaining the necessary distance to detail.

Psychoanalytic treatment can be characterized in many ways. A wide variety of metaphors have been used to delineate the characteristic and essential features of psychoanalysis. We have discussed Freud's comparison of the analytic process with chess, as well as the analogies that he saw between the analyst's activities and those of the archaeologist, painter, and sculptor (Chaps. 7 and 8). Although Freud left no doubt that the analyst can decisively influence the course of analysis, either for better or for worse, he placed more emphasis on the autonomous course of analysis:

> The analyst ... sets in motion a process, that of the resolving of existing repressions. He can supervise this *process*, further it, remove obstacles in its way, and he can undoubtedly vitiate much of it. But on the whole, once begun, it goes its own way and does not allow either the direction it takes or the order in which it picks up its points to be prescribed for it. (1913c, p. 130, emphasis added)

Implicit in these metaphors are theories and models which we now want to identify. Sandler's (1983) demand that the dimension of private meaning in concepts be worked out in order to achieve real progress is also directed at the practicing analyst:

> Research should be directed toward making explicit the implicit concepts of practising psychoanalysts, and it is suggested that this process will result in the accelerated development of psychoanalytic theory. The essentials of that theory must be those aspects which relate to the work the psychoanalyst has to do, and therefore its main emphasis needs to be clinical. (p. 43)

To aid in accomplishing this task, the following sections contain discussions of the function of process models (Sect. 9.1) and of the features essential for evaluating them (Sect. 9.2), and a description of various conceptions of the process (Sect. 9.3), including our own (Sect. 9.4).

## 9.1 Function of Process Models

If we focus our attention on the therapeutic process, i.e., on the entire distance that the patient and analyst together cover between the initial interview and the termination of analysis, it is necessary to relegate the vast majority of the events that occur to the background. We have to restrict ourselves to essentials, otherwise we run the risk of not seeing the woods for the trees. The heart of the matter with regard to the function *and* general difficulties of process models is that events are not essential per se, but are made essential by the *significance* that we attach to them. What the psychoanalyst considers to be of great significance during the course of therapy depends on the pattern of meanings he has internalized regarding the organization and course of the psychoanalytic process. We can postpone answering the question of how explicit and differentiated the ideas about the analytic process are or should be. At this juncture we wish solely to emphasize that no therapist can conduct or evaluate treatment without having a model of the possible courses of therapy which provides him with instructions for action and with criteria to use in evaluation.

The analyst's conception of the process fulfills an important regulatory function in the transformation of his goals into interventions. The understanding of the process is thus not merely abstract and theoretical. On the contrary, it is, in a more or less elaborated form, a component of every therapist's daily activity. Yet this is the point where the qualitative differences between the more implicit views of the analytic process and the detailed models begin to emerge. The less explicitly or more generally a model is formulated, the more easily it evades critical reflection. For this reason, the models handed down from one generation of analysts to the next are often formulated in such general terms that it is impossible for them to be refuted by observation. It is dubious, however, whether such models are adequate for the object they refer to.

One of the factors decisive in determining whether analysts' ideas about the analytic process are adequate is the position these ideas occupy on the scales "degree of complexity" and "degree of inference." We attribute the status of a model to a conception located near the poles "complex" (in contrast to "undifferentiated") and "inferential" (in contrast to "observable").

According to Klaus and Buhr (1972, p. 729), a model is

> an object which is introduced and used by a subject on the basis of a structural, functional, or behavioral analogy in order to be able to solve a certain task .... The use of a model is especially necessary in certain situations in order to gain new knowledge about the original object.

This definition is based on an understanding of "model" that originated in the fields of science and technology, as Klaus and Buhr made clear:

> A common feature of all models is that they cannot be arbitrarily created (chosen or produced) by a subject, but instead are subordinated to their own inner regularity, which is the real object of analysis in the subject's model experiment, cognition, behavioral adaption etc. (p. 730)

This definition of the concept of the model does not apply to models of the psychoanalytic process. The act of cognition as practiced by an analyst during treatment, in his role as participant observer, is clearly different from that in the sciences, where the object is not altered by the researcher's observations. The scientific researcher influences the object only as part of a controlled experiment. Most importantly, however, the researcher himself, as a person exerting influence, is not part of the object being studied (see also Sect. 3.1). Although this epistemological view of science is increasingly being questioned, for instance in modern physics, qualitative differences nonetheless remain between the modes of cognition of a scientist and a psychoanalyst. The analyst who approaches his object, the analytic process, with a specific conception of a model *influences, by means of his expectations, the occurrence of events* which agree with his model. Thus, an analyst who views therapy as a sequence of predetermined phases looks carefully for signs marking the transition to the next phase. He will, at the same time, selectively pursue those of the patient's utterances which fit his model of the analytic process. He may thus actually determine the direction the process takes, although he believes that he has only observed it. In this way, he transforms his model of the process, which he takes to be *descriptive*, into therapeutic action in a *prescriptive* manner.

The reason that we have emphasized this aspect is not that we consider such a procedure to be reprehensible. On the contrary, the analyst has no choice but to understand the therapeutic process on the basis of his model of it, to derive hypotheses from this model, and to conduct therapy according to these hypotheses. The critical question is not whether the analyst derives his course of action from his model, but whether he follows this course of action in a strictly prescriptive way.

In our discussion of therapeutic rules and strategies (see Chaps. 7 and 8), we have placed great value on the distinction between stereotypical and heuristic strategies. Process models can also be used by the analyst in a stereotypical way, i.e., as if they were algorithms. An algorithm lays down a precise sequence of individual steps which lead inevitably to the prescribed goal if followed exactly. Process models cannot adopt such a prescriptive function; they must always be employed in a heuristic and creative manner (Peterfreund 1983). A model can be used as an algorithm only if it is all-encompassing, a condition that will probably never be satisfied with regard to the psychoanalytic process. Process models provide suggestions as to how the highly complex, dyad-specific information accumulated over a long period of time can be organized. Even after this form of organization has been chosen, it must still be tested over and over again as to whether it can integrate new information.

The analyst must pay special attention to information that does *not* fit his model. He will always be able to find items among the wealth of material which confirm his model; however, this says little about the utility of his understanding of the analytic process. Information which cannot be integrated serves, in contrast, as an incentive for him to modify his understanding of the analytic process in such a way as to make it compatible with the new information. In this way, the analyst's image gradually becomes a more accurate approximation of the object.

We realize how great a mental effort is required and how much of an emotional burden it is on the analyst to admit that the conception of the analytic process that he has used is inappropriate, and thus consciously to create the insecurity which inevitably results. An essential function of process models is, after all, to introduce order into the multiplicity of information, to steer the therapist's perception and behavior, and thus to ensure continuity in his therapeutic measures. It is understandable that nobody likes to lose such support, even if only temporarily. Such a short-term loss of orientation is easier to tolerate if the analyst has resisted the seductive idea that there is a true model of the psychoanalytic process. In our opinion, the notion of a true process model is just as fictive as that of a true psychoanalytic process which follows natural laws and immanent regularities as long as the analyst's interventions do not disturb it. Process models have a direct impact on therapy. Whether an analyst adheres to the fiction of a natural process, or rather views treatment as a dyad-specific, psychosocial process of negotiation, thus has very real consequences for the patient. An analyst holding the latter view must repeatedly determine whether his assumptions regarding the analytic process are still compatible with his observations of the interaction in each individual case.

It is primarily up to the individual analyst whether he (erroneously) takes his process model for reality, and consequently directs his interventions in a stereotypical way, or whether he views it as a tool in the organization of the process which must be revised as soon as information incompatible with it is acquired by means of heuristic strategies. Of course, certain characteristics of models tend to lead to *stereotypical* interpretations, while others tend to promote the use of *heuristic* strategies. We would now like to discuss different characteristics of process models from this point of view.

## 9.2 Features of Process Models

As we have explained above, the issue is not to distinguish between true and false process models. At issue is rather the suitability of different process models to provide effective therapeutic strategies. The central criterion in this regard seems to us to be whether a model presumes the psychoanalytic process to follow a quasi-natural course. Such models do not inevitably lead to a stereotypical application by the analyst, but they do support any tendency he may have to orient himself rigidly on the expected, natural course. Observations that do not fit into a course conforming with the model are often ignored or interpreted as manifestations of resistance.

This can be seen particularly clearly in the way analysts deal with utterances by patients which indicate that they either have failed to understand or do not accept particular interpretations. If a patient's rejection of an interpretation is then interpreted on the basis of the very hypothesis that the patient did not understand or accept, and is thus understood as resistance, the analyst will remain a captive of his preconception and the patient will be deprived of a possibility to make major corrections to it. Although the concept of resistance is well founded, as we discuss in Chap. 4, it must still be possible in the everyday communicative situation in analysis for a patient's rejection of an interpretation to be accepted as valid (see also Thomä and Houben 1967; Wisdom 1967).

Prominent among the models suggesting a quasi-natural course of treatment is the widespread view that the process of therapy is analogous to development in early childhood. In Sect. 9.3 we will discuss Fürstenau's (1977) process model as a typical example of this type. The most common assumption in such models is that the patient progresses from early to later stages of development in the course of therapy. That this is not inevitably the case can be seen in Balint's account of "a peculiar phase in the analytic treatment of patients." He described it in the following way:

> My clinical experience was briefly this: At times when the analytic work has already progressed a long way, i.e. towards the end of a cure, my patients began — very timidly at first — to desire, to expect, even to demand certain simple gratifications, mainly, though not exclusively, from their analyst. (Balint 1952, p. 245)

The patients Balint refers to here are not in a position to examine their basal pathogenic assumptions (in the sense described by Weiss and Sampson 1984) during therapy until after the primarily oedipal conflicts have been dealt with and the patients experience the resulting increase in ego strength and security. A.E. Meyer (personal communication) suggests calling this "the chronological retrograde model."

Patients' process models also have a place in this discussion; they are an accurate reflection of how patients experience the process. Patients often speak of analysis as the exploration of their own house. This metaphor invites reflections on the interior structure of the building. Even if careful observation from the outside can give an experienced architect some clues to the interior design, knowledge about the layout, use, and furnishings of the rooms can only be gained by seeing inside. Of course, houses have many things in common that we can infer on the basis of our knowledge of their construction and function. Similarly, human psychic development takes each of us inevitably through certain stages, as has been described by many authors (e.g., Erikson 1959). We acquire our psychic structure in grappling with the developmental tasks facing every one of us: separation from symbiosis, triangulation, Oedipus configuration, adolescence, etc. The accessibility of these structures to therapeutic work depends on a multitude of different factors which interact with the treatment technique and which we grasp as intrapsychic defense and acts of psychosocial adjustment (see Mentzos' [1982, p. 109] description of his three-dimensional model of diagnosis).

Viewing the process of therapy and development in early childhood as parallel phenomena is certainly often accurate and may provide a fruitful guide for intervention. Yet this approach becomes problematic if applied inflexibly, e.g., if the analyst overlooks the fact that the therapeutic process, as formed together with the adult patient, differs from early childhood experiences in some essential aspects, not the least of which is the quality of subjective experience. Early experiences *cannot* be reexperienced authentically; the therapeutic process is always concerned with the overdetermined experiences of an adult.

A process model oriented toward psychological development must also do justice to these experiences.

The seductive element of these models is, as described above, the implication that the individual phases follow an inevitable sequence. The result can be that the analyst considers and uses only information which fits into the current phase, disregarding the rest. Thus one phase after the other may be *created* interactively, while their sequence is interpreted as a process-immanent regularity. In models based on the idea that the psychoanalytic process follows a natural course, the patient's development is logically at the center of attention. If, in contrast, the psychoanalytic treatment is considered to be a dyad-specific, interactional process (see Sect. 9.4), the therapist's contribution is very important.

Another, essential criterion for the evaluation of process models is provided by the answers to the questions: What does a model say about the analyst's role? Which function in the formation of the process is attributed to him? Generally it is possible to assume that the more "natural" or autonomous a process is conceived to be, the less there is to say about the analyst's role (and about the responsibility he assumes for it). In the extreme case, he fulfills his function merely by being aware of the process regularities postulated by his model and not disturbing their course. In this case, the employment of heuristic strategies by the analyst is neither necessary nor desirable. His behavior is in any case not oriented primarily around the patient, but rather around his "natural" view of the process, which he as a rule attempts to support with neutrality and interpretations.

In such an approach an important role is logically played by the question of whether a patient the analyst has just seen for an initial interview is at all suited for this process, since its course is determined by the "nature of things." An adaptive indication, in the sense we propose (see Chap. 6), is not possible in this framework because it demands great flexibility on the part of the analyst, who has to offer himself in changing roles as a partner for interaction.

We have described an extreme case in order to clarify a risk that becomes greater the more "naturally" the analyst views the analytic process, namely the danger that he will evade his obligation to see that the therapeutic process is structured in a responsible and flexible way. We believe he may thus incorrectly classify a growing number of patients as nonanalyzable.

We would like to describe the view put forward by Menninger and Holzman (1958) as an example of an understanding of the analytic process which hardly specifies the analyst's role. These authors propose a process model according to which a suitable patient makes a contract with the analyst and, at the end of a typical process, has changed his psychic structure and resolved his transference. This view is, by the way, refuted by the follow-up studies conducted by Schlessinger and Robbins (1983). According to them the resolution of transference at the end of successful therapy is a myth; on the contrary, even successfully analyzed patients soon showed clear manifestations of transference in follow-up interviews. For Menninger and Holzman the analyst seems to be not much more than a usually silent companion whose patience and friendliness convince the analysand that his love and hate transferences lack all positive and negative foundation in the present.

This fiction of a psychoanalytic process purified of the real person of the analyst presumes the existence of an average analyst and a suitable patient. Disregarding the fact that there is no such patient-analyst pair, this conception also prevents the findings of social science research commensurate with the essence of the therapeutic relationship from entering the psychoanalytic situation. The pressing problems of psychoanalytic technique cannot be solved by upholding — as a kind of counterreaction to the identity crisis — an increasingly rigid conception of treatment. On the contrary, we assign the analyst a central role in codetermining the structure of the therapeutic process. He fulfills this role in a dyad-specific way which depends on his own personality and on the patient. This view of the therapist's role cannot be reconciled with the conception of the psychoanalytic process as a natural event.

Each of these two opposing conceptions of the psychoanalytic process is at first nothing more than a statement of belief. Information on the suitability of process models can ultimately only be provided by the observation of psychoanalytic processes. A precondition for this is that the models be formulated in a way which makes it possible to validate or refute them by observation. We consider this question of the empirical validation of process models to be an important criterion for the evaluation of different models; it is in fact the only way to determine their utility.

This precondition requires that models be made as explicit as currently possible. The closer to the level of observation the models are formulated, the more clearly operational hypotheses can be derived which then can be tested on observable events in interviews. It must be possible to test hypotheses and especially to collect data incompatible with the model. This means that a model which can effortlessly explain an outcome diametrically opposed to the original prognosis is useless. Yet precisely in the formation of psychoanalytic theories, there is a widespread tendency to devise such irrefutable models. This is certainly due partly to the initial helplessness which inevitably overcomes analysts when they are confronted with the highly complex subject matter. It is risky to make prognoses if human behavior is overdetermined, if the struggle between wish and defense is undecided. The uncertainty increases with the length of time for which the prognosis is supposed to be valid. Thus the formulation of process models is always an uncertain undertaking. This is especially true if the models are supposed, ideally, to provide a grid enabling the analyst to classify a large number of interactive, interdependent events without detailed knowledge about the nature of the relationship between them.

There are two conceivable ways out of this difficulty. One is to formulate process models in such an abstract manner that they become universally valid and thus irrefutable. This form of theorizing is a dead end and distorts, rather than sharpens, one's eye for new material. An expression of such abstract generalization is the apparent ability of some analysts to fit a case into a comprehensive theoretical framework after only a short presentation, a fact that is a frequent source of wonder at clinical seminars. The case is forced into the Procrustean bed of a theory, and information which does not fit is passed over, while information which is lacking is presumed to be compatible with the theory.

The other way of coping with the complexity of the psychoanalytic process is to limit the model's claim to provide a comprehensive conception of the process. A fruitful approach is initially to propose hypotheses in the form of if-then statements concerning various events which commonly recur in the course of therapy. Both the "if" and the "then" components should be specified as exactly as possible in order to ensure the refutability of the hypotheses.

## 9.3 Models of the Psychoanalytic Process

Freud's technical recommendations for the conducting of treatment, and thus for the process, are rather cursory, intentionally vague, and indefinite with regard to the overall course of treatment. Although a whole series of rules (Chap. 7) and strategies (Chap. 8) can be compiled, no understanding of the process can be discerned which does more than simply label the initial, middle, and concluding phases of analysis, as Glover (1955) noted. We have already mentioned Menninger and Holzman's understanding of the process; regardless of how the substance of their position is evaluated, their attempt to outline an understanding of the entire process is an expression of awareness of the problem and was warmly welcomed upon its publication in 1958. The development of a theory of psychoanalytic therapy which is more than a loose collection of technical principles has been an unsolved task since Bibring's presentation at the Marienbad congress in 1936. The number of coherent process models which have collected statements about individual issues in order to provide an overall understanding nonetheless remains small. This is probably related both to the preference of most analysts for an essayistic presentation of case studies (Kächele 1981) and to the complexity of the subject matter. The following descriptions of several of the attempts to formulate process models reflect this state of development.

One common feature of thinking about the process is the concept of *phase*. The differentiation of individual stages of treatment according to the accepted substantive patterns is a feature both of the case descriptions by candidates in training, characterized by the frequent use of headings rich in images, and of the approach taken by Meltzer (1967), who describes the following phases of the typical processes in children's analyses conducted according to Klein:

1. The gathering of transference
2. The sorting of geographical confusions
3. The sorting of zonal confusions
4. The threshold of the depressive position
5. The weaning process

According to Meltzer (1967, p. 3), this sequence of phases expresses a truly natural, *organic process* which originates when a treatment is conducted strictly according to Klein's methods. The sequence of stages from early to later development is obvious in the understanding of child analysis, but becomes problematic if used in an attempt to understand the analytic process in adults. This is illustrated by Fürstenau's (1977) model of the "progressive structure of nonfocal psychoanalytic treatment." This progressive structure results from the interplay of dynamic factors in the analytic situation which we have already described in numerous ways.

In the psychoanalytic process it is important to distinguish two interwined dimensions which together constitute the progressive structure. According to Fürstenau (1977, p. 858), these two partial processes are:

1. The process of the gradual structuring and normalization of the self, with recurrent phases of severe structurally formative relapses in regressive crises, and of the analyst's manner of dealing with it in a substitutive and supportive way.
2. The process of the scenic unravelling and processing of fixations, layer by layer, through the analysis of transference and countertransference.

We will now briefly describe the seven phases of Fürstenau's progressive model and mention the problems it brings. According to Fürstenau, each phase is described from the general points of view of "working through the rigid patterns which the patient carries over" and "constructing a new pattern of relationships."

In the first phase the analyst fulfills a maternal role for the patient; he behaves in a way intended to provide security.

In the second phase the patient unravels his symptoms; he still has little interest in understanding unconscious connections, but makes important discoveries with regard to the analyst's reliability and firmness.

In the third phase negative aspects of the early relationship to the mother are dealt with.

In the fourth phase a turn to oneself takes place by handling the concealed aggressions and affronts from the early mother-child relationship; this is accompanied by improvement in the diffuse depressive symptoms. In the analytic relationship, the patient learns that the analyst is interested in his secret fantasies without being obtrusive or making him feel guilty because of his narcissistic withdrawal.

In the fifth phase the patient's sexual identity is defined; analysis takes different courses for male and female patients. This theme is continued in the sixth phase, the phase of oedipal triangularity.

The termination of treatment in the seventh phase is facilitated by newly developed relationships which the patient has been able to establish both to himself and to partners. The working through of mourning is the focus of attention.

Fürstenau distinguishes between two classes of psychic disturbances, which he calls the relatively ego-intact neuroses and the structural ego disturbances. The latter class includes psychotic, narcissistically withdrawn, asocial, addicted, perverted, and psychosomatic patients. In contrast to the therapy of ego-intact patients, which proceeds in the described manner throughout the phases, especially in the first of the two partial processes outlined above, in the nonfocal psychoanalytic treatment of patients with structural ego disturbances the partial processes become intimately entwined. In addition, for the latter group there are changes especially in the first three phases of treatment. For instance, in the first phase the analyst must increasingly assume substitutive functions. Furthermore, there is no clear transition to the fourth phase, and the second half of the process is dominated by the patient's alternating occupation with himself and with others. "Corresponding to this, there is a continuous *alternation* in the analyst's interventions between working on transference and resistance, on the one hand, and strengthening the patient's self, on the other" (Fürstenau 1977, p. 869).

In contrast to our own process model (Sect. 9.4), Fürstenau's progressive structure is characterized by fixed content. This has a therapeutic function in itself because it provides the analyst security. Fürstenau developed this model structure on the basis of his experience in clinical supervision. One important aspect of agreement with our own view is the idea that the treatment process consists of phases characterized by different themes. Less accurate, in our opinion, is the assumption that the sequence of phases in every process is organized in the sense of a linear reworking of ontogenetic development. From the point of view of the social sciences, it is improbable that this model's claim to generality can be achieved; yet the establishment of a model of a typical course of treatment would certainly represent a great advance in the description of the course and outcome of psychoanalysis.

The advantage of such a model is that it adapts the psychoanalytic method to the real characteristics of two large groups of patients. This obviates continuous redefinition of the range of a more or less narrowly defined understanding of "classical technique." Consequently, it eliminates the source of the controversies — neither advantageous for psychoanalysis nor helpful to patients — which generally result in limiting the application of the so-called classical technique to patients with intrapsychic conflicts at the oedipal level, referring everyone else to analytic psychotherapy or so-called psychodynamic psychotherapies, or founding a new school of therapy for their treatment. Orientation on the method's potential could ultimately still lead to the differentiation according to type of illness which Freud (1919 a) called for. This implies the necessity for a certain degree of flexibility, in the sense of adjustment to the individual patient's needs, which has not yet been achieved. It is not difficult to recognize that Fürstenau's model of therapeutic activity also refers to the area of so-called narcissistic disturbances, in that it includes the partial process "of the gradual structuring and normalization of the self."

Kohut, in his later writings (1971, 1977), makes a fundamental distinction between a technique based on instinct theory and ego psychology, and his understanding of analysis and the restoration of the self. The process model in Kohut's theory of restoration of the self is determined by the following theses:

1. The selfobject seeks itself in others.
2. There is a lack of empathic resonance by the mother. The degree to which the empathic resonance is absent ultimately determines the deficit in the self. Empathic resonance is composed of several stages determined by development: mirror transference, twinship transference, and idealizing self transference. These determine the form taken by empathic resonance and are described as man's basic needs.

3. Deficits in self provide the decisive basis for all disturbances. In his later works Kohut (1984, p. 24) considers even oedipal pathology as an emanation of the nonempathic mother or father. In his view, if there were no primary self damage, there would be no castration anxiety with its *pathological* consequences.
4. After the resistances directed against renewed selfobject frustrations (frustrations because the other is not how we would like) have been overcome, there is a mobilization of "selfobject transferences" in the therapeutic process, with inevitable conflicts in the analytic relationship. The conflict is between the constant need for appropriate selfobject reactions on the one hand, and the patient's fear of injury of the self on the other. If the patient feels he has been understood, archaic, disavowed needs are revived on the selfobject in the selfobject transference.
5. The relationship between the analysand's self and the selfobject, i.e., the analyst's self function, is inevitably incomplete. Since the attempt to establish complete empathic harmony with the analysand is doomed to failure, there are self regressions with symptoms which are understood as disintegration products.
6. By means of his empathic resonance, the analyst senses the patient's legitimate needs for his selfobject function, which are buried under distorted manifestations. He clarifies the sequence of events and corrects his own misunderstandings.
7. The goal of therapy is the transformation of the "selfobject function of the selfobject analyst to a function of the analysand's self" (Wolf 1982, p. 312). This is known as transmuting internalization. What is significant is that the increase in self structure does not mean any independence from selfobjects; on the contrary, it means a greater capacity to find and to use them.

The application of these theses to the process of a classical transference neurosis, which by definition can be limited to oedipal conflicts, leads to the following structure of phases (Kohut 1984, p. 22):

1. A phase of "generally severe resistances"
2. A phase of "oedipal experiences in the traditional sense dominated by the experience of severe castration anxiety" (Oedipus complex)
3. A renewed phase of severe resistances
4. A phase of disintegration anxiety
5. A phase of "mild anxiety, alternating with joyous anticipation"
6. A final phase, for which Kohut suggests the term "oedipal stage in order to indicate its significance as a healthy, joyfully undertaken developmental step, the beginning of a gender-differentiated firm self that points to a fulfilling creative-productive future"

Kohut himself points out that the "one theoretical assumption" underlying this classification of phases is that "the process of analysis generally leads from the surface to the depth," from which he concludes that "transference sequences generally repeat developmental sequences *in the reverse order*" (1984, p. 22). The goal and motor of this process is to show the patient that "the sustaining echo of empathic resonance is indeed available in this world" (1984, p. 78).

In his last, posthumously published study, Kohut no longer shied away from using the well-known but disreputable expression "corrective emotional experience" to describe his position. As he points out, the controversy originally surrounding the expression arose from the manipulative use of the emotional experience as a replacement for working through. At the end of his life, Kohut considered his position to be firmly anchored in the classical technique, despite all changes, inasmuch as neutrality and abstinence constituted his basic position, supplemented by "dynamic (transference) interpretations and genetic reconstructions."

Critical evaluation of the theory of self must orient itself on the fact that the explanatory device which Kohut employs throughout his work is a contemporary version of the principle of security. Instinctual desire has been replaced by the regulation of the relationship to the meaningful other, which, however, is conceived according to the theory of narcissism.

Balint's early work on primary love intersects here with the social psychological theses of Cooley and Mead. Kohut rejected symbolic interactionism, even in the form represented by Erikson, to the great disadvantage of his own theory and practice. In this context mention must also be made of the first efforts to integrate Piaget's process of adaptation and accommodation into the psychoanalytic theory of development (see Wolff 1960; Greenspan 1979, 1981). Psychoanalytic object relationship psychologies do not do justice to the capacity for social interaction. In its first 6 months a baby learns "how to invite his mother to play and then initiate an interaction with her" (Stern 1977). Applying this new perspective to the psychoanalytic process, the question of regulatory competence becomes the focus of all considerations and leads to an understanding of process which possibly overcomes Kohut's one-sidedness and unnecessary generalizations, and which yet makes it apparent that Kohut discovered an important central factor: that the regulation of well-being and security is hierarchically superior to the realization of particular desires.

Our discussion of Moser et al.'s process model (which we outline below) is limited by the fact that the sphere of cognitive psychology (see Holt 1964) is still foreign to many psychoanalysts, and thus by the difficulty in presenting the conceptions in a manner compatible with a textbook. Moser et al. (1981) presented a theory of the regulation of mental processes in which they described object relationships, affects, and defense processes using the terminology normally employed in the development of computer simulation models. In their model, the analyst-analysand relationship is understood as the interaction of two process systems according to explicit or implicit rules. It is important to be able to imagine the concept of process systems in order to understand the following discussion. It might be helpful to refer to the familiar psychoanalytic structural model as a process system in which three regulatory contexts — ego, superego, and id — interact. "Context" refers to a loose grouping of affective cognitive functions whose interaction is (more or less) tense, comparable with Waelder's (1960) image of border traffic which is normal in peacetime but prohibited in times of war. Von Zeppelin (1981) emphasizes that the main assumption of the process model is that analyst and patient continuously make images (models) of the state of the regulatory system, both of their own and the other's, and of the presumed interaction. An important characteristic of the model is that a special regulatory context is established for the creation and maintenance of relationships, and that the context contains the wishes and rules for the realization of the relationships. The rules governing relationships also include those which belong to the communicative "hardware" of interaction regulation and have to be classified as part of, for instance, Habermas' theory of universal pragmatism. Such rules are not of interest in the therapeutic process unless they are severely disturbed and manifest themselves as pathological phenomena. Of general clinical significance are the so-called self-relevant rules of the relationship, which are important for maintaining the stability of the entire regulatory system. Subordinate to them are the (object-) relevant rules, which follow the given social rules of relationship. A first understanding of transference results from the distinction between these two sets of rules: transference occurs only where self-relevant rules are involved.

The therapeutic process is set in motion when the analysand seeks the help of the analyst's regulatory competence. He does this in his own typical way as determined by his development. It is the task of the therapeutic process to clarify the unconsciously introduced expectations which the analysand places on the analyst's assistance. For this purpose, the model defines four main functions of the therapeutic relationship (von Zeppelin 1981):

1. The extension of the cognitive affective search process with regard to regulatory activity, especially the extension of self-reflective capabilities
2. The preparation and introduction of an ad hoc model of the relationship between analyst and analysand; a better interactive competence is thus acquired in the here-and-now, which then must be transferred to the real relationships outside the analysis
3. The gradual modification of the therapeutic interaction in the sense of a revised distribution of regulation between analyst and analysand
4. The modification of the analysand's regulatory system by means of greater differentiation of self-reflective functions

The analysis of transference and countertransference originates in the application of these four main functions to the therapeutic relationship. The resulting processes pass through various phases in which different focal points are worked through again and again (see Sect. 9.4). Insight can be described as the construction of progressively more exact modes, which have to be sought in an iterative manner.

Without being able to go further into the differentiated descriptive and representative possibilities offered by this formalized model, we would like to emphasize the central significance of the concept of regulatory competence, whose strategic and tactical task is at the center of the hypothetical "subject processor." Although the images of the terminology employed here appear foreign, they accurately describe the concept of *security* that we can also identify in the process model of the Mount Zion Psychotherapy Research Group led by Weiss and Sampson, which we will now outline.

In a series of studies since 1971, this group has devised, on the basis of a clinically and theoretically elaborated conceptualization of the analysis of defense, new empirical approaches to verification. Without here going into the details of individual, empirically described psychodynamic configurations, the group characterizes the course of psychoanalytic treatment as a conflict between the patient's need to express his unconscious pathogenic beliefs and the analyst's efforts to pass these critical situations (called "tests") in such a way that the patient does not experience any confirmation of his negative expectations. If the outcome of the test is positive, the patient can acquire the security afforded by knowing that there is no longer any justification for his systems of beliefs consisting of infantile wish-defense patterns, and can therefore inactivate their regulatory function. This view, derived from the critical analysis of Freud's early (instinctual) and later (ego psychological) theories of defense, can be found in the works of Loewenstein (1969, p. 587), Kris (1950, p. 554), Loewald (1975, p. 284), and Greenson (1967, p. 178). A precursor of this concept of test was Freud's statement that the ego interpolates, "between the demand made by an instinct and the action that satisfies it, the activity of thought which, after taking its bearings in the present and assessing earlier experiences, endeavours by means of experimental actions to calculate the consequences of the course of action proposed" (1940 a, p. 199). This was applied by Weiss (1971), the Mount Zion Group's theorist, to the transference situation; Rangell (1971) and Dewald (1978) have expressed similar considerations.

The course of a psychoanalytic treatment is consequently viewed as a sequence of tests in which the themes specific to individual patients are tried out and worked through. Weiss and Sampson's special achievement was to have tested this process hypothesis empirically against the frustration thesis. Although both positions take the same segments of treatment to be decisive, the prognostic power of the Weiss-Sampson thesis proves to be far superior to that of the frustration thesis. The progress in treatment can in fact be viewed as the consequence of the successful refutation of unconscious pathogenic assumptions. It was further shown that if the analytic climate offers the security which the patient feels is necessary, repressed contents can manifest themselves without anxiety even if there is no explicit interpretation (Sampson and Weiss 1983).

A central theme has thus been conceptualized and empirically tested, although the processes studied by the Mount Zion Group account for only one section of the complex of events. A more comprehensive model still cannot be devised because there has been no explicit elaboration of the goal of the entire process; only individual steps of the process have been considered. One could perhaps assume that a satisfactory conclusion of therapy has been reached according to this process model when all of the patient's pathogenic assumptions have been refuted. This utopian goal raises the question of which of the patient's pathogenic assumptions are actualized in a concrete process in such a way that they stumble into the cross fire of transference.

According to Sampson and Weiss, the formal steps characterizing the course of therapy take place at every point in time in every therapy and are independent of whether the analyst follows this theory. The model thus claims a general validity regardless of the patient's particular illness, the stage of therapy, or the therapist's technique. And it is only concerned with one aspect out of the entire course of therapy: the patient's attempt to induce the analyst to act in a particular way and the analyst's reaction. The entire process is apparently viewed as a series of such sequences, and no consideration is given to the possibility that there might be a change in the sequences in the course of therapy. The only distinction is between the short-term and long-term effects of the refutation of assumptions. An immediate effect is that the patient's anxiety decreases; he is more relaxed, takes a more active role in the analytic work, and is more courageous in confronting his problems. The manifestation of new memories is considered, in contrast, more as a long-term effect.

It can be expected that the more the authors attempt to integrate further clinical observations and the results of process research into their model, the more necessary it will be for the model to be made more specific and supplemented with further assumptions. This might well make the model better able to describe the complexity of the psychoanalytic process, although its compelling simplicity would probably suffer as a result.

## 9.4 The Ulm Process Model

The development of the psychoanalytic technique has from its very beginnings been the object of two antagonistic tendencies, one toward methodological uniformity and the other toward syndrome-specific variation of the technique. On the subject of *therapeutic activity*, for example, Freud mentions technical modifications for phobias and compulsion neuroses: "another quite different kind of activity is necessitated by the gradually growing appreciation that the various forms of disease treated by us cannot all be dealt with by the same technique" (1919a, p. 165). In the general and specific theories of neurosis, hypotheses of the genesis of psychiatric and psychosomatic illnesses have been developed which are empirically more or less well founded. By making diagnoses and prognoses we apply our imprecise knowledge of what would have to happen in the psychoanalysis of anxiety neurosis, anorexia nervosa, or depressive reaction, to name just a few examples, in order to achieve an improvement in the symptoms or a cure.

The therapeutic process begins before the first session of treatment. The very fact that a potential patient approaches the analyst, and the way he establishes contact and makes an appointment are factors which themselves establish patterns influencing the beginning of treatment and determine whether the initiation of treatment is successful. Even at this early stage the question is raised as to how much openness and flexibility the analyst may use in shaping the situation so that an analytic situation results. The termination of a therapeutic process is another occasion for handling the topics of separation and parting in such a way that the specific relationship can be favorably concluded. We comprehend the transference neurosis as an *interactional representation* (Thomä and Kächele 1975) in the therapeutic relationship of the patient's inner psychic conflicts, the concrete arrangement of which is a function of the analytic process. This is unique for each dyad, and thus psychoanalysis can legitimately be called a historical science; on the other hand, at a higher level of abstraction it permits the identification of typical patterns of the course of analysis. Implicit in the simplifications that this involves, however, is the danger that the contribution of the therapist's *personal equation* and theoretical orientation to this development might be overlooked. Whether the intended, syndrome-specific strategy of treatment can be achieved depends, of course, on numerous imponderables beyond the influence of the analyst. Thus, events which take place in a patient's life often create new situations requiring a modification in strategy.

A serviceable process model must therefore combine flexibility in approaching the individual patient with regularity structured around the therapeutic task. In trying to do justice to this requirement, we base our process model on the following set of axioms:

1. The patient's free association does not lead by itself to the discovery of the unconscious portions of conflicts.
2. The psychoanalyst makes a selection according to his tactical (immediate) and strategic (long-term) goals.
3. Psychoanalytic theories serve to generate hypotheses, which must constantly be tested by trial and error.
4. The utility of therapeutic instruments can be judged by whether the desired change is achieved; if the change fails to occur, the treatment must be varied.
5. Myths of uniformity in psychoanalysis and psychotherapy lead to self-deceptions.

This list clearly outlines our conception of psychoanalytic therapy as a process of treatment regulated according to strategic considerations. This point of view is definitely unusual inasmuch as our call for *evenly suspended attention* on the one hand and for *free association* on the other seems to express just the opposite of a plan of treatment. In order not to create an objectively unnecessary contradiction it is advisable to refer to Freud's justification for his recommendation on evenly suspended attention: it is an excellent means for correcting theoretical prejudices and for more easily discovering the origin (focus) of each individual illness. Evenly suspended attention and focussing thus fulfill complementary functions: the functional state of gaining a maximal amount of information (the evenly suspended attention) and the organization of this information according to the most significant points of view (the focussing) alternate at the forefront of the analyst's mind.

We have now introduced a central concept of the Ulm process model: the focus. Before examining the numerous meanings attached to this term in the psychoanalytic literature, we would like to refer to its etymology. Focussing means bringing rays of light together at one point, and at the focus it burns. The fact that we assign focussing an important position in our conception of the analytic process does not mean a rigid commitment to one topic. Rather, we would like to call attention to man's limited capacity to absorb and process information, which permits no more than selective perception and, consequently, focussed attention.

At the beginning we mentioned that process models should enable us to make rule-like statements about the course of treatment. A focal conception of the process fulfills this function. Although ultimately we can do justice to psychotherapeutic activity (regardless of its orientation) only by ideographic means, i.e., by considering individual dyads, we still find regularly recurring topics in the psychoanalytic process. If the patient speaks about his anxieties, for instance, this topic then becomes the psychodynamic focus if

1. The analyst can generate hypotheses about unconscious motives which seem sensible to the patient
2. The analyst succeeds in leading the patient to this topic by using appropriate interventions
3. The patient can develop active emotional and cognitive interest in this topic

Our response to the question of whether a focus leads an existence in the patient independent of the analyst's structuring interventions is affirmative in that the patient has after all developed his own symptoms, but at the same time negative in terms of treatment technique. In view of the high degree of interrelatedness of unconscious structures of motivation, it is hardly possible for any focal diagnostic activity not to influence the interactional form of the focus activity (see the empirical results reported by Gabel et al. 1981). The analyst's cognitive processes, which regulate his reactions and selections and are discussed under terms such as "empathy" and "trial identification" (Heimann 1969), presumably take place largely below the threshold of conscious perception. They only become accessible to the analyst as a result of his work on his affective and cognitive reactions. For our understanding it is generally unimportant whether the analyst reaches his formulation of the focus in a largely intuitive, empathic manner, or whether he derives it to a greater extent from theoretical considerations. It is vital for focussing to be understood as a heuristic process which must demonstrate its utility in the progress of analysis. An indication for a correct formulation of focus is the thematization of a general focal topic, e.g., unconscious separation anxiety, in numerous forms. These different manifestations in the patient's everyday life are the object of the detailed interpretive work, which must be oriented around ideographic knowledge, i.e., around the detailed knowledge of the individual course of treatment.

In working through a focus we expect, in a favorable case, that the manner in which the patient (and perhaps even the analyst) deals with the focal topic will change in a specific way. More exact statements about this process of change can be made during analysis only if the constellation of transference and resistance, the working relationship, and the capacity for insight are also taken into consideration in a differentiated manner. If the same focus reappears at a later point in time, the questions raised are in principle the same. It can be expected, however, that the progress achieved earlier has not been lost and that the treatment can be continued at a higher level.

The result can be summarized as follows: We consider the interactionally formed focus to be the axis of the analytic process, and thus conceptualize psychoanalytic therapy as an *ongoing, temporally unlimited focal therapy with a changing focus.*

This model adequately reflects the clinical experience that the course of *transference neurosis* is a variable largely dependent on the analyst. There are a large number of studies in psychotherapy research on the influence of different *therapist variables*, and these variables have to be considered within the framework of an understanding of the psychoanalytic process (see Parloff et al. 1978; Luborsky and Spence 1978). We cannot return to the state prior to the discovery that the psychoanalytic process is constituted and develops interactively. Thus, in contrast to several of the models discussed above, we believe the sequence of the focusses to be the result of an unconscious exchange between the patient's needs and the possibilities open to the analyst. A change of analyst leads as a rule to completely new experiences. While this phenomenon has frequently been reported orally, it has only rarely found its way into the psychoanalytic literature (for example, in Guntrip 1975). The process that a patient and his analyst experience together comes to a standstill when their productivity is exhausted, even if the treatment continues indefinitely. Some processes never really get going because the two participants are not successful in establishing this interactional meshing in working through focal topics (see Huxter et al. 1975).

The analyst's process model, and not just his personality, exerts an influence on the course of therapy. If an analyst assumes, for instance, that the treatment must proceed according to a supposedly natural sequence of particular developmental phases, he will structure the treatment accordingly. The intensity and quality of the work on individual topics are also influenced by the importance the analyst attaches to the topics within the framework of his particular view of the analytic process.

Our view of the process does not exclude the possibility that therapy may proceed according to a regular developmental scheme (see Sect. 9.3).

Before beginning our detailed presentation of the Ulm process model, we would like to discuss the historical predecessors of the focal concept which have obviously influenced and motivated us. French (1952) first conceived of his idea of focus within the context of his systematic dream analyses:

We think of the cognitive structure of a dream as a constellation of related problems. In this constellation, there is usually one problem on which deeper problems converge and from which more superficial problems radiate. *This was the dreamer's focal problem* at the moment of dreaming. Every focal conflict is a reaction to some event or emotional situation of the preceding day which served as a "precipitating stimulus." (French 1970, p. 314)

This model, developed as a paradigm to help understand dreams, was employed in the well-known consensus study carried out at the Chicago Institute to record the dominant conflicts in individual treatment sessions, in which Kohut was one of the participants (Seitz 1966, p. 212). The assumption was that preconscious thinking tends in every interview to concentrate on a central (admittedly, highly condensed and overdetermined) problem. A multitude of associations capable of entering consciousness are concentrated at one point; similarly, "associated, unconscious, genetic conflicts are activated .... the emotional charges of which are characteristically transferred to the single, hypercathected, *focal* conflict in the preconscious." Seitz (1966, p. 212) suggests, following Freud, that

the focal conflict usually consists of the current transference to the analyst, and is best understood theoretically in terms of the dynamics of day-residues. Because these hypercathected, preconscious conflicts constitute points of convergence of dynamic forces within the mind, they provide a useful focus for unifying and integrating interpretive formulations of the complex, seemingly heterogeneous associational material of individual interviews.

According to Seitz, the focal conflict is identical to the dominant transference in the interview. The further development of the concept of focus in the Focal Therapy Workshop, described by Malan (1963), led to the crystallization of a focus. This concept was intended to express the idea that the focus is not chosen by the analyst, but gradually develops out of the joint work of patient and therapist.

Balint's ideas on these issues, as reflected in his report on the focal therapy of patient B. (Balint et al. 1972), were themselves influenced by the "flash" experiences of the Focal Therapy Workshop. Balint, however, goes further and demands that no focal plan may be designed without a precise formulation of the focus, which itself is a translation into words of the flash experience. The formulation of the focus as a guideline for treatment was supposed to be "specific (not a general idea like 'homosexuality' or the 'Oedipus complex'), sharply delineated (not as vague as 'the patient's relationship with his mother'), and unambiguous" (Balint et al. 1972, p. 152). This demand for specific formulations appears to us to be necessary, even outside this context. The customary case discussions are very unsatisfactory if the participants stop at overly general and consequently almost meaningless descriptions such as "oedipal" or "preoedipal." Such terms neither help us to understand an individual pathogenesis, nor provide instructions for appropriate action.

The choice of the appropriate level of abstraction seems to us to be the problem most easily solved in focal therapy. It involves bridging the gap between diagnosis and therapy, so that we can go from one to the other. The demand that the focus should be expressed in the form of an interpretation seems to reflect the wishful thinking of many analysts. Even Balint seems to have succumbed to this idea when he advised "that the focus should be expressed in the form of an interpretation that could be given meaningfully to the patient towards the end of the treatment" (Balint et al. 1972, p. 152).

Our understanding of focus, following Balint's Workshop formulation, goes beyond French's conception inasmuch as it refers to a structure which extends over a longer period of time. There is, of course, no reason not to formulate a focus for individual interviews, but from the point of view of treatment strategy it is desirable to work through a basic topic continuously over a longer period of time. What period of time is best, and whether it is better defined by a specific number of sessions or by the rate of the patient's progress are clinical questions and must be decided empirically.

Indications for a suitable division of the treatment process into segments can be found in the final reports of candidates in training, who as a rule break the treatment process into four to five phases with thematic headings. These reports, however, also illustrate that the length of the phases depends on the analyst's technical procedure to a significant degree. We therefore have to distinguish our understanding of focus from Balint's description of the focal conflict as the focal plan which the analyst formulates for conducting treatment. It may appear convincing that in a psychoanalytic short therapy *one* focus is selected and that *only* this one is worked through, although the experience in the Hamburg focal therapy project (Meyer 1981b; especially Gabel et al. 1981) raises some doubts. We, however, put more emphasis on the cooperative aspect, the continuous work of patient and analyst, whose efforts to establish a focus reflect a creative process of agreement and disagreement.

In the controversy surrounding the work of Alexander and French (1946), one constant point was the criticism that the therapist manipulates the patient in the focus-centered procedure. This objection is unfounded with regard to our understanding because of the emphasis we put on joint work on the focus. On the contrary, there is more openness in our approach than in the standard technique, in which the analyst proceeds in a concealed way and often manipulates without sufficient reflection. Peterfreund (1983, pp. 7-50) has provided several instructive examples of this procedure from his own work and the literature.

In the following we describe the course of treatment for a hypothetical patient in order to illustrate our ideas about the analytic process. As is by now clear, we use "focus" to refer to the major interactionally created theme of the therapeutic work, which results from the material offered by the patient and the analyst's efforts at understanding. We assume that the patient can offer different material within a certain period of time, but that the formation of a focus is only achieved by selective activity on the part of the analyst. With regard to the process, we expect the joint work on a focus to lead to further major points of substance, which can only be formed on the basis of the preceding work.

Let us consider an example in which the patient offers four different topics in the initial phase. We understand these four offers in the sense of French's "nuclear conflicts" (1952, 1970), as infantile conflict constellations which are unconscious, psychogenetically acquired structures determining the patient's symptoms and character.

The designation of a certain number of initial offers is arbitrary inasmuch as a large number of infantile conflicts have been conceptualized in psychoanalytic theory. We will identify more, fewer, or different core conflicts according to where we direct our attention, which itself depends on our theory. The expected number of nuclear conflicts will probably fall with increasing specificity of the disturbance, and rise with increasing severity of the disturbance. In the diagnostic phase of the initial interview (time $T_0$; see Chap. 6), the analyst attempts to gain a first impression of possible conflicts, at this point independent of therapeutic interventions. When first therapeutic steps are tried in the further course of the initial interview (time $T_1$), a first focal constellation ($F_1$) is formed; its utility must be demonstrated in the first phase of treatment. In the identification of the substance of this constellation, we closely follow French's criteria for the description of the *focal conflict*, which require information about the source (unconscious, infantile stimuli), precipitating causes (recent and current events), principal forms of defense, and attempted solutions.

In contrast to French, we would not like to make a quantitative statement about the period of time a given focal theme is dominant. At some point — we do not dare to be more precise — the work on the first focus makes a second focus ($F_2$) accessible. The work on this second focus leads in our example back to the first focus, which then again becomes the center of work, although in a qualitatively different form ($F_{1'}$).

In our example, the initial and diagnostically founded focus $F_1$ also represents a major motif of the entire process. This corresponds to the well-verified clinical finding that the individual focusses are linked to one another via a central conflict. A schematic example is hysterical disturbance; in an uncomplicated case the primary conflict is in the area of the positive oedipal relationship. At the same time, however, the disturbance may implicate the negative oedipal area ($F_2$) or anal ($F_3$) and oral ($F_4$) conflict themes, which might, and depending on the structure of the analytic process probably will, appear as a secondary focus in the analysis.

In this regard we follow a suggestion made by Luborsky (1984), who was able to demonstrate empirically that this classification of conflict themes is accurate. He termed this major transference issue the core conflictual relationship theme. This theoretically and practically well-grounded conception of a central conflictual dynamic which guides therapy also provides the foundation for a focal procedure (Balint et al. 1972; Klüwer 1985; Malan 1963; Strupp and Binder 1984) whose object is the handling of such a main conflict, which supposedly can be grasped in the first interview (see also Leuzinger-Bohleber 1985). The other focusses in our example ($F_2$, $F_3$, $F_4$) are, as is easy to imagine, encountered and handled in the course of treatment, each providing a new means of access to the major transference issue $F_1$.

We have chosen a relatively crude example of the course of treatment for didactic reasons. Using our model it is possible to describe the process at different degrees of differentiation, depending on the purpose.

To return to the metaphor of psychoanalysis as the exploration of a house, exploration of the interior revolves primarily around a room which by virtue of its central position controls the access to the other rooms, but which itself can also be entered from various neighboring rooms.

We do not want to go into detail on the wealth of further assumptions which are part of our model. Our sole intention was to present a scheme for conceptualizing the psychoanalytic process which satisfies a number of the criteria we believe to be relevant. It should have become clear that a stereotypical view of the process introduces unnecessary rigidity into the psychoanalytic work. Our model provides a framework for understanding psychodynamic processes in very different settings, and can be applied to both short- and long-term therapies. It is compatible with various theoretical approaches in psychoanalysis which are used to help gain an understanding of the material the patient initially offers. We consider our conception of process to be genuinely social scientific, and to be in complete opposition to those process theories which start from a view that the process is a naturally occurring phenomenon and which develop where the formation of schools and a tendency to ideology go hand in hand.

The psychoanalytic process as we understand it lives from a diversity and openness which leaves room for creativity, but which has to restrict itself whenever it becomes concrete. The model therefore does not dictate whether the next session will continue the same topic or whether another focus will be revived as a result of situational stimuli. In every session a situation inevitably arises in which a decision must be made as to which direction to take. The analytic process lives in the dialectic tension between the conception that "the way is the goal" (von Blarer and Brogle 1983, p. 71) and the fact that there is no such thing as aimless wandering. There will always be times when the two wanderers pause and become engrossed in a topic which appears significant to both of them. Von Blarer and Brogle's attractive metaphor of the psychoanalytic process as a path that analyst and analysand "have taken since the first interview" can be adopted if the path leads from problems to their solutions.

We would like to contrast the conception of the process as an ongoing, temporally unlimited focal therapy with qualitatively changing focus to the fictive notion of a puristic psychoanalytic process. We strongly favor a flexible process model, i.e., a technique which is heuristically oriented, suitable for searching, finding, and discovering, and directed at creating the best possible conditions for change. We are convinced that the traditional rules of psychoanalytic procedure contain much that is useful but which becomes counterproductive when the method is cultivated as an end in itself. The same is true of conceptions of process. They have the function of providing orientation, and are primarily instruments to help the analyst organize his own work and to facilitate the necessary communication between analysts. They become a threat to therapy if they are taken for unchallengable reality and are thus no longer subjected to the constant reexamination which is necessary.

# 10 Relationship Between Theory and Practice

## 10.1 Freud's Prize Question

Sixty years ago Ferenczi and Rank (1924) attempted to clarify "the relationship between analytic technique and analytic theory" and to investigate "the extent to which the technique has influenced theory and the extent to which each currently assists or obstructs the other" — Freud's prize question (1922d, pp. 267-270). It is now time to compare today's problems with those of that time. A few general observations have survived the passage of time. For example, Ferenczi and Rank pleaded the case for both an inductive empirical procedure and a deductive procedure to test hypotheses when they wrote:

> It is perhaps not an exaggeration to assert that this mutual control of cognition by experience (given facts, induction) and of experience by previous knowledge (systematization, deduction) is the only kind which can keep a science from erring. A discipline which utilized only one or the other of these paths of research or which prematurely attempted to forgo control by a countercheck would be condemned to lose the solid ground under its feet: pure facts because they lack the fructifying idea, pure theory because its premature omniscience would cause it to lose the motivation for further research. (Ferenczi and Rank 1924, p. 47)

In evaluating the interaction of theory and practice, it is essential to distinguish the growing treasure of knowledge and its systematization in the general and specific theories of neurosis from its appropriate therapeutic application. The fact that the theoretical phase (in which Ferenczi and Rank included, for example, knowledge of unconscious emotional mechanisms) raced ahead of therapeutic skill led analysts to place great emphasis on remembering and on rational reconstruction of the past. Thus the object of criticism was a therapeutically ineffective "interpretation fanaticism" derived from etiological theory.

Another aspect of this problem can be illustrated using the examples of the therapeutic function of remembering and interpreting and of the reconstruction of a child's early life history. Etiological theory always started from the assumption that the emotional and affective portion of repressed memories is essential for the genesis of emotional illnesses. Thus in interpretation fanaticism, theoretical knowledge was translated into therapeutic practice in a one-sided and incomplete manner. We would like to clarify a general point here by quoting from Goethe's *Dichtung und Wahrheit*: "Theory and practice always affect each other; it is possible to see what people think in their deeds, and predict what they will do from their opinions."

Ferenczi and Rank used the expression "interpretation fanaticism" in criticizing the therapeutically unfavorable way in which theoretical knowledge was transformed. They obviously believed that the knowledge that had already been systematized was applied by many of their colleagues in a technically incomplete fashion, even though these colleagues' theoretical opinions about an unconscious psychic context may have been completely correct.

To describe the present range of opinions, we can refer to the discussion by a panel of prominent analysts on the relationship between psychoanalytic theory and technique. Richards' (1984) comprehensive report on Wallerstein's introductory presentation, the papers by Rangell, Kernberg, and Ornstein, and the comments of the panel members provides a representative cross section of today's views.

Ferenczi and Rank had spoken of a *circulus benignus*, i.e., of a "mutually beneficial influence of theory on practice and of practice on theory" (Ferenczi and Rank 1924, p. 47). However, they put equal emphasis on the *circulus vitiosus*. Rangell now views progress as the "progressive elaboration of the therapeutic process in a sequence linked directly with the incremental expansion of the theory of etiology" (quoted in Richards 1984, p. 588). Ego psychology is cited as an example; it "placed the analysis of defences on a par with the analysis of drive contents" (Richards 1984, p. 588). Since according to his account all theoretical assumptions, including the most abstruse metapsychological ones, are linked in some way to treatment technique, Rangell is able to create a seemingly close and unproblematic connection. Even if theory should at some point develop more rapidly than technique, each still seems to be in a constant process of growth described in evolutionary terms.

Rangell accordingly sees problems only where the comprehensive view is restricted by theoretical or practical one-sidedness. In an ideal relationship, theory and technique complement each other perfectly. One thus gets the impression that psychoanalysis would have progressed even further along the spiral line of evolution of the *circulus benignus* if the familiar foundation had continued to serve as the basis for development. A. Freud (1954a) held a similar opinion. Rangell attributes mistakes on the technical or the theoretical side to personal or school-determined one-sidedness, to over-emphasis, or to negligence, the very mistakes previously criticized by Ferenczi and Rank.

Unexplained, however, is what is to be classified as a mistake. Rangell does not even raise the question of what characterizes the scientific validity of a theory. He also neither discusses the problem of therapeutic effectiveness, nor asks to what degree theory and practice support or inhibit each other. He thus does not touch on the central problems, but conveys the impression of wonderful harmony. The most abstract components of metapsychology appear to be related to clinical observations just as much as, conversely, immediate analytic experience seems to fall under the guidelines of the supposedly established theory. Rangell does not mention that, despite decades of effort, the cleverest analysts have not succeeded in determining rules of correspondence between the different levels of abstraction of theory, or that both Hartmann et al.'s (1953) attempts to improve the inner consistency of theory in a way relevant to practice and Rapaport's large-scale systematization (1960) were failures. Since

Rangell starts from the idea of a continuous development in theory and technique, in close interdependence, he does not need to look for disturbances resulting from disproportionate development on one side or the other. For Rangell, such disruptions are rooted almost exclusively in individual or school-specific misunderstandings with regard to technique or theory. At issue for him are not the truth of psychoanalytic theories and the effectiveness and optimization of technique; the weaknesses and faults lie elsewhere, namely in the analyst who — because of his personal equation — fails to attain the realizable standards of technical and theoretical knowledge. Certain though it is that each psychoanalyst can embody only a certain portion of the entire theoretical and technical knowledge which has been accumulated in the active psychoanalytic community and in the literature in a century, Rangell's ad hominem argument is equally out of date. This argument has always made the scientific clarification of difficult problems even harder, sometimes impossible.

Wallerstein (see Richards 1984), in contrast, doubts the truth of the dogma that technique and theory are so closely associated that each alteration in theory must also lead to modifications of technique. In his opinion, theory has changed significantly within a century but it is very difficult to demonstrate how technique has changed as a consequence. The degree of correspondence between theory and technique is thus much smaller than usually asserted, which leads Wallerstein to recommend that the relationship between them be considered in an unprejudiced way.

To do this, it is necessary to go to the level of practice and investigate those problems which were avoided in large measure as a result of the assertion that theory and technique promote each other in a perpetual *circulus benignus*. The naive view that it is possible to assume the existence of a *circulus benignus* without empirical investigation prevents genuine progress because it overlooks the demands that must be placed on practice if theory and technique are to be mutually beneficial.

To avoid any chance of being misunderstood, we emphasize that significant developments and changes have, of course, taken place in recent decades. An excellent example of the interrelated development of theory and technique is Kohut's self psychology, which was Ornstein's starting point in the panel reported by Richards (1984). Mutually dependent development must not be equated, however, with the assertion that technique and theory promote each other in the sense of mutual progress making theory *truer* and technique *more effective*. Kohut, like many other psychoanalysts, claims that practical application and theory form an exclusive "functional unit" when he says:

> In most sciences there exists a more or less clear separation between the area of practical, empirical application and the area of concept formation and theory. In analysis, however, these two areas ... are merged into a single functional unit. (Kohut 1973, p. 25)

The naive conception that increase in the effectiveness of a technique and increase in the truth of a theory are mutually dependent has been fostered by Freud's legacy of an inseparable bond linking therapy and research. The inseparable bond links the promotion of a cure to that of knowledge, and thus effectiveness to truth. In the following sections we will try to demonstrate the questions and problems this inseparable bond raises. We believe that we can propose general descriptions of the relationship between theory and technique by referring to the theses that form the context of the inseparable bond concept in Freud's works.

Ferenczi and Rank's failure becomes more comprehensible in light of our current knowledge that it was based solely on familiar processes of group dynamics. The "increasing disorientation of analysts, especially in regard to practical, technical questions," which the authors hoped to clarify definitively, forms part of the history of the psychoanalytic paradigm. For many reasons, the transformation of the therapeutic paradigm into a research method appropriate to psychoanalysis — in Kuhn's (1962) sense of normal science — could take place only gradually. It now appears that the validity of the psychoanalytic theory of the genesis of illnesses that are at least in part psychic in origin cannot be evaluated according to the same criteria as the theory of treatment technique.

## 10.2 Psychoanalytic Practice in Light of the Inseparable Bond

Freud described the relationship between therapy and theory, between practice and research, with the following three theses:

> In psychoanalysis there has existed from the very first an *inseparable bond between cure and research.* Knowledge brought therapeutic success. It was impossible to treat a patient without learning something new; it was impossible to gain fresh insight without perceiving its beneficent results. Our analytic procedure is the only one in which this precious conjunction is assured. It is only by carrying on our analytic *pastoral work* that we can deepen our dawning *comprehension* of the human mind. This prospect of scientific gain has been the proudest and happiest feature of analytic work. (Freud 1927a, p. 256, emphasis added)

> Analyses which lead to favourable conclusion in short time are of value in ministering to the therapeutist's self-esteem and substantiate the *medical importance* of psycho-analysis; but they remain for the most part insignificant as regards the *advancement of scientific knowledge.* Nothing new is learnt from them. In fact they only succeed so quickly because everything that was necessary for their accomplishment was already known. Something new can only be gained from analyses that present special difficulties, and to the overcoming of these a great deal of time has to be devoted. Only in such cases do we succeed in descending into the deepest and most primitive strata of mental development and in gaining from there solutions for the problems of the later formations. And we feel afterwards that, strictly speaking, *only an analysis which has penetrated so far deserves the name.* (Freud 1918b, p. 10, emphasis added)

> I have told you that psycho-analysis began as a method of treatment; but I did not want to commend it to your interest as a method of treatment but on account of the *truths it contains,* on account of the information it gives us about what concerns human beings most of all — their own nature — and on account of the connections it discloses between the most different of their activities. As a method of treatment it is one among many, though, to be sure, *primus inter pares.* If it was without therapeutic value it would not have been discovered, as it was, in connection with sick people and would not have gone on developing for more than thirty years. (Freud 1933a, pp. 156-157, emphasis added)

These passages reveal the high demands Freud placed on "true" analysis. The inseparable bond thesis can only be upheld if the reason for the therapeutic effectiveness of psychoanalytic practice lies in the truth of the knowledge that has been gained. This assertion is not easily proven because the inseparable bond does not simply occur of itself. Such an idea is an illusion which sees each analysis as an enterprise in therapy and in research. The precious conjunction of effective therapy and true cognition as a product of the psychoanalytic method cannot be considered an innate trait of psychoanalytic practice. Certain conditions must be satisfied before the claim that there is an inseparable bond can be justified. We would like to attempt to determine these conditions by means of a rational reconstruction of the relationship between theory and practice.

One aspect of Freud's inseparable bond assertion concerns the conditions under which psychoanalytic cognition takes place — the context of discovery, i.e., everything associated with the discovery and acquisition of knowledge. With regard to practice, the context in which psychoanalytic knowledge is discovered is a matter of psychoanalytic heuristics, which deals with the questions of how interpretations arise in the analyst and of which inferential processes form the basis of an analyst's discovery of dyad-specific relationships. Clinical discussions revolve primarily around the heuristics. This is concerned primarily with the discovery of unconscious wishes which result in conflicts when they confront the realities of life. For this reason the pleasure principle, although transformed somewhat, continues to play a central role in psychoanalysis even after the death of metapsychology. Openness becomes essential in psychoanalytic heuristics in order to do justice to the multiplicity of possible interrelations.

> The cases of illness which come under a psychoanalyst's observations are of course of unequal value in adding to his knowledge. There are some on which he has to bring to bear all that he knows and from which he learns nothing; and there are others which show him what he already knows in a particularly clearly marked manner and in exceptionally revealing isolation, so that he is endebted to them not only for a confirmation but for an extension of his knowledge. (Freud 1913h, p. 193)

At this point it is appropriate to comment on the problem of the contexts of discovery and justification, a distinction introduced by von Reichenbach (1938). Although this distinction is useful, we do not view it as a radical dichotomy and therefore, in contrast to Popper (1969), do not relegate the question of how something arises in the clinician and scientist — and thus the entire heuristics of discoveries of all kinds — to the sphere of irrational mysticism. In our opinion, Spinner (1974) has shown convincingly that the strict differentiation between a context of discovery and a context of justification is not adequate either for heuristics or for the justification and foundation in the research process (Spinner 1974, pp. 118, 174ff., 262ff.). Of course, we have to acknowledge that this differentiation is by and large not made at all in psychoanalysis. In contrast to Freud's scientific credo, the function that most analysts attribute to heuristics, to the context of discovery, goes far beyond dyad-specific truths.

In the dyad the therapist is also a researcher only inasmuch as he conducts his research with genuinely psychoanalytic means (e.g., free associations, recognition of countertransference, and interpretive interventions). Such research is the "home-ground" of psychoanalytic theory formation. Thus, in his 34th lecture to an imagined audience Freud said:

> As you know, psychoanalysis originated as a method of treatment; it has far outgrown this, but it has not abandoned its home-ground and it is still linked to its contact with patients for increasing its depth and for its further development. The accumulated impressions from which we derive our theories could be arrived at in no other way. (Freud 1933a, p. 151)

Psychoanalytic research within the dyad consists in the analyst's acquisition of knowledge about the patient and his relationship to the therapist. In the following we describe such knowledge as *dyad-specific*. The cure results from the fact that the analyst communicates his impressions — including the affective interactional processes (transference and countertransference) — to the patient according to the rules of the art, i.e., in the form of interpretations. This dyad-specific communication of knowledge in treatment stimulates the patient to further reflection about his experiences and especially about his unconscious motivations. A circumscribed form of reflection by the patient is called insight. A consequence of the insight process itself is that new material can be brought to the surface, which in turn means a growth in knowledge, enabling the patient to attain new insights conducive to cure. The kind of knowledge communicated to the patient in interpretations must be strictly distinguished from that resulting from "accumulated impressions," which, in its general formulation as psychoanalytic knowledge, constitutes the *theory* of psychoanalysis.

Although dyad-specific knowledge is acquired against the backdrop of hypotheses stemming from psychoanalytic theory, it can lead to an extension and modification of existing suppositions. Knowledge thus evolves to a more general form, which in turn provides the theoretical backdrop for the acquisition of new dyad-specific insights. The acquisition of psychoanalytic knowledge follows a *hermeneutic circle*. Freud's assertion of the existence of an inseparable bond in analytic practice is thus not related to general theory immediately but via dyad-specific knowledge.

The differentiation of the concept of research implicit here is a source of help and relief. A field ethologist conducts research without being burdened by the necessity of simultaneous general theorizing. Like the psychoanalyst, he develops his theories at a desk, not in the field. Dyad-specific cognition thus constitutes a special step in research; this step can, however, be taken only in the psychoanalytic situation. One branch of this knowledge goes in the direction of general theorizing, another in the direction of effective communication. Viewed in this manner, a special kind of knowledge — dyad-specific knowledge — is acquired by employing a uniform procedure that is at one and the same time a method of research and a method of treatment. The inseparable bond thesis thus means that:

1. The cure results from the dyad-specific knowledge communicated to the patient, i.e., from the affective and intellectual experiences in the dyad that coalesce into knowledge.
2. Knowledge must be conveyed in the technically correct way, i.e., according to the rules of the art of therapy.

3. The therapeutic technique leads to further and deeper insights into the psychic activity of the patient and his relationship to the analyst, i.e., the therapeutic technique produces increased dyad-specific knowledge.

Psychoanalytic practice orients itself around the accumulated psychoanalytic knowledge. To further illuminate the relationship between theory and practice in light of the inseparable bond assertion, we want to differentiate psychoanalytic knowledge in order to be able to describe more exactly which knowledge governs activities of analytic research and treatment.

*Descriptive and classificatory knowledge* provides an answer to the question of *what* something is, but not *why* it is. It serves to describe and classify, and puts the facts required for a map of the subject matter at the disposal of psychoanalysis. Assertions about relationships belonging to this kind of knowledge are only correlative; they do not provide any information on the dependent or conditional nature of relationships. An example in the clinical area is knowledge about forms of behavior and experience which are typical and specific for certain psychic illnesses, e.g., the knowledge that a strong need for control is often observed in obsessional neuroses and that attachment needs, separation anxieties, and more or less concealed aggressions are often observed in neurotic depressions. In this sense the entire field of symptomatology can be considered as belonging to the realm of descriptive and classificatory knowledge.

*Causal knowledge* answers the question of *why* something is, how things are related, which dependent relationships exist between given facts, and how they influence each other. This kind of knowledge thus provides the foundation for psychoanalytic explanations. The following two assertions from the clinical sphere are examples of causal knowledge: First, patients who have been made aware of the aggressive components of their personalities by interpretations, but who have shut them out of their consciousness, will deny their aggressive impulses when certain marginal conditions are satisfied. Second, if thoughts, feelings, and sensations are appealed to which are beyond the realm of the subject's conscious awareness, he reacts defensively. The second of these hypotheses, which both belong to the theory of defenses, is formulated at a higher level of abstraction than the first. In this sense, clinical knowledge of the etiology and pathogenesis of psychic illnesses can be considered causal knowledge.

*Treatment and change knowledge* (Kaminski 1970, pp. 45-46) is claimed to be useful in *practice*. This kind of knowledge is defined by its relationship to action, and includes statements about the capacity to create the phenomena and conditions that have to be satisfied before certain goals can effectively be reached. This knowledge therefore concerns phenomena and facts that do not yet exist, and thus goals which can be reached with its help. In contrast to causal knowledge, described above, knowledge of treatment and change does not say anything about the conditional nature of the relationships of given circumstances, but rather about the production of certain circumstances through action. The following statements are examples of this form of knowledge, which for the sake of clarity we refer to as action knowledge: (a) Consequences undesirable for the psychoanalytic process result if the analyst returns all of the patient's questions. (b) The furtherance of the patient's perception of reality is unfavorably affected if the analyst simply disregards, rather than acknowledges, the plausibility of the patient's comments. (c) If the patient's resistance to the conscious realization of certain contents grows at an increasing rate as a consequence of previous interpretations of these contents, and if the analyst fears the patient may completely close up and remain silent, then it is advisable for the analyst to drop content-related interpretations and to discuss the resistance instead. Thus, such statements, especially concerning the psychoanalytic treatment technique, can be classified as treatment and change knowledge.

On the basis of this differentiation we can say that clinical psychoanalytic research and treatment in divers spheres are governed by change (treatment) knowledge, for example by mutative knowledge. In contrast, the descriptive (classificatory) and causal forms of knowledge, while also originating in the clinical situation, do not originate exclusively or *specifically* there; they have to be produced by the analyst's processes of reflection outside the clinical situation. The causal knowledge which constitutes the theoretical subject matter of psychoanalysis can only result from the hardly explicit operation of reflectively processing experience. On the one hand, descriptive (classificatory) knowledge stands in opposition to the causal and change (treatment) types of knowledge, since descriptive knowledge does not make statements about cause and effect. On the other hand, change knowledge, as a technical form of knowledge, contrasts with descriptive and causal knowledge, which are theoretical forms of knowledge. Technical knowledge tells us how we can act; theoretical knowledge provides us with an insight into the nature of things. How are these two forms of knowledge related? For example, can technical knowledge (change or treatment knowledge) be derived from theoretical knowledge (descriptive or classificatory knowledge and causal knowledge)? These questions lead us to the issues usually discussed within the framework of the *context of justification.*

## 10.3 The Context of Justification of Change Knowledge

In the framework of the context of justification a question is generally asked regarding the accuracy of the assertions that have been made, i.e., the justification of the assertion that a statement is accurate (true). There are at least two kinds of justification. First, we can justify the accuracy of a statement by deriving the statement from an existing body of knowledge which has already been established as true. Second, the accuracy of a statement (an item of knowledge) can be confirmed empirically by consulting one's experience to see whether the assertion reflects reality. When considering change knowledge within the context of justification in the following, we are interested in the first of these two approaches. We inquire whether the accuracy and established effectiveness of its recommendations for action can be derived logically from psychoanalytic causal knowledge, or whether recourse to another form of knowledge is necessary. We ask, for example, whether the assertion that a patient's resistance can be resolved effectively by interpreting it can be explained and justified by psychoanalytic causal knowledge (and thus theoretical knowledge). We will present in detail the two approaches which seem to us to be most important.

The *continuity assumption*, as Westmeyer called it (1978, p. 111), is widespread. In the theory of science its proponents include Albert (1960), Weber (1968), and Prim and Tilmann (1973), in psychiatry Möller (1976), in psychoanalysis Reiter (1975), and in behavior therapy Eysenck and Rachman (1968) and Schulte (1976).

Characteristic is Weber's (1968, p. 267) assertion that it is only necessary to reverse the order of statements about relationships and conditions in order to obtain information about how something can be changed. It is also said that effective knowledge of change results from reversing true assertions about relationships. Assume that the following psychoanalytic assertion is accurate: "If a patient becomes conscious of unconscious processes, the pathogenic conflicts based on them are resolved." Then the following effective knowledge of change would have to result: "In order to resolve pathogenic conflicts the patient should be made aware of the unconscious processes on which they are based." The following statements are to be understood in this sense: "If someone has understood something correctly, then he can make it." "If someone can make something, then he has understood it correctly." In these statements, understanding and doing are assumed to be interconnected from the very beginning. Insight into the nature of something is allegedly sufficient to enable someone to make it, and if someone is able to make something, people think they can assume that he has understood it. In that case, the correct understanding of a thing would go hand in hand with its successful production; correct understanding and successful production would constitute a continuum. This is a mistake for several reasons, and we will now comment on the two most important of these.

In general, statements about connections and conditional relationships apply only under ideal conditions, i.e., the sphere to which these assertions claim to apply has significantly fewer variables than reality. For example, there are fewer variables in a controlled laboratory situation than in real life. We find enormous idealization and abstraction regarding the features to be considered (parameters and variables) in, for example, Skinner's experiments. There are considerable differences between human learning in a real-life situation and that of a rat in a Skinner box, and they must be taken into consideration if, for example, a teacher wants to intervene in his pupil's learning processes. What is sufficient for the theorist to explain behavior under restricted (ideal) circumstances may by no means be sufficient for the practitioner to intervene in a complex real-life situation to modify behavior. The difference between the idealized sphere and the practitioner's real sphere of activity is one of the reasons that behavior therapy, according to its original self-understanding, failed as applied learning theory and was not able to demonstrate that the laws of learning shown to be accurate in laboratory experiments are a sufficient basis for effective practice.

Causal knowledge provides information about which facts are the prerequisites for other facts, but not about which actions bring about which facts. It is asserted, for example, that a certain state A leads to a different state B. In the position of the practitioner, I have to ask how I can create state A so that it can lead to state B. The analyst thus has to ask himself how he can make unconscious processes conscious in order to resolve pathogenic conflicts. In practice, it is not sufficient to know the prerequisites and the consequences — the *what* and *why*. The agent must know *how* he can create the necessary conditions.

For these reasons the continuity assumption cannot be used in the attempt to explain and justify hypotheses about effective action (which belong to knowledge of change) by appeal to the truth of causal knowledge.

Bunge's (1967) *foundations approach* heeds the legitimate objections to the continuity assumption. The major differences between his approach and the continuity assumption are that the transition from causal knowledge to knowledge of change does not take place immediately, but by means of an intermediate step, and that this transition has more of a heuristic than a justificatory quality.

A typical starting point is the proposition: "When repressed conflicts threaten to reach consciousness, there is increased resistance to these conflicts." This can be transformed into a nomopragmatic proposition by expanding it to include concepts related to action: "When the analyst interprets a patient's repressed conflicts, the patient's defenses are strengthened." Yet interpretation of a patient's repressed conflicts does not mean the same as the threat that such conflicts will reach the level of consciousness. It is also impossible to derive the first proposition from the second, because the concepts of the former are not contained in the latter. The proposition about the interpretation of repressed conflicts cannot be directly derived from causal knowledge. Concepts of action, such as "interpret," must also be brought in.

In order finally to establish a rule for practice, the nomopragmatic proposition is inverted: "If the patient's defenses are to be strengthened, it is advisable to interpret his repressed conflicts," or "If the patient's defenses are to be weakened, it is advisable not to interpret repressed conflicts." This inversion also cannot be established rigorously and thus remains problematic (Perrez 1983, p. 154).

Since neither step 1 (from causal knowledge to pragmatic proposition) nor step 2 (from a nomopragmatic proposition to a rule of treatment) can be established rigorously, Bunge's foundations approach also fails to ground change knowledge in causal knowledge. Bunge even raises the consideration that it is quite possible for ineffective rules of action to be derived from established theories (concerning causal knowledge), and vice versa. Although it is only by coincidence that a completely inaccurate assessment of certain conditional relationships can lead to their effective management, even with a true theory it would be impossible to give a strict explanation and foundation for effective practice (e.g., the cure of a neurosis with the psychoanalytic treatment technique), because of the above-mentioned relationship between causal knowledge and knowledge of change. Bunge discusses both the idealization problem — less relevant for psychoanalysis because psychoanalytic theory develops in close association with practice — and the difference between knowing what and why and knowing how, and shows that the difficulties cannot be solved in this manner. He offers in their place another possibility for the treatment knowledge, using technological theories or technology instead of causal knowledge. Wisdom (1956), a psychoanalytically trained philosopher, founded an early and original form of a similar "psychoanalytic technology."

Technologies are also theories, yet they differ from those mentioned above, which are constituted by descriptive knowledge, in that they have the character of applied instead of pure science, i.e., they are related directly to acts which are suited to create particular circumstances. Technologies encompass the more general technical knowledge (in contrast to the concrete rules of change or treatment knowledge), that is suitable both for acquisition of treatment knowledge and for the effectiveness of the rules of action furnished by treatment knowledge. They refer to what can and should be done in a particular case in order to be able to produce, avoid, change, or improve something.

Bunge (1967) distinguishes two kinds of technological theories, substantive and operative. The former refer to the objects of action and include, for example, statements about typical transference patterns or forms of resistance for certain groups of patients. In other words, they include statements about those theoretical statements designed to transmit knowledge relevant to practice, i.e., they convey the knowledge necessary for mastering the everyday tasks of therapeutic practice, not that necessary for a detailed explanation of what and why. Substantive technological theories are usually the fruit of the theories of pure science and adopt from them structural elements which, while regularly subject to conceptual coarsening and impoverishment, thereby gain in practical utility.

Operative technological theories, on the other hand, refer to the practical act itself. They lend themselves to the development of strategies for the formulation of recommendations for effective action. These recommendations take the form of global rules and refer to the special circumstances of the concrete therapeutic situation, i.e., lead directly to "know-how."

The advantage of technological theories lies in the fact that they are able to model practice significantly more effectively and to provide better explanations and justifications of the effectiveness of practice because of their ties to applicability.

Thus there are two opposing spheres of knowledge, neither of which is derived directly and immediately from the other: the pure scientific theory of psychoanalysis — including the descriptive and causal forms of knowledge and the theory they constitute — and the applied scientific theory of psychoanalysis — substantive and operative technological theories and change (treatment) knowledge. Different demands are placed on these two types of scientific theories (see also Eagle 1984).

## 10.4 The Differing Requirements for Theories of Pure and Applied Science

Truth and practical utility are the two criteria by which pure and applied scientific theories have to be evaluated (Herrmann 1979, pp. 138-140). "Truth" means here that hypotheses and statements (including explanations) about a range of objects have been shown by experience to be accurate. Practical utility means that these statements lead to effective acts, i.e., to acts by which the desired goals are achieved.

Pure scientific theories may be (indeed, are supposed to be) bold, original, and innovative. Surprises during the testing of a theory are often of great heuristic value. For example, the psychoanalytic hypothesis regarding the etiology of a given illness may turn out not to be valid for that illness, but to be true of another illness where this etiology had not even been suspected. On the basis of the existing theory, the attempt is made to explain this surprise. New assumptions result, producing an extended (or corrected) form of the theory with the resultant new attempts at verification. In this example, the unexpected has been decisive in the growth of knowledge — understood in the sense of an ever more successful explanation of the world of facts.

The demand is placed on the pure scientific theory of psychoanalysis that it possess depth, range, precision, and sufficient degree of validity (Stegmüller 1969). For example, it is expected that the general hypotheses of clinical psychoanalytic theory represent as close an approximation to clinical reality as possible. Thus they are supposed to be able to adequately and comprehensively describe the genesis, development, and course of psychic illnesses, or to be able to sufficiently explain all the significant factors and the interdependence of psychic processes.

The truth of pure scientific theories (including in psychoanalysis the theories of development, personality, and neuroses) consists in the accurate and sufficient explanation of the reality they are making statements about. Thus, if scientific theories are not to describe reality merely in an abridged and consequently inadequate way, they have to be a maximal approximation to the complexity of reality. In the empirical sciences, the degree to which this approximation is successful is tested by observation and experiment. Thus the dilemma is created that complex (and thus parameter-rich) theories, such as psychoanalytic theory, are difficult to test empirically, while theories which are easier to test often have very few parameters and are thus usually abridged representations of reality.

Technologies are expected above all else to be reliable. Those which are original and bold, which lead to surprises, and which do not guarantee to keep practice firmly under control are of no value. Simple and rough representations of reality are often precisely the ones which provide the technological advantages expected and demanded of them, by making it possible to formulate recommendations for effective action (treatment rules) to accomplish current tasks in concrete problem situations under specific circumstances.

A fully formulated technology of psychoanalysis — as yet there is none — would have to demonstrate a sufficient degree of applicability, usefulness, and reliability for therapeutic practice (Lenk 1973, p. 207). All of this implies the demand for the practical utility (efficiency) of technological theories. From the point of view of efficiency, it is a matter not of how well the psychoanalytic technology explains clinical reality, but rather of how well it is able to master the routine tasks of clinical psychoanalysis. The theories concerning technique must be investigated in order to determine which approaches are especially useful for therapeutic practice. The effectiveness of a psychoanalytic technology is judged by the success of the therapeutic practice employing the technology. The distinctive feature of psychoanalytic technology is without doubt interpretation. In this sense it is possible to speak of a technological hermeneutics differing in essential features from theological and philological hermeneutics (Thomä and Kächele 1975; Thomä et al. 1976; Eagle 1984). Psychoanalytic interpretations are made not for texts, but for patients with therapeutic expectations. Blight (1981) therefore stressed that psychoanalysts cannot merely retreat inside the hermeneutic circle. The attempt to prove the therapeutic effectiveness of psychoanalytic interpretations forces analysts to take at least one step outside the hermeneutic circle and confront questions regarding the empirical proof of change. Thus, even Ricoeur cannot escape viewing the effectiveness of therapy as the decisive criterion for the hermeneutic psychoanalytic method of proving the existence of unconscious motivations: "The guarantee that the reality of the unconscious is not just a pure figment of psychoanalysts' imagination is provided finally only by therapeutic success" (Ricoeur 1974, p. 19). In general, however, it is precisely the hermeneutic school of psychoanalysis which has paid no more than lip service to effectiveness. With surprising modesty, analysts are satisfied with subjective evidence, that is, with dyad-specific truths within the hermeneutic circle (Lorenzer 1970).

Even a high degree of effectiveness (the main criterion) does not guarantee the truth of the technology, i.e., the accuracy of the technological explanation, which is another important consideration. A technological rule might specify, for example, that the analyst interpret resistance instead of unconscious conflicts if he wants to resolve the resistance resulting from repeatedly addressing a repressed conflict in various interpretations. Assuming that the effectiveness of this rule has been shown, we now ask why this recommendation for action is effective. The answer is provided by technological assumptions in the form of a technological explanation. The factor to be explained and founded is the connection between the condition established by the analyst (e.g., via interpretation) and the effect it has on the patient (reaction). The effectiveness of this rule can be explained in the following way: The unconscious conflict is repressed for specific reasons, i.e., there is a motive for the repression (e.g., avoiding the guilt feelings that arise when the conflict becomes conscious). For this reason the motive for repression is strengthened when the analyst ignores the patient's resistance and interprets the unconscious content of the conflict directly. The repression then expresses itself as the patient's increased resistance to insight into the unconscious content of the conflict. The motive for repression is also unconscious, and causes the patient's resistance as long as it remains so. The automatic nature of this mechanism can be overcome if the resistance is interpreted. Here, interpretation of resistance means that the patient is made aware, not of the unconscious content of the conflict, but rather of the motive for repression, which is closer to the ego. This destroys the automatic mechanism, removing the basis for the formation of resistance.

The validity of this explanation is tested in the course of research into the therapeutic process following the usual methods of empirical research, i.e., in the same way that the statements and hypotheses in pure scientific theories are tested. It is quite possible that the mechanisms asserted in the technological assumptions, and alleged to explain the effectiveness of the rule, are inadequate for the facts, i.e., the explanation is insufficient. It may nevertheless still be possible to formulate effective rules using these assumptions. The reverse is also possible: the therapeutic process, in contrast to the preparation of a list of effective rules, might be satisfactorily explained by the assumptions of a given technology. Technologies can thus have two faces. First (the explanation), they can be treated as pure scientific theories and consequently have to satisfy the requirement of such theories. Alternatively (the generation), they remain theories of applied science and are expected to demonstrate practical utility, i.e., effectiveness in practice. Satisfying the requirements of pure science is neither necessary nor sufficient for satisfying the requirements of applied science, and vice versa

This fact can be explained by the difference which exists between verbal expressions and the actions a person actually performs. Inasmuch as it is already possible to speak of psychoanalytic technology (since, at best, the statements on treatment technique can be regarded as operative technological theory), in therapeutic practice this technology is transformed by the psychoanalyst into a therapist-specific (personal) theory that might lead to effective therapy even if the objective technology is not completely valid. The opposite is the case if the technology is sufficiently "true" yet its operative conditions are different from those of therapeutic practice, or if the therapist's subjective adaptation of it produces an ineffective result.

A refined technology which takes all the special circumstances of a real, complex situation into consideration is lacking in psychoanalysis, as indeed it is in the applied social sciences as a whole. Such a technology would be able, if it were sufficiently valid, to provide recommendations in the form of rules for the appropriate action in every specific situation. If an analyst wanted to use such a utopian technology in the course of therapy, he would have to master a wealth of parameters exceeding the limits of his cognitive capacity. Even if such mastery were possible, the analyst's personal degree of adroitness would still come between his technological knowledge and his actual performance. The fact that the subjective adaptation of objective technology is an inevitable problem in the translation of theory into practice is a reference to the practice of psychoanalytic therapy as an art. The translation is ultimately a skill, and the practice of therapy an art. Mastering this art is a question of training and personality.

## 10.5 Consequences for Therapeutic Action and for the Scientific Justification of Theory

The consequence of the distinction made above between the truth of knowledge and the effectiveness of action is to separate these two factors which were so closely linked in psychoanalytic practice by Freud's inseparable bond thesis. Their relationship is not a priori such that one is the prerequisite or consequence of the other. In the analytic situation, research is not automatically linked with therapeutic acts, or vice versa. The bond has to be produced each time through concrete action. The analyst must ask himself whether his daily psychoanalytic activity not only leads to true individual insights into the patient's psychic processes, but also promotes the patient's eventual cure. In other words, the question is whether his technique is equally suited to gain new insights and to achieve therapeutic success. The inseparable bond must be created, it is no law inevitably governing psychoanalytic practice. The assertion that a *circulus benignus* exists in practice, i.e., that (true) theory and (effective) therapy promote each other, is not justified until the inseparable bond has been established. Therapy research conducted by third parties not directly involved in therapeutic activity has the task of determining whether this has been achieved in practice in more than just individual cases (see also Sampson and Weiss 1983; Neudert et al. 1985; and Chap. 9).

In view of the fact that neither effectiveness nor truth necessarily determines or results from the other, in attempts to validate psychoanalytic hypotheses it is essential that there be clarity with regard to whether the hypotheses are understood in the sense of pure science or applied science. If the latter is the case, it is also necessary to clarify whether the object of discussion is their explanatory value and/or their generative value (their usefulness in formulating effective rules). The testing criteria and procedure vary accordingly.

The divergence of truth and effectiveness is not given sufficient consideration even if, for example, the "tally" argument, as it was named by Grünbaum, is used to prove the correctness of psychoanalytic hypotheses. This argument is based on the following statement by Freud:

> After all, his conflicts will only be successfully solved and his resistances overcome if the *anticipatory ideas* he is given *tally* with what is real in him [i.e., the patient]. Whatever in the doctor's conjectures is inaccurate drops out in the course of the analysis; it has to be withdrawn and replaced by something more correct. (Freud 1916/17, p. 452, emphasis added)

Here Freud expresses the opinion that therapy can be successful only if the patient achieves accurate insight into the historical truth of his life and his suffering. The tally argument describes a problem of correspondence and not a claim to truth, as Freud has supposed.

Grünbaum, who has dealt in detail with the problem of testing psychoanalytic theory on the couch (i.e., in and through practice; see especially Grünbaum 1984), calls the assertion that true insight leads to success in therapy the "necessary condition thesis." This thesis is the most important assumption for the tally argument, that is for the argument that therapeutically successful analyses speak for the truth of the analytic (dyadic) knowledge gained in these analyses and communicated to the patient. Grünbaum raises the following doubts about the therapeutic effect of true insight: The therapeutic effect might actually be due to the analyst's suggestion, e.g., could be based on untrue insights and pseudoexplanations; it might be a placebo effect due to the analyst's and patient's faith in the truth and effectiveness of insight gained through interpretation; or it could result from yet other aspects of the psychoanalytic situation, such as from the experience of a new kind of interpersonal relationship, and not from "true insight."

In contrast, Edelson (1984) continues to support the claim that a patient's true insight is a necessary prerequisite for changes which are valued as therapeutically positive in the framework of a psychoanalysis. At the same time, he admits that true insight is not a sufficient precondition for achieving therapeutic changes in psychoanalysis. Edelson argues that analysis-specific goals and changes are all tied to the patient's true insight, and that it is only possible to speak of a successful and effective psychoanalytic treatment if these goals and changes are achieved.

It is not difficult to recognize that the controversy about the correctness of the necessary condition thesis is actually about the question of whether Freud's assertion of an inseparable bond is valid for psychoanalytic practice or not. Anyone who simply accepts the inseparable bond as a given fact in his arguments (e.g., in the form of the tally argument) treats the bond as a law of nature. It is often forgotten that the role of true insight has not been sufficiently studied in empirical research into the therapeutic process, and that the conception of insight is tied to serious methodological difficulties (see the survey in Roback 1974). It would therefore be premature to accept assertions about the association of true insight with therapeutic success as valid (as in natural law). This caution is justified in view of the fact that empirical research into the therapeutic process has acknowledged that a whole series of conditions beyond true insight play a significant role (Garfield and Bergin 1978).

Grünbaum's contamination thesis had previously been put forward by Farrell (see Farrell 1981), and specifically addressed by Cheshire (1975, Chap. 4), who convincingly defended psychoanalysis against it. The decision as to the correctness of this thesis must be made on the basis of empirical research into the therapeutic process, and not within the framework of philosophical discussions. The same is true of the allegation regarding suggestion, the legitimacy of which would have to be substantiated empirically with regard to psychoanalytic practice before it could be asserted with the certainty which often characterizes it (Thomä 1977). It must therefore be demanded, first, that the forms of changes specific to psychoanalysis be described exactly and be distinguished from other processes; second, that research seek indicators for the changes in question, since the changes, inasmuch as they concern dispositions, can only be observed indirectly via these indicators; and third, that not only the conditions for true insight be specified and examined, but also what is necessary in addition to true insight in order to achieve the personality changes envisaged by the goals specific to psychoanalysis (Edelson 1984). Freud's leitmotif "Where id was, ego shall be" (Freud 1933a, p. 80) sets an ambitious goal, which in another form coincides with the aim of structural changes. Everyone who has attempted systematic research in this field knows that our task is difficult to discharge if we want to go beyond clinically confirmed knowledge. In the previous chapter we described examples making it clear that modifications of our theoretical ideas are also to be expected which will have beneficial effects on our clinical activity.

Based on the previous results of process-oriented therapy research, it is possible to predict that in future, more sophisticated studies the umbrella concepts of suggestion and insight will dissolve into a broad spectrum of communicative processes. Psychoanalytic therapy also takes life, even though in a particularly refined manner, from the general ingredients of helpful therapy, as Luborsky (1984) has shown empirically for the "helping alliance." Furthermore, psychoanalytic forms of therapy exhibit specific characteristics which distinguish them more or less clearly from other approaches to therapy. We tend to the view that exact exploration of the processes of change in psychoanalytic therapy is just beginning and that numerous detailed studies at different levels of research and using different theoretical approaches will have to be conducted. Tape recordings make it possible to verify observations concerning changes, creating a third area between experimental and clinical psychoanalysis, namely the systematic clinical study of the treatment material (Kächele 1981; Leuzinger and Kächele 1985; Gill and Hoffman 1982).

We would term these approaches "technological research" in the sense described above, i.e., research into psychoanalytic technique and technology. We question whether verification of the basic science theories of psychoanalysis is possible in the treatment room, and agree with the demand, repeated by Grünbaum (1984), that the numerous hypotheses brought to light in the course of treatment be made the object of systematic research by empirical social science and psychology (Kline 1972; Fisher and Greenberg 1977). There has, of course, been an ever growing corpus of just such objective, nonclinical studies since Sears' pioneering work appeared a few years after Freud's death (see Fisher and Greenberg 1977). In our opinion, the psychoanalyst's observations in the therapeutic situation make a significant contribution to studying the etiology of psychopathology or the theory of personality development by generating numerous hypotheses. Yet they can contribute to a theory of therapy in a much more comprehensive manner, i.e., to

> an understanding of the relationship between certain kinds of operations and interventions and the occurrence or failure of occurrence of certain kinds of specific changes. It seems to me ironic that psychoanalytic writers attempt to employ clinical data for just about every purpose but the one for which they are most appropriate — an evaluation and understanding of therapeutic change. (Eagle 1984, p. 163)

We agree with Grünbaum (1984) that the office is not the place where the analyst can test basic science theories. However, while Grünbaum considers the phenomena in the clinical situation to be useless as a basis for the verification and testing of psychoanalytic hypotheses, in our opinion these data make an excellent touchstone for use in scientific evaluation by uninvolved third parties testing the validity of the hypotheses (Luborsky et al. 1985). Supplementing

Eagle's position, we think these data are relevant for the generation and testing of both technological and basic science assumptions. We agree with Edelson (1984), who demonstrated this for two examples — his interpretation of the case of "Miss X," reported by Luborsky and Mintz (1974), and Glymour's (1980) argumentation concerning Freud's Rat Man (1909 d).

The test in this case is not based on a postulated link between effectiveness and truth, but directly on clinical data. Eagle (1984) also correctly emphasizes that diagnostic knowledge, i.e., that gained from observation of the specific ways in which syndromes develop, represents an independent field relying neither on dyad-specific truth nor on therapeutic effectiveness. For example, Thomä's (1967 a) descriptions of anorexia nervosa in psychodynamic terms have proven to be correct in their essentials despite the changes in therapeutic strategies which have occurred both within and without psychoanalysis.

The basic science hypotheses of psychoanalysis have a wide field of reference (e.g., development, personality, and illness) and can move at a variety of levels (see, e.g., Waelder 1962). It is necessary for analysts, when preparing to test psychoanalytic assumptions on the clinical data, to ask themselves which assumptions the clinical data can serve as a touchstone for, and what degree of reliability can be attributed to the clinical data. It is clear from both theoretical considerations (Wallerstein and Sampson 1971; Thomä and Kächele 1975) and empirical investigations (Luborsky and Spence 1978; Kiener 1978) that metapsychological assumptions are useless for this task. It is necessary in this regard that the (often distorting) influence of metapsychological assumptions on clinical experience and interpretation be judged very critically (see Chap. 1). There have been numerous discussions of the real difficulties regarding the use of clinical data to validate basic science hypotheses, and of the controversial possible solutions; we will therefore limit ourselves here to a few references to the literature (Thomä and Kächele 1975; Möller 1978; Grünbaum 1982; Eagle 1984; Edelson 1984).

In closing, we would like to plead for the consideration of psychoanalytic practice both as the core of therapy and as an essential component of the research process in psychoanalysis. Psychoanalytic practice is the sphere where the process of cure takes place and heuristically valuable knowledge is gained. The inclusion of uninvolved third parties is essential and decisive in the testing of this knowledge, whether it be from basic science or applied science. We have to restrict the psychoanalytic research referred to in the inseparable bond assertion, in the sense that its results can be used only for the discovery and development of preliminary hypotheses, not for testing them. The analyst in his daily therapeutic routine must ask himself whether his treatment technique is appropriate both for establishing new hypotheses and widening psychoanalytic knowledge and for promoting the process of cure.

For reasons of methodological principle, the individual analyst is not in a position to do justice to this triad. Who indeed would claim — as Freud did — not only to have gained something new, but also, by means of strict analysis, to have descended into the deepest strata *and* to have proven that he had thus gained solutions for later configurations? In addition, according to Freud's scientific credo, the increase in generalizable, objectified knowledge of psychic connections can, indeed must, lead to an acceleration of the process of cure if the knowledge is communicated in the course of therapy in an appropriate manner.

Within the psychoanalytic system, short therapies are thus a necessary consequence of scientific progress. In any case, a practical and theoretical foundation is required for descent into the deepest mental strata as well as for analyses which have favorable results in a short time. Only then can it be proven that interpretive therapy is also a treatment promoting the patient's knowledge of himself. This self-knowledge, however, does not have to have an innovative character with regard to the basic and applied science theory of psychoanalysis. Its primary value consists in the fact that, along with other factors, it exercises a positive influence on the process of cure. It is thus very ambitious to want to connect psychoanalytic research in the psychoanalytic situation (i.e., gaining new psychoanalytic hypotheses, which must be distinguished from the research carried out by uninvolved third parties to test the hypotheses) with the interest in achieving a cure. Freud's theory of technique requires that the analyst distinguish between the following components: *curing*, *gaining* new hypotheses, *testing* hypotheses, the *correctness* of explanations, and the *utility* of knowledge.

# References

Freud's works are cited by year and indicating letter according to the complete Freud bibliography given in volume XXIV of the *Standard Edition* (SE), published by the Hogarth Press, London. Dates given in square brackets refer to the year a work was originally published should this diverge considerably from the date of the edition cited.


Abraham K (1953[1913]) Should patients write down their own dreams. In: Jones E (ed) Selected papers of Karl Abraham M. D., vol I (Internat psycho-analytical library, no 13). Basic Books, New York, pp 33—35

Abraham K (1953[1919]) A particular form of neurotic resistance against the psychoanalytic method. In: Jones E (ed) Selected papers of Karl Abraham M. D., vol I (Internat psychoanalytical library, no 13). Basic Books, New York, pp 303—311

Abraham K (1953[1920]) The applicability of psycho-analytic treatment to patients at an advanced age. In: Jones E (ed) Selected papers of Karl Abraham M. D., vol I (Internat psycho-analytical library, no 13). Basic Books, New York, pp 312—317

Adler R (1979) Anamneseerhebung in der psychosomatischen Medizin. In: Uexküll T von (ed) Lehrbuch der psychosomatischen Medizin. Urban & Schwarzenberg, Munich Vienna Baltimore, pp 329—348

Adorno TW (1952) Zum Verhältnis von Psychoanalyse und Gesellschaftstheorie. Psyche 6:1—18

Adorno TW (1972[1955]) Zum Verhältnis von Soziologie und Psychologie. In: Tiedemann R (ed) Theodor W. Adorno. Gesammelte Schriften, vol 8: Soziologische Schriften I. Suhrkamp, Frankfurt am Main, pp 42—85

Adorno TW, Dirks W (eds) (1957) Freud in der Gegenwart. Frankfurter Beiträge zur Soziologie, vol 6. Europäische Verlagsanstalt, Frankfurt am Main

Albert H (1960) Wissenschaft und Politik. Zum Problem der Anwendbarkeit einer wertfreien Sozialwissenschaft. In: Topitsch E (ed) Probleme der Wissenschaftstheorie. Festschrift für Victor Kraft. Springer, Berlin Heidelberg New York

Alexander F (1935) The problem of psychoanalytic technique. Pschoanal Q 4:588—611

Alexander F (1937) Five-year report of the Chicago Institute for Psychoanalysis, 1933—1937 (unpublished report)

Alexander F (1950) Psychosomatic medicine. Its principles and application. Allen & Unwin, London

Alexander F (1956) Two forms of regression and their therapeutic implications. Psychoanal Q 25:178—196

Alexander F, French TM (1946) Psychoanalytic therapy. Ronald Press, New York

Altman L (1976) Discussion of G. Epstein's "A note on a semantic confusion in the fundamental rule of psychoanalysis". J Philadelphia Assoc Psychoanal 3:58—59

Angst W (1980) Aggression bei Affen und Menschen. Springer, Berlin Heidelberg New York

Apel KO (1955) Das Verstehen. Arch Begriffsgesch 1:142—199

Appelbaum SA (1975) The idealization of insight. Int J Psychoanal Psychother 4:272—302

Appelbaum SA (1976) The dangerous edge of insight. Psychother Theory Res Pract 13:202—206

Argelander H (1966) Zur Psychodynamik des Erstinterviews. Psyche 20:40—53

Argelander H (1967) Das Erstinterview in der Psychotherapie. Psyche 21:341—368, 429—467, 473—512
Argelander H (1970) Das Erstinterview in der Psychotherapie (Erträge der Forschung, vol 2). Wissenschaftliche Buchgesellschaft, Darmstadt
Argelander H (1979) Die kognitive Organisation psychischen Geschehens. Ein Versuch zur Systematisierung der kognitiven Organisation in der Psychoanalyse. Klett-Cotta, Stuttgart
Argelander H, Eckstaedt A, Fischer R, Goldschmidt O, Kennel K (1973) Das Sprechstundeninterview. Psyche 27:1001—1066
Arlow JA (1979) Metaphor and the psychoanalytic situation. Psychoanal Q 48:363—385
Arlow JA (1982) Psychoanalytic education. A psychoanalytic perspective. Annu Psychoanal 10:5—20
Arlow JA, Brenner C (1964) Psychoanalytic concepts and the structural theory. International University Press, New York
Asch SS (1976) Varieties of negative therapeutic reaction and problems of technique. J Am Psychoanal Assoc 24:383—407
Austin JL (1962) How to do things with words. Clarendon Press, Oxford
Bachrach HM (1983) On the concept of analyzability. Psychoanal Q 52:180—204
Bacon F (1960[1620]) The new organon. In: Anderson FH (ed) The new organon and related writings. Liberal Arts Press, New York
Bakan D (1958) Sigmund Freud and the Jewish mystical tradition. Van Nostrand, Princeton
Balint A (1936) Handhabung der Übertragung auf Grund der Ferenczischen Versuche. Int Z Psychoanal 22:47—58
Balint A, Balint M (1939) On transference and countertransference. Int J Psychoanal 20:223—230
Balint M (1934) Charakteranalyse und Neubeginn. Int Z Psychoanal 20:54—63. Engl (1952) Character analysis and new beginning. In Balint M (ed) Primary love and psycho-analytic technique. Hogarth, London, pp 159—173o
Balint M (1935) Zur Kritik der Lehre von den prägenitalen Libidoorganisationen. Int Z Psychoanal 21:525—543. Engl: (1952) Critical notes on the theory of pregenital organisation of the libido. In: Balint M (ed) Primary love and psycho-analytic technique. Hogarth, London, pp 49—72
Balint M (1948) On the psychoanalytic training system. Int J Psychoanal 29:163—173
Balint M (1950) Changing therapeutical aims and techniques in psycho-analysis. Int J Psychoanal 31:117—124
Balint M (1952) Primary love and psycho-analytic technique. Hogarth, London
Balint M (1954) Analytic training and training analysis. Int J Psychoanal 35:157—162
Balint M (1957) Problems of human pleasure and behaviour. Hogarth, London
Balint M (1959) Thrills and regressions. Hogarth, London
Balint M (1968) The basic fault. Therapeutic aspects of regression. Tavistock, London
Balint M, Balint E (1961) Psychotherapeutic techniques in medicine. Tavistock, London
Balint M, Ornstein PH, Balint E (1972) Focal psychotherapy. An example of applied psychoanalysis. Tavistock, London
Balint M, Tarachow pp (1950) General concepts and theory of psychoanalytic therapy. In: Frosch J (ed) The annual survey of psychoanalysis, vol I. Allen & Unwin, London, pp 227—240
Balter L, Lothane Z, James H, Spencer JR (1980) On the analysing instrument. Psychoanal Q 49:474—504
Bartels M (1979) Ist der Traum eine Wunscherfüllung? Psyche 33:97—131
Basch MF (1984) Selfobjects and selfobject transference. Theoretical implications. In: Stepansky PE, Goldberg A (eds) Kohut's legacy. Contributions to self psychology. Analytic Press, Hillsdale London, pp 21—41
Bateson G, Jackson DD, Haley J, Weakland JH (1963) A note on the double bind - 1962. Family Process 2:154—161
Baumann U (ed) (1981) Indikation zur Psychotherapie. Perspektiven für Forschung und Praxis (Fortschritte der klinischen Psychologie, vol 25). Urban & Schwarzenberg, Munich
Baumann U (ed) (1984) Psychotherapie. Makro- / Mikroperspektive. Hogrefe, Göttingen Toronto Zürich

Baumann U, Wedel B von (1981) Stellenwert der Indikationsfrage im Psychotherapiebereich. In: Baumann U (ed) Indikation zur Psychotherapie. Perspektiven für Praxis und Forschung (Fortschritte der klinischen Psychologie, vol 25). Urban & Schwarzenberg, Munich Vienna Baltimore, pp 1—36
Baumeyer F (1971) Zur Geschichte der Psychoanalyse in Deutschland. 60 Jahre Deutsche Psychoanalytische Gesellschaft. Z Pschosom Med Psychoanal 17:203—240
Beckermann A (1977) Handeln und Handlungserklärungen. In: Beckermann A (ed) Analytische Handlungstheorie. vol 2: Handlungserklärungen. Suhrkamp, Frankfurt am Main, pp 7—84
Beckmann D (1974) Der Analytiker und sein Patient. Untersuchungen zur Übertragung und Gegenübertragung. Huber, Bern Stuttgart Vienna
Beigler JS (1975) A commentary on Freud's treatment of the rat man. Annu Psychoanal 3:271—285
Beland H (1978) Überlegungen zum Problem der finanziellen Selbständigkeit des Patienten als Heilungsfaktor. In: Die Einflüsse der Kassenreglung auf die psychoanalytische Behandlung. Referate und Protokolle der Arbeitstagung der DPV in Berlin vom 16—18 November 1978, pp 3—10 (unpublished report)
Bellak L (1961) Free association. Conceptual and clinical aspects. Int J Psychoanal 42:9—20
Bergin AE, Lambert MJ (1978) The evalutation of therapeutic outcomes. In: Garfield SL, Bergin AE (eds) Handbook of psychotherapy and behavior change: An empirical analysis, 2nd edn. Wiley, New York, pp 139—189
Berman L (1949) Countertransferences and attitudes of the analyst in the therapeutic process. Psychiatry 12:159—166
Bernfeld S (1934) Die Gestalttheorie. Imago 20:32—77
Bernfeld S (1935) Über die Einteilung der Triebe. Imago 21:125—142
Bernfeld S, Feitelberg S (1929) Das Prinzip von Le Chatelier und der Selbsterhaltungstrieb. Imago 15:289—298
Bernfeld S, Feitelberg S (1930) Über psychische Energie, Libido und deren Meßbarkeit. Imago 16:66—118
Bertalanffy L von (1958) Comments on aggression. Bull Menn Clin 22:50—57
Bettelheim B (1982) Freud and man's soul. Knopf, New York
Bibring E (1937) Versuch einer allgemeinen Theorie der Heilung. Int Z Psychoanal 23:18—42
Bibring E (1941) The development and problems of the theory of instincts. Int J Psychoanal 22:102—131
Bibring E (1947) The so-called English school of psychoanalysis. Psychoanal Q 16:69—93
Bibring E (1954) Psychoanalysis and the dynamic psychotherapies. J Am Psychoanal Assoc 2:745—770
Binswanger L (1955[1920]) Psychoanalyse und klinische Psychiatrie. In: Binswanger L (ed) Ausgewählte Vorträge und Aufsätze. vol II: Zur Problematik der psychiatrischen Forschung und zum Problem der Psychiatrie. Francke, Bern, pp 40—66
Binswanger L (1962) Erinnerungen an Freud. Francke, Bern
Bion WR (1955) Language and the schizophrenic. In: Klein M, Heimann P, Money-Kyrle RE (eds) New directions in psycho-analysis. Basic Books, New York, pp 220—239
Bion WR (1970) Attention and interpretation. A scientific approach to insight in psychoanalysis and groups. Tavistock, London
Birbaumer N (ed) (1973) Neuropsychologie der Angst (Fortschritte der Klinischen Psychologie 3). Urban & Schwarzenberg, Munich
Blacker KH (1981) Insight. Clinical conceptualizations. J Am Psychoanal Assoc 29:659—671
Blanck G, Blanck R (1974) Ego psychology. Theory and practice. Columbia University Press, New York
Blanck G, Blanck R (1979) Ego psychology, vol 2. Columbia University Press, New York Guilford
Blanton S (1971) Diary of my analysis with Sigmund Freud. Hawthorn Books, New York

Blarer A von, Brogle I (1983) Der Weg ist das Ziel. Zur Theorie und Metatheorie der psychoanalytischen Technik. In: Hoffmann SO (ed) Deutung und Beziehung. Kritische Beiträge zur Behandlungskonzeption und Technik in der Psychoanalyse. Fischer, Frankfurt am Main, pp 71—85

Bleuler E (1910) Die Psychoanalyse Freuds. Verteidigung und kritische Bemerkungen. Jahrb Psychoanal Psychopath Forsch 2:623—730

Blight J (1981) Must psychoanalysis retreat to hermeneutics? Psychoanalytic theory in the light of Popper's evolutionary epistemology. Psychoanal Contemp Thought 4:127—206

Blos P (1963) The concept of acting out in relation to the adolescent process. J Am Acad Child Psychiatry 2:118—143

Blos p (1985) Son and father. Before and beyond the Oedipus complex. Free Press, New York London

Blum HP (1971) On the conception and development of the transference neurosis. J Am Psychoanal Assoc 19:41—53

Blum HP (1973) The concept of erotized transference. J Am Psychoanal Assoc 21:61—76

Blum HP (1976) Acting out, the psychoanalytic process, and interpretation. Annu Psychoanal 4:163—184

Blum HP (1979) The curative and creative aspects of insight. J Am Psychoanal Assoc 27 [Suppl]:41—69

Boden MA (1977) Artificial intelligence and natural man. Basic Books, New York

Boesky D (1982) Acting out. A reconsideration of the concept. Int J Psychoanal 63:39—55

Bolk-Weischedel D (1978) Veränderungen beim unbehandelten Partner des Patienten während einer analytischen Psychotherapie. Z Psychosom Med Psychoanal 24:116—128

Bonaparte M (1940) Time and the unconscious. Int J Psychoanal 21:427—468

Boor C de, Künzler E (1963) Die psychosomatische Klinik und ihre Patienten. Klett, Stuttgart

Boor C de, Moersch E (1978) Stellungnahme zu P. Parins "Kritischer Glosse". Psyche 32:400—402

Bowlby J (1969) Attachment and loss. Vol I: Attachment. Basic Books, New York

Bracher KD (1982) Zeit der Ideologien. Deutsche Verlagsanstalt, Stuttgart

Bräutigam W (1983) Bemerkungen zur psychoanalytischen Behandlungsführung in der Eröffnungs- und Abschlußphase. In: Hoffmann SO (ed) Deutung und Beziehung. Kritische Beiträge zur Behandlungskonzeption und Technik in der Psychoanalyse. Fischer, Frankfurt am Main, pp 119—131

Bräutigam W (1984) Rückblick auf das Jahr 1942. Betrachtungen eines psychoanalytischen Ausbildungskandidaten des Berliner Instituts der Kriegsjahre. Psyche 38:905—914

Brandchaft B, Stolorow RD (1984) A current perspective on difficult patients. In: Stepansky PE, Goldberg A (eds) Kohut's legacy. Contributions to self psychology. Analytic Press, Hillsdale London, pp 93—116

Brandt LW (1961) Some notes on English Freudian terminology. J Am Psychoanal Assoc 9:331—339

Brandt LW (1972) Mindless psychoanalysis. Contemp Psychol 17:189—191

Brandt LW (1977) Psychoanalyse versus psychoanalysis: traduttore, traditore. Bedeutungsunterschiede zwischen psychoanalytischen Grundbegriffen im Englischen und im Deutschen. Psyche 31:1045—1051

Brazelton TB, Als H (1979) Four early stages in the development of mother-infant interaction. Psychoanal Study Child 34:349—369

Brenner C (1976) Psychoanalytic technique and psychic conflict. International University Press, New York

Brenner C (1979a) Working alliance, therapeutic alliance and transference. J Am Psychoanal Assoc 27:137—157

Brenner C (1979b) The components of psychic conflict and its consequences in mental life. Psychoanal Q 48:547—567

Brenner C (1980) Metapsychology and psychoanalytic theory. Psychoanal Q 49:189—214

Brenner C (1982) The mind in conflict. International University Press, New York

Breuer J, Freud S (1936) Studies in hysteria (Nervous and mental disease monograph series no 61). Nervous and Mental Disease Publishing Co, New York

Brierley M (1937) Affects in theory and practice. Int J Psychoanal 18:256—268
Buber M (1974[1923]) Ich und Du, 8th edn. Schneider, Heidelberg
Bubner R (1976) Handlung, Sprache und Vernunft. Suhrkamp, Frankfurt am Main
Bunge M (1967) Scientific research, vol 2: The search for truth. Springer, New York Berlin Heidelberg
Bush M (1978) Preliminary considerations for a psychoanalytic theory of insight. Historical perspective. Int Rev Psychoanal 5:1—13
Buxbaum E (1950) Technique of terminating analysis. Int J Psychoanal 31:184—190
Calder KT (1980) An analyst's self-analysis. J Am Psychoanal Assoc 28:5—2
Calef V (1971) On the current concept of the transference neurosis. Introduction. J Am Psychoanal Assoc 19:137—157
Calogeras RC (1967) Silence as a technical parameter in psycho-analysis. Int J Psychoanal 48:536—558
Cantor MB (1957) The initial interview. Am J Psychoanal 17:39—44; 121—126
Caruso IA (1972) Soziale Aspekte der Psychoanalyse. Rowohlt, Reinbek bei Hamburg
Carveth DL (1984a) Psychoanalysis and social theory. The Hobbesian problem revisited. Psychoanal Contemp Thought 7:43—98
Carveth DL (1984b) The analyst's metaphors. A deconstructionist perspective. Psychoanal Contemp Thought 7:491—560
Cheshire NM (1975) The nature of psychodynamic interpretation. Wiley, London New York Sidney Toronto
Cheshire NM, Thomä H (eds) (1987) The self. Symptoms and psychotherapy. Wiley, London
Cocks GC (1983) Psychoanalyse, Psychotherapie und Nationalsozialismus. Psyche 37:1057—1106
Cocks GC (1984) Psychotherapy in the Third Reich. The Göring Institute. Oxford University Press, New York
Cohen DB (1976) Dreaming: Experimental investigation of representational and adaptive properties. In: Schwartz GE, Shapiro D (eds) Consciousness and self-regulation, vol 1. Plenum Press, New York London, pp 313—360
Cohen MB (1952) Countertransference and anxiety. Psychiatry 15:231—243
Cohler BJ (1980) Developmental perspectives on the psychology of the self in early childhood. In: Goldberg A (ed) Advances in selfpsychology. International University Press, New York, pp 69—115
Colby K (1960) Experiment on the effects of an observer's presence on the imago system during free association. Behav Sci 5:216—232
Collingwood RG (1946) The idea of history. Oxford University Press, London
Cooley CH (1964[1902]) Human nature and the social order. Schocken, New York
Cooper AM (1984a) Psychoanalysis at one hundred. Beginnings of maturity. J Am Psychoanal Assoc 32:245—267
Cooper AM (1984b) Columbia Center celebrates 40th anniversary. Am Psychoanal Assoc Newsletter 18 (4):10—15
Cremerius J (1969) Schweigen als Problem der psychoanalytischen Technik. Jahrb Psychoanal 6:69—103
Cremerius J (1977a) Ist die "psychosomatische Struktur" der französischen Schule krankheitsspezifisch? Psyche 31:293—317
Cremerius J (1977b) Grenzen und Möglichkeiten der psychoanalytischen Behandlungstechnik bei Patienten mit Über-Ich-Störungen. Psyche 31:593—636
Cremerius J (1978) Einige Überlegungen über die kritische Funktion des Durcharbeitens in der Geschichte der psychoanalytischen Technik. In: Drews S et al (eds) Provokation und Toleranz. Alexander Mitscherlich zu ehren. Festschrift für Alexander Mitscherlich zum 70. Geburtstag. Suhrkamp, Frankfurt am Main, pp 196—214
Cremerius J (1979) Gibt es zwei psychoanalytische Techniken? Psyche 33:577—599
Cremerius J (1981a) Die Präsenz des Dritten in der Psychoanalyse. Zur Problematik der Fremdfinanzierung. Psyche 35:1—41
Cremerius J (1981b) Freud bei der Arbeit über die Schulter geschaut. Seine Technik im Spiegel von Schülern und Patienten. In: Ehebald U, Eickhoff FW (eds) Humanität und Technik

in der Psychoanalyse. Jahrb Psychoanal, Beiheft 6. Huber, Bern Stuttgart Vienna, pp 123–158
Cremerius J (1982) Kohuts Behandlungstechnik. Eine kritische Analyse. Psyche 36:17–46
Cremerius J (1984) Die psychoanalytische Abstinenzregel. Vom regelhaften zum operativen Gebrauch. Psyche 38:769–800
Cremerius J, Hoffmann SO, Trimborn W (1979) Psychoanalyse, Über-Ich und soziale Schicht. Die psychoanalytische Behandlung der Reichen, der Mächtigen und der sozial Schwachen. Kindler, Munich
Curtis HC (1979) The concept of therapeutic alliance. Implications for the widening scope. J Am Psychoanal Assoc 27 [Suppl]:159–192
Dahl H (1978) A new psychoanalytic model of motivation. Emotion as appetites and messages. Psychoanal Contemp Thought 1:373 408
Dahmer H (1983) Kapitulation vor der "Weltanschauung". Zu einem Aufsatz von Carl Müller-Braunschweig aus dem Herbst 1933. Psyche 37:1116–1135
Dallet J (1973) Theories of dream function. Psychol Bull 79:408–416
Dantlgraber J (1982) Bemerkungen zur subjektiven Indikation für Psychoanalyse. Psyche 36:191–225
Darwin CR (1872) The expressions of the emotions in men and animals. J Murray, London
Deutsch F (1957) A footnote to Freud's "fragment of an analysis of a case of hysteria". Psychoanal Q 26:159–167
Deutsch F, Murphy WF (1955) The clinical interview, 2 vols. International University Press, New York
Deutsch H (1926) Okkulte Vorgänge während der Psychoanalyse. Imago 12:418–433
Deutsch H (1932) Psychoanalysis of the neuroses. Hogarth, London
Devereux G (1951) Some criteria for the timing of confrontations and interpretations. Int J Psychoanal 32:19–24
Devereux G (1967) From anxiety to method in the behavioral sciences. Mouton, Den Haag Paris
Dewald PA (1972) The psychoanalytic process. A case illustration. Basic Books, New York London
Dewald PA (1978) The psychoanalytic process in adult patients. Psychoanal Study Child 33:323–331
Dewald PA (1982) The clinical importance of the termination phase. Psychoanal Inquiry 1:441–461
Dilman I (1984) Freud and the mind. Blackwell, Oxford
Dollard JA, Miller NE, Doob LW, Mowrer OH, Sears RR (1967[1939]) Frustration and aggression. Yale University Press, New Haven
Doolittle H (1956) Tribute to Freud. Pantheon Books, New York
Dräger K (1971) Bemerkungen zu den Zeitumständen und zum Schicksal der Psychoanalyse und der Psychotherapie in Deutschland zwischen 1933 und 1949. Psyche 25:255–268
Drigalski D von (1979) Blumen auf Granit. Eine Irr- und Lehrfahrt durch die deutsche Psychoanalyse. Ullstein, Frankfurt am Main Berlin Vienna
Dührssen A (1953) Katamnestische Untersuchungen bei Patienten nach analytischer Psychotherapie. Z Psychother Med Psychol 3:167–170
Dührssen A (1962) Katamnestische Ergebnisse bei 1004 Patienten nach analytischer Psychotherapie. Z Psychosom Med 8:94–113
Dührssen A (1972) Analytische Psychotherapie in Theorie, Praxis und Ergebnissen. Vandenhoek & Ruprecht, Göttingen
Dührssen A (1981) Die biographische Anamnese unter tiefenpsychologischem Aspekt. Vandenhoek & Ruprecht, Göttingen
Eagle M (1973) Sherwood on the logic of explanation in psychoanalysis. Psychoanal Contemp Sci 2:331–337
Eagle M (1984) Recent developments in psychoanalysis. A critical evaluation. McGraw-Hill, New York
Earle JB (1979) An approach to the study of analyzability and analysis: The course of forty consecutive cases selected for supervised analysis. Psychoanal Q 48:198–228
Edelson JT (1983) Freud's use of metaphor. Psychoanal Study Child 38:17–59

Edelson M (1983) Is testing psychoanalytic hypotheses in the psychoanalytic situation really impossible? Psychoanal Study Child 38:61–109

Edelson M (1984) Hypothesis and evidence in psychoanalysis. University of Chicago Press, Chicago

Ehebald U (1978) Der Psychoanalytiker und das Geld – oder die Ideologie vom persönlichen finanziellen Opfer des Patienten. In: Drews S et al. (eds) Provokation und Toleranz. Alexander Mitscherlich zu ehren. Festschrift für Alexander Mitscherlich zum 70. Geburtstag. Suhrkamp, Frankfurt am Main, pp 361–386

Ehlers W (1983) Die Abwehrmechanismen. Definitionen und Beispiele. Praxis Psychother Psychosom 28:55–66

Ehlich K, Rehbein J (1979) Sprachliche Handlungsmuster. In: Soeffner HG (ed) Interpretative Verfahren in den Sozial- und Textwissenschaften. Metzler, Stuttgart

Eibl-Eibesfeldt I (1970) Liebe und Haß. Zur Naturgeschichte elementarer Verhaltensweisen. Piper, Munich

Eibl-Eibesfeldt I (1980) Die Entwicklung der destruktiven Aggression. Mater Med Nordmark 32:16–29

Eissler KR (ed) (1949) Searchlights on delinquency. New psychoanalytic studies dedicated to Professor August Aichhorn on the occasion of his seventieth birthday, July 27, 1948. International University Press, New York

Eissler KR (1950) The Chicago Institute of Psychoanalysis and the sixth period of the development of psychoanalytic technique. J Gen Psychol 42:103–157

Eissler KR (1953) The effect of the structure of the ego on psychoanalytic technique. J Am Psychoanal Assoc 1:104–143

Eissler KR (1958) Remarks on some variations in psychoanalytic technique. Int J Psychoanal 39:222–229

Eissler KR (1963a) Notes on the psychoanalytic concept of cure. Psychoanal Study Child 18:424–463

Eissler KR (1963b) Goethe. A psychoanalytic study, 1775–1786. Wayne State University Press, Detroit

Eissler KR (1965) Medical orthodoxy and the future of psychoanalysis. International University Press, New York

Eissler KR (1971) Death drive, ambivalence, and narcissism. Psychoanal Study Child 26:25–78

Eissler KR (1974) One some theoretical and technical problems regarding the payment of fees for psychoanalytic treatment. Int Rev Psychoanal 1:73–101

Ekstein R, Friedman SW (1959) On the meaning of play in childhood psychosis. In: Jessner L, Pavenstedt E (eds) Dynamics of psychopathology in childhood. Grune & Stratton, New York, pp 269–292

Emde RN (1981) Changing models of infancy and the nature of early development. Remodeling the foundation. J Am Psychoanal Assoc 29:179–219

Emde RN, Robinson J (1979) The first two month. Recent research in developmental psychobiology and the changing view of the new born. In: Noshpitz JD (ed) Basic handbook of child psychiatry, vol 1. Basic Books, New York, pp 72–105

Engel GL (1962) Psychological development in health and disease. Saunders, Philadelphia

Engel GL, Schmale AH jr (1967) Psychoanalytic theory of somatic disorder. J Am Psychoanal Assoc 15:344–365

Engelman E (1976) Berggasse 19. Sigmund Freud's home and offices, Vienna 1938. Basic Books, New York

Epstein G (1976) A note on a semantic confusion in the fundamental rule of psychoanalysis. J Philadelphia Assoc Psychoanal 3:54–57

Erikson EH (1954) The dream specimen of psychoanalysis. J Am Psychoanal Assoc 2:5–56

Erikson EH (1959) Identity and the life cycle. Selected papers (Psychological issues, vol 1, no 1, monograph 1). International University Press, New York

Erikson EH (1962) Reality and actuality. An address. J Am Psychoanal Assoc 11:451–474

Erikson EH (1964) Insight and responsibility. Lectures on the ethical implications of psychoanalytic insight. Norton, New York

Erikson EH (1968) Identity youth and crisis. Norton, New York

Etchegoyen RH (1982) The relevance of the "here and now" transference interpretation for the reconstruction of early psychic development. Int J Psychoanal 63:65—75

Eysenck HJ, Rachman S (1968) Neurosen. Ursachen und Heilmethoden, 2nd edn. Springer, Berlin Heidelberg New York

Ezriel H (1963) Experimentation within the psycho-analytic session. In: Paul L (ed) Psychoanalytic clinical interpretation. Free Press of Glencoe, London, pp 112—142

Faber FR (1981) Der Krankheitsbegriff in der Reichsversicherungsordnung. Psychother Med Psychol 31:179—182

Farell BA (1961) Can psychoanalysis be refuted ? Inquiry 4:16—36

Farell BA (1964) The status of psychoanalytic theory. Inquiry 7:104—123

Farrell BA (1981) The standing of psychoanalysis. Oxford University Press, Oxford

Farrow EP (1942) A practical method of self-analysis. Allen & Unwin, London

Federn P (1932) The reality of death instinct, especially in melancholia. Remarks on Freud's book "Civilisation and its discontents". Psychoanal Rev 19:129—151

Federn P (1952) Ego psychology and the psychoses. Basic Books, New York

Fenichel O (1930) Statistischer Bericht über die therapeutische Tätigkeit 1920—1930. In: Rad& S, Fenichel O, Müller-Braunschweig C (eds) Zehn Jahre Berliner Psychoanalytisches Institut. Poliklinik und Lehranstalt. Int Psychoanal Verlag, Vienna

Fenichel O (1934) Besprechung von T. Reik: "New ways in psycho-analytic technique". Int Z Psychoanal 20:399—400

Fenichel O (1941) Problems of psychoanalytic technique. Psychoanal Quart Inc, Albany New York

Fenichel O (1945) The psychoanalytic theory of neurosis. Norton, New York

Fenichel O (1953[1935a]) Concerning the theory of psychoanalytic technique. In: The collected papers of Otto Fenichel, first series. Norton, New York, pp 332—348

Fenichel O (1953[1935b]) A critique of the death instinct. In: The collected papers of Otto Fenichel, first series. Norton, New York, pp 636—372

Ferenczi S (1950[1919a]) On the technique of psycho-analysis. In: Jones E, Rickman J (eds) Further contributions to the theory and technique of psycho-analysis by Sandor Ferenczi M. D. Hogarth, London, pp 177—189

Ferenczi S (1950[1919b]) Technical difficulties in a case of hysteria. In: Jones E, Rickman J (eds) Further contributions to the theory and technique of psycho-analysis by Sandor Ferenczi M. D. Hogarth, London, pp 189—197

Ferenczi S (1950[1925]) Psychoanalysis of sexual habits. In: Jones E, Rickman J (eds) Further contributions to the theory and technique of psycho-analysis by Sandor Ferenczi M. D. Hogarth, London, pp 259—297

Ferenczi S (1955[1912]) Dirigible dreams. In: Balint M (ed) Final contributions to the problems and methods of psycho-analysis by Sandor Ferenczi M. D. Hogarth, London, pp 313—315

Ferenczi S (1955[1927]) The problem of the termination of analysis. In: Balint M (ed) Final contributions to the problems and methods of psycho-analysis by Sandor Ferenczi M. D. Hogarth, London, pp 77—86

Ferenczi S (1955[1928]) The elasticity of psychoanalytic technique. In: Balint M (ed) Final contributions to the problems and methods of psycho-analysis by Sandor Ferenczi M. D. Hogarth, London, pp 87—101

Ferenczi S (1955[1933]) The confusion of tongues between adults and the child. In: Balint M (ed) Final contributions to the problems and methods of psycho-analysis by Sandor Ferenczi M. D. Hogarth, London, pp 156—167

Ferenczi S, Rank O (1924) Entwicklungsziele der Psychoanalyse. Int Psychoanal Verlag, Vienna

Ferguson M (1981) Progress and theory change. The two analyses of Mr. Z. Annu Psychoanal 9:133—160

Fine BD, Joseph ED, Waldhorn HF (eds) (1971) Recollection and reconstruction. Reconstruction in psychoanalysis (The Kris study group of the New York Psychoanalytic Institute, monograph 4). International University Press, New York

Fine BD, Waldhorn HF (eds) (1975) Alterations in defences during psychoanalysis. Aspects of psychoanalytic intervention (The Kris study group of the New York Psychoanalytic Institute, monograph 6). International University Press, New York
Fingarette H (1977) Self-deception. Routledge & Kegan Paul, London
Firestein SK (1982) Termination of psychoanalysis. Theoretical, clinical, and pedagogic considerations. Psychoanal Inquiry 2:473—497
Fisher C (1965) Psychoanalytic implications of recent research on sleep and dreaming. J Am Psychoanal Assoc 13:197—270
Fisher S, Greenberg RP (1977) The scientific credibility of Freud's theories and therapies. Basic Books, New York
Flader D, Grodzicki WD (1978) Hypothesen zur Wirkungsweise der psychoanalytischen Grundregel. Psyche 32:545—594
Flader D, Grodzicki WD (1982) Die psychoanalytische Deutung. Eine diskursanalytische Fallstudie. In: Flader D, Grodzicki WD, Schröter K (eds) Psychoanalyse als Gespräch. Interaktionsanalytische Untersuchungen über Therapie und Supervision. Suhrkamp, Frankfurt am Main, pp 138—193
Fliess R (1953) Counter-transference and counter-identification. J Am Psychoanal Assoc 1:268—284
Foppa K (1968) Lernen, Gedächtnis, Verhalten. Ergebnisse und Probleme der Lernpsychologie. Kiepenheuer & Witsch, Cologne Berlin
Fosshage JL (1983) The psychological function of dreams. A revised psychoanalytic perspective. Psychoanal Contemp Thought 6:641—669
Foulkes D (1977) Children's dreams. Ages changes and sex differences. Waking and Sleeping 1:171—174
Foulkes D (1979) Children's dreams. In: Wolman BB (ed) Handbook of dreams. Van Nostrand, New York, pp 131—167
Foulkes D (1982) Children's dreams. Longitudinal studies. Wiley, New York
Frank A (1979) Two theories or one? Or none? J Am Psychoanal Assoc 27:169—207
French TM (1933) Interrelations between psychoanalysis and the experimental work of Pavlov. Am J Psychiatry 89:1165—1203
French TM (1936) A clinical study of learning in the course of psychoanalytic treatment. Psychoanal Q 5:148—194
French TM (1952) The integration of behaviour. Vol I: Basic postulates. University of Chicago Press, Chicago
French TM (1970) Psychoanalytic interpretations. The selected papers of Thomas M. French, M.D. Quadrangle, Chicago
French TM, Fromm E (1964) Dream interpretation. Basic Books, New York
Freud A (1927) Einführung in die Technik der Kinderanalyse. Internationaler Psychoanalytischer Verlag, Leipzig. Engl edn: (1948) Introduction to the technique of child analysis. Imago, London
Freud A (1937) The ego mand the mechanisms of defence. Hogarth, London
Freud A (1954a) The widening scope of indications for psychoanalysis. Discussion. J Am Psychoanal Assoc 2:607—620
Freud A (1954b) Problems of technique in adult analysis. Bulletin of the Philadelphia Association for Psychoanalysis 4:44—69.
Freud A (1971) The ideal psychoanalytic institute. A utopia. In: Freud A (ed) The writings of Anna Freud, vol VII, pp 73—93. International University Press, New York
Freud A (1972a) Child analysis as a sub-speciality of psychoanalysis. Int J Psychoanal 53:151—156
Freud A (1972b) Comments on aggression. Int J Psychoanal 53:163—171
Freud A (1983) Some observations. In: Joseph ED, Widlöcher D (eds) The identity of the psychoanalyst (Int Psychoanal Assoc, monograph series no 2). International University Press, New York, pp 257—263
Freud S (1895d) Studies on hysteria. SE vol II
Freud S (1900a) The interpretation of dreams. SE vol VI/V, pp 1—625
Freud S (1901a) On dreams. SE vol V, pp 629—686
Freud S (1904a) Freud's psychoanalytic procedure. SE vol VII, pp 247—254

Freud S (1905 a) On psychotherapy. SE vol VII, pp 255—268
Freud S (1905 d) Three essays on the theory of sexuality. SE vol VII, pp 123—245
Freud S (1905 e) Fragment of an analysis of a case of hysteria. SE vol VII, pp 1—122
Freud S (1906 c) Psycho-analysis and the establishment of facts in legal proceedings. SE vol IX, pp 97—114
Freud S (1909 b) Analysis of a phobia in a five-year-old boy. SE vol X, pp 1—149
Freud S (1909 d) Note upon a case of obsessional neurosis. SE vol X, pp 151—318
Freud S (1910 a) Five lectures on psycho-analysis. SE vol XI, pp 1—55
Freud S (1910 d) The future prospects of psycho-analytic therapy. SE vol XI, pp 139—151
Freud S (1910 k) 'Wild' psycho-analysis. SE vol XI, pp 219—227
Freud S (1911 b) Formulations on the two principles of mental functioning. SE vol XII, pp 213—226
Freud S (1911 e) The handling of dream-interpretation in psycho-analysis. SE vol XII, pp 89—96
Freud S (1912 b) The dynamics of tranference. SE vol XII, pp 97—108
Freud S (1912 e) Recommandations to physicians practising psycho-analysis. SE vol XII, pp 109—120
Freud S (1913 c) On beginning the treatment. SE vol XII, pp 121—144
Freud S (1913 h) Observations and examples from analytic practise. SE vol XIII, pp 189—198
Freud S (1914 d) On the history of the psycho-analytic movement. SE vol XIV, pp 1—66
Freud S (1914 g) Remembering, repeating, and working through SE vol XII, pp 145—156
Freud S (1915 a) Observations on transference-love. SE vol XII, pp 157—171
Freud S (1915 c) Instincts and their vicissitudes. SE vol XIV, pp 109—140
Freud S (1915 e) The unconscious. SE vol XIV, pp 159—215
Freud S (1916 a) On transience. SE vol XIV, pp 303—307
Freud S (1916/17) Introductory lectures on psycho-analysis. SE vol XV/XVI
Freud S (1917 d) A metapsychological supplement to the theory of dreams. SE vol XIV, pp 217—235
Freud S (1917 e) Mourning and melancholia. SE vol XIV, pp 237—258
Freud S (1918 b) From the history of an infantile neurosis. SE vol XVII, pp 1—122
Freud S (1919 a) Lines of advance in psycho-analytic therapy. SE vol XVII, pp 157—168
Freud S (1919 e) 'A child is being beaten'. SE vol XVII, pp 175—204
Freud S (1919 j) On the teaching of psycho-analysis in universities. SE vol XVII, pp 169—173
Freud S (1920 a) The psychogenesis of a case of homosexuality in a woman. SE vol XVII, pp 145—172
Freud S (1920 g) Beyond the pleasure principle. SE vol XVIII, pp 1—64
Freud S (1921 c) Group psychology and the analysis of the ego. SE vol XVIII, pp 65—143
Freud S (1922 d) Publications and prizes. SE vol XVII, p 269
Freud S (1923 a) Two encyclopaedia articles. SE vol XVIII, pp 233—259
Freud S (1923 b) The ego and the id. SE vol XIX, pp 1—66
Freud S (1923 c) Remarks on the theory and practise of dream-interpretation. SE vol XIX, pp 107—121
Freud S (1925 d) An autobiographical study. SE vol XX, pp 1—74
Freud S (1926 c) Prefatory note to a paper by E. Pickworth Farrow. SE vol XX, p 280
Freud S (1926 d) Inhibitions, symptoms, and anxiety. SE vol XX, pp 75—174
Freud S (1926 e) The question of lay analysis. SE vol XX, pp 177—250
Freud S (1926 f) Psycho-analysis. SE vol XX, pp 259—270
Freud S (1927 a) Postscript to the question of lay analysis. SE vol XX, pp 251—258
Freud S (1930 a) Civilisation and its discontents. SE vol XXI, pp 57—145
Freud S (1930 b) Preface to "Ten years of the Berlin Psychoanalytic Institute". SE vol XXI, p 257
Freud S (1931 d) The expert opinion of the Halsmann case. SE vol XXI, pp 251—253
Freud S (1933 a) New introductory lectures on psycho-analysis. SE vol XXII, pp 1—182
Freud S (1933 b) Why war? SE vol XXII, pp 195—215
Freud S (1937 c) Analysis terminable and interminable. SE vol XXII, pp 209—253

Freud S (1937 d) Constructions in analysis. SE vol XXIII, pp 255–269

Freud S (1940 a) An outline of psycho-analysis. SE vol XXIII, pp 139–207

Freud S (1950 a) Project for a scientific psychology. SE vol I, pp 281–397

Freud S (1960 a) In: Freud E, Freud L (eds) Letters of Sigmund Freud. Basic Books, New York

Friedman L (1978) Trends in the psychoanalytic theory of treatment. Psychoanal Q 47:524–567

Fürstenau P (1964) Ich-Psychologie und Anpassungsproblem. Eine Auseinandersetzung mit Heinz Hartmann. Jahrb Psychoanal 3:30–55

Fürstenau P (1977) Praxeologische Grundlagen der Psychoanalyse. In: Pongratz LJ (ed) Klinische Psychologie. Hogrefe, Göttingen Toronto Zürich (Handbuch der Psychologie, vol 8/1, pp 847–888)

Gabel H, Deneke F, Meyer AE, Bolz W, Stuhr U (1981) Our focus formulations. Practicability for therapy. Content analyses and relation to outcome and other variables. Psychother Psychosom 35:110–133

Gabel J (1975) False consciousness. An essay on reification. Basil Blackwell, Oxford

Gadamer HG (1965) Wahrheit und Methode. Anwendungen einer philosophischen Hermeneutik. Mohr Tübingen

Gardiner M (1971) The wolf-man. Basic Books, New York

Garfield SL, Bergin AE (eds) (1978) Handbook of psychotherapy and behaviour change. An empirical analysis, 2nd edn. Wiley, New York

Gaskill HS (1980) The closing phase of the psychoanalytic treatment of adults and the goals of psychoanalysis. "The myth of perfectibility". Int J Psychoanal 61:11–23

Geist WB, Kächele H (1979) Zwei Traumserien in einer psychoanalytischen Behandlung. Jahrb Psychoanal 11:138–165

Gill HS (1982) The life-context of the dreamer and the setting of dreaming. Int J Psychoanal 63:475–482

Gill MM (1976) Metapsychology is not psychology. In: Gill MM, Holzman PS (eds) Psychology versus metapsychology. Psychoanalytic essays in memory of George S. Klein (Psychological issues, vol 9, no 4, monograph 36). Basic Books, New York, pp 71–105

Gill MM (1977) Psychic energy reconsidered. Discussion. J Am Psychoanal Assoc 25:581–597

Gill MM (1979) The analysis of the transference. J Am Psychoanal Assoc 27 (Suppl):263–288

Gill MM (1982) Analysis of transference. Vol I: Theory and technique. International University Press, New York

Gill MM (1983) The point of view of psychoanalysis. Energy discharge or person. Psychoanal Contemp Thought 6:523–551

Gill MM, Hoffman IZ (1982) Analysis of transference. Vol II: Studies of nine audio-recorded psychoanalytic sessions. International University Press, New York

Gill MM, Holzman PS (eds) (1976) Psychology versus metapsychology. Psychoanalytic essays in memory of George S. Klein (Psychological issues, vol 9, no 4, monograph 36). International University Press, New York

Gill MM, Klein GS (1964) The structuring of drive and reality. David Rapaport's contribution to psychoanalysis and psychology. Int J Psychoanal 45:483–498

Gill MM, Newman R, Redlich FC (1954) The initial interview in psychiatric practice. International University Press, New York

Gillespie WH (1971) Aggression and instinct theory. Int J Psychoanal 52:155–160

Gilman RD (1982) The termination phase in psychoanalytic practice. A survey of 48 completed cases. Psychoanal Inquiry 2:463–472

Giora Z (1981) Dream styles and the psychology of dreaming. Psychoanal Contemp Thought 4:291–381

Giovacchini PL (1972) Interpretation and definition of the analytic setting. In: Giovacchini PL (ed) Tactics and techniques in psychoanalytic therapy. Hogarth, London

Gitelson M (1952) The emotional position of the analyst in the psychoanalytic situation. Int J Psychoanal 33:1–10

Gitelson M (1962) The curative factors in psycho-analysis I. The first phase of psychoanalysis. Int J Psychoanal 43:194—205
Gitelson M (1964) On the identity crisis in American psychoanalysis. J Am Psychoanal Assoc 12:451—476
Glover E (1937) On the theory of the therapeutic results of psycho-analysis. Int J Psychoanal 18:125—132
Glover E (1945) Examination of the Klein system of child psychology. Psychoanal Study Child 1:75—118
Glover E (1955) The technique of psychoanalysis. Baillière Tindall & Cox, London
Glymour C (1980) Theory and evidence. Princeton University Press, Princeton
Göring MH (ed) (1934) Deutsche Seelenheilkunde. Hirzel, Leipzig
Görres A, Heiss R, Thomä H, Uexküll T von (1964) Denkschrift zur Lage der ärztlichen Psychotherapie und der Psychosomatischen Medizin. Steiner, Wiesbaden
Goffman E (1961) Asylums. Essays on the social situation of mental patients and other inmates. Doubleday, New York
Goldberg A (1981) One theory or more? Contemp Psychoanal 17:626—638
Grassi E (1979) Die Macht der Phantasie. Zur Geschichte abendländischen Denkens. Athenäum, Königstein im Taunus
Green A (1977) Conceptions of affect. Int J Psychoanal 58:129—156
Greenacre P (1950) General problems of acting out. Psychoanal Q 19:455—467
Greenacre P (1954) The role of transference. Practical considerations in relation to psychoanalytic therapy. J Am Psychoanal Assoc 2:671—684
Greenacre P (1956) Re-evaluation of the process of working through. Int J Psychoanal 37:439—444
Greenberg JR, Mitchell SA (1983) Object relations in psychoanalytic theory. Harvard University Press, Cambridgeusetts
Greenberg R, Pearlman C (1975) A psychoanalytic dream continuum. The source and function of dreams. Int Rev Psychoanal 2:441—448
Greene TA (1979) C.G. Jung's theory of dreams. In: Wolman BB (ed) Handbook of dreams. Van Nostrand, New York, pp 298—318
Greenson RR (1960) Empathy and its vicissitudes. Int J Psychoanal 41:418—424
Greenson RR (1965) The problem of working through. In: Schur M (ed) Drives, affects, behavior, vol 2. International University Press, New York, pp 277—314
Greenson RR (1967) The technique and practice of psychoanalysis, vol I. International University Press, New York
Greenson RR (1974) The decline and fall of the 50-minute hour. J Am Psychoanal Assoc 22:785—791
Greenson RR (1978) On transitional objects and transference. In: Grolnick SA, Barkin L, Muensterberger W (eds) Between reality and fantasy. Transitional objects and phenomena. Aronson, New York, pp 205—209
Greenson RR, Heimann P, Wexler M (1970) Discussion of the "non-transference relationship in the psychoanalytic situation" (Plenary session of the 26th International Psychoanalytical Congress, Rome 28 July 1969). Int J Psychoanal 51:143—150
Greenspan SI (1979) Intelligence and adaption. An integration of psychoanalytic and Piagetian developmental psychology. International University Press, New York
Greenspan SI (1981) The clinical interview of the child. McGraw-Hill, New York
Greenspan SI, Pollock GH (eds) (1980a) The course of life. Psychoanalytic contributions toward understanding personality development. Vol I: Infancy and early childhood. US Department of Health and Human Services, Washington DC
Greenspan SI, Pollock GH (eds) (1980b) The course of life. Psychoanalytic contribution toward understanding personality development. Vol II: Latency, adolescence and youth. US Department of Health and Human Services, Washington DC
Greenspan SI, Pollock GH (eds) (1981) The course of life. Psychoanalytic contribution toward understanding personality development. Vol III: Adulthood and aging process. US Department of Health and Human Services, Washington DC
Grice HP (1975) Logic and conversation. In: Cole P, Morgan JL (eds) Speech acts. Seminar Press, New York (Syntax and semantics, vol 3, pp 41—58)

Grinberg L (1979) Projective counteridentification and countertransference. In: Epstein L, Feiner AH (eds) Countertransference. Aronson, New York, pp 169—191

Groen-Prakken H (1984) Government and psychoanalytic training. Psychoanalysis in Europe. Bull Eur Psychoanal Fed (Engl edn) 23:77—84

Grossman WI, Simon B (1969) Anthropomorphism. Motive, meaning, and causality in psychoanalytic theory. Psychoanal Study Child 24:78—111

Grotjahn M (1950) About the "third ear" in psychoanalysis. Psychoanal Rev 37:56—65

Grotstein JS (1982) Newer perspectives in object relation theory. Contemp Psychoanal 18:43—91

Grünbaum A (1982) Can psychoanalytic theory be cogently tested "on the couch"? Psychoanal Contemp Thought 5:155—255, 311—436

Grünbaum A (1984) The foundations of psychoanalysis. A philosophical critique. University of California Press, Berkeley Los Angeles London

Grunberger B (1958) Über-Ich und Narzißmus in der analytischen Situation. Psyche 12:270—290

Grunert J (1984) Zur Geschichte der Psychoanalyse in München. Psyche 38:865—904

Grunert U (1979) Die negative therapeutische Reaktion als Ausdruck einer Störung im Loslösungs- und Individuationsprozeß. Psyche 33:1—28

Grunert U (1982) Selbstdarstellung und Selbstentwicklung im manifesten Traum. Jahrb Psychoanal 14:179—209

Guntrip H (1961) Personality structure and human interaction. International University Press, New York

Guntrip H (1968) Schizoid phenomena, object relation, and the self. Hogarth, London

Guntrip H (1971) Psychoanalytic theory, therapy, and the self. Basic Books, New York

Guntrip H (1975) My experience of analysis with Fairbairn and Winnicott. Int Rev Psychoanal 2:145—156

Haarstrick R (1976) Kommentierung der Psychotherapie-Vereinbarungen. Dtsch Ärztebl 73:2084—2087

Habermas J (1971) Knowledge and human interests. Beacon Press, Boston

Habermas J (1981) Theorie des kommunikativen Handelns. Suhrkamp, Frankfurt am Main

Habermas J (1985) Theory of communicative action, vol 1. Beacon Press, Boston

Häfner H (1985) Sind psychische Krankheiten häufiger geworden? Nervenarzt 56:120—133

Hall CS, Lindzey G (1968) The relevance of Freudian psychology and related viewpoints for the social sciences. In: Lindzey G, Aronson E (eds) Historical introduction. Systematic positions. Addison-Wesley, Reading Menlo Park London Don Mills (The handbook of social psychology, 2nd edn, vol 1, pp 245—319)

Harlow HF (1958) The nature of love. Am Psychol 13:673—685

Harlow HF (1962) The heterosexual affectional system in monkeys. Am Psychol 17:1—9

Hartmann H (1927) Die Grundlagen der Psychoanalyse. Thieme, Leipzig

Hartmann H (1955) Notes on the theory of sublimation. Psychoanal Study Child 10:9—29

Hartmann H (1958[1939]) Ego psychology and the problem of adaption. International University Press, New York

Hartmann H, Kris E, Loewenstein RM (1949) Notes on the theory of aggression. Psychoanal Study Child 3—4:9—36

Hartmann H, Kris E, Loewenstein RM (1953) The function of theory in psychoanalysis. In: Loewenstein RM (ed) Drives, affects, behaviour. International University Press, New York, pp 13—37

Hartocollis P (1980) Time and the dream. J Am Psychoanal Assoc 28:861—877

Hartocollis P (1985) Time and timelessness. A psychoanalytic exploration of the varieties of temporal experience. International University Press, New York

Hatcher RL (1973) Insight and self-observation. The development of the concept of insight in psychoanalysis. J Am Psychoanal Assoc 21:377—398

Hayman A (1969) What do we mean by "Id"? J Am Psychoanal Assoc 17:353—380

Heigl FS, Triebel A (1977) Lernvorgänge in psychoanalytischer Therapie. Die Technik der Bestätigung. Eine empirische Untersuchung. Huber, Bern Stuttgart

Heimann P (1950) On countertransference. Int J Psychoanal 31:81—84
Heimann P (1956) Dynamics of transference interpretations. Int J Psychoanal 37:303—310
Heimann P (1960) Counter-transference. Br J Med Psychol 33:9—15
Heimann P (1966) Bemerkungen zum Arbeitsbegriff in der Psychoanalyse. Psyche 20:321—361
Heimann P (1969) Gedanken zum Erkenntnisprozeß des Psychoanalytikers. Psyche 23:2—24
Heimann P (1970) Opening and closing remarks of the moderator. Plenary Session of the 26th international congress, Rome, 28 July 1969. Discussion of the "non-transference relationship in the psychoanalytic situation". Int J Psychoanal 51:145—147
Heimann P (1977) Further observations on the analyst's cognitive process. J Am Psychoanal Assoc 25:313—333
Heimann P (1978) Über die Notwendigkeit für den Analytiker mit seinen Patienten natürlich zu sein. In: Drews S et al (eds) Provokation und Toleranz. Alexander Mitscherlich zu ehren. Festschrift für Alexander Mitscherlich zum 70. Geburtstag. Suhrkamp, Frankfurt am Main, pp 215—230
Hendrick I (1942) Instinct and the ego during infancy. Psychoanal Q 11:33—58
Hendrick I (1943a) Work and the pleasure principle. Psychoanal Q 12:311—329
Hendrick I (1943b) The discussion of the "instinct to master". A letter to the editors. Psychoanal Q 12:561—565
Henseler H (1974) Narzißtische Krisen. Zur Psychodynamik des Selbstmords. Rowohlt, Reinbek bei Hamburg
Hermann I (1963) Die Psychoanalyse als Methode, 2nd edn. Westdeutscher Verlag, Cologne Opladen
Herrmann T (1979) Psychologie als Problem. Klett-Cotta, Stuttgart
Hesse MB (1966) Models and analogies in science. University Press, Notre Dame
Hoffer W (1950) Three psychological criteria for the termination of treatment. Int J Psychoanal 31:194—195
Hoffmann SO (1979) Charakter und Neurose. Suhrkamp, Frankfurt am Main
Hoffmann SO (1983) Die niederfrequente psychoanalytische Langzeittherapie. Konzeption, Technik und Versuch einer Abgrenzung gegenüber dem klassischen Verfahren. In: Hoffmann SO (ed) Deutung und Beziehung. Kritische Beiträge zur Behandlungskonzeption und Technik in der Psychoanalyse. Fischer, Frankfurt am Main, pp 183—193
Hohage R, Klöss L, Kächele H (1981) Über die diagnostisch-therapeutische Funktion von Erstgesprächen in einer psychotherapeutischen Ambulanz. Psyche 35:544—556
Hohage R, Thomä H (1982) Über das Auftauchen von Erinnerungen als Ergebnis fokussierter Traumdeutung. Z Psychosom Med 28:385—392
Holt RR (1964) The emergence of cognitive psychology. J Am Psychoanal Assoc 12:650—655
Holt RR (1967a) David Rapaport. A memoir. In: Holt RR (ed) Motives and thought. Psychoanalytic essays in honor of David Rapaport (Psychological issues, vol 5, no 2—3, monograph 18—19). International University Press, New York, pp 7—17
Holt RR (1967b) The development of the primary process. A structural view. In: Holt RR (ed) Motives and thought. Psychoanalytic essays in honor of David Rapaport (Psychological issues, vol 5, no 2—3, monograph 18—19). International University Press, New York, pp 344—383
Holt RR (1976) Drive or wish? A reconsideration of the psychoanalytic theory of motivation. In: Gill MM, Holzman PS (eds) Psychology versus metapsychology. Psychoanalytic essays in memory of George S. Klein (Psychological issues, vol 9, no 4, monograph 36). International University Press, New York, pp 158—197
Holt RR (1981) The death and transfiguration of metapsychology. Int Rev Psychoanal 8:129—143
Holt RR (1982) The manifest and latent meanings of metapsychology. Annu Psychoanal 10:233—255
Holt RR (1984) Biographical sketch. Merton M. Gill. Psychoanal Inquiry 4:315—323
Holzman PS (1976) The future of psychoanalysis and its institutes. Psychoanal Q 45:250—273

Home H (1966) The concept of mind. Int J Psychoanal 47:42—49

Hurvich M (1970) On the concept of reality testing. Int J Psychoanal 51:299—312

Huxter H, Lower R, Escoll P (1975) Some pitfalls in the assessment of analyzability in a psychoanalytic clinic. J Am Psychoanal Assoc 23:90—106

Isaacs S (1939) Criteria for interpretation. Int J Psychoanal 20:148—160

Jacobson E (1964) The self and the object world. International University Press, New York

Jaspers K (1963) General psychopathology. University of Chicago Press, Chicago

Jones E (1920) Treatment of the neuroses. Baillière Tindall & Cox, London

Jones E (1936) Results of treatment. In: Decennial report of the Londom Clinic of Psychoanalysis, May 1926—May 1936, pp 12—14 (unpublished report)

Jones E (1959) Free associations. Basic Books, New York

Jones E (1954) Sigmund Freud. Life and work, vols I - III. Hogarth, London

Joseph ED, Widlöcher D (eds) (1983) The identity of the psychoanalyst (Int Psychoanal Assoc, monograph series no 2). International University Press, New York

Jung CG (1981[1906]) Experimental researches. In: The collected works of C. G. Jung, vol 2. Bollingen, Princeton

Jung CG (1972[1912]) The psychology of the unconscious. In: The collected works of C. G. Jung, vol 7. Bollingen, Princeton, pp 3—117

Jung CG (1964[1928]) The relations between the ego and the unconscious. In: The collected works of C. G. Jung, vol 7. Bollingen, Princeton, pp 202—507

Junker H, Waßner T (1984) Psychotherapeutisch denken. Patient und Therapeut in der analytischen Arbeit. Springer, Berlin Heidelberg New York Tokyo

Kächele H (1981) Zur Bedeutung der Krankengeschichte in der klinisch-psychoanalytischen Forschung. Jahrb Psychoanal 12:118—177

Kächele H (1985) Zwischen Skylla und Charybdis. Erfahrungen mit dem Liegungsrückblick. Psychother Med Psychol 35:306—309

Kächele H, Schors R (1981) Ansätze und Ergebnisse psychoanalytischer Therapieforschung. In: Baumann U, Berbalk H, Seidenstücker G (eds) Klinische Psychologie. Trends in Forschung und Praxis, vol 4. Huber, Bern Stuttgart Vienna, pp 209—257

Kafka E (1979) On examination dreams. Psychoanal Q 48:426—447

Kafka JS (1977) On reality. An examination of object constancy, ambiguity, paradox and time. Psychiatry Human 2:133—158

Kaiser H (1934) Probleme der Technik. Int Z Psychoanal 20:490—522

Kaminski G (1970) Verhaltenstheorie und Verhaltensmodifikation. Entwurf einer integrativen Theorie psychologischer Praxis am Individuum. Klett, Stuttgart

Kandel ER (1979) Psychotherapy and the single synapse. The impact of psychiatric thought on neurobiologic research. N Engl J Med 301:1028—1037

Kandel ER (1983) From metapsychology to molecular biology. Explorations into the nature of anxiety. Am J Psychiatry 140:1277—1293

Kanzer M (1955) The communicative function of the dream. Int J Psychoanal 36:260—266

Kanzer M (1961) Verbal and nonverbal aspects of free association. Psychoanal Q 30:327—350

Kanzer M (1966) The motor sphere of transference. Psychoanal Q 35:522—539

Kanzer M (1972) Superego aspects of free association and the fundamental rule. J Am Psychoanal Assoc 20:246—266

Kanzer M (1979) Object relations theory. An introduction. J Am Psychoanal Assoc 27:313—325

Kanzer M, Glenn J (eds) (1980) Freud and his patients. Aronson, New York

Kemper WW (1950) Die Honorarfrage in der Psychotherapie. Psyche 4:201—221

Kemper WW (1969) Übertragung und Gegenübertragung als funktionale Einheit. Jahrb Psychoanal 6:35—68

Kemper WW (1973) Werner W. Kemper. In: Pongratz LJ (ed) Psychotherapie in Selbstdarstellungen. Huber, Bern Stuttgart Vienna, pp 259—345

Kernberg OF (1965) Notes on countertransference. J Am Psychoanal Assoc 13:38—56

Kernberg OF (1972) Critique of the Kleinian school. In: Giovacchini PL (ed) Tactics and techniques in psychoanalytic therapy. Hogarth, London, pp 62—93

Kernberg OF (1975) Borderline conditions and pathological narcissism. Aronson, New York
Kernberg OF (1977) The structural diagnosis of borderline personality organization. In: Hartocollis P (ed) Borderline personality disorders. International University Press, New York, pp 87—121
Kernberg OF (1979) Some implications of object relations theory for psychoanalytic technique. J Am Psychoanal Assoc 27 [Suppl]:207—239
Kernberg OF (1981) Structural interviewing. Psychiatr Clin North Am 4:169—195
Kernberg OF (1982) To teach or not to teach psychotherapy techniques in psychoanalytic education. In: Joseph ED, Wallerstein RS (eds) Psychotherapy. Impact on psychoanalytic training. The influence of practice and theory of psychotherapy on education in psychoanalysis (Int Psychoanal Assoc, monograph series no 1). International University Press, New York, pp 1—37
Kernberg OF (1984) Severe personality disorders. Psychotherapeutic strategies. Yale University Press, New Haven London
Kernberg OF (1985) Changes in the nature of psychoanalytic training, structure of training, and standards of training. In: Wallerstein RS (ed) Changes in analysts and their training (Int Psychoanal Assoc, monograph series no 4). International Psychoanalytic Association, London, pp 56—61
Kernberg OF, Bursteine ED, Coyne L, Appelbaum A, Horwitz L, Voth H (1972) Psychotherapy and psychoanalysis. Final report of the Menninger Foundation's psychotherapy research project. Bull Menn Clin 36:3—275
Kerz JP (1985) Das wiedergefundene "Es". Zu Bernd Nitzschkes Aufsatz über die Herkunft des "Es". Psyche 85:125—149
Khan MMR (1969) On the clinical provision of frustrations, recognitions, and failures in the analytic situation. Int J Psychoanal 50:237—248
Kiener F (1978) Empirische Kontrolle psychoanalytischer Thesen. In: Pongratz LJ (ed) Klinische Psychologie. Hogrefe, Göttingen Toronto Zürich (Handbuch der Psychologie, vol 8/2, pp 1200—1241)
King P (1983) Paula Heimann and the British Psychoanalytical Society. Her quest for her own identity as a psycho-analyst. Br Psychoanal Soc Bull 6:20—30
Klauber J (1968) On the dual use of historical and scientific method in psychoanalysis. Int J Psychoanal 49:80—88
Klauber J (1972a) On the relationship of transference and interpretation in psychoanalytic therapy. Int J Psychoanal 53:385—391
Klauber J (1972b) Psychoanalytic consultation. In: Giovacchini PL (ed) Tactics and techniques in psychoanalytic therapy. Hogarth, London, pp 99—112
Klauber J (1981) Difficulties in the analytic encounter. Aronson, New York London
Klaus G, Buhr M (1972) Philosophisches Wörterbuch, vol 2. Das europäische Buch, Berlin
Klein GS (1969) Freud's two theories of sexuality. In: Breger L (ed) Clinical-cognitive psychology. Models and integrations. Prentice Hall, Englewood Cliffs, pp 136—181
Klein GS (1970) Two theories or one? Bull Menn Clin 37:102—132
Klein GS (1973) Is psychoanalysis relevant? Psychoanal Contemp Sci 2:3—21
Klein GS (1976) Psychoanalytic theory. An exploration of essentials. International University Press, New York
Klein M (1935) A contribution to the psychogenesis of manic-depressiv states. Int J Psychoanal 16:145—174
Klein M (1945) The Oedipus complex in the light of early anxieties. Int J Psychoanal 26:11—33
Klein M (1946) Notes on some schiziod mechanisms. Int J Psychoanal 27:99—110
Klein M (1948) Contributions to psycho-analysis, 1921—1945. Hogarth, London
Klein M (1957) Envy and gratitude. A study of unconscious sources. Basic Books, New York
Klein Milton (1981) On Mahler's autistic and symbiotic phases. An exposition and evaluation. Psychoanal Contemp Thought 4:69—105
Kline P (1972) Fact and fantasy in Freudian theory. Methuen, London

Klüwer R (1983) Agieren und Mitagieren. In: Hoffmann SO (ed) Deutung und Beziehung. Kritische Beiträge zur Behandlungskonzeption und Technik in der Psychoanalyse. Fischer, Frankfurt am Main, pp 132—145

Klüwer R (1985) Versuch einer Standortbestimmung der Fokaltherapie als psychoanalytische Kurztherapie. In: Leuzinger-Bohleber M (ed) Psychoanalytische Kurztherapien. Westdeutscher Verlag, Opladen, pp 54—93

Knight RP (1941) Evaluation of the results of psychoanalytic therapy. Am J Psychiatry 98:434—446

Köhler-Weisker A (1978) Freuds Behandlungstechnik und die Technik der klienten-zentrierten Gesprächspsychotherapie nach Rogers. Psyche 32:827—847

Kohl RN (1962) Pathologic reactions of marital partners to improvement of patient. Am J Psychiatry 118:1036—1041

Kohut H (1959) Introspection, empathy, and psychoanalysis an examination of the relationship between mode of observation and theory. J Am Psychoanal Assoc 7:459—483

Kohut H (1971) The analysis of the self. A systematic approach to the psychoanalytic treatment of narcissistic personality disorders. International University Press, New York

Kohut H (1973) Psychoanalysis in a troubled world. Annu Psychoanal 1:3—25

Kohut H (1977) The restoration of the self. International University Press, New York

Kohut H (1979) The two analyses of Mr. Z. Int J Psychoanal 60:3—27

Kohut H (1984) How does analysis cure? University of Chicago Press, Chicago London

Kordy H, Rad M von, Senf W (1983) Success and failure in psychotherapy: Hypotheses and results from the Heidelberg follow-up project. Psychother Psychosom 40:211—227

Koukkou M, Lehmann D (1980) Psychophysiologie des Träumens und der Neurosentherapie. Das Zustands-Wechsel-Modell, eine Synopsis. Fortschr Neurol Psychiatr 48:324—350

Koukkou M, Lehmann D (1983) Dreaming. The functional stateshift hypothesis, a neuropsychophysiological model. Br J Psychiatry 142:221—231

Kramer MK (1959) On the continuation of the analytic process after psychoanalysis. A self-observation. Int J Psychoanal 40:17—25

Krause R (1983) Zur Onto- und Phylogenese des Affektsystems und ihrer Beziehungen zu psychischen Störungen. Psyche 37:1016—1043

Krause R (1985) Über die psychoanalytische Affektlehre am Beispiel der Einsicht. In: Eckensberger LH, Lantermann ED (eds) Emotion und Reflexivität. Urban & Schwarzenberg, Munich Vienna Baltimore, pp 267—290

Kris AO (1982) Free association. Method and process. Yale University Press, New Haven

Kris E (1936) The psychology of caricature. Int J Psychoanal 17:285—303

Kris E (1950) On preconscious mental processes. Psychoanal Q 19:540—560

Kris E (1951) Ego psychology and interpretation in psychoanalytic therapy. Psychoanal Q 20:15—30

Kris E (1956a) On some vicissitudes of insight in psychoanalysis. Int J Psychoanal 37:445—455

Kris E (1956b) The recovery of childhood memories in psychoanalysis. Psychoanal Study Child 11:54—88

Kris E (1975[1947]) The nature of psychoanalytic propositions and their validation. In: Newman LM (ed) Selected papers of Ernst Kris. Yale University Press, New Haven, pp 3—23

Krohn A (1978) Hysteria, the elusive neurosis. International University Press, New York

Kubie LS (1935) Über die Beziehung zwischen dem bedingten Reflex und der psychoanalytischen Technik. Imago 21:44—49

Kubie LS (1947) The fallacious use of quantitative concepts in dynamic psychology. Psychoanal Q 16:507—518

Künzler E, Zimmermann I (1965) Zur Eröffnung des Erstinterviews. Psyche 19:68—79

Kuhn TS (1962) The structure of scientific revolutions. University of Chicago Press, Chicago

Kuiper PC (1968) Indications and contraindications for psychoanalytic treatment. Int J Psychoanal 49:261—264

Kunz H (1946a) Die anthropologische Bedeutung der Phantasie. Recht und Gesellschaft, Basel

Kunz H (1946b) Die Aggressivität und die Zärtlichkeit. Zwei psychologische Studien. Francke, Bern
Lacan J (1968) The language of the self. The function of language in psychoanalysis. Johns Hopkins Press, Baltimore
Lampl-de Groot J (1976) Personal experience with psychoanalytic technique and theory during the last half century. Psychoanal Study Child 37:283—296
Langs RJ (1976) The bipersonal field. Aronson, New York
Laplanche J, Pontalis JB (1973) The language of psycho-analysis. Hogarth, London
Lasch C (1979) Haven in a heartless world. The family besieged. Basic Books, New York
Laufer M (1982) The cost of psychoanalytic training and the future psychoanalyst. Int Psychoanal Assoc Newsletter 14 (2):1
Lebovici S, Soule M (1970) La connaissance de l'enfant par la psychanalyse. Presses Universitaires de France, Paris
Leeuw PJ van der (1965) Zur Entwicklung des Begriffs der Abwehr. Psyche 19:161—171
Leider RJ (1984) The neutrality of the analyst in the analytic situation. J Am Psychoanal Assoc 32:573—585
Lenk H (1973) Zu neueren Ansätzen der Technikphilosophie. In: Lenk H, Moser S (eds) Techne, Technik, Technologie. Verlag Dokumentation, Pullach
Leupold-Löwenthal H (1984) Zur Geschichte der "Frage der Laienanalyse". Psyche 38:97—120
Leuzinger M (1981) Kognitive Prozesse bei der Indikationsstellung. In: Baumann U (ed) Indikation zur Psychotherapie. Perspektiven für Praxis und Forschung (Fortschritte der klinischen Psychologie, vol 25). Urban & Schwarzenberg, Munich Vienna Baltimore, pp 103—121
Leuzinger M (1984) Psychotherapeutische Denkprozesse. Kognitive Prozesse bei der Indikation psychotherapeutischer Verfahren. PSZ-Verlag, Ulm
Leuzinger M, Kächele H (1985) Veränderte Wahrnehmung von Traumgestalten im psychoanalytischen Behandlungsprozeß. In: Czogalik D, Ehlers W, Teufel R (eds) Perspektiven der Psychotherapieforschung. Einzelfall, Gruppe, Institution. Hochschulverlag, Freiburg im Breisgau, pp 94—119
Leuzinger-Bohleber M (1985) Psychoanalytische Fokaltherapie. Eine klassische psychoanalytische Kurztherapie in Institutionen. In: Leuzinger-Bohleber M (ed) Psychoanalytische Kurztherapien. Westdeutscher Verlag, Opladen, pp 54—93
Lewin BD (1946) Sleep, the mouth, and the dream screen. Psychoanal Q 15:419—434
Lewin BD (1950) The psychoanalysis of elation. Norton, New York
Lichtenberg JD (1983) Psychoanalysis and infant research. Analytic Press, Hillsdale
Lichtenstein H (1974) Some considerations regarding the phenomenology of the repetition compulsion and the death instinct. Annu Psychoanal 2:63—84
Lidz T (1968) The person. His development throughout the life cycle. Basic Books, New York
Lidz T, Fleck S (1985) Schizophrenia and the family, rev edn. International University Press, New York
Lidz T, Fleck S, Cornelison AR (1965) Schizophrenia and the family. International University Press, New York
Lifton RJ (1985) Review of the book "Psychotherapy in the Third Reich. The Göring Institute" by Geoffry Cocks. The New York Times 27 January 1985, pp 1 and 28
Limentani A (1981) On some positive aspects of negative therapeutic reaction. Int J Psychoanal 62:379—390
Lindsay PH, Norman DA (1977) Human information processing. An introduction to psychology, 2nd edn. Academic Press, New York
Lipton SD (1982) Essays on Paul Dewald's "The psychoanalytic process". Contemp Psychoanal 18:349—372
Little M (1951) Counter-transference and the patient's response to it. Int J Psychoanal 32:32—40
Loch W (1963) Regression. Über den Begriff und seine Bedeutung in einer allgemeinen psychoanalytischen Neurosentheorie. Psyche 17:516—545

Loch W (1965 a) Übertragung - Gegenübertragung. Anmerkungen zur Theorie und Praxis. Psyche 19:1—23

Loch W (1965 b) Voraussetzungen, Mechanismen und Grenzen des psychoanalytischen Prozesses. Huber, Bern Stuttgart

Lockot R (1985) Erinnern und Durcharbeiten. Zur Geschichte der Psychoanalyse und Psychotherapie im Nationalsozialismus. Fischer, Frankfurt am Main

Loevinger J (1966) Three principles for a psychoanalytic psychology. J Abnorm Psychol 71:432—443

Loewald HW (1960) On the therapeutic action of psychoanalysis. Int J Psychoanal 41:16—33

Loewald HW (1971) The transference neurosis: Comments on the concept and the phenomenon. J Am Psychoanal Assoc 19:54—66

Loewald HW (1975) Psychoanalysis as an art and the phantasy character of the psychoanalytic situation. J Am Psychoanal 23:277—299

Loewald HW (1980) Papers on psychoanalysis. Yale University Press, New Haven London

Loewenstein RM (1940) The vital or somatic instincts. Int J Psychoanal 21:377—400

Loewenstein RM (1951) The problem of interpretation. Psychoanal Q 20:1—14

Loewenstein RM (1958) Remarks on some variations in psychoanalytic technique. Int J Psychoanal 39:202—210

Loewenstein RM (1969) Developments in the theory of transference in the last fifty years. Int J Psychoanal 50:583—588

Lohmann HM (1980) Psychoanalyse in Deutschland — eine Karriere im Staatsapparat? Ansichten von jenseits des Rheins. Psyche 34:945—957

Lorenz K (1963) Das sogenannte Böse. Zur Naturgeschichte der Aggression. Borotha-Schoeler, Vienna

Lorenz K (1973) Die Rückseite des Spiegels. Versuch einer Naturgeschichte menschlichen Erkennens. Piper, Munich Zürich

Lorenzer A (1970) Sprachzerstörung und Rekonstruktion. Vorarbeiten zu einer Metatheorie der Psychoanalyse. Suhrkamp, Frankfurt am Main

Lorenzer A (1974) Die Wahrheit der psychoanalytischen Erkenntnis. Ein historisch-materialistischer Entwurf. Suhrkamp, Frankfurt am Main

Lowy S (1967) New research results in practical dream interpretation. Psychoanal Rev 54:510—526

Luborsky L (1984) Principles of psychoanalytic psychotherapy. A manual for supportive-expressive treatment. Basic Books, New York

Luborsky L, Mintz J (1974) What sets off momentary forgetting during a psychoanalysis? Psychoanal Contemp Sci 3:233—268

Luborsky L, Spence DP (1978) Quantitative research on psychoanalytic therapy. In: Garfield SL, Bergin AE (eds) Handbook of psychotherapy and behavior change. An empirical analysis. Wiley, New York, pp 331—368

Luborsky L, Mellon J, Cohen KD, Ravenswaay P van, Hole AV, Childress AR, Crits-Christoph P, Levine FJ, Alexander K (1985) A verification of Freud's grandest clinical hypothesis. The transference. Clin Psychol Rev 5:231—246

Luborsky L, Mintz J, Auerbach A, Christoph P, Bachrach H, Todd T, Johnson M, Cohen M, O'Brien CP (1980) Predicting the outcomes of psychotherapy. Findings of the Penn psychotherapy project. Arch Gen Psychiatry 37:471—481

Lüders W (1982) Traum und Selbst. Psyche 36:813—829

Lytton SM (1983) A brief historical survey on the influence of value judgements on psychoanalytic theory and practice. Psychoanal Inquiry 3:573—576

Macalpine I (1950) The development of the transference. Psychoanal Q 19:501—539

Mahler MS (1969) On human symbiosis and the vicissitudes of individuation. Hogarth, London

Mahler MS (1971) A study of the separation-individuation process and its possible application to borderline phenomena in the psychoanalytic situation. Psychoanal Study Child 26:403—424

Mahler MS, Pine F, Bergmann A (1975) The psychological birth of the human infant. Basic Books, New York

Mahony P (1979) The boundaries of free association. Psychoanal Contemp Thought 2:151–198
Malan DH (1963) A study of brief psychotherapy. Tavistock, London
Malan DH (1976) The frontier of brief psychotherapy. An example of the convergence of research and clinical practice. Plenum Press, New York
Malmcolm J (1980) Psychoanalysis: The impossible profession. Knopf, New York
Mannoni M (1979) La thêorie comme fiction. Freud, Groddeck, Winnicot, Lacan. Seuil, Paris
McDevitt JB (1979) The role of internalization in the development of object relations during the separation-individuation phase. J Am Psychoanal Assoc 27:327–343
McLaughlin JT (1981) Transference, psychic reality, and countertransference. Psychoanal Q 50:639–664
McReynolds P (1976) Assimilation and anxiety. In: Zuckermann M, Spielberger CD (eds) Emotions and anxiety. New concepts, methods, and application. Erlbaum, Hillsdale, pp 35–86
Mead GH (1913) The social self. J Philosophy 10:374–380
Mead GH (1934) Mind, self, and society. From the standpoint of a social behaviorist. University of Chicago Press, Chicago
Meissner WW (1979) Internalization and object relations. J Am Psychoanal Assoc 27:345–360
Meissner WW (1981) Metapsychology—who needs it? J Am Psychoanal Assoc 29:921–938
Meltzer D (1967) The psychoanalytical process. Heinemann, London
Menne K, Schröter K (1980) Soziale Herkunft — ein Hindernis für die psychoanalytische Behandlung? In: Menne K, Schröter K (eds) Psychoanalyse und Unterschicht. Suhrkamp, Frankfurt am Main, pp 7–34
Menninger KA, Holzman PS (1958) Theory of psychoanalytic technique. Basic Books, New York
Mentzos S (1976) Interpersonale und institutionalisierte Abwehr. Suhrkamp, Frankfurt am Main
Mentzos S (1982) Neurotische Konfliktverarbeitung. Einführung in die psychoanalytische Neurosenlehre unter Berücksichtigung neuer Perspektiven. Kindler, Munich
Merloo J (1952) Free association, silence, and multiple function of speech. Psychiatr Q 26:21–31
Meyer AE (1981a) Psychoanalytische Prozessforschung zwischen der Skylla der "Verkürzung" und der Charybdis der "systematischen akustischen Lücke". Z Psychosom Med Psychoanal 27:103–116
Meyer AE (ed) (1981b) The Hamburg short psychotherapy comparison experiment. Psychother Psychosom 35:77–270
Michaelis W (1976) Verhalten ohne Aggression. Versuch zur Integration der Theorien. Kiepenheuer & Witsch, Cologne
Miller I (1975) A critical assessment of the future psychoanalysis. A view from within. J Am Psychoanal Assoc 23:139–153
Minkowski E (1933) Le temps vêcu. D'Artrey, Paris
Mitscherlich A (1967) Krankheit als Konflikt. Studien zur psychosomatischen Medizin, vol 2. Suhrkamp, Frankfurt am Main
Modell AH (1981) Does metapsychology still exist? Int J Psychoanal 63:391–402
Modell AH (1984) Psychoanalysis in a new context. International University Press, New York
Moeller ML (1977) Zur Theorie der Gegenübertragung. Psyche 31:142–166
Möller HJ (1976) Methodische Grundprobleme der Psychiatrie. Kohlhammer, Stuttgart
Möller HJ (1978) Psychoanalyse — erklärende Wissenschaft oder Deutungskunst? Wilhelm Fink, Munich
Monchaux C de (1978) Dreaming and the organizing function of the ego. Int J Psychoanal 59:443–453
Money-Kyrle RE (1956) Normal countertransference and some of its deviations. Int J Psychoanal 37:360–366

Moore MS (1980) The nature of psychoanalytic explanation. Psychoanal Contemp Thought 3:459—543
Morgenthaler F (1978) Technik. Zur Dialektik der psychoanalytischen Praxis. Syndikat, Frankfurt am Main
Moser U (1962) Übertragungsprobleme in der Psychoanalyse eines chronisch schweigenden Charakterneurotikers. Psyche 15:592—624
Moser U (1978) Affektsignal und aggressives Verhalten. Zwei verbal formulierte Modelle der Aggression. Psyche 32:229—258
Moser U, Zeppelin I von, Schneider H (1981) Objektbeziehungen, Affekte und Abwehrprozesse. Aspekte einer Regulierungstheorie mentaler Prozesse. Berichte der interdisziplinären Konfliktforschungsstelle der Universität Zürich, no 9 (unpublished report)
Mowrer OH (1960) Learning theory and the symbolic processes. Wiley, New York
M'Uzan M de (1977) De l' art à la mort. Gallimard, Paris
Myerson PG (1965) Modes of insight. J Am Psychoanal Assoc 13:771—792
Nacht S (1964) Silence as an integrative factor. Int J Psychoanal 45:299—303
Nedelmann C (1980) Behandlungsziel und Gesundheitsbegriff der Psychoanalyse. In: Bach H (ed) Der Krankheitsbegriff in der Psychoanalyse. Bestimmungsversuche auf einem Psychoanalytiker-Kongreß der Deutschen Gesellschaft für Psychotherapie, Psychosomatik und Tiefenpsychologie 1980. Vandenhoeck & Ruprecht, Göttingen, pp 55—67
Neisser U (1976) Cognition and reality. Principles and implications of cognitive psychology. Freeman, San Francisco
Nerenz K (1983) Eine Legende zum Begriff der Gegenübertragung. In: Hoffmann SO (ed) Deutung und Beziehung. Kritische Beiträge zur Behandlungskonzeption und Technik in der Psychoanalyse. Fischer, Frankfurt am Main, pp 146—151
Neudert L, Kübler C, Schors R (1985) Die inhaltsanalytische Erfassung von Leiden im psychotherapeutischen Prozeß. In: Czogalik D, Ehlers W, Teufel R (eds) Perspektiven der Psychotherapieforschung. Einzelfall, Gruppe, Institution. Hochschulverlag, Freiburg im Breisgau, pp 120—134
Neyraut M (1974) Le transfert. Etude psychoanalytique. Presses Universitaires de France, Paris
Norman HF, Blacker KH, Oremland JD, Barett WG (1976) The fate of the transference neurosis after termination of a satisfactory analysis. J Am Psychoanal Assoc 24:471—498
Noy P (1978) Insight and creativity. J Am Psychoanal Assoc 26:717—748
Nunberg H (1931) The synthetic function of the ego. Int J Psychoanal 12:123—140
Nunberg H (1951) Transference and reality. Int J Psychoanal 32:1—9
Olinick SL (1964) The negative therapeutic reaction. Int J Psychoanal 45:540—548
Olinick SL (1970) Negative therapeutic reaction. J Am Psychoanal Assoc 18:655—672
Ornstein RE (1969) On the experience of time. Penguin Books, Baltimore
Ornston D (1982) Strachey's influence. A preliminary report. Int J Psychoanal 63:409—426
Ornston D (1985a) Freud's conception is different from Strachey's. J Am Psychoanal Assoc 33:379—412
Ornston D (1985b) The invention of "cathexis" and Strachey's strategy. Int Rev Psychoanal 12:391—412
Orr WD (1954) Transference and countertransference. A historical study. J Am Psychoanal Assoc 2:621—670
Palombo SR (1973) The associative memory tree. Psychoanal Contemp Sci 2:205—219
Papoušek H, Papoušek M (1983) Interactional failures. Their origins and significance in infant psychiatry. In: Call JD, Galenson E, Tyson RL (eds) Frontiers of infant psychiatry. Basic Books, New York, pp 31—37
Papoušek H, Papoušek M, Giese R (1984) Die Anfänge der Eltern-Kind Beziehung. In: Frick-Bruder V, Platz P (eds) Psychosomatische Probleme in der Gynäkologie und Geburtshilfe. Springer, Berlin Heidelberg New York Tokyo
Parin P (1978) Warum die Psychoanalytiker so ungern zu brennenden Zeitproblemen Stellung nehmen. Eine ethnologische Betrachtung. Psyche 32:385—399
Parin P, Parin-Matthèy G (1983a) Medicozentrismus in der Psychoanalyse. Eine notwendige Revision der Neurosenlehre und ihre Relevanz für die Theorie der Behandlungstechnik. In:

Hoffmann SO (ed) Deutung und Beziehung. Kritische Beiträge zur Behandlungskonzeption und Technik in der Psychoanalyse. Fischer, Frankfurt am Main, pp 86—106
Parin P, Parin-Matthàey G (1983b) Gegen den Verfall der Psychoanalyse. Gespräch mit A. Messerli. Tell 15:9—15
Parkin A (1980) On masochistic enthralment. A contribution to the study of moral masochism. Int J Psychoanal 61:307—314
Parloff MB, Waskow IE, Wolfe BE (1978) Research on therapist variables in relation to process and outcome. In: Garfield SL, Bergin AE (eds) Handbook of psychotherapy and behaviour change. An empirical analysis, 2nd edn. Wiley, New York Chichester Brisbane, pp 233—282
Parsons T (1964) Social structure and personality. Free Press, London
Perrez M (1983) Wissenschaftstheoretische Probleme der klinischen Psychologie. Psychotherapeutische Methoden — zum Stand ihrer metatheoretischen Diskussion. In: Minsel WR, Scheller R (eds) Forschungskonzepte der klinischen Psychologie. Kösel, Munich (Brennpunkte der klinischen Psychologie, vol 6, pp 148—163)
Peterfreund E (1975) How does the analyst listen? On models and strategies in the psychoanalytic process. Psychoanal Contemp Sci 4:59—101
Peterfreund E (1980) On information and systems models for psychoanalysis. Int Rev Psychoanal 7:327—345
Peterfreund E (1983) The process of psychoanalytic therapy. Models and strategies. Analytic Press, Hillsdale
Pfeffer AZ (1959) A procedure for evaluating the results of psychoanalysis. A preliminary report. J Am Psychoanal Assoc 7:418—444
Pfeffer AZ (1961) Follow-up study of a satisfactory analysis. J Am Psychoanal Assoc 9:698—718
Pfeffer AZ (1963) The meaning of the analyst after analysis. A contribution to the theory of therapeutic results. J Am Psychoanal Assoc 11:229—244
Piaget J (1954) The construction of reality in the child. Basic Books, New York
Pines M (1985) On the question of revision of the Standard Edition of Freud's writing. Int J Psychoanal 66:1—2
Polanyi M (1958) Personal knowledge. Towards a post-critical philosophy. Routledge & Kegan Paul, London
Pontalis JB (1965) Après Freud. Julliard, Paris
Popper KR (1969) Logik der Forschung, 3rd edn. Mohr, Tübingen
Popper KR, Eccles JC (1977) The self and its brain. An argument for interactionism. Springer, Berlin Heidelberg New York
Pressman MD (1969) The cognitive function of the ego in psychoanalysis. I. The search for insight. Int J. Psychoanal 50:187—196
Pribram KH, Gill MM (1976) Freud's project reassessed. Hutchinson, London
Prim R, Tilmann H (1973) Grundlagen einer kritisch-rationalen Sozialwissenschaft. Quelle & Meyer, Heidelberg
Pulver SE (1978) Survey of psychoanalytic practice 1976. Some trends and implications. J Am Psychoanal Assoc 26:615—631
Quint H (1984) Der Zwang im Dienst der Selbsterhaltung. Psyche 38:717—737
Racker H (1957) The meanings and uses of countertransference. Psychoanal Q 26:303—357
Racker H (1968) Transference and countertransference. International University Press, New York
Radebold H (1982) Probleme der psychotherapeutischen Technik bei neurotischen und reaktiven Erkrankungen im höheren und hohen Lebensalter. In: Helmchen H, Linden M, Rüger U (eds) Psychotherapie in der Psychiatrie. Springer, Berlin Heidelberg New York, pp 303—309
Radô S, Fenichel O, Müller-Braunschweig C (eds) (1930) Zehn Jahre Berliner Psychoanalytisches Institut. Poliklinik und Lehranstalt. Internationaler Psychoanalytischer Verlag, Vienna
Ramzy I (1974) How the mind of the psychoanalyst works. An essay on psychoanalytic inference. Int J Psychoanal 55:543—550

Rangell L (1966) An overview of the ending of an analysis. In: Litman RE (ed) Psychoanalysis in the Americas. Original Contributions from the First Pan-American Congress for Psychoanalysis. International University Press, New York, pp 141—165
Rangell L (1968) A point of view on acting out. Int J Psychoanal 49:195—201
Rangell L (1971) The decision making process. A contribution from psychoanalysis. Psychoanal Study Child 26:425—452
Rangell L (1981) Psychoanalysis and dynamic psychotherapy. Similarities and differences twenty-five years later. Psychoanal Q 50:665—693
Rangell L (1984) The analyst at work. The Madrid congress. Synthesis and critique. Int J Psychoanal 65:125—140
Rapaport D (1953) On the psycho-analytic theory of affects. Int J Psychoanal 34:177—198
Rapaport D (1959) A historical survey of psychoanalytic ego psychology. In: Klein GS (ed) Identity and the life cycle. Selected papers by Erik H Erikson (Psychological issues, vol 1, no 1, monograph 1).International University Press, New York, pp 5—17
Rapaport D (1960) The structure of psychoanalytic theory. A systematizing attempt (Psychological issues, vol 2, no 2, monograph 6). International University Press, New York
Rapaport D (1967) The collected papers of David Rapaport. Basic Books, New York
Rapaport D (1974) The history of the concept of association of ideas. International University Press, New York
Rapaport D, Gill MM (1959) The points of view and assumptions of metapsychology. Int J Psychoanal 40:153—162
Rappaport EA (1956) The management of an erotized transference. Psychoanal Q 25:515—529
Redlich FC (1968) Psychoanalyse und soziale Verantwortung. Psyche 22:658—671
Redlich FC, Freedman DX (1966) The theory and practice of psychiatry, 3rd edn. Basic Books, New York.
Reich A (1951) On counter-transference. Int J Psychoanal 32:25—31
Reich W (1933) Charakteranalyse. Technik und Grundlagen für studierende und praktizierende Analytiker. Reich, Vienna. Engl edn: (1958) Character analysis. Vision Press, London
Reichenbach H (1938) Experience and prediction. Univ of Chicago Press, Chicago
Reid JR, Finesinger JE (1952) The role of insight in psychotherapy. Am J Psychiatry 108:726—734
Reik T (1949) The inner experience of a psychoanalyst. Allen & Unwin, London
Reis WJ (1970) Formen der freien Assoziation zu Träumen. Psyche 24:101—115
Reiser MF (1985) Converging sectors of psychoanalysis and neurobiology. Mutual challenges and opportunity. J Am Psychoanal Assoc 33:11—34
Reiss D (1983) Illusion as a tool in psychoanalytic investigation. Psychoanal Contemp Thought 6:331—402
Reiter L (1975) Wissenschaftstheoretische Probleme der Psychotherapie. In: Strotzka H (ed) Psychotherapie. Grundlagen, Verfahren, Indikationen. Urban & Schwarzenberg, Munich, pp 7—31
Richards AD (1980) Technical consequences of object relations theory. J Am Psychoanal Assoc 28:623—636
Richards AD (1984) The relation between psychoanalytic theory and psychoanalytic technique. J Am Psychoanal Assoc 32:587—602
Richfield J (1954) An analysis of the concept of insight. Psychoanal Q 23:390—408
Richter HE (1970) Patient Familie. Entstehung, Struktur und Therapie von Konflikten in Ehe und Familie. Rowohlt, Reinbek bei Hamburg
Richter HE (1984) Sterbeangst und Destruktivität. Psyche 38:1105—1123
Richter HE (1985) Als Psychoanalytiker in der Friedensbewegung. Psyche 39:289—300
Rickman J (1957) Selected contributions to psychoanalysis. Basic Books, New York
Ricoeur P (1970) Freud and philosophy. Yale University Press, New Haven London. Fr: (1965) De l'interpretation. Seuil, Paris
Ricoeur P (1974) Hermeneutik und Psychoanalyse. Kösel, Munich. Fr: (1969) Le conflit des interpretations. Essais d'hermeneutique. Seuil, Paris

Riemann F (1973) Fritz Riemann. In: Pongratz LJ (ed) Psychotherapie in Selbstdarstellungen. Huber, Bern Stuttgart Vienna, pp 346—376

Riviere J (1936) On the genesis of psychical conflict in earliest infancy. Int J Psychoanal 17:395—422

Roback HB (1974) Insight. A bridging of the theoretical and research literature. Canadian Psychologist 15:61—88

Robbins WS (1975) Termination: Problems and techniques. J Am Psychoanal Assoc 23:166—176

Rochlin G (1973) Man's aggression. The defence of the self. Gambit, Boston

Roland A (1971) The context and unique function of dreams in psychoanalytic therapy. Clinical approach. Int J Psychoanal 52:431—439

Rosenblatt AD, Thickstun JT (1977) Energy, information, and motivation. A revision of psychoanalytic theory. J Am Psychoanal Assoc 25:537—558

Rosenfeld H (1955) Notes on the psycho-analysis of the super-ego conflict in an acute schizophrenic patient. In: Klein M, Heimann P, Money-Kyrle RE (eds) New directions in psycho-analysis. Basic Books, New York, pp 180—219

Rosenfeld H (1971) A clincal approach to the psychoanalytic theory of the life and death instincts. An investigation into the aggressive aspects of narcissism. Int J Psychoanal 52:169—178

Rosenfeld H (1972) A critical appreciation of James Strachey's paper on the nature of the therapeutic action of psychoanalysis. Int J Psychoanal 53:455—461

Rosenfeld H (1975) Negative therapeutic reaction. In: Giovacchini PL (ed) Tactics and techniques in psychoanalytic therapy, vol 2. Hogarth, London, pp 217—228

Rosenkötter L (1973) Die psychoanalytische Situation als Grundlage der psychoanalytischen Therapie. Psyche 27:989—1000

Rosenkötter L (1983) Alexander Mitscherlich als Chef und Lehrer. Psyche 37:346—351

Ross M (1973) Some clinical and theoretical aspects of working through. Int J Psychoanal 54:331—343

Rothenberg A (1984) Creativity and psychotherapy. Psychoanal Contemp Thought 7:233—268

Rothstein A (1983) The structural hypothesis. An evolutionary perspective. International University Press, New York

Rubinstein BB (1967) Explanation and mere description. A metascientific examination of certain aspects of the psychoanalytic theory of motivation. In: Holt RR (ed) Motives and thought. Psychoanalytic essays in honor of David Rapaport (Psychological issues, vol 5, no 2—3, monograph 18—19). International University Press, New York, pp 18—77

Rubinstein BB (1972) On metaphor and related phenomena. Psychoanal Contemp Sci 1:70—108

Rubinstein BB (1976) On the possibility of a strictly clinical psychoanalytic theory. An essay in the philosophy of psychoanalysis. In: Gill MM, Holzman PS (eds) Psychology versus metapsychology. Psychoanalytic essays in memory of George S. Klein (Psychological issues, vol 9, no 4, monograph 36) International University Press, New York, pp 229—264

Rubinstein BB (1980) The self and its brain. An argument for interactionism. By Karl Popper and John C Eccles. J Am Psychoanal Assoc 28:210—219

Ruffler G (1957) Zur Bedeutung der Anamnese für die psychosomatische Fragestellung, dargestellt an einer Anfallskranken. Psyche 11:416—458

Rycroft C (1966) Psychoanalysis observed. Constable, London

Russell HN, Dugan RS, Stewert JQ (1945) Astronomy. A revision of Young's manual of astronomy. Ginn, Boston

Sabshin M (1985) Psychoanalysis and psychiatry. Models for potential future relations. J Am Psychoanal Assoc 33:473—491

Sager CJ, Grundlach R, Kremer M, Lenz R, Royce JR (1968) The married in treatment. Effects of Psychoanalysis on the marital state. Arch Gen Psychiatry 19:205—217

Sampson H, Weiss J (1983) Testing hypotheses. The approach of the Mount Zion Psychotherapy Research Group. In: Greenberg L, Pinsof W (eds) The psychotherapeutic process. A research handbook. Guilford, New York

Sand R (1964) A systematic error in the use of free association (unpublished paper)

Sander LW (1980) Investigation of the infant and its care giving environment as a biological system. In: Greenspan SI, Pollock GH (eds) The course of life, vol 1. US Department of Health and Human Services, Washington DC, pp 177—201

Sandler J (1960) The background of safety. Int J Psychoanal 41:352—356

Sandler J (1976) Countertransference and role-responsiveness. Int Rev Psychoanal 3:43—47

Sandler J (1982) Psychoanalysis and psychotherapy. The training analyst's dilemma. In: Joseph ED, Wallerstein RS (eds) Psychotherapy. Impact on psychoanalytic training. The influence of practice and theory of psychotherapy an education in psychoanalysis (Int Psychoanal Assoc, monograph series, no 1). International University Press, New York, pp 39—47

Sandler J (1983) Reflections on some relations between psychoanalytic concepts and psychoanalytic practice. Int J Psychoanal 64:35—45

Sandler J, Dare C, Holder A (1973) The patient and the analyst: The basis of the psychoanalytic process. International University Press, New York

Sargent HD, Horwitz L, Wallerstein RS, Appelbaum A (1968) Prediction in psychotherapy research. Method for the transformation of clinical judgements into testable hypothesis (Psychological issues, vol 6, no 1, monograph 21). International University Press, New York

Sashin JI, Eldred SH, Amerongen ST van (1975) A search for predictive factors in institute supervised cases. A retrospective study of 183 cases from 1959—1966 at the Boston Psychoanalytic Society and Institute. Int J Psychoanal 56:343—359

Saul LJ (1962) The erotic transference. Psychoanal Q 31:54—61

Schacht L (1973) Subjekt gebraucht Subjekt. Psyche 27:151—168

Schachtel EG (1947) On memory and childhood amnesia. Psychiatry 10:1—26

Schafer R (1968) Aspects of internalization. International University Press, New York

Schafer R (1973) The idea of resistance. Int J Psychoanal 54:259—285

Schafer R (1976) A new language for psychoanalysis. Yale University Press, New Haven

Schafer R (1981) Action language and the psychology of the self. Annu Psychoanal 8:83—92

Schafer R (1982) The relevance of the "here and now" transference interpretation to the reconstruction of early development. Int J Psychoanal 63:77—82

Schafer R (1985) Wild analysis. J Am Psychoanal Assoc 33:275—299

Schepank H (1982) Epidemiologie psychogener Erkrankungen. Ein Beitrag zur Grundlagenforschung aus einer Feldstudie. Z Psychosom Med Psychoanal 28:104—125

Scheunert G (1973) Über das "Agieren" als theoretisches und praktisches Problem in der Psychoanalyse. In: Hahn P, Herdieckerhoff E (eds) Materialien zur Psychoanalyse und analytisch orientierten Psychotherapie. Sektion B: Schriften zur Technik, Heft 1. Vandenhoeck & Ruprecht, Göttingen Zürich

Scheunert G (1984) Von den Anfängen der Deutschen Psychoanalytischen Vereinigung. Erinnerungen eines Beteiligten. Int Psychoanal Assoc Newsletter 16, no 4 (German edn):4—5

Schilder P (1935a) The image and appearance of the human body. Studies in the constructive energies of the psyche. Kegan Paul, London

Schilder P (1935b) Psychoanalyse und bedingte Reflexe. Imago 21:50—66

Schleiermacher FDE (1959[1819]) Hermeneutik. In Kimmerle H (ed) Fr. D. E. Schleiermacher Hermeneutik. Nach den Handschriften neu herausgegeben und eingeleitet von Heinz Kimmerle (Abhandlungen der Heidelberger Akademie der Wissenschaften, philosophisch-historische Klasse, Jg 1959, 2. Abh). Winter, Heidelberg, pp 78—109

Schimek JG (1983) The construction of the transference. The relativity of the here and now and the there and then. Psychoanal Contemp Thought 6:435—456

Schleiermacher FDE (1959[1819]) Hermeneutik. In Kimmerle H (ed) Fr. D. E. Schleiermacher Hermeneutik. Nach den Handschriften neu herausgegeben und eingeleitet von Heinz Kimmerle (Abhandlungen der Heidelberger Akademie der Wissenschaften, philosophisch-historische Klasse, Jg 1959, 2. Abh). Winter, Heidelberg

Schlesinger HJ (1974) Problems of doing research on the Therapeutic process. J Am Psychoanal Assoc 22:3—13

Schlessinger N, Robbins FP (1983) A developmental view of the psychoanalytic process. Follow-up studies and their consequences. International University Press, New York

Schlieffen H von (1983) Psychoanalyse ohne Grundregel. Psyche 37:481—486

Schmale HT (1966) Working through. J Am Psychoanal Assoc 14:172—182

Schott HG (1981) "Traumdeutung" und "Infantile Cerebrallähmung". Überlegungen zu Freuds Theoriebildung. Psyche 35:97—110

Schott HG (1983) Die Selbstanalyse als eine praktische Methode bei Freud. Freiburger Universitätsblätter 22:67—77

Schröter K (1979) Einige formale Aspekte des psychoanalytischen Dialogs. In: Flader D, Wodak-Leodolter R (eds) Therapeutische Kommunikation. Ansätze zur Erforschung der Sprache im psychoanalytischen Prozeß. Scriptor, Königstein im Taunus, pp 179—185

Schröter K (1980) Spezifische Reaktionen auf das Behandlungsverfahren und die soziale Distanz zum Therapeuten. In: Menne K, Schröter K (eds) Psychoanalyse und Unterschicht. Soziale Herkunft — ein Hindernis für die psychoanalytische Behandlung? Suhrkamp, Frankfurt am Main, pp 59—72

Schulte D (1976) Psychodiagnostik zur Erklärung und Modifikation von Verhalten. In: Pawlik K (ed) Diagnose der Diagnostik. Klett, Stuttgart

Schultz-Hencke H (1951) Lehrbuch der analytischen Psychotherapie. Thieme, Stuttgart

Schur M (1966) Some additional "day residues" on the specimen dream of psychoanalysis. In: Loewenstein RM et al (eds) Psychoanalysis. A general psychology. International University Press, New York, pp 45—85

Searles HF (1965) Collected papers on schizophrenia and related subjects. International University Press, New York

Sedler MJ (1983) Freud's concept of working through. Psychoanal Q 52:73—98

Segal H (1964) Introduction to the work of Melanie Klein, 1st edn. Basic Books, New York

Segal H (1973) Introduction to the work of Melanie Klein, rev edn. Hogarth, London

Segal H (1982) Early infantile development as reflected in the psychoanalytic process. Steps in integration. Int J Psychoanal 63:15—22

Seidenberg H (1971) The basic rule. Free association. A reconsideration. J Am Psychoanal Assoc 19:98—109

Seitz P (1966) The consensus problem in psychoanalysis. In: Gottschalk LA, Auerbach AH (eds) Methods of research in psychotherapy. Appleton Century Crofts, New York, pp 209—225

Shane M (1980) Countertransference and the developmental orientation and approach. Psychoanal Contemp Thought 3:195—212

Shane M, Shane E (1980) Psychoanalytic developmental theories of the self. An integration. In: Goldberg A (ed) Advances in selfpsychology. International University Press, New York, pp 23—46

Shapiro SH (1984) The initial assessment of the patient. A psychoanalytic approach. Int Rev Psychoanal 11:11—25

Shapiro T (1984) On neutrality. J Am Psychoanal Assoc 32:269—282

Sharpe EF (1950) The technique of psychoanalysis. Seven lectures. In: Brierley M (ed) Collected papers on psychoanalysis by Ella Freeman Sharpe. Hogarth, London, pp 9—106

Sherwood M (1969) The logic of explanation in psychoanalysis. Academic Press, New York

Siebenthal W von (1953) Die Wissenschaft vom Traum. Ergebnisse und Probleme. Eine Einführung in die allgemeinen Grundlagen. Springer, Berlin Göttingen Heidelberg

Simmel E (1930) Zur Geschichte und sozialen Bedeutung des Berliner Psychoanalytischen Instituts. In: Rad& S, Fenichel O, Müller-Braunschweig C (eds) Zehn Jahre Berliner Psychoanalytisches Institut. Poliklinik und Lehranstalt. Internationaler Psychoanalytischer Verlag, Vienna

Slap JW (1976) A note on the drawing of dream details. Psychoanal Q 45:455—456

Slap JW, Levine FJ (1978) On hybrid concepts in psychoanalysis. Psychoanal Q 47:499—523

Snyder F (1970) The phenomenology of dreaming. In: Madow L, Snow LH (eds) The psychodynamic implications of physiological studies on dreams. Thomas, Springfield, pp 124—151

Solnit AJ (1982) Early psychic development as reflected in the psychoanalytic process. Int J Psychoanal 63:23—37

Specht EK (1981) Der wissenschaftstheoretische Status der Psychoanalyse. Das Problem der Traumdeutung. Psyche 35:761—787
Spence DP (1981) Toward a theory of dream interpretation. Psychoanal Contemp Thought 4:383—405
Spence DP (1982a) Narrative truth and historical truth. Meaning and interpretation in psychoanalysis. Norton, New York
Spence DP (1982b) On some clinical implications of action language. J Am Psychoanal Assoc 30:169—184
Spence DP (1984) Perils and pitfalls of free floating attention. Contemp Psychoanal 20:37—59
Spinner H (1974) Pluralismus als Erkenntnismodell. Suhrkamp, Frankfurt am Main
Spitz RA (1956) Countertransference. Comments on its varying role in the analytic situation. J Am Psychoanal Assoc 4:256—265
Spitz RA (1957) No and Yes. On the genesis of human communication. International University Press, New York
Spitz RA (1965) The evolution of dialogue. In: Schur M (ed) Drives, affects, behavior, vol 2. International University Press, New York, pp 170—190
Spruiell V (1983) Kuhn's "paradigm" and psychoanalysis. Psychoanal Q 52:353—363
Stegmüller W (1969) Probleme und Resultate der Wissenschaftstheorie und analytischen Philosophie. vol II: Theorie und Erfahrung. Springer, Berlin Heidelberg New York
Stein MH (1981) The unobjectionable part of the transference. J Am Psychoanal Assoc 29:869—892
Stendhal [Beyle H] (1975) Love. Penguin Books, Harmondsworth
Sterba RF (1934) The fate of the ego in the analytic therapy. Int J Psychoanal 15:117—126
Sterba RF (1936) Zur Theorie der Übertragung. Imago 22:456—470
Sterba RF (1940) The dynamics of the dissolution of the transference resistance. Psychoanal Q 9:363—379
Stern A (1924) On countertransference in psychoanalysis. Psychoanal Rev 11:166—174
Stern D (1977) The first relationship. Mother and infant. Fontana Open Books, London
Stern DN, Beebe B, Jaffe J, Bennett SL (1977) The infant's stimulus world during social interaction. A study of caregiver behaviours with particular reference to repetition and timing. In: Schaffer HR (ed) Studies of mother-infant interaction. Academic Press, London, pp 177—202
Stern H (1966) The truth as resistance to free association. Psychoanal Rev 53:642—646
Steury S, Blank ML (eds) (1981) Readings in psychotherapy with older people. US Department of Health and Human Services, Washington DC
Stewart WA (1963) An inquiry into the concept of working through. J Am Psychoanal Assoc 11:474—499
Stone L (1961) The psychoanalytic situation. An examination of its development and essential nature. International University Press, New York
Stone L (1971) Reflections on the psychoanalytic concept of aggression. Psychoanal Q 40:195—244
Stone L (1973) On resistance to the psychoanalytic process. Some thoughts on its nature and motivations. Psychoanal Contemp Sci 2:42—73
Stone L (1981a) Notes on the noninterpretive elements in the psychoanalytic situation and process. J Am Psychoanal Assoc 29:89—118
Stone L (1981b) Some thoughts on the "here and now" in psychoanalytic technique and process. Psychoanal Q 50:709—733
Strachey J (1934) The nature of the therapeutic action of psycho-analysis. Int J Psychoanal 15:127—159
Strachey J (1937) On the theory of the therapeutic results of psycho-analysis. Int J Psychoanal 18:139—145
Strauch I (1981) Ergebnisse der experimentellen Traumforschung In: Baumann U, Berbalk H, Seidenstücker G (eds) Klinische Psychologie, vol 4. Huber, Bern, pp 22—47
Straus E (1935) Vom Sinn der Sinne. Ein Beitrag zur Grundlegung der Psychologie. Springer, Berlin

Strotzka H (1969a) Psychotherapy for the working class patient. In: Redlich FC (ed) Social psychiatry. Williams & Wilkins, Baltimore
Strotzka H (1969b) Psychotherapie und soziale Sicherheit. Huber, Bern Stuttgart Vienna
Strotzka H (ed) (1980) Der Psychotherapeut im Spannungsfeld der Institutionen. Erfahrungen, Forderungen, Fallbeispiele. Urban & Schwarzenberg, Munich Vienna Baltimore
Strupp HH (1973) Psychotherapy. Clinical research, and theoretical issues. Aronson, New York
Strupp HH (1978) Suffering and psychotherapy. Contemp Psychoanal 14:73—97
Strupp HH (1982) Psychoanalytic failure. Reflections on an autobiographical account. Contemp Psychoanal 18:235—258
Strupp HH, Binder J (1984) Psychotherapy in a new key. A guide to time-limited dynamic psychotherapy. Basic Books, New York
Strupp HH, Hadley SW, Gommes-Schwartz B (1977) Psychotherapy for better or worse. Jason Aronson, New York
Sullivan HS (1953) The interpersonal theory of psychiatry. Norton, New York
Sulloway FJ (1979) Freud, biologist of the mind. Beyond the psychoanalytic legend. Basic Books, New York
Sutherland JD (1980) The British object relations theorists. Balint, Winnicott, Fairbairn, Guntrip. J Am Psychoanal Assoc 28:829—860
Swaan A de (1980) On the sociogenesis of the psychoanalytic situation. Psychoanal Contemp Thought 3:381—413
Tafertshofer A (1980) Latente Funktionen psychoanalytischer Verfahrensregeln. Psychoanalyse 1:280—320
Tenzer A (1983) Piaget and psychoanalysis. Some reflections on insight. Contemp Psychoanal 19:319—339
Tenzer A (1984) Piaget and psychoanalysis II. The problem of working through. Contemp Psychoanal 20:421—436
Thomä H (1963) Die Neo-Psychoanalyse Schultz-Henckes. Eine historische und kritische Betrachtung. Psyche 17:44—128
Thomä H (1964) Einige Bemerkungen zur Geschichte der Psychoanalyse in Deutschland von 1933 bis heute. In: Sigmund-Freud-Institut (ed) Ansprachen und Vorträge zur Einweihung des Institutsneubaues am 14. Oktober 1964. Sigmund-Freud-Institut, Frankfurt am Main, pp 31—39
Thomä H (1967a) Anorexia nervosa. International University Press, New York
Thomä H (1967b) Konversionstheorie und weiblicher Kastrationskomplex. Psyche 21:827—847
Thomä H (1969) Some remarks on psychoanalysis in Germany, past and present. Int J Psychoanal 50:683—692
Thomä H (1977) Psychoanalyse und Suggestion. Z Psychosom Med Psychoanal 23:35—55
Thomä H (1978) Von der "biographischen Anamnese" zur "systematischen Krankengeschichte". In: Drews S et al (eds) Provokation und Toleranz. Alexander Mitscherlich zu ehren. Festschrift für Alexander Mitscherlich zum 70. Geburtstag. Suhrkamp, Frankfurt am Main, pp 254—277
Thomä H (1980) Über die Unspezifität psychosomatischer Erkrankungen am Beispiel einer Neurodermitis mit zwanzigjähriger Katamnese. Psyche 34:589—624
Thomä H (1981) Schriften zur Praxis der Psychoanalyse: Vom spiegelnden zum aktiven Psychoanalytiker. Suhrkamp, Frankfurt am Main
Thomä H (1983a) Erleben und Einsicht im Stammbaum psychoanalytischer Techniken und der "Neubeginn" als Synthese im "Hier und Jetzt". In: Hoffmann SO (ed) Deutung und Beziehung. Kritische Beiträge zur Behandlungskonzeption und Technik in der Psychoanalyse. Fischer, Frankfurt am Main
Thomä H (1983b) The position of psychoanalysis within and outside the German university. Psychoanalysis in Europe. Bull Eur Psychoanal Fed 20—21:181—199
Thomä H (1983c) Conceptual dimensions of psychoanalyst's identity. In: Joseph ED, Widlöcher D (eds) The identity of the psychoanalyst (Int Psychoanal Assoc, monograph series, no 2). International University Press, New York, pp 93—134
Thomä H (1984) Der "Neubeginn" Michael Balints aus heutiger Sicht. Psyche 38:516—543

Thomä H (1986) Psychohistorische Hintergründe typischer Identitätsprobleme deutscher Analytiker. Forum Psychoanal 2:59—68
Thomä H, Grünzig HJ, Böckenförde H, Kächele H (1976) Das Konsensusproblem in der Psychoanalyse. Psyche 30:978—1027
Thomä H, Houben A (1967) Über die Validierung psychoanalytischer Theorien durch die Untersuchung von Deutungsaktionen. Psyche 21:664—692
Thomä H, Kächele H (1975) Problems of metascience and methodology in clinical psychoanalytic research. Annu Psychoanal 3:49—119
Thomä H, Kächele H (1976) Bemerkungen zum Wandel neurotischer Krankheitsbilder. Psychother Med Psychol 26:183—190
Thomä H, Thomä B (1968) Die Rolle der Angehörigen in der psychoanalytischen Technik. Psyche 22:802—822
Thomae H (1968) Das Individuum und seine Welt. Eine Persönlichkeitstheorie. Hogrefe, Göttingen
Thomson PG (1980) On the receptive function of the analyst. Int Rev Psychoanal 7:183—205
Ticho EA (1971) Probleme des Abschlusses der psychoanalytischen Therapie. Psyche 25:44—56
Ticho GR (1967) On self-analysis. Int J Psychoanal 48:308—318
Ticho GR (1971) Selbstanalyse als Ziel der psychoanalytischen Behandlung. Psyche 25:31—43
Ticho EA, Ticho GR (1969) Das Behandlungsbündnis und die Übertragungsneurose. Jahrb Psychoanal 6:19—34
Tower L (1956) Countertransference. J Am Psychoanal Assoc 4:224—265
Treurniet N (1983) Psychoanalysis and self psychology. A metapsychological essay with a clinical illustration. J Am Psychoanal Assoc 31:59—100
Trevarthen C (1977) Descriptive analyses of infant communicative behaviour. In: Schaffer HR (ed) Studies in mother-infant interaction. Academic Press, New York, pp 227—270
Tyson Rl, Sandler J (1971) Problems in the selection of patients for psychoanalysis: Comments on the application of concepts of "indications", "suitability", and "analysability". Br J Med Psychol 44:211—228
Valenstein AF (1962) The psycho-analytic situation. Affects, emotional reliving, and insight in the psychoanalytic process. Int J Psychoanal 43:315—324
Valenstein AF (1979) The concept of "classical" psychoanalysis. J Am Psychoanal Assoc 27 (Suppl):113—136
Viderman S (1979) The analytic space. Meaning and problems. Psychoanal Q 48:257—291
Wachtel PL (1977) Psychoanalysis and behaviour therapy. Toward an integration. Basic Books, New York
Wachtel PL (1980) Transference, schema, and assimilation. The relevance of Piaget to the psychoanalytic theory of transference. Annu Psychoanal 8:59—76
Wachtel PL (1982) Vicious circles. The self and the rhetoric of emerging and unfolding. Contemp Psychoanal 18:259—273
Waelder R (1936) The principle of multiple function. Observations on over-determination. Psychoanal Q 5:45—62
Waelder R (1937) The problem of genesis of psychical conflict in earliest infancy. Remarks on a paper by Joan Riviere. Int J Psychoanal 18:406—473
Waelder R (1956) Introduction to the discussion on problems of transference. Int J Psychoanal 37:367—368
Waelder R (1960) Basic theory of psycho-analysis. International University Press, New York
Waelder R (1962) Psychoanalysis, scientific method and philosophy. J Am Psychoanal Assoc 10:617—637
Waldhorn HF (1959) The silent patient. Panel report. J Am Psychoanal Assoc 7:548—560
Waldhorn HF (1960) Assessment of analysability. Technical and theoretical observations. Psychoanal Q 29:478—506
Wallerstein RS (1973) Psychoanalytic perspectives on the problem of reality. J Am Psychoanal Assoc 21:5—33

Wallerstein RS (1983) Self psychology and "classical" psychoanalytic psychology. The nature of their relationship. Psychoanal Contemp Thought 6:553—595

Wallerstein RS (ed) (1985) Changes in analysts and their training (Int Psychoanal Assoc, monograph series, no 4) International Psychoanalytic Association, London

Wallerstein RS (1986) Forty-two lives in treatment. Guilford, New York

Wallerstein RS, Sampson H (1971) Issues in research in the psychoanalytic process. Int J Psychoanal 52:11—50

Watzlawick P, Beavin JH, Jackson DD (1967) Pragmatics of human communication. A study of interactional patterns, pathologies, and paradoxes. Norton, New York

Weber JJ, Bachrach HM, Solomon M (1985) Factors associated with the outcome of psychoanalysis. Report of the Columbia Psychoanalytic Center Research Project (II). Int Rev Psychoanal 12:127—141

Weber M (1968) Methodologische Schriften. Fischer, Frankfurt am Main

Wehler HU (ed) (1971) Geschichte und Psychoanalyse. Kohlhammer, Stuttgart Berlin Cologne Mainz

Wehler HU (ed) (1972) Soziologie und Psychoanalyse. Kohlhammer, Stuttgart Berlin Köln Mainz

Weigert E (1952) Contribution to the problem of terminating psychoanalyses. Psychoanal Q 21:465—480

Weiner H (1979) Freud's project reassessed. By Karl H Pribram and Merton M Gill. J Am Psychoanal Assoc 27:215—223

Weinrich H (1968) Die Metapher. Poetica 2:100—130

Weinshel E (1966) Severe regressive states during analysis. A panel report. J Am Psychoanal Assoc 14:538—568

Weiss J (1971) The emergence of new themes. A contribution to the psycho-analytic theory of therapy. Int J Psychoanal 52:459—467

Weiss J, Sampson H (1984) The psychotherapeutic process. Guilford, New York

Weiss J, Sampson H (1985) Testing alternative psychoanalytic explanations of the therapeutic process. In: Masling JM (ed) Empirical studies of psychoanalytic theories, vol 2. Erlbaum, New Jersey

Weiss SS, Fleming J (1980) On teaching and learning of termination in psychoanalysis. Annu Psychoanal 8:37—55

Weizsäcker R von (1985) Ansprache in der Gedenkstunde im Plenarsaal des Deutschen Bundestages am 8. Mai 1985. In: Presse- und Informationsamt der Bundesregierung (ed) Erinnerung, Trauer und Versöhnung. Presse- und Informationsamt der Bundesregierung, Bonn, pp 63—82

Weizsäcker V von (1943) Klinische Vorstellungen. Hippokrates, Stuttgart

Weizsäcker V von (1977[1954]) Natur und Geist. Erinnerungen eines Arztes, 3rd edn. Kindler, Munich

Westerlundh B, Smith G (1983) Perceptgenesis and the psychodynamics of perception. Psychoanal Contemp Thought 6:597—640

Westmeyer H (1978) Wissenschaftstheoretische Grundlagen klinischer Psychologie. In: Baumann U, Berbalk H, Seidenstücker G (eds) Klinische Psychologie. Trends in Forschung und Praxis, vol 1. Huber, Bern Stuttgart Vienna, pp 108—132

White RW (1959) Motivation reconsidered. The concept of competence. Psychol Rev 66:297—333

White RW (1963) Ego and reality in psychoanalytic theory. A proposal regarding independend ego energies (Psychological issues, vol 3, no 3, monograph 11). International University Press, New York

Winnicott DW (1949) Hate in the countertransference. Int J Psychoanal 30:69—74

Winnicott DW (1965) The maturational processes and the facilitating environment. Studies in the theory of emotional development. International University Press, New York

Winnicott DW (1971) Playing and reality. Tavistock, London

Wisdom JO (1956) Psycho-analytic technology. Br J Philosophy Sci 7:13—28

Wisdom JO (1967) Testing an interpretation within a session. Int J Psychoanal 48:44—52

Wisdom JO (1970) Freud and Melanie Klein. Psychology, ontology, Weltanschauung. In: Hanly C, Lazerowitz M (eds) Psychoanalysis and philosophy. International University Press, New York, pp 327–362

Wisdom JO (1984) What is left of psychoanalytic theory? Int Rev Psychoanal 11:313–326

Wittgenstein L (1953) Philosophische Untersuchungen – philosophical investigations, bilingual edn. Basil Blackwell, Oxford

Wolf E (1982) Empathische Resonanz. Psychoanalyse 3:306–314

Wolff PH (1960) The developmental psychologies of Jean Piaget and psychoanalysis. International University Press, New York

Wolff PH (1971) Review of psychoanalytic theory in the light of current research in child development. J Am Psychoanal Assoc 19:565–576

Wollheim R, Hopkins J (eds) (1982) Philosophical essays on Freud. Cambridge University Press, Cambridge

Wolman BB (1979) Preface. In: Wolman BB (ed) Handbook of dreams. Van Nostrand, New York

Wurmser L (1977) A defense of the use of metaphor in analytic theory formation. Psychoanal Q 46:466–498

Wurmser L (1981) The mask of shame. A psychoanalytic study of shame affects and shame conflicts. Johns Hopkins University Press, Baltimore

Wyatt F (1984) Unnötige Widersprüche und notwendige Unterscheidungen. Überlegungen zur Differenzierung von Psychoanalyse und psychoanalytischer Psychotherapie. Psychother Psychosom Med Psychol 34:91–96

Wyss D (1958) Die Bedeutung der Assoziationstheorien für die Psychoanalyse. Confin Psychiatr 1:113–132

Zeligs MA (1957) Acting in. A contribution to the meaning of some postural attitudes observed during analysis. J Am Psychoanal Assoc 5:685–706

Zeligs MA (1960) The role of silence in transference, countertransference, and the psychoanalytic process. Int J Psychoanal 41:407–412

Zeppelin I von (1981) Skizze eines Prozeßmodells der psychoanalytischen Therapie. Berichte aus der Abteilung Klinische Psychologie, Psychologisches Institut der Universität Zürich, no 14 (unpublished paper)

Zetzel ER (1956) Current concepts of transference. Int J Psychoanal 37:369–376

Zetzel ER (1965) The theory of therapy in relation to a developmental model of the psychic apparatus. Int J Psychoanal 46:39–52

Zetzel ER (1970) The capacity for emotional growth. Hogarth, London

Zilboorg G (1952) Precursors of Freud in free association. Some sidelights on free association. Int J Psychoanal 33:489–497

# Name Index

## G

# Subject Index

L



M



N



O



P

## T

MIX
Papier aus verantwortungsvollen Quellen
Paper from responsible sources
FSC® C105338

If you have any concerns about our products,
you can contact us on
**ProductSafety@springernature.com**

In case Publisher is established outside the EU,
the EU authorized representative is:
**Springer Nature Customer Service Center GmbH**
**Europaplatz 3, 69115 Heidelberg, Germany**

Printed by Libri Plureos GmbH
in Hamburg, Germany